Informatik aktuell

Herausgeber: W. Brauer
im Auftrag der Gesellschaft für Informatik (GI)

T0137795

Thomas Tolxdorff   Thomas M. Deserno
Heinz Handels   Hans-Peter Meinzer (Hrsg.)

Bildverarbeitung für die Medizin 2012

Algorithmen – Systeme – Anwendungen

Proceedings des Workshops
vom 18. bis 20. März 2012 in Berlin

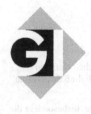

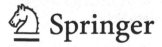 Springer

Herausgeber

Thomas Tolxdorff
Charité – Universitätsmedizin Berlin
Institut für Medizinische Informatik
Hindenburgdamm 30, 12200 Berlin

Thomas Martin Deserno, geb. Lehmann
Rheinisch-Westfälische Technische Hochschule Aachen
Universitätsklinikum Aachen
Institut für Medizinische Informatik
Pauwelsstraße 30, 52074 Aachen

Heinz Handels
Universität zu Lübeck
Institut für Medizinische Informatik
Ratzeburger Allee 160, 23562 Lübeck

Hans-Peter Meinzer
Deutsches Krebsforschungszentrum
Abteilung für Medizinische und Biologische Informatik
Im Neuenheimer Feld 280, 69120 Heidelberg

CR Subject Classification (1998):
A.0, H.3, I.4, I.5, J 3, H.3.1, I.2.10, I.3.3, I.3.5, I.3.7, I.3.8, I.6.3

ISSN 1431-472-X

ISBN 978-3-642-28501-1   e-ISBN 978-3-642-28502-8
DOI 10.1007/978-3-642-28502-8
Springer Heidelberg Dordrecht London New York

Die Deutsche Nationalbibliothek verzeichnet diese Publikation in der Deutschen National-
bibliografie; detaillierte bibliografische Daten sind im Internet über http://dnb.d-nb.de abrufbar.

Einbandentwurf: WMXDesign GmbH, Heidelberg

Gedruckt auf säurefreiem Papier

Springer ist Teil der Fachverlagsgruppe Springer Science+Business Media
(www.springer.com)

Bildverarbeitung für die Medizin 2012

Veranstalter

IMI   Institut für Medizinische Informatik
Charité – Universitätsmedizin Berlin
mit Unterstützung durch die Fachgesellschaften:

BVMI   Berufsverband Medizinischer Informatiker
CURAC Deutsche Gesellschaft für Computer- und Roboterassistierte Chirurgie
DGBMT Fachgruppe Medizinische Informatik
der Deutschen Gesellschaft für Biomedizinische Technik im VDE
GI   Fachgruppe Imaging und Visualisierungstechniken
der Gesellschaft für Informatik
GMDS   Arbeitsgruppe Medizinische Bild- und Signalverarbeitung
der Deutschen Gesellschaft für Medizinische Informatik,
Biometrie und Epidemiologie
IEEE   Joint Chapter Engineering in Medicine and Biology, German Section

Tagungsvorsitz

Prof. Dr. Thomas Tolxdorff

Institut für Medizinische Informatik, Charité – Universitätsmedizin Berlin

Lokale Organisation

Dr. Jürgen Braun
Dr. Egbert Gedat
Prof. Dr. Dagmar Krefting
Dr. Thorsten Schaaf
Sabine Sassmann
Dagmar Stiller
u.v.m.

Institut für Medizinische Informatik, Charité – Universitätsmedizin Berlin

Verteilte BVM-Organisation

Prof. Dr. Thomas M. Deserno, Christoph Classen, Adrian Menzel
Rheinisch-Westfälische Technische Hochschule Aachen (Tagungsband)

Prof. Dr. Heinz Handels, Dr. Jan-Hinrich Wrage
Universität zu Lübeck (Begutachtung)

Prof. Dr. Hans-Peter Meinzer, Dipl. Inform. Alexander Seitel
Deutsches Krebsforschungszentrum Heidelberg (Anmeldung)

Prof. Dr. Thomas Tolxdorff, Dagmar Stiller
Charité – Universitätsmedizin Berlin (Internetpräsenz)

Programmkomitee

Prof. Dr. Til Aach, Rheinisch-Westfälische Technische Hochschule Aachen
Prof. Dr. Dr. Johannes Bernarding, Universität Magdeburg
Priv.-Doz. Dr. Jürgen Braun, Charité – Universitätsmedizin Berlin
Prof. Dr. Oliver Burgert, Hochschule Reutlingen
Prof. Dr. Thorsten M. Buzug, Universität zu Lübeck
Prof. Dr. Thomas M. Deserno, Rheinisch-Westfälische
                        Technische Hochschule Aachen
Prof. Dr. Hartmut Dickhaus, Universität Heidelberg
Dr. Jan Ehrhardt, Universität zu Lübeck
Dr. Thomas Elgeti, Charité – Universitätsmedizin Berlin
Prof. Dr. Dr. Karl-Hans Englmeier, Helmholtz-Zentrum München
Prof. Dr. Bernd Fischer, Fraunhofer MEVIS, Lübeck
Dr. Klaus Fritzsche, Harvard Medical School, USA
Dr. Egbert Gedat, Charité – Universitätsmedizin Berlin
Prof. Dr. Horst Hahn, Fraunhofer MEVIS, Bremen
Prof. Dr. Heinz Handels, Universität zu Lübeck
Priv.-Doz. Dr. Peter Hastreiter, Universität Erlangen-Nürnberg
Dr. Tobias Heimann, Deutsches Krebsforschungszentrum Heidelberg
Prof. Dr. Joachim Hornegger, Universität Erlangen-Nürnberg
Prof. Dr. Alexander Horsch, Technische Universität München
                        & Universität Tromsø, Norwegen
Prof. Dr. Erwin Keeve, Charité – Universitätsmedizin Berlin
Prof. Dr. Dagmar Krefting, Hochschule für Technik und Wirtschaft Berlin
Prof. Dr. Frithjof Kruggel, University of Carlifornia Irvine, USA
Dr. Lena Maier-Hein, Deutsches Krebsforschungszentrum Heidelberg
Prof. Dr. Hans-Peter Meinzer, Deutsches Krebsforschungszentrum Heidelberg
Prof. Dr. Heinrich Müller, Universität Dortmund
Prof. Dr. Henning Müller, Université Sierre, Schweiz
Prof. em. Dr. Heinrich Niemann, Universität Erlangen-Nürnberg
Prof. Dr. Dietrich Paulus, Universität Koblenz-Landau
Prof. Dr. Heinz-Otto Peitgen, Fraunhofer MEVIS, Bremen
Prof. Dr. Dr. Siegfried J. Pöppl, Universität zu Lübeck
Prof. Dr. Bernhard Preim, Universität Magdeburg
Prof. Dr. Karl Rohr, Universität Heidelberg
Prof. Dr. Ingolf Sack, Charité – Universitätsmedizin Berlin
Prof. Dr. Thomas Tolxdorff, Charité – Universitätsmedizin Berlin
Dr. Gudrun Wagenknecht, Forschungszentrum Jülich
Prof. Dr. Herbert Witte, Universität Jena
Priv.-Doz. Dr. Thomas Wittenberg, Fraunhofer IIS, Erlangen
Prof. Dr. Ivo Wolf, Hochschule Mannheim

Industrieaussteller und Sponsoren

AGFA   Agfa HealthCare GmbH
Konrad-Zuse-Platz 1-3, 53227 Bonn

CHILI   Chili GmbH Digital Radiology
Burgstraße 61, 69121 Heidelberg

DEKOM   DEKOM Engineering GmbH
Hoheluftchaussee 108, 20253 Hamburg

DGBMT   Deutsche Gesellschaft für Biomedizinische Technik im VDE
Stresemannallee 15, 60596 Frankfurt

GE   GE Healthcare
Information Technologies GmbH & Co. KG
Lerchenbergstraße 15, 89160 Dornstadt

GMDS   Deutsche Gesellschaft für Medizinische Informatik,
Biometrie und Epidemiologie e.V.
Industriestraße 154, 50996 Köln

HP   Hewlett-Packard GmbH
Herrenberger Straße 140, 71034 Böblingen

ID   Information und Dokumentation
im Gesundheitswesen GmbH & Co. KGaA
Platz vor dem Neuen Tor 2, 10115 Berlin

IEEE   IEEE Joint Chapter Engineering in Medicine and Biology
German Section
3 Park Avenue, 17th Floor, New York, YN, 10016-5995 USA

INFINITT   INFINITT Europe GmbH
Gaugrafenstraße 34, 60489 Frankfurt am Main

ITERNITY   iTernity GmbH
Bötzinger Straße 60, 79111 Freiburg im Breisgau

MCS   MCS Labordatensysteme GmbH & Co. KG
Im Kappelhof 1, 65343 Eltville

NDI   NDI Europe GmbH
Fritz-Reichle-Ring 2, 78315 Radolfzell

SIEMENS   Siemens AG
Siemens Deutschland Healthcare Sector – GER H BD&S MC
Karlheinz-Kaske-Straße 2, 91052 Erlangen

SPRINGER   Springer Science & Business Media Deutschland GmbH
Heidelberger Platz 3, 14197 Berlin

VIII

Preisträger des BVM-Workshops 2011 in Lübeck

Der BVM-Award für eine herausragende Diplom-, Bachelor-, Master- oder Doktorarbeit aus dem Bereich der Medizinischen Bildverarbeitung ist mit 1.000 € dotiert und wurde im Jahre 2011 gesplittet. Die je mit einem Preisgeld von 250 € dotierten BVM-Preise zeichnen besonders hervorragende Arbeiten aus, die auf dem Workshop präsentiert wurden.

BVM-Award 2011 für eine herausragende Dissertation

Dr. rer. nat. Klaus Fritsche (Deutsches Krebsforschungszentrum Heidelberg)
Quantification of Structural Changes in the Brain using Magnetic Resonance Imaging

Dr.-Ing. Christopher Rohkohl (Universität Erlangen-Nürnberg)
Motion Estimation and Compensation for Interventional Cardiovascular Image Reconstruction

BVM-Preis 2011 für die beste wissenschaftliche Arbeit

Nils D. Forkert mit *Alexander Schmidt-Richberg, Jan Ehrhardt, Jens Fiehler, Heinz Handels, Dennis Säring* (Universitätsklinikum Hamburg-Eppendorf)
Vesselness-geführte Level-Set Segmentierung von zerebralen Gefäßen

BVM-Preis 2011 für die zweitbeste wissenschaftliche Arbeit

Tim Becker mit *Daniel H. Rapoport, Amir Madany Mamlouk* (Universität zu Lübeck)
Adaptive Mitosis Detection in Large in vitro Stem Cell Populations using Time-lapse Microscopy

BVM-Preis 2011 für die drittbeste wissenschaftliche Arbeit

Andreas Mang mit *Stefan Becker, Alina Toma, Thomas Polzin, Tina A. Schütz, Thorsten M. Buzug* (Universität zu Lübeck)
Modellierung tumorinduzierter Gewebedeformation als Optimierungsproblem mit weicher Nebenbedingung

BVM-Preis 2011 für den besten Vortrag

Michael Schwenke mit *Anja Hennemuth, Bernd Fischer, Ola Friman* (Fraunhofer MEVIS, Bremen)
Blood Particle Trajectories in Phase-Contrast-MRI as Minimal Paths Computed with Anisotropic Fast Marching

BVM-Preis 2011 für die beste Posterpräsentation

Veronika Zimmer mit *Nils Papenberg, Jan Modersitzki, Bernd Fischer* (Fraunhofer MEVIS, Lübeck)
Bildregistrierung zur Verbrennungsanalyse

Vorwort

Die digitale Bildverarbeitung in der Medizin hat sich nach vielen Jahren rasanter Entwicklung als zentraler Bestandteil diagnostischer und therapeutischer Verfahren fest etabliert. Von der Industrie kontinuierlich fortentwickelte Gerätetechnik sorgt für eine stetig steigende Datenkomplexität. Diese Informationsvielfalt, gepaart mit ständig wachsender Verarbeitungsgeschwindigkeit von Rechnersystemen, verlangt neue Methoden, um die möglich gewordenen Vorteile zum Wohl von Patienten erschließen zu können. Die computergestützte Bildverarbeitung wird mit dem Ziel eingesetzt, Strukturen automatisch zu erkennen und insbesondere pathologische Abweichungen aufzuspüren und zu quantifizieren, um so beispielsweise zur Qualitätssicherung in der Diagnostik beizutragen.

Doch die Anforderungen sind hoch, um die visuellen Fähigkeiten eines Experten bei der Begutachtung von medizinischem Bildmaterial nachzubilden. Dennoch gelingt die wichtige Unterscheidung von Strukturen durch zielgerichtete Algorithmen in Kombination mit der Leistungsfähigkeit moderner Computer. So wird es möglich, die Algorithmen und Technologien der medizinischen Bildverarbeitung zur Unterstützung der Medizin und zum Nutzen des Patienten einzusetzen. Der Workshop Bildverarbeitung für die Medizin (BVM) bietet hier ein Podium zur Präsentation und Diskussion neuer Algorithmen, Systeme und Anwendungen.

Die BVM konnte sich durch erfolgreiche Veranstaltungen in Aachen, Berlin, Erlangen, Freiburg, Hamburg, Heidelberg, Leipzig, Lübeck und München als ein zentrales interdisziplinäres Forum für die Präsentation und Diskussion von Methoden, Systemen und Anwendungen der medizinischen Bildverarbeitung etablieren. Ziel ist die Darstellung aktueller Forschungsergebnisse und die Vertiefung der Gespräche zwischen Wissenschaftlern, Industrie und Anwendern. Die BVM richtet sich dabei erneut ausdrücklich auch an Nachwuchswissenschaftler, die über ihre Bachelor-, Master-, Promotions- oder Habilitationsprojekte berichten wollen.

Die auf Fachkollegen aus Aachen, Berlin, Heidelberg und Lübeck verteilte Organisation hat sich auch diesmal wieder bewährt. Die webbasierte Einreichung und Begutachtung der Tagungsbeiträge wurde von den Kollegen in Lübeck durchgeführt und ergab nach anonymisierter Bewertung durch jeweils drei Gutachter die Annahme von 76 Beiträgen: 48 Vorträge, 25 Poster und 3 Softwaredemonstrationen. Die Qualität der eingereichten Arbeiten war insgesamt sehr hoch. Die besten Arbeiten werden auch in diesem Jahr mit BVM-Preisen ausgezeichnet. Die schriftlichen Langfassungen werden im Tagungsband erscheinen, der von den Aachener Kollegen aufbereitet und vom Springer-Verlag in der bewährten Reihe „Informatik Aktuell" der Gesellschaft für Informatik (GI) – erstmals elektronisch – publiziert wird. Die LaTeX-Vorlage zur BVM wurde erneut verbessert und der gesamte Erstellungsprozess ausschließlich über das Internet abgewickelt, ebenso wie die von den Heidelberger Kollegen organisierte Tagungsanmeldung. Die Internetpräsentation des Workshops wird in Berlin gepflegt und bietet ausführliche Informationen über das Programm und organisatorische Details rund um die BVM 2012. Sie sind abrufbar unter der Adresse

http://www.bvm-workshop.org

Am Tag vor dem wissenschaftlichen Programm werden zwei Tutorien angeboten:

- *Prof. Dr. Dagmar Krefting* von der Hochschule für Technik und Wirtschaft, Berlin, erläutert neue Entwicklungen in der medizinischen Bildverarbeitung im Zusammenhang mit GRID-Technologien. Verteilte IT-Systeme, sogenannte wissenschaftliche GRIDS, ermöglichen den Zugriff auf Rechenleistung, Daten und Algorithmen über die eigenen institutionellen Grenzen hinaus. In der medizinischen Forschung können solche Health-GRIDS zum einen für die Entwicklung von eigenen Algorithmen eingesetzt werden, beispielsweise bei großen Parameterstudien und bei Evaluation mit existierenden Goldstandards. Zum anderen können aber auch mit existierenden Algorithmen große Datenmengen, beispielsweise bei Bildserien, effizient berechnet werden.
- *Prof. Dr. Erwin Keeve* von der Charité – Universitätsmedizin Berlin stellt Lösungen zur Bildgebung und -verarbeitung im Operationssaal vor. In diesem Tutorial werden integrierte und hybride Informationssysteme und moderne intraoperativ einsetzbare Bildgebungsgeräte und deren Anwendungsspektren vorgestellt. Es werden Workflow-Analysen für integrierte und hybride Operationssäle und die daraus ableitbaren Nutzungskonzepte dargestellt. Fragen und Lösungsstrategien zur dynamischen Vernetzung bildgebender Geräte im OP werden aufgezeigt und ausführlich diskutiert.

An dieser Stelle möchten wir allen, die bei den umfangreichen Vorbereitungen zum Gelingen des Workshops beigetragen haben, unseren herzlichen Dank für ihr Engagement bei der Organisation des Workshops aussprechen: den Referenten der Gastvorträge, den Autoren der Beiträge, den Referenten der Tutorien, den Industrierepräsentanten, dem Programmkomitee, den Fachgesellschaften, den Mitgliedern des BVM-Organisationsteams und allen Mitarbeitern des Instituts für Medizinische Informatik der Charité.

Wir wünschen allen Teilnehmerinnen und Teilnehmern des Workshops BVM 2012 lehrreiche Tutorials, viele interessante Vorträge, Gespräche an den Postern und bei der Industrieausstellung sowie spannende neue Kontakte zu Kolleginnen und Kollegen aus dem Bereich der medizinischen Bildverarbeitung.

Januar 2012

Thomas Tolxdorff (Berlin)
Thomas Deserno (Aachen)
Heinz Handels (Lübeck)
Hans-Peter Meinzer (Heidelberg)

Inhaltsverzeichnis

Die fortlaufende Nummer am linken Seitenrand entspricht den Beitragsnummern, wie sie im endgültigen Programm des Workshops zu finden sind. Dabei steht V für Vortrag, P für Poster und S für Softwaredemonstration.

Eingeladene Vorträge

V1   *Braun J, Sack I:* Magnetresonanzelastografie 1

V2   *Curio G:* Brain-Computer Interfaces 2

Segmentierung I

V3   *Tzschätzsch H, Elgeti T, Hirsch S, Krefting D, Klatt D, Braun J, Sack I:* Direct Magnetic Resonance Elastography 3

V4   *Eck S, Rohr K, Müller-Ott K, Rippe K, Wörz S:* Combined Model-Based and Region-Adaptive 3D Segmentation and 3D Co-localization Analysis of Heterochromatin Foci 9

V5   *Gollmer ST, Buzug TM:* Formmodellbasierte Segmentierung des Unterkiefers aus Dental-CT-Aufnahmen 15

V6   *Katouzian A, Karamalis A, Laine A, Navab N:* A Systematic Approach Toward Reliable Atherosclerotic Plaque Characterization in IVUS Images 21

V7   *Stucht D, Yang S, Schulze P, Danishad A, Kadashevich I, Bernarding J, Maclaren J, Zaitsev M, Speck O:* Improved Image Segmentation with Prospective Motion Correction in MRI 27

Motion & Tracking

V8   *Bögel M, Maier A, Hofmann HG, Hornegger J, Fahrig R:* Diaphragm Tracking in Cardiac C-Arm Projection Data 33

XII

V9   *Groch A, Haase S, Wagner M, Kilgus T, Kenngott H,*
Schlemmer H-P, Hornegger J, Meinzer H-P, Maier-Hein L:
Optimierte endoskopische Time-of-Flight Oberflächenrekonstruktion
durch Integration eines Struktur-durch-Bewegung-Ansatzes 39

V10   *Reichl T, Gergel I, Menzel M, Hautmann H, Wegner I,*
Meinzer H-P, Navab N: Motion Compensation for Bronchoscope
Navigation Using Electromagnetic Tracking, Airway Segmentation,
and Image Similarity 45

V11   *Ruthotto L, Gigengack F, Burger M, Wolters CH, Jiang X,*
Schäfers KP, Modersitzki J: A Simplified Pipeline for Motion
Correction in Dual Gated Cardiac PET 51

V12   *Scherf N, Ludborzs C, Thierbach K, Kuska J-P, Braumann U-D,*
Scheibe P, Pompe T, Glauche I, Roeder I: FluidTracks 57

Methoden I

V13   *Mang A, Toma A, Schütz TA, Becker S, Buzug TM:* Eine effiziente
Parallel-Implementierung eines stabilen Euler-Cauchy-Verfahrens für
die Modellierung von Tumorwachstum 63

V14   *Wessel N, Riedl M, Malberg H, Penzel T, Kurths J:* Symbolic
Coupling Traces for Coupling Analyses of Medical Time Series 69

V15   *Gedat E, Mohajer M, Foert E, Meyer B, Kirsch R, Frericks B:*
Hybride Multi-Resolutions *k*-Raum Nachbearbeitung für
Gadofosveset-verstärkte hochaufgelöste arterielle periphere
MR-Angiographie 75

V16   *Köhler B, Neugebauer M, Gasteiger R, Janiga G, Speck O,*
Preim B: Surface-Based Seeding for Blood Flow Exploration 81

V17   *Friedl S, Herdt E, König S, Weyand M, Kondruweit M,*
Wittenberg T: Determination of Heart Valve Fluttering by
Analyzing Pixel Frequency 87

3D

V18   *Graser B, Hien M, Rauch H, Meinzer H-P, Heimann T:*
Automatische Detektion des Herzzyklus und des Mitralannulus
Durchmessers mittels 3D Ultraschall 92

V19 *Krüger J, Ehrhardt J, Bischof A, Barkhausen J, Handels H:*
Automatische Bestimmung von 2D/3D-Korrespondenzen in
Mammographie- und Tomosynthese-Bilddaten 99

V20 *Bauer S, Wasza J, Hornegger J:* Photometric Estimation of 3D
Surface Motion Fields for Respiration Management 105

V21 *Haase S, Forman C, Kilgus T, Bammer R, Maier-Hein L,*
Hornegger J: ToF/RGB Sensor Fusion for Augmented 3D
Endoscopy using a Fully Automatic Calibration Scheme 111

V22 *Fortmeier D, Mastmeyer A, Handels H:* GPU-Based Visualization of
Deformable Volumetric Soft-Tissue for Real-Time Simulation of
Haptic Needle Insertion 117

Methoden II

P1 *Toma A, Régnier-Vigouroux A, Mang A, Schütz TA, Becker S,*
Buzug TM: In-silico Modellierung der Immunantwort auf
Hirntumorwachstum 123

P2 *Wagner T, Lüttmann SO, Swarat D, Wiemann M, Lipinski H-G:*
Pfadbasierte Identifikation von Nanopartikel-Agglomerationen in
vitro 129

P3 *Jonas S, Deniz E, Khokha MK, Deserno TM, Choma MA:*
Microfluidic Phenotyping of Cilia-Driven Mixing for the Assessment
of Respiratory Diseases 135

P4 *Wu H, Hornegger J:* Sparsity Level Constrained Compressed
Sensing for CT Reconstruction 141

P5 *Kleine M, Müller J, Buzug TM:* L1-Regularisierung für die
Computertomographie mit begrenztem Aufnahmewinkel 147

P6 *Röttger D, Denter C, Müller S:* Advanced Line Visualization for
HARDI 153

P7 *Ritschel K, Dekomien C, Winter S:* Modellfunktion zur
Approximation von Ultraschallkontrastmittelkonzentration zur
semi-quantitativen Gewebeperfusionsbestimmung 159

Softwaredemo

S1   *Bremser M, Mittag U, Weber T, Rittweger J, Herpers R:* Diameter
Measurement of Vascular Structures in Ultrasound Video
Sequences 165

S2   *Gutbell R, Becker M, Wesarg S:* Ein Prototyp zur Planung von
Bohrpfaden für die minimal-invasive Chirurgie an der Otobasis 171

S3   *Neher PF, Stieltjes B, Reisert M, Reicht I, Meinzer H-P,
Fritzsche KH:* Integration eines globalen Traktographieverfahrens in
das Medical Imaging Interaction Toolkit 177

S4   *Fetzer A, Meinzer H-P, Heimann T:* Interaktive 3D Segmentierung
auf Basis einer optimierten Oberflächeninterpolation mittels radialer
Basisfunktionen 183

Segmentierung II

P8   *Scheibe P, Wüstling P, Voigt C, Hierl T, Braumann U-D:*
Inkrementelle lokal-adaptive Binarisierung zur Unterdrückung von
Artefakten in der Knochenfeinsegmentierung 189

P9   *Gross S, Morariu CA, Behrens A, Tischendorf JJ, Aach T:*
Farbbasierte Entfernung von Artefakten bei der
Blutgefäßsegmentierung auf Dickdarmpolypen 195

P10   *Schmidt-Richberg A, Ehrhardt J, Wilms M, Werner R, Handels H:*
Evaluation of Algorithms for Lung Fissure Segmentation in CT
Images 201

Registrierung I

V23   *Furtado H, Gendrin C, Bloch C, Spoerk J, Pawiro SA, Weber C,
Figl M, Bergmann H, Stock M, Georg D, Birkfellner W:* Real-Time
Intensity Based 2D/3D Registration for Tumor Motion Tracking
During Radiotherapy 207

V24   *Faltin P, Chaisaowong K, Kraus T, Aach T:* Registration of Lung
Surface Proximity for Assessment of Pleural Thickenings 213

V25 Strehlow J, Rühaak J, Kluck C, Fischer B: Effiziente Verpunktung
     pulmonaler MR-Bilder zur Evaluierung von
     Registrierungsergebnissen 219

V26 Forkert ND, Schmidt-Richberg A, Münchau A, Fiehler J,
     Handels H, Boelmans K: Automatische atlasbasierte Differenzierung
     von klassischen und atypischen Parkinsonsyndromen 225

Visible Light

V27 Jaiswal A, Godinez WJ, Eils R, Lehmann MJ, Rohr K: Tracking
     Virus Particles in Microscopy Images Using Multi-Frame
     Association 231

V28 Libuschewski P, Weichert F, Timm C: Parameteroptimierte und
     GPGPU-basierte Detektion viraler Strukturen innerhalb
     Plasmonen-unterstützter Mikroskopiedaten 237

V29 Harder N, Batra R, Gogolin S, Diessl N, Eils R, Westermann F,
     König R, Rohr K: Cell Tracking for Automatic Migration and
     Proliferation Analysis in High-Throughput Screens 243

V30 Greß O, Posch S: Model Dependency of RBMCDA for Tracking
     Multiple Targets in Fluorescence Microscopy 249

Segmentierung III

V31 Gross S, Klein M, Behrens A, Aach T: Segmentierung von
     Blutgefäßen in retinalen Fundusbildern 256

V32 Kadas EM, Kaufhold F, Schulz C, Paul F, Polthier K, Brandt AU:
     3D Optic Nerve Head Segmentation in Idiopathic Intracranial
     Hypertension 262

V33 Habes M, Kops ER, Lipinski H-G, Herzog H: Skull Extraction from
     MR Images Generated by Ultra Short TE Sequence 268

V34 Egger J, Dukatz T, Freisleben B, Nimsky C: Ein semiautomatischer
     Ansatz zur Flächenbestimmung von Wirbeln in
     MRT-Aufnahmen 274

V35　*Fränzle A, Bendl R:* Automatische Segmentierung und
Klassifizierung von Knochenmarkhöhlen für die Positionierung von
Formmodellen 280

Methoden III

V36　*Mastmeyer A, Fortmeier D, Handels H:* Anisotropic Diffusion for
Direct Haptic Volume Rendering in Lumbar Puncture
Simulation 286

V37　*Köhler T, Hornegger J, Mayer M, Michelson G:* Quality-Guided
Denoising for Low-Cost Fundus Imaging 292

V38　*Boero F, Ruppertshofen H, Schramm H:* Femur Localization Using
the Discriminative Generalized Hough Transform 298

V39　*Cordes A, Levakhina YM, Buzug TM:* Mikro-CT basierte
Validierung digitaler Tomosynthese Rekonstruktion 304

V40　*Hamer J, Kratz B, Müller J, Buzug TM:* Modified Eulers Elastica
Inpainting for Metal Artifact Reduction in CT 310

Bildanalyse & Klassifizierung

V41　*Wasza J, Bauer S, Haase S, Hornegger J:* Sparse Principal Axes
Statistical Surface Deformation Models for Respiration Analysis and
Classification 316

V42　*Dolnitzki J-M, Winter S:* Merkmale aus zweidimensionalen
Orientierungshistogrammen zur Beurteilung von Tremorspiralen ... 322

V43　*Kirschner M, Wesarg S:* Regularisierung lokaler Deformation im
probabilistischen Active Shape Model 328

V44　*Friedrich D, Jin C, Zhang Y, Demin C, Yuan L, Berynskyy L,
Biesterfeld S, Aach T, Böcking A:* Identification of Prostate Cancer
Cell Nuclei for DNA-Grading of Malignancy 334

OP-Unterstützung & Gerätetechnik

V45   Seitel A, Servatius M, Franz AM, Kilgus T, Bellemann N,
      Radeleff BR, Fuchs S, Meinzer H-P, Maier-Hein L: Markerlose
      Navigation für perkutane Nadelinsertionen 340

V46   Gaa J, Gergel I, Meinzer H-P, Wegner I: Kalibrierung
      elektromagnetischer Trackingsysteme 346

V47   Barendt S, Modersitzki J: SPECT Reconstruction with a
      Transformed Attenuation Prototype at Multiple Levels 352

V48   Erbe M, Grüttner M, Sattel TF, Buzug TM: Experimentelle
      Realisierungen einer vollständigen Trajektorie für die magnetische
      Partikel-Bildgebung mit einer feldfreien Linie 358

Methoden IV

P11   Fehlner A, Hirsch S, Braun J, Sack I: Fast 3D Vector Field
      Multi-Frequency Magnetic Resonance Elastography of the Human
      Brain 363

P12   Swarat D, Sudyatma N, Wagner T, Wiemann M, Lipinski H-G:
      Bildgestützte Formanalyse biomedizinisch relevanter Gold
      Nanorods 369

P13   Schnaars A, Tietjen C, Soza G, Preim B: Auffaltung von
      Gefäßbäumen mit Hilfe von deformierbaren Oberflächen 375

P14   Alassi S, Kowarschik M, Pohl T, Köstler H, Rude U: Estimating
      Blood Flow Based on 2D Angiographic Image Sequences 380

Anwendungen

P15   Kurzendorfer T, Brost A, Bourier F, Koch M, Kurzidim K,
      Hornegger J, Strobel N: Cryo-Balloon Catheter Tracking in Atrial
      Fibrillation Ablation Procedures 386

P16   Franz AM, Servatius M, Seitel A, Hummel J, Birkfellner W,
      Bartha L, Schlemmer H-P, Sommer CM, Radeleff BA,
      Kauczor H-U, Meinzer H-P, Maier-Hein L: Elektromagnetisches
      Tracking für die interventionelle Radiologie 392

P17   *Mersmann S, Guerrero D, Schlemmer H-P, Meinzer H-P,*
      Maier-Hein L: Effect of Active Air Conditioning in Medical
      Intervention Rooms on the Temperature Dependency of
      Time-of-Flight Distance Measurements 398

P18   *Birr S, Mönch J, Sommerfeld D, Preim B:* A novel Real-Time
      Web3D Surgical Teaching Tool based on WebGL 404

Registrierung II

P19   *Ahmadi S-A, Klein T, Plate A, Boetzel K, Navab N:* Rigid US-MRI
      Registration Through Segmentation of Equivalent Anatomic
      Structures 410

P20   *Huppert A, Ihme T, Wolf I:* Parallelisierung intensitätsbasierter
      2D/3D-Registrierung mit CUDA 416

P21   *Mang A, Schütz TA, Toma A, Becker S, Buzug TM:* Ein
      dämonenartiger Ansatz zur Modellierung tumorinduzierter
      Gewebedeformation als Prior für die nicht-rigide
      Bildregistrierung 422

Klassifikation

P22   *Hetzheim H, Hetzheim HG:* Image Processing for Detection of Fuzzy
      Structures in Medical Images 428

P23   *Harmsen M, Fischer B, Schramm H, Deserno TM:* Support Vector
      Machine Classification using Correlation Prototypes for Bone Age
      Assessment 434

P24   *Piesch T-C, Müller H, Kuhl CK, Deserno TM:* IRMA Code II 440

Kategorisierung der Beiträge 447

Autorenverzeichnis 449

Stichwortverzeichnis 453

Magnetresonanzelastografie
Grundlagen, Methoden und erste klinische Erfahrungen

Jürgen Braun[1], Ingolf Sack[2]

[1]Institut für Medizinische Informatik
[2]Institut für Radiologie und Neuroradiologie
Charité – Universitätsmedizin Berlin
juergen.braun@charite.de

Die Magnetresonanzelastografie (MRE) ist ein neues nichtinvasives Verfahren zur quantitativen Bestimmung mechanischer Gewebeeigenschaften. Diese Technik kann als bildgestützter, quantitativer Tastbefund angesehen werden. Die hohe Sensitivität des seit Jahrhunderten erfolgreich in der Diagnostik angewandten Tastbefundes geht auf die oft drastische Änderung der mechanischen Eigenschaften von Geweben aufgrund von Erkrankungen zurück. Auch heutzutage ist der Tastbefund ein wichtiger Bestandteil der klinischen Diagnose von oberflächennahen, krankhaften Gewebeveränderungen.

Mit Hilfe der MRE lassen sich erstmals elastische und viskose Kenngrößen auch von mechanisch abgeschirmten oder tiefliegenden Geweben quantitativ bestimmen. Dazu wird das Fortschreiten mechanischer Wellen durch bewegungssensitive MR Aufnahmetechniken aufgenommen. Die MRE umfasst insgesamt drei grundlegende Schritte:

1. Erzeugung niederfrequenter harmonischer Scherwellen in Gewebe,
2. Kodierung der Gewebebewegung in MR Phasenbildern und
3. Berechnung quantitativer Karten elastischer Kenngrößen.

Das Verfahren wird inzwischen klinisch zur Graduierung von Leberfibrose eingesetzt. Neue Forschungsergebnisse zeigen das Potenzial der MRE zum Nachweis neurodegenerativer Prozesse, wie sie beispielsweise bei Multipler Sklerose oder Normaldruckhydrozephalus auftreten. Weitere wichtige Anwendungen liegen in der mechanischen Charakterisierung von Tumoren in Gehirn, Brust, Prostata oder Leber. Zusätzlich kann die MRE zur Bestimmung von Druckgrößen eingesetzt werden. Dies erlaubt unter anderem Aussagen zur Herzfunktion durch direkte, nichtinvasive Druckmessungen in den Herzkammern.

Der Vortrag umfasst eine Einführung in die Grundlagen der MRE, Darstellung aktueller Ergebnisse an ausgewählten Anwendungen sowie erste Modelle, mit denen ein Zusammenhang zwischen makroskopisch bestimmten Elastizitätskenngrößen und krankheitsbedingter Änderungen auf zellulärer Ebene hergestellt werden kann.

Brain-Computer Interfaces

Prinzip und Perspektiven einer neuen Mensch-Maschine Schnittstelle

Gabriel Curio

Klinik für Neurologie, Charité – Universitätsmedizin Berlin
`gabriel.curio@charite.de`

Maschinen allein durch die Kraft der Gedanken steuern – was gestern wie Science Fiction klang, ist heute ein rasch expandierendes Forschungsfeld der klinischen und angewandten Neurowissenschaft. Brain-Computer Interfaces (BCIs) können tetraplegischen Patienten, z.B. im locked-in Syndrom, neue Handlungsmöglichkeiten eröffnen oder in der industriellen Neuroergonomie kritische Mensch-Maschine Interaktionen monitoren und ggfs. in Echtzeit optimieren.

Das Berliner BCI (http://www.bbci.de) integriert dafür das nicht-invasiv messbare Oberflächen-EEG mit der algorithmischen Technologie des Maschinellen Lernens. Dabei kommt ein mehrschrittiges Verfahren zur Anwendung: Zunächst werden neokortikale Aktivierungen, z.B. während verschiedener intendierter Bewegung, mittels eines Multikanal-EEGs aufgezeichnet, dann extrahieren auf den einzelnen Nutzer adaptierte Klassifikationsalgorithmen Intentionsspezifische, raumzeitliche Aktivierungsmuster, mit denen anschließend technische Geräte und Hilfsmittel gesteuert werden können. Nach einer Kalibrationsphase von nur 20 Minuten können EEG-Signale schon heute so genau klassifiziert werden, dass untrainierte Probanden Übertragungsraten bis 35 bit/min erreichen. Untersuchungen an Patienten mit lange zurückliegenden Amputationen haben gezeigt, dass derartige EEG-Signale auch dann noch nachweisbar sind, wenn beispielsweise nur eine „Phantom-Hand" bewegt werden soll.

Mit BCIs können Computer-Cursor gesteuert und „mentale Schreibmaschinen" bedient, Prothesen oder Computerspiele kontrolliert, sowie Wachheit und Konzentration an sicherheitsrelevanten Arbeitsplätzen erfasst werden. Aktuelle technologische Innovationen betreffen kapazitiv koppelnde („berührungsfreie") sowie im Alltagseinsatz „unsichtbare" EEG-Elektroden. BCIs werden medizinisch und industriell von Bedeutung sein, werden jedoch auch hinsichtlich militärischer Einsatzbereiche erforscht. Deshalb sollten in der öffentlichen Diskussion sowohl methodeninhärente Grenzen wie auch ethische Implikationen dieser Technologie Beachtung finden.

Direct Magnetic Resonance Elastography
Feasibility for Measuring Myocardial Elasticity Changes

Heiko Tzschätzsch[1], Thomas Elgeti[1], Sebastian Hirsch[1], Dagmar Krefting[2],
Dieter Klatt[1], Jürgen Braun[2], Ingolf Sack[1]

[1]Department of Radiology, Charité–Universitätsmedizin Berlin
[2]Institute of Medical Informatics, Charité–Universitätsmedizin Berlin
heiko.tzschaetzsch@gmx.de

Abstract. Direct cardiac magnetic resonance elastography (MRE) based on harmonically oscillating tissue interfaces is introduced. This method exploits cardiac triggered cine imaging synchronized to extrinsic harmonic motion of 22.83 Hz frequency for displaying oscillatory tissue deformations in the magnitude image. Oscillations are analyzed by intensity-threshold based image processing for delineating wave amplitude variations over the cardiac cycle. Initial results showed that endocardial wave amplitudes during systole (0.13 ± 0.07) mm were significantly lower than during diastole (0.34 ± 0.14) mm. Wave amplitudes were found to decrease (117 ± 40) ms before myocardial contraction and to increase (75 ± 31) ms prior to myocardial relaxation. Not requiring extra motion-encoding gradients the introduced method enables short-TR vibration imaging and therewith improves the time resolution in cardiac MRE.

1 Introduction

Cardiac function is determined by the alteration of myocardial elasticity during the cardiac cycle. Therefore, measurement of myocardial elasticity may support the diagnosis of cardiac relaxation abnormalities. Several groups have tackled cardiac elasticity imaging by developing a variety of dedicated elastography methods [1, 2, 3]. Cardiac magnetic resonance elastography (MRE) uses mechanical oscillations for mechanically stimulating the heart through the chest wall.

Compression waves penetrate the body widely undamped. Due to elastic wave scattering compression waves are converted to shear waves. At drive frequencies below 25 Hz those shear deflections are in the order of millimeters imposing signal shifts to the morphological contrast of an MR image. The oscillatory response of the heart's morphology to external stimuli depends on the variation of the myocardial shear modulus over the cardiac cycle. The myocardial shear modulus is synchronize with the heart's tension. As has been shown by phase-based MRE [1] the oscillation amplitude during systole is smaller than during diastole. More over, the alteration of the oscillation amplitude precedes cardiac motion due to isovolometric contraction and relaxation. This could be measured by standard MRI and may provide elastodynamic information without phase image processing, motion-encoding gradients (MEG) and wave inversion. Hence this approach is called direct MRE. The resulting echo time shortening reduces signal losses due to relaxation and improves temporal resolution in direct MRE.

The aim of the study was to analyze the timing and the degree of wave amplitude alterations over the cardiac cycle and to compare the results with values reported by echocardiography and phase-based cardiac MRE.

2   Methods

Ten healthy volunteers were included in this study. None of them had any history of cardiac events.

An extended piston driver was placed on the anterior chest wall. It was used to stimulate the heart with $f = 22.83$ Hz acoustic oscillations by a remote loudspeaker [1]. The oscillations were synchronized to a pulse-triggered balanced steady-state imaging sequence (bSSFP) in a short cardiac axis (Fig. 1).

An echo time (TE) of 1.51 ms and a repetition time (TR) of 3.65 ms was achieved. One image was acquired in a short-axis view with a 1.56 mm in-plane resolution and 5 mm slice thickness.

For post-processing, a vector $\mathbf{r}$ running from the anterior chest wall through the short axis of the left ventricle was manually selected in each volunteer (Fig. 2a).

The intensity profiles $I(\mathbf{r})$ were combined in a space-time matrix $I(\mathbf{r},t)$ (Fig. 2b). Vibrations in the direction of $\mathbf{r}$ (Fig. 3) were delineated by a processing routine applied to the space-time matrix $I(\mathbf{r},t)$, which included i) manual raw selection of the interface of interest (endocardial region of the left ventricle) and ii) automatic tracing of isolines of equal intensity I_0: $u(t) = I(\mathbf{r},t)\big|_{I=I_0}$. The

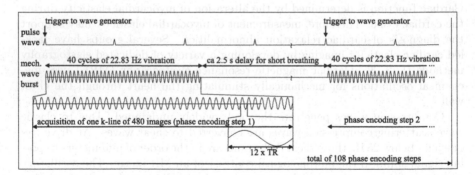

Fig. 1. Basic scheme of the direct MRE imaging technique. Here, a pulse-wave triggered and k-space segmented balanced steady state free precession (bSSFP) imaging sequence is synchronized with the external vibration, so that 12 TR match one vibration period. Alternatively, bSSFP can be replaced by any imaging technique which provides appropriate blood/myocardium contrast and which supports a temporal resolution in the range of (3 to 4) ms

assumption was that the total deflection $u(t)$ is a superposition of the cardiac motion $u_{card}(t)$ and the vibration $u_{vib}(t) = U(t) \sin(2 \pi f t)$.

As a result, a 1D vibration amplitude function $U(t)$ was obtained, which was analyzed twofold: For determining the amplitude of the vibration, first a 5 Hz bandpass filter centered at the vibration frequency was applied to $u(t)$. Secondly, the complex vibration signal $u_{vib}^*(t)$ was calculated by means of the Hilbert transformed of $u_{vib}(t)$: $u_{vib}^*(t) = u_{vib}(t) + \mathrm{i}\,H\{u_{vib}(t)\}$. The absolute value of this signal was taken as the vibration magnitude $U(t) = |u_{vib}^*(t)|$. For determining cardiac motion $u_{card}(t)$, the vibration was eliminated from $u(t)$ applying a low-pass filter with 10 Hz cutoff frequency. The wave amplitudes $U(t)$ had to be corrected by the cosine of the effective angle ϕ to $U'(t) = \cos(\phi)\,U(t)$ (Fig. 3). This correction is based on the assumption that planar waves emanate from the actuator plate towards the heart with wave vector $\mathbf{k}$ collinear to the anterior-posterior axis (the y-axis) (Fig. 3). Corrected wave amplitudes were measured at the body surface (U'_{surf}) encompassing a region close to the position of the piston driver and in the endocardial region of the left ventricle (U'_{LV}). Systolic phases of the cardiac cycle were defined as inward movement of the left ventricular wall, whereas an outward movement characterized diastolic phases.

To estimate the temporal relationship between wave amplitude variation and motion of the myocardial wall, isovolumetric cardiac times were manually assessed from $u_{card}(t)$ and $U_{LV}(t)$ similar to the method described in [4]: the

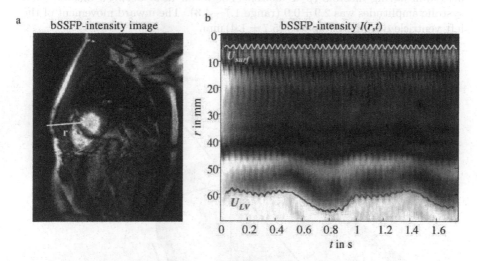

Fig. 2. a) Systolic short axis view of the heart using a magnitude image derived from a bSSFP acquisition to display cardiac anatomy and the position of profile $\mathbf{r}$. b) Profile $\mathbf{r}$ shown in 2a plotted over time using a M-mode like view. Vibrations due to the externally induced 22.83 Hz motion are well visible in the chest wall, the anterior heart boundary of the right ventricle, and in the septum. In this study we focused on vibrations of the endocardium (U_{LV}) in relation to systolic heart motion as well as vibrations delineated at the thorax surface (U_{surf})

isovolumetric contraction (IVC) was estimated by measuring the delay between descending branches of $u_{card}(t)$ and $U(t)$. Correspondingly, isovolumetric relaxation (IVR) was determined from the delay between the ascending branches of $u_{card}(t)$ and $U(t)$.

The isovolumetric times derived from direct MRE and spin-phase based MRE were compared by a two-sample Kolmogorov-Smirnov test.

3   Results

Vibrations induced by the external actuator were visible in the thoracic wall and left ventricular myocardium (Fig. 2b). The contrast-to-noise ratio of the myocardium-blood interface averaged in all volunteers was on the order of 11.6. A change in the gray value of a pixel on the myocardium-blood boundary by 11.6 would indicate a deflection of $1.56\,mm/11.6 = 0.134\,mm$ which we consider here as the in-plane resolution limit in our direct MRE experiment.

At the surface of the thoracic wall the corrected vibration amplitude was $(0.68 \pm 0.39)\,mm$ (0.25 to 1.45) mm. No change in amplitude related to the periodicity of the cardiac cycle was observed.

The wave amplitude in the left ventricular myocardium showed a time varying difference between systolic and diastolic phase of the cardiac cycle (Fig. 4).

The mean wave amplitude was $(0.13 \pm 0.07)\,mm$ during systole and $(0.34 \pm 0.14)\,mm$ during diastole ($p < 0.001$). The mean ratio between diastolic and systolic amplitudes was 2.9 ± 0.9 (range $1.7 - 4.3$). The inward movement of the left ventricle during systole was $(5.7 \pm 1.4)\,mm$.

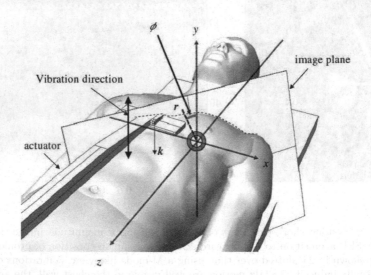

Fig. 3. For estimating the relative angle between profile **r** and wave vector k, a wave propagation direction along y (the anterior-posterior axis) was assumed. **r** is within in the image plane which intersects the heart in the short anatomical axis

The alteration in myocardial wave amplitude was (117 ± 40) ms before myocardial contraction, and (75 ± 31) ms before diastolic dilatation. Using phase-based cardiac MRE isovolumetric times of (130 ± 19) ms during contraction and (83 ± 22) ms during relaxation were measured. The IVC- and IVR-time are not significantly different in direct MRE and phase-based MRE ($p = 0.68$ and $p = 0.31$, respectively).

4   Discussion

This study shows that externally induced low-frequency acoustic waves inside the thoracic wall and the left ventricular myocardium can be measured without phase-contrast motion sensitization by using a cine imaging sequence synchronized to the periodicity of the motion. It was shown that minor oscillatory deflections far below voxel size can cause changes in partial volumes, resulting in changes in the magnitude signal analyzed by direct MRE. This high sensitivity of direct MRE to oscillatory deflections is due to the integrated signal of partial volumes within a voxel. In our experience, direct MRE requires steady wave amplitudes at least in the order of one tenth of the in-plane image resolution, which is still about a factor of ten higher than what is needed in conventional phase-based MRE. Of note, direct MRE depends on the amplitude and not on the wave number of the induced tissue vibration and displays coherent oscillatory shifts whose frequency can be arbitrarily low. Low frequencies are beneficial

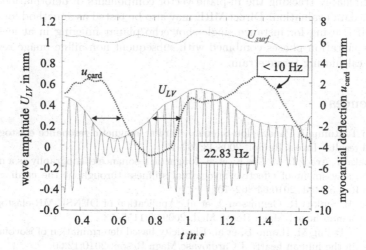

Fig. 4. Time course of wave amplitudes detected at the surface (green) and in the left ventricular myocardium (blue). The movement of the left ventricular wall is displayed in red. On the surface of the thoracic wall no alteration of wave amplitudes periodic to the heart cycle is seen. The wave amplitude in the left ventricle changes with respect to the cardiac phase. The change in wave amplitude is ahead of heart motion, giving rise to isovolumetric contraction and relaxation times (indicated by arrows)

as high wave amplitudes are achievable without exceeding the vibration safety limits [5].

Our main finding is that a change in wave amplitude $U_{LV}(t)$ can be observed ahead of cardiac motion $u_{card}(t)$. Low vibration amplitudes for $U'_{LV}(t)$ during systole were preceded and followed by higher wave amplitudes during diastole. The observed delay between alteration of wave amplitudes and myocardial motion strongly indicates that direct MRE can separate myocardial elastodynamics from heart morphology. The isovolumetric times measured by direct MRE are not significantly different from phase-contrast based steady-state cardiac MRE with a mean IVC-time of (136 ± 36) ms and an IVR-time of (75 ± 31) ms in healthy volunteers. The MRE-derived isovolumetric contraction time is considerable longer than the echocardiographic isovolumetric contraction time of (63 ± 14) ms. This might be attributable to the fact that the elastic properties of muscle tissue are nonlinear under large deformation, rendering the measured MRE wave response stretch-dependent.

The variation of systolic and diastolic wave amplitude in direct MRE was 2.9 ± 0.9. Assuming a plane shear wave model and a constant flux of wave energy allows to calculate a relative change of the shear modulus by $2.9^4 = 70.7$ ($\mu \propto U'^{-4}$, with the shear modulus μ) [6]. This value is in good agreement with the ratio derived by phase-based MRE [1, 6]. Future studies have to be conducted to determine which diagnostic parameters can be derived by direct MRE.

For further improvements, a two-dimensional cross-correlation method capable of reliably tracking the in-plane vector components of deformation could facilitate data evaluation. Direct MRE may also be tested as a method for quasi-static MRE using for instance single-shot echo planar imaging in at least two different vibration phases combined with subsequent non-affine image registration for calculating tissue strain.

References

1. Elgeti T, Rump J, Papazoglou S, et al. Cardiac magnetic resonance elastography: initial results. Invest Radiol. 2008;43:762–72.
2. Kolipaka A, Araoz P, McGee K, et al. Magnetic resonance elastography as a method for the assessment of effective myocardial stiffness throughout the cardiac cycle. Magn Reson Med. 2010;64:862–70.
3. Robert B, Sinkus R, Gennisson J, et al. Application of DENSE-MR-elastography to the human heart. Magn Reson Med. 2009;62:1155–63.
4. Elgeti T, Beling M, Hamm B, et al. Elasticity-based determination of isovolumetric phases in the human heart. J Cardiovasc Magn Reson. 2010;12:60.
5. Ehman E, Rossman P, Kruse S, et al. Vibration safety limits for magnetic resonance elastography. Phys Med Biol. 2008;53:925–35.
6. Sack I, Rump J, Elgeti T, et al. MR elastography of the human heart: Noninvasive assessment of myocardial elasticity changes by shear wave amplitude variations. Magn Reson Med. 2009;61:862–70.

Combined Model-Based and Region-Adaptive 3D Segmentation and 3D Co-Localization Analysis of Heterochromatin Foci

Simon Eck[1], Karl Rohr[1], Katharina Müller-Ott[2], Karsten Rippe[2], Stefan Wörz[1]

[1]Biomedical Computer Vision Group, Univ., BioQuant, IPMB, and DKFZ Heidelberg
[2]Research Group Genome Organization & Function, DKFZ and BioQuant, Heidelberg
simon.eck@bioquant.uni-heidelberg.de

Abstract. The nuclear organization of euchromatin and heterochromatin is important for genome regulation and cell function. Therefore, the analysis of heterochromatin formation and maintenance is an important topic in biological research. We introduce an automatic approach for analyzing heterochromatin foci in 3D multi-channel fluorescence microscopy images. The approach combines model-based segmentation with region-adaptive segmentation and performs a 3D co-localization analysis in different nuclear regions. Our approach has been successfully applied to 275 3D two-channel fluorescence microscopy images of mouse fibroblast cells.

1 Introduction

Heterochromatin, in contrast to euchromatin, is densely packed within the nucleus and responsible, e.g., for nuclear organization and centromere function [1]. In mouse fibroblast cells heterochromatin localizes to distinct foci and thus can be distinguished from euchromatic regions. Using DAPI (4',6-diamidino-2-phenylindole) and immunofluorescent staining, high concentrations of heterochromatin and associated proteins can be visualized as fluorescent foci in light microscopy images (Fig. 1). Investigation of these foci under different experimental conditions provides important information about heterochromatin formation and maintenance. Since biological studies typically involve large amounts of image data and since manual analysis of such images is time-consuming and error-prone, automatic image analysis is essential.

In previous work, only few approaches for 3D analysis of heterochromatin foci from fluorescence microscopy images have been proposed. Previous approaches usually depend on global thresholds [2, 3, 4, 5] and require manual interaction [3, 5]. For denoising and illumination correction, median and Gaussian filters [2, 3] as well as the top-hat transform [4, 5] have been applied. In [6], segmentation is performed by local maxima search and energy minimization within image regions. However, the approach is bound to the pixel raster and thus not accurate for small foci, and a co-localization analysis was not performed.

In this work, we introduce a new approach for automatic 3D segmentation of heterochromatin foci and 3D co-localization analysis in multi-channel microscopy images. Our approach combines accurate model-based segmentation based on 3D parametric intensity models for small foci and regularly shaped foci with region-adaptive segmentation for large foci of irregular shape. To characterize the 3D shape of foci, we use a shape regularity measure. Based on the segmentation results, we determine and exploit the 3D geometry of segmented foci to detect and classify 3D co-localizations between different image channels. Furthermore, co-localizations are determined separately in different nuclear regions. Note that model-based approaches using 3D parametric intensity models have previously been applied to microscopy images [7, 8] and for co-localization analysis [8]. However, application to heterochromatin images was not considered, foci of irregular shape were not addressed, and a co-localization analysis was not performed in different nuclear regions. Our approach is fully automatic and has been applied to 275 3D two-channel fluorescence microscopy images of mouse fibroblast cells.

2   Materials and methods

Our approach for analyzing heterochromatin foci in 3D multi-channel fluorescence microscopy images consists of 3D cell nuclei segmentation, 3D foci segmentation, and 3D co-localization analysis. 3D cell nuclei segmentation is required since individual intensity histograms of the nuclei are needed during foci segmentation. For 3D foci segmentation, we propose a two-step approach. The idea is to distinguish between different types of foci and select an appropriate segmentation scheme. In the first step, we use region-adaptive segmentation. Based on a shape regularity measure and size information we distinguish large irregularly shaped foci from small foci and regularly shaped foci. In the second step, small foci and regularly shaped foci are refined by model-based segmentation. Based on the 3D geometry of segmented foci, we detect and classify 3D

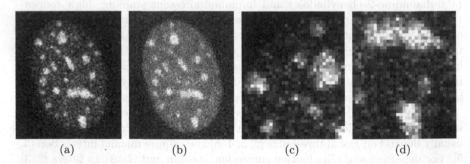

| (a) | (b) | (c) | (d) |

Fig. 1. Maximum intensity projections (MIPs) of a 3D two-channel fluorescence microscopy image: (a) Heterochromatin protein 1 (HP1α), (b) DAPI stained heterochromatin, (c) and (d) are enlarged sections of (a) showing regular and irregular HP1α foci, respectively

co-localizations. Note that in our experiments, we perform 3D foci segmentation on both the HP1α and the DAPI channel (Fig. 1), and 3D cell nuclei segmentation is carried out on a third channel which is generated based on the two other channels.

2.1   3D cell nuclei segmentation

One challenge in the considered two-channel microscopy image data is that the segmentation of nuclei is difficult due to staining artifacts and weak nuclei boundaries. To cope with this problem, we combine the information from the two image channels g_1 and g_2 by generating a third channel g_3 which is computed by $g_3(\mathbf{x}) = \max(g_1(\mathbf{x}), g_2(\mathbf{x}))$, where $\mathbf{x} = (x, y, z)$ denotes the 3D position and $g(\mathbf{x})$ denotes the intensity value at $\mathbf{x}$. For denoising g_3 we apply a 3D Gaussian filter and for labeling nuclei we use 3D Otsu thresholding. To determine the 3D positions of foci relative to the cell nucleus, we partition the nucleus into shells of equal volume (iso-volumetric shells). The shells are computed by first iteratively removing N thin shells from a segmented nucleus volume by erosion until no voxel remains. Then, the N thin shells are combined to M iso-volumetric shells so that the volume variance $\sigma^2 = \sum_{s=1}^{M} \left(V_s - \overline{V} \right)^2$ is minimal, where V_s denotes the volume of shell s and $\overline{V}$ denotes the mean volume of the shells (Fig. 2c).

2.2   3D region-adaptive segmentation of irregular foci

In the first step of our 3D foci segmentation approach, we concentrate on large foci of irregular shape. Since the intensity histograms vary strongly between images (e.g., depending on the number and size of nuclei in an image) and also the contrast of foci varies between different nuclei, we use a region-adaptive segmentation approach. An optimal threshold T_i is computed based on the 3D intensity histogram h_i for the i-th nucleus by

$$T_i = \overline{h_i} + c \cdot \sigma_i \tag{1}$$

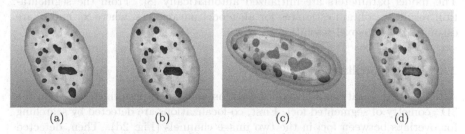

(a)   (b)   (c)   (d)

Fig. 2. Visualization of 3D foci segmentation results in (a) HP1α and (b) DAPI channel using combined model-based (red) and region-adaptive (blue) segmentation, (c) 3D localization of HP1α foci using iso-volumetric shells, and (d) 3D co-localization between HP1α (yellow) and DAPI (blue)

where $\overline{h}_i$ and σ_i denote the mean and the standard deviation of h_i, respectively, and c is a constant which can be adapted to the biological application. After denoising with a 3D Gaussian filter, foci of the i-th nucleus are segmented by thresholding with T_i. In our experiments, we used $c = 1.9$ and $c = 1.4$ in the HP1α and the DAPI channel, respectively, and $\sigma = 1$ for the 3D Gaussian filter in both channels. To distinguish whether foci are regular or irregular, we compute a shape regularity measure r, which is a 3D extension of the 2D circularity factor in [9] and is given by

$$r = \frac{|F \cap S|}{|F|}, r \in [0, 1] \tag{2}$$

where F denotes the segmented region of a focus and S denotes a sphere located at the center of F with the same volume as F. For example, $r \approx 1$ characterizes regular foci with a 3D shape very similar to a sphere. Values of $r \ll 1$ characterize very irregular foci. Foci with a high value of r or a small volume are excluded from the result, since they can be segmented more accurately by model-based segmentation (see below). In our experiments, foci with $r > 0.8$ are regarded as regular foci and foci with a volume of $V < 50$ voxels are regarded as small.

2.3   3D model-based segmentation of regular foci

For segmentation of small foci and regular foci, we employ a 3D model-based approach. In our application, the 3D intensity profile of small foci and regular foci can be well represented by a 3D Gaussian function

$$g_{\text{Gaussian3D}}(\mathbf{x}) = \exp\left(-\frac{x^2}{2\sigma_x^2} - \frac{y^2}{2\sigma_y^2} - \frac{z^2}{2\sigma_z^2}\right) \tag{3}$$

where $\boldsymbol{\sigma} = (\sigma_x, \sigma_y, \sigma_z)$ are the standard deviations. By including intensity levels a_0 (background) and a_1 (focus) as well as a 3D rigid transform $\mathcal{R}$ with rotation $\boldsymbol{\alpha} = (\alpha, \beta, \gamma)$ and translation $\mathbf{x}_0 = (x_0, y_0, z_0)$, we obtain the 3D intensity model $g_M(\mathbf{x}) = a_0 + (a_1 - a_0)\, g_{\text{Gaussian3D}}(\mathcal{R}(\mathbf{x}, \mathbf{x}_0, \boldsymbol{\alpha}))$ [8]. To fit the model to the image data, we use the non-linear optimization scheme of Levenberg/Marquardt. The model parameters are initialized automatically [8]. From the segmentation result, we obtain estimates for all model parameters, where $\mathbf{x}_0$ and $\boldsymbol{\sigma}$ are estimated at subvoxel resolution.

2.4   3D co-localization analysis

After 3D segmentation, a 3D co-localization analysis is performed based on the 3D geometry of segmented foci. First, co-localizations are detected by searching for overlaps between foci in the two image channels (Fig. 2d). Then, detected co-localizations are classified based on the amount of overlap, the size, and the shape of foci. Furthermore, the number and type of co-localizations in different nuclear regions (e.g., the nuclear periphery or the center) are quantified based on the iso-volumetric shells generated during nuclei segmentation (Sect. 2.1).

Table 1. Number of foci in different iso-volumetric shells (n_{s_i}) (s_1 is the outermost shell) and in all nuclei (n_{total}), mean number per nucleus (n_{mean}), and mean foci volume (V_{mean})

	n_{s_1}	n_{s_2}	n_{s_3}	n_{total}	n_{mean}	V_{mean}
HP1α foci	1280	11528	24252	37060	43.81	57.48
DAPI foci	236	6301	20528	27065	31.99	104.80

3 Results

We have successfully applied our combined approach to 275 3D two-channel images of NIH 3T3 mouse fibroblast cells. The images were acquired by a confocal laser scanning microscope with $512 \times 512 \times 49$ voxels resolution. Image analysis was performed fully automatically and with fixed parameter settings for all images. The approach successfully distinguished between regular and irregular foci, and achieved good segmentation results (Fig. 2a,b). We also compared the results with those from a pure model-based approach and a pure region-adaptive segmentation approach, and found that the combined approach yields the best results w.r.t. ground truth (HP1α and DAPI foci in five nuclei segmented by an expert). For example, Fig. 3 shows ground truth and segmentation results of HP1α foci for the nucleus in Fig. 1.

Table 1 shows for all 275 3D images the number n_{s_i} of segmented foci located in different shells s_i, the total number n_{total} of segmented foci, the mean number of foci per nucleus n_{mean}, and the mean foci volume V_{mean}. It can be seen that the majority of segmented foci localizes near the nucleus center (n_{s_3}). Considering co-localizations, we found that about 62% of DAPI foci co-localize with HP1α foci (about 54%, 64%, and 62% of DAPI foci located in the shells s_1, s_2, and s_3 co-localize with HP1α foci, respectively).

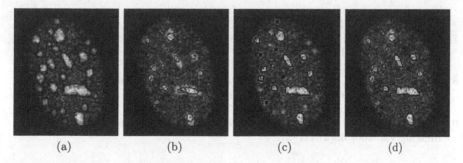

(a)   (b)   (c)   (d)

Fig. 3. MIPs of 3D foci segmentation results: (a) ground truth, (b) pure model-based approach, (c) pure region-adaptive segmentation approach, and (d) combined model-based (red) and region-adaptive (blue) segmentation approach

4   Discussion

We developed an approach for automatic analysis of heterochromatin foci in 3D multi-channel fluorescence microscopy images. Our approach combines region-adaptive segmentation for large foci of irregular shape with model-based segmentation for small foci and regular foci. A 3D co-localization analysis is performed based on the 3D geometry of segmented foci. Furthermore, co-localizations are detected and classified separately in different nuclear regions. We have successfully applied our approach to 275 3D two-channel images of mouse fibroblast cells. In future work, we will apply our approach to images from new experiments to compare, e.g., heterochromatin formation between different cell types.

Acknowledgement. This work has been funded by the BMBF (SysTec) project EpiSys.

References

1. Müller KP, Erdel F, Caudron-Herger M, et al. Multiscale analysis of dynamics and interactions of heterochromatin protein 1 by fluorescence fluctuation microscopy. Biophys J. 2009;97(11):2876–85.
2. Jost KL, Haase S, Smeets D, et al. 3D-Image analysis platform monitoring relocation of pluripotency genes during reprogramming. Nucleic Acids Res. 2011;39(17):e113.
3. Andrey P, Kieu K, Kress C, et al. Statistical analysis of 3D images detects regular spatial distributions of centromeres and chromocenters in animal and plant nuclei. PLoS Comput Biol. 2010;6(7):e1000853.
4. Ivashkevich AN, Martin OA, Smith AJ, et al. H2AX foci as a measure of DNA damage: A computational approach to automatic analysis. Mutat Res. 2011;711(1-2):49–60.
5. Böcker W, Iliakis G. Computational methods for analysis of foci: Validation for radiation-induced y-H2AX foci in human cells. Radiat Res. 2006;165(1):113–24.
6. Dzyubachyk O, Essers J, van Cappellen WA, et al. Automated analysis of time-lapse fluorescence microscopy images: from live cell images to intracellular foci. Bioinformatics. 2010;26(19):2424–30.
7. Thomann D, Rines DR, Sorger PK, et al. Automatic fluorescent tag detection in 3D with super-resolution: application to the analysis of chromosome movement. J Microsc. 2002;208:49–64.
8. Wörz S, Sander P, Pfannmöller M, et al. 3D geometry-based quantification of colocalizations in multichannel 3D microscopy images of human soft tissue tumors. IEEE Trans Med Imaging. 2010;29(8):1474–84.
9. Ritter N, Cooper J. New resolution independent measures of circularity. J Math Imaging Vis. 2009;35(2):117–27.

Formmodellbasierte Segmentierung des Unterkiefers aus Dental-CT-Aufnahmen
Ein vollautomatischer Ansatz

Sebastian T. Gollmer, Thorsten M. Buzug

Institut für Medizintechnik, Universität zu Lübeck
gollmer@imt.uni-luebeck.de

Kurzfassung. Dental-CT-Aufnahmen leiden unter einer vergleichsweise schlechten Bildqualität bezüglich des Signal-zu-Rausch Verhältnisses. Aus diesem Grund benutzen wir ein statistisches Formmodell (SFM) zur robusten Segmentierung des Unterkiefers. Im Gegensatz zu bisherigen Arbeiten ist das von uns vorgestellte Verfahren vollautomatisch - sowohl was die Korrespondenzfindung angeht, als auch bezüglich der Segmentierung an sich. Obwohl unsere Trainingspopulation weniger als 30 % des Umfangs ähnlicher Arbeiten aufweist, erzielen wir vergleichbare Ergebnisse. Ein wesentlicher Grund hierfür ist die Korrespondenzfindung mittels Optimierung einer modellbasierten Zielfunktion: Unsere Ergebnisse zeigen, dass dies eine deutliche Verbesserung der Segmentierungsergebnisse erlaubt und belegen damit erstmals die Bedeutung dieses Ansatz unmittelbar in einer Anwendung zur Segmentierung.

1 Einleitung

Hochauflösende Cone-Beam-CT (CBCT) Geräte werden zunehmend für die Erstellung von Übersichtsaufnahmen vor dental-chirurgischen Eingriffen eingesetzt. Deren Planung mit Hilfe eines individuellen Modells der Knochenanatomie erfordert zunächst eine entsprechende Segmentierung. Diese muss aus Zeit- und Kostengründen automatisch erfolgen. Hierbei sieht man sich jedoch einem, für die i.d.R. mit geringer Strahlenintensität betriebenen Geräte charakteristischen, hohen Bildrauschen und vermehrten Auftreten von Artefakten konfrontiert. Das Sichtfeld ist zudem auf ein die Kieferregion eng umschließendes Volumen begrenzt, an dessen Rändern (z.B. Kondylen) die Bildqualität zusätzlich leidet.

Ausschließlich auf der Bildinformation basierende Algorithmen liefern deswegen meist keine brauchbaren Ergebnisse, wohingegen das Einbringen von Vorwissen über die zu segmentierende Struktur bessere Resultate erwarten lässt. Statistische Formmodelle (SFM) integrieren die zu erwartende Formvariabilität einer bestimmten Objektklasse [1] und erlauben somit die Trennung benachbarter Strukturen mit ähnlichen Intensitätswerten, die Verbesserung der Robustheit gegenüber Bildrauschen sowie die Extrapolation bei fehlender Bildinformation.

Die Anpassung des SFM an das Bild erfolgt auf der Basis lokaler Bildmerkmale. Voraussetzungen für die lokale Suche ist das Wissen, ausgehend von welchen Punkten des Modells dies zu tun ist (Korrespondenzfindung) und an welcher globalen Position im Bild die Suche gestartet werden soll (Initialisierung). Bisherige Arbeiten zur SFM basierten Segmentierung des Unterkiefers kommen nicht ohne manuelle Interaktion in mindestens einer dieser Komponenten aus. In [2] werden Korrespondenzen semi-automatisch in 2D-Schnittbildern ermittelt. [3] bestimmen Korrespondenzen in 3D, benötigen dafür jedoch ebenfalls eine manuelle Interaktion. Dagegen bestimmen wir die Korrespondenzen vollautomatisch durch Optimierung einer modellbasierten Kostenfunktion, dem derzeitigen Quasi-Standard bezüglich Korrespondenzfindung ([4]). Zudem ist unser Verfahren zur automatischen Lokalisation des Unterkiefers sehr effizient während [3] die vergleichsweise aufwändige generalisierte Hough-Transformation benutzen.

2   Material und Methoden

2.1   Statistische Formmodelle

Die $n_s \in \mathbb{N}^+$ Formen $\{S_i \subset \mathbb{R}^3, \ i = 1, \ldots, n_s\}$ der Trainingspopulation lassen sich durch Abtastung mit n_p korespondierenden Landmarken als sogenannte Formvektoren $x_i \in \mathbb{R}^{3n_p}$ repräsentieren. Zur Berechnung der Durchschnittsform $\bar{x} = n_s^{-1} \sum_{i=1}^{n_s} x_i$ sowie der $n_m \in \mathbb{N}$ Eigenwerte $\{\lambda_m, \ m = 1, \ldots, n_m\}$ und Eigenvektoren $P = (p_1 \ldots p_{n_m})$ der Kovarianzmatrix der Formvektoren, werden diese in einem gemeinsamen Koordinatensystem ausgerichtet. Das lineare SFM repräsentiert die Formen $\{x = \bar{x} + Pb \mid b \in \mathbb{R}^{n_m}, b^{(m)} \in [-3\sqrt{\lambda_m}, 3\sqrt{\lambda_m}]\}$.

2.2   Korrespondenzfindung

Die Etablierung von Punktkorrespondenzen kann z.B. durch Abbildung der Formen $\{S_i\}$ in eine geeignete Parameterdomäne und äquidistante Abtastung der Parametrisierungen erfolgen. Im Unterschied zu [3] verwenden wir die Einheits-2-Sphäre $\mathbb{S}^2$ als Parameterdomäne (Abb. 2(a),(b)). Für eine solche $\mathbb{S}^2$-Parametrisierung gibt es etablierte Algorithmen ([4]) welche die Korrespondenzen durch iterative Optimierung einer modellbasierten Kostenfunktion verbessern.

Wir verwenden die distmin-Abbildung [5] zur Erstellung initialer Parametrisierungen $\{\omega_i : \mathbb{S}^2 \to S_i, \ i = 1, \ldots, n_s\}$. Diese liefert einen guten Kompromiss zwischen der Minimierung der Verzerrungen innerhalb einzelner Abbildungen ω_i einerseits (Abb. 1) und einer hohen Konsistenz zwischen allen Abbildungen $\{\omega_i\}$ andererseits und damit eine geeignete Initialisierung der anschließenden Korrespondenzoptimierung. Letztere basiert auf dem Algorithmus in [6], wir ersetzen die dort verwendete Kostenfunktion jedoch durch die sogenannte detcov-Kostenfunktion [7], da diese in unseren Experimenten bessere Ergebnisse lieferte. Im Unterschied zu [7] setzen wir den Regularisierungsparameter ϵ_{detcov} nicht auf einen zuvor festgelegten kleinen Wert, sondern berechnen diesen (in Anlehnung an [6]) in Abhängigkeit vom mittleren Radius $\bar{r}$ der $\{S_i\}$ zu $\epsilon_{detcov} = (\sigma_n / \bar{r})^2$, wobei $\sigma_n = 0{,}3$ die Standardabweichung des Rauschen ist (hier: $\bar{r} = 48$ mm).

Abb. 1. Exemplarische Trainingsform S_i (a), deren sphärische Parametrisierung ω_i (b) (gleiche Farben identifizieren 1-zu-1 Korrespondenzen zwischen S_i und ω_i) und mittels äquidistanter Abtastung von ω_i rekonstruierter Formvektor x_i (c) (Reduktion der Vertexzahl um 83 %, Farben geben den Abstand gegenüber S_i an). Das quadratische Mittel des durch Parametrisierung und Abtastung induzierten Rekonstruktionsfehlers liegt mit $0{,}18 + 0{,}03$ mm unter der Auflösung der CBCT-Aufnahmen von 0,3 mm

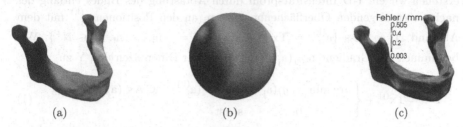

(a)   (b)   (c)

2.3 Initialisierung

Im Unterschied zu [3] benutzen wir kein aufwändiges Suchverfahren, sondern lokalisieren den Unterkiefer unter Ausnutzung der Verteilung der Intensitätswerte und ihres Gradienten im Bildvolumen $I(u)$, $u \in \Omega \subset \mathbb{R}^3$. Wir definieren zunächst eine Region of Interest (ROI) Ω^*, welche lediglich den Unterkieferkörper beinhaltet. Dabei nutzen wir aus, dass die Menge der zum Zahnschmelz beitragenden Voxel $V_t = \{I(u) \mid I(u) \in [t_{\min}, t_{\max}], u \in \Omega\}$ sehr robust durch Festlegung eines Grauwertintervalls $[t_{\min}, t_{\max}] \in \mathbb{Z}^2$ geschätzt werden kann. Aus der Projektion von V_t auf die y-z-Ebene und anschließende Akkumulation über diese beiden Achsen leiten wir die Ausdehnung des Gebisses und damit des Unterkieferkörpers in y- und z-Richtung ab. Innerhalb der ROI Ω^* (orange markierter Bereich in Abb. 2 links) klassifizieren wir die Pixel bezüglich ihres Intensitätswertes sowie ihres Gradienten, um die zur Kortikalis des Unterkieferknochens beitragenden Voxel $V_m = \{I(u) \mid I(u) \in C \wedge \partial I(u)/\partial u \geq g_{\max}/10, u \in \Omega^*\}$ zu bestimmen. Dabei sind $C = [c_{\min}, c_{\max}] \in \mathbb{Z}^2$ ein Grauwertintervall und $g_{\max} \in \mathbb{R}$ der maximale, mittels Sobel-Operator bestimmte Bildgradient. Anschließende Dilatation der V_m liefert eine zusammenhängende binäre Repräsentation der Kortikalis. Deren Oberfläche tasten wir mit ca. 10.000 Punken zufällig ab und registrieren die resultierende Punktmenge mit Hilfe des Iterative Closest Point Algorithmus [8] rigide mit dem im Zentrum von Ω platzierten $\bar{x}$ (Abb. 2).

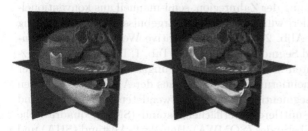

Abb. 2. Links: Initiale Platzierung von $\bar{x}$ (gelb) durch rigide Registrierung mit der, die Unterkieferkortikalis repräsentierende Punktewolke (blau). Rechts: Resultat der anschießenden Unterkiefersegmentierung

2.4 Segmentierung

Wir bestimmen die Positions- und Formparameter T bzw. b durch iterative Minimierung von $\mathcal{L} = \sum_{j=1}^{n_p} \left\| Y^{(j)} - Tx^{(j)} \right\|_2^2$ [1], wobei Y eine Schätzung der gesuchten Segmentierung ist. Für jede Landmarkenposition $x^{(j)} \in \mathbb{R}^3, j = 1, \ldots, n_p$ erstellen wir ein 1-D Intensitätsprofil durch Abtastung des Bildes entlang der nach außen zeigenden Oberflächennormale n_j an den Positionen $a_j^{(k)}$ mit dem Abstand Δ, so dass $\{a_j^{(k)} = Tx^{(j)} + k\Delta n_j, k = -n_l, \ldots, n_l, n_l \in \mathbb{N}^+\}$. Wir bestimmen den Gradienten $g_j(a_j^{(k)})$ mittels finiter Differenzen und Y zu

$$Y^{(j)} = Tx^{(j)} + \begin{cases} \arg\min_{a_j^{(k)}} g_j(a_j^{(k)}) & \text{falls } I'(a_j^{(k)}) \in C \wedge g_j(a_j^{(k)}) < g_{\min} \\ 0 & \text{sonst} \end{cases} \qquad (1)$$

Dabei ist $I'(a_j^{(k)})$ der Intensitätswert nach gerichteter Gaussglättung entlang von n_j, $C = [c_{\min}, c_{\max}]$ und $g_{\min} \in \mathbb{R}$ ein Schwellwert für den Gradienten.

In jeder Iteration verwenden wir (1) zunächst zur Bestimmung von T [9], wobei wir die $Y^{(j)}$, deren Abstand $d_j = \left\| Y^{(j)} - Tx^{(j)} \right\|_2$ größer als $1/n_p \sum_{j=1}^{n_p} d_j$ ist, mit $0{,}5\,d_j^{-2}$ bestrafen. Anschließend bestimmen wir die Formparameter b wie in [1]. Dabei wird eine Multi-Resolutions-Bildpyramide benutzt, um die Größe des Suchradius um $x^{(j)}$ nach und nach zu verkleinern.

2.5 Experimente

Neben der Frage nach der Güte der von uns erstellten Segmentierungen, interessiert uns die bereits in [4] aufgeworfene Frage, in welchem Maße die Korrespondenzfindung die Segmentierung beeinflusst und inwiefern Korrespondenz- und Segmentierungsgüte in Zusammenhang stehen. Aus diesem Grund lösen wir das Korrespondenzproblem zum einen mittels Optimierung (Abschnitt 2.2), zum anderen verwenden wir den distmin- [5] und den spharm- [10] Ansatz für die SFM-Erstellung. Wir berechnen zunächst die Korrespondenzgüte für die drei SFM und verwenden diese anschließend für die automatische Segmentierung.

3   Ergebnisse

Unsere Trainingspopulation umfasst 30 Formen (13 weibl., 17 männl., Alter: 18-72 Jahre), die, unter Auslassung der Zahnregion, semi-manuell aus konventionellen CT-Aufnahmen segmentiert wurden. Qualitativ Ergebnisse der Initialisierung bzw. Segmentierung zeigen Abb. 2 bzw. 3. Quantitative Werte der Korrespondenzgüte, Initialisierung und Segmentierung enthält Tab. 1. Die Korrespondenzgüte entspricht dem bekannten Maß der Generalisierungsfähigkeit, die Güte der Initialisierung und der Segmentierung ergeben sich aus der Abweichung von den manuell erstellten Referenzsegmentierungen. Die verwendeten Distanzmaße sind der (jeweils symmetrische) mittlere Oberflächenabstand (SMA), quadratische Mittelwert des Oberflächenabstandes (SQMWA), Hausdorff-Abstand (SHA) und

Tabelle 1. Korrespondenzgüte, Lokalisations-, und Segmentierungsergebnisse (von oben nach unten) für die drei verschiedenen SFM (jew. Mittelw.±Standardabw.)

	SMA/mm	SQMWA/mm	SHA/mm	VUF/%
distmin-SFM	$0,8 \pm 0,1$	$1,0 \pm 0,2$	$4,7 \pm 1,3$	$21,3 \pm 3,4$
spharm-SFM	$0,8 \pm 0,1$	$1,0 \pm 0,2$	$4,7 \pm 0,9$	$21,6 \pm 3,6$
detcov-SFM	$\mathbf{0,6 \pm 0,1}$	$\mathbf{0,8 \pm 0,1}$	$\mathbf{4,2 \pm 1,2}$	$17,4 \pm 2,9$
Initialisierung	$2,0 \pm 0,4$	$2,7 \pm 0,5$	$13,2 \pm 2,6$	$47,5 \pm 8,7$
distmin-SFM	$0,9 \pm 0,2$	$1,4 \pm 0,4$	$\mathbf{9,3 \pm 2,9}$	$24,1 \pm 7,7$
spharm-SFM	$0,9 \pm 0,2$	$1,4 \pm 0,3$	$11,1 \pm 3,9$	$22,9 \pm 4,6$
detcov-SFM	$\mathbf{0,8 \pm 0,1}$	$\mathbf{1,2 \pm 0,3}$	$9,9 \pm 3,7$	$\mathbf{20,7 \pm 4,2}$

die sich aus dem Jaccard-Index ergebende Abweichung in der Volumenüberlagerung (VUF). Für sämtliche Ergebnisse wurde n_m so gewählt, dass das jeweilige SFM 98% der gesamten Formvariabilität der Trainingspopulation beschreibt.

Die automatische Segmentierung wurde auf sechs Dental-CT-Aufnahmen angewendet, wobei $t_{min}/t_{max} = 1500/2700$, $\Delta = 1,0/0,5/0,25$ mm für die drei Auflösungen der Bildpyramide, $n_l = 4$, $c_{min}/c_{max} = 400/1200$ und $g_{min} = -100/$mm. Initialisierung und Segmentierung benötigen auf einem modernen Desktoprechner insgesamt $60 - 70$ s pro Datensatz unter Verwendung von $20/20/40$ Iterationen auf den drei Stufen der Bildpyramide und $n_p = 4002$ Landmarken.

4   Diskussion

Aus Tab. 1 ist ersichtlich, dass das mittels modellbasierter Korrespondenzoptimierung erstellte detcov-SFM sowohl bezüglich der Korrespondenz- als auch der Segmentierungsgüte überlegen ist. Interessanterweise liefert das spharm-SFM außer für den SHA etwas bessere Segmentierungs-Ergebnisse als das distmin-SSM bei gleicher Korrespondenzgüte, bleibt aber hinter dem detcov-SFM zurück

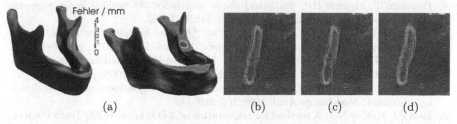

(a)   (b)   (c)   (d)

Abb. 3. Ergebnisse der Segmentierung für zwei CBCT Datensätze (a), die Farben geben den Abstand zur Referenzsegmentierung an. Die größten Abweichungen treten im Bereich der Zähne und der Kondylen auf. (b)-(d): Ergebnisse für das distmin-, spharm und detcov-SFM jeweils im Vergleich zur Referenzsegmentierung (grün). Das detcov-SFM zeigt die beste Anpassung an die Knochenkontur

(Abb. 3(b)-(d)). Dessen kompaktere Beschreibung der Formvariabilität verbessert die Robustheit gegenüber fälschlicherweise detektierten Bildmerkmalen. Ein solch direkter Vergleich des Einflusses der Korrespondenzfindung auf die Segmentierungsergebnisse ist unseres Wissens bislang nicht erfolgt und stellt somit eine neuartige, anwendungsbezogene Erweiterung von [5] dar.

In [2, 3] sind die einfachen Abstände der Segmentierung zur Referenzoberfläche angegeben. Diesbezüglich erzielen wir für das detcov-SFM $0,7 \pm 0,1$ mm, $1,0 \pm 0,2$ mm bzw. $6,1 \pm 2,5$ mm für den MA, QMWA bzw. HA und liegen damit unter den in [3] aufgeführten und nur geringfügig über den in [3] berichteten Werten. Dies dürfte zu großen Teilen daran liegen, dass unsere Trainingspopulation nur ca. 28% des Umfangs in [3] aufweist. Zudem birgt die gradientenbasierte Kostenfunktion (1) Verbesserungspotenzial. Hierbei ist zu betonen, dass wir im Gegensatz zu [3] auf deren heuristische Feinabstimmung bewusst verzichten, da wir erst durch das Lernen von Intensitäts- und/oder Gradientenprofilen ([4]) eine signifikante Verbesserung bei der Detektion lokaler Bildmerkmale erwarten. Neben einer dahingehenden Erweiterung unseres Modells, sowie der Vergrößerung unserer Test- und Trainingspopulation, ist die Einbringung zusätzlicher Freiheitsgrade bei der Segmentierung Gegenstand aktueller Arbeit.

Trotz der genannten Limitierungen wurde erstmals eine formmodellbasierte Segmentierung des Kiefers vorgestellt, die bei Modellerstellung und Segmentierung ohne manuelle Interaktion auskommt. Das mit Korrespondenzoptimierung erstellte SFM liefert bessere Segmentierungsergebnisse und ermöglicht die Erstellung eines genaueren individuellen Modells dieser Anatomie.

Literaturverzeichnis

1. Cootes TF, Taylor CJ, Cooper DH, et al. Active shape models: their training and application. Comput Vis Image Underst. 1995;61(1):38–59.
2. Rueda S, Gil JA, Pichery R, et al. Automatic segmentation of jaw tissues in CT using active appearance Models and Semi-automatic Landmarking. In: Proc MICCAI; 2006. p. 167–74.
3. Kainmueller D, Lamecker H, Seim H, et al. Automatic extraction of mandibular nerve and bone from cone-beam CT data. In: Proc MICCAI; 2009. p. 76–83.
4. Heimann T, Meinzer HP. Statistical shape models for 3D medical image segmentation: a review. Med Image Anal. 2009;13(4):5431–563.
5. Kirschner M, Gollmer ST, Wesarg S, et al. Optimal initialization for 3D correspondence optimization: an evaluation study. In: Proc IPMI; 2011. p. 308–19.
6. Heimann T, Wolf I, Williams T, et al. 3D active shape models using gradient descent optimization of description length. In: Proc IPMI; 2005. p. 566–77.
7. Kotcheff ACW, Taylor CJ. Automatic construction of eigenshape models by direct optimization. Med Image Anal. 1998;2(4):303–14.
8. Besl PJ, McKay ND. A method for registration of 3-D shapes. IEEE Trans Pattern Anal Mach Intell. 1992;14(2):239–56.
9. Horn BKP. Closed-form solution of absolute orientation using unit quaternions. J Opt Soc Am A. 1987;4(4):629–42.
10. Brechbühler C, Gerig G, Kübler O. Parametrization of closed surfaces for 3-D shape description. Comput Vision Image Understanding. 1995;61(2):154–70.

A Systematic Approach Toward Reliable Atherosclerotic Plaque Characterization in IVUS Images

Amin Katouzian[1,2], Athanasios Karamalis[1], Andrew Laine[2], Nassir Navab[1]

[1]Computer Aided Medical Procedures, Technical University of Munich, Germany
[2]Biomedical Engineering Department, Columbia University, New York, USA
amin.katouzian@cs.tum.edu

Abstract. Intravascular ultrasound (IVUS) is the most favorable imaging modality that often used in coronary artery catheterization procedures and provides cross-sectional images of arterial wall structures and extend of atherosclerosis. Although several techniques have been developed to classify atherosclerotic tissues, deploying IVUS radiofrequency (RF) backscattered signals and/or grayscale images their clinical applications have seen limited success. In this paper, we propose a unified methodological framework from data collection, histology preparation, registration, feature extraction, and classification to achieve a reliable in vitro trained tissue characterization classifier for in vivo applications. Finally, the results from proposed algorithm is compared with state of the art virtual histology (VH) technique.

1 Introduction

The importance of atherosclerotic disease in coronary artery has been a subject of study for many researchers in the past decade. In brief, the aim is to understand progression of such disease and provide interventional cardiologists with reliable clinical tools so they can identify vulnerable plaques [1], choose the most appropriate drugs or implant devices (i.e. stent), and stabilize plaques at risks during and after catheterization procedures. Among all medical imaging modalities, IVUS provides real-time images with fairly good resolution and sufficient penetration. Hence, researchers employed intravascular ultrasound (IVUS) radiofrequency (RF) signals [2, 3] and grayscale images [4, 5] and extracted spectral and/or textural features to characterize atherosclerotic plaques in a supervised classification framework [6]. Although existing algorithms have their own advantages there is not a reliable atherosclerotic tissue characterization method yet. This could be due to stringent behavior of tissues in response to ultrasound signal and heterogeneity of tissues that make it more sophisticated than a classical classification problem.

The main contribution of this work is development of a systematic framework from data collection toward classification. For the first time, we study registration among IVUS and histology images, consistency among extracted features and compare our results with state of the art virtuall histology (VH) images.

2   Data collection, histology preparation, and IVUS-histology matching procedure

We collected IVUS data in vitro using 40 MHz transducer from arteries dissected from autopsied or transplanted hearts (24 hour postmortem or surgery) with circulating saline as well as human blood followed by formalin fixation, decalcification, slicing and staining to obtain histology images. Fig. 1 illustrates our experimental setup, a grayscale IVUS image with corresponding Hematoxylin

Fig. 1. Experimental setup (a), artery cage fixture (b), a grayscale IVUS image (c), and corresponding H&E histology image (d). Manually traced lumen (red) and media-adventitia (green) borders. The white star on histology image marks the location of necrotic core. Registered IVUS-histology images via non-rigid deformable method (e)

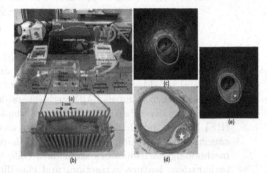

and eosin (H&E) histology image. The main advantage of this methodology is that the orientation of artery is not changed throughout the whole procedure. Therefore, more reliable IVUS-histology pairs could be obtained and the number of cross sections of interest (CSIs) per vessel is significantly increased (average of 25 regions).

The histology images are then used to find IVUS images counterparts and construction of one-to-one IVUS-histology matched database that is deployed for feature extraction, validation, and quantification of constructed tissue color maps. Traditionally, an expert manually selects regions corresponding to each tissue types, visually imposes them on IVUS image, and labels them to retrieve corresponding signals/textures for building training dataset prior to feature extraction. However, due to heterogeneity of tissues as well as visual registration of IVUS-histology plaque regions, manual-visual labeling produces unreliable training dataset and therefore inconsistency among extracted features, resulting deficiency in classification performance. The challenge is more sensible when one tries to manually label the most homogenous regions on histology image, Fig. 1(d) and visually impose them on corresponding IVUS frame in Fig. 1(c).

As described above, the experimental setup ensures an anatomical correspondence between IVUS and histology images. However, the images need to be registered in the same coordinate space to properly assess their corresponding structures. Such a registration becomes challenging not only because of underlying differences between two imaging modalities, but also because of deformations introduced during histology preparation as well as acquisition process (i.e. shrinkage). A direct non-rigid registration of two modalities is challenging and outside the scope of this paper. Nevertheless, a registration of intermediate image representations is feasible. Hence, we generated segmentation masks corresponding to lumen and media-adventitia borders for both histology and IVUS images and employed non-rigid registration with discrete Markov-Random-Field (MRF) objective function and approximate curvature penalty for smoothness regularization [7]. The resulting deformation field was applied to the original histology image to transfer it to IVUS coordinate system. As we can see, the registered image, Fig. 1(e), is easier and more reliable to be used for labeling and extracting features corresponding to each tissue type.

3   Feature extraction and classification methodologies

We projected IVUS signals on spatial-frequency-localized orthogonal functions such as Lemarie-Batlle that were symmetric and quadrature mirror filters (QMF) and its generalization to two-dimension (2D) through tensor product extension to discern textural patterns on IVUS images while geometrically oriented features were provided at this dimension. Due to heterogeneity of atherosclerotic tissues, the projections were performed, employing discrete orthogonal wavelet packet frames, in an overcomplete fashion to preserve as much textural information as possible. The envelopes of features are then extracted at the bottom of decomposition tree and an unsupervised ISODATA clustering was deployed to classify tissues. Complete description of feature extraction and classification methodologies can be found in [8]. Unlike existing algorithms, we design our framework upon unsupervised characterization of tissues for two reasons. First, it is infeasible to build a reliable training dataset due to heterogeneity of atherosclerotic tissues. Secondly, we hypothesized that, in an unsupervised classifier, if extracted signatures represent true characteristics of atherosclerotic tissues, then they could be more reliably used for supervised classification. In fact, we can use the result of our unsupervised classifier, as labels for feature extraction and construction of training dataset.

4   Results

We performed our algorithm on 83 CSIs collected from 51 segments of 32 hearts and tissues into calcified, fibrotic, lipidic and "no tissues". Fig. 2 demonstrates a CSI, corresponding H&E histology image, and constructed tissue colormap or so we called prognosis histology (PH) image. The blue, yellow and pink colors represent calcified, fibrotic, and lipidic tissues, respectively. We evaluated the

Fig. 2. IVUS grayscale image (left), corresponding H&E histology image (middle), and constructed PH image (right)

Table 1. Confusion matrix showing the percentages of correct and misclassification for each tissue type

	Calcified	Fibrotic	Lipidic	No Tissue
Calcified	99.60	0.32	0.08	0.00
Fibrotic	7.00	87.75	5.10	0.15
Lipidic	1.89	6.50	90.87	0.74

accuracy of characterization through composite rating for each tissue type by asking two histopathologists to visually contrast between PH images and corresponding histology images. Table 1 demonstrates the average values for correct and miss-classified tissues in 83 CSIs. For example, the first row shows that 99.60% of calcified tissues in histology images were correctly classified as calcified while 0.32% and 0.07% of them were misclassified as fibrotic and lipidic, respectively. The overall classification performance has been evaluated to be 99.60%, 87.75%, and 90.87% for calcified, fibrotic, and lipidic tissues, respectively.

The best way to examine the consistency among extracted features is to examine the PH images in adjacent frames. We know that the local properties of lesions are gradually changed during pullback and abrupt changes among successive tissue colormaps are not expected. Fig. 3 demonstrates the grayscale images and corresponding changes in plaque constituents in constructed PH images for 4 consecutive frames. Contrary to IVUS-VH algorithm that deploys gating protocol and provides the VH images for every other 30 frames, our technique generates the PH images for all acquired frames. We counted number of pixels corresponding to every tissue types in each frame and Fig. 3(b) shows the Box- Whisker plot of counted pixels for 15 consecutive frames. Since Lipidic tissue appears in outer boundaries, some of the differences for this particular tissue are due to manual tracing of luminal borders by expert specially for the last few frames.

We also evaluated our technique in comparison with state of the art VH method [3] and performed our algorithm on 62 in vivo images acquired with 20 MHz 64-elements phased array transducer from 2 patients. Fig. 4 illustrates resulting tissue colormaps from VH algorithm and our proposed technique. We quantified our results using VH images as gold standard since histology images were not available for in vivo cases. Table 2 demonstrates classification accuracy, specificity, and sensitivity of PH results.

5   Conclusion and discussion

The main contribution of this work is that the generated PH images through unsupervised classification represent atherosclerotic tissues with high correlation with histology images and also can be used as labels for feature extraction and training a supervised classifier. For the first time we registered IVUS and

Table 2. Classification statistics of resulting tissue colormaps from our proposed technique in comparison with VH algorithm for each tissue type

Tissue type	Accuracy (%)	Specificity (%)	Sensitivity (%)
Calcified	95.60±3.3	99.24±1.5	8.10±6.3
Necrosis	91.54±5.8	92.63±6.1	25.52±8.1
Fibrotic	85.41±10.7	90.62±11.3	22.60±10.5
Fibro-fatty	79.60±15.3	78.32±13.2	28.90±11.3

histology images, investigated consistency among successive PH images, and performed a comparison study with state of the art VH algorithm. Previously, we studied effects of flowing blood and change of pressure on tissue colormaps [9], and reliability of classified tissues behind arc of calcified plaques [9, 10] that had not been considered by any group before. The primary goal of recent attempt was to attract attentions toward crucial factors such as IVUS-histology registration that impacts labeling, construction of training dataset and therefore consistency among extracted features. Secondly, we observed that our algorithm could generate almost the same results as VH algorithm without using any spectral features and only from signatures driven from image domain. From technical point of view, this validated the reliability of our proposed technique. From clinical perspective, we observed that excessive detection of necrotic tissues needs to be further investigated and requires special attention since histopathological studies confirm that necrotic core is a rare tissue. The immediate conclusion is that neither our proposed algorithm nor VH technique detects necrosis tissue reliably. Alternatively, combination of textural and spectral features may resolve this challenging issue.

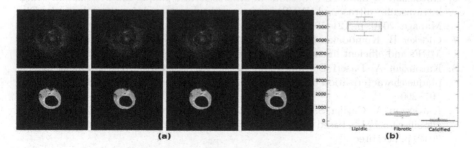

Fig. 3. Four consecutive in vivo IVUS grayscale images acquired with a 40MHz single-element Boston scientific transducer (top row) and corresponding generated PH images (bottom row) (a), Box-Whisker plot of number of pixels for each tissue type in 15 consecutive frames (b)

Fig. 4. Grayscale images from two distinct in vivo cases (left column). Resulting tissue colormaps form VH algorithm (middle column) and our proposed technique (right column). White, red, light green, and dark green represent calcified, necrosis, fibro-fatty, and fibrotic tissues, respectively

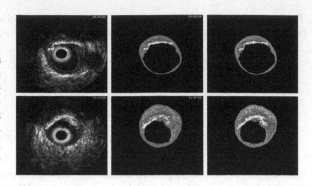

References

1. Virmani R, Burke AP, Kolodgie FD, et al. Pathology of the thin-cap fibroatheroma: a type of vulnerable plaque. J Inteven Cardiol. 2003;16(3):2672.
2. Kawasaki M, Takatsu H, Noda T, et al. In vivo quantitative tissue characterization of human coronary arterial plaques by use of integrated backscatter intravascular ultrasound and comparison with angioscopic findings. Circulation. 2002;105(21):2487–92.
3. Nair A, Kuban BD, Tuzcu M, et al. Coronary plaque classification with intravascular ultrasound radiofrequency data analysis. Circulation. 2002;106:2200–6.
4. Escalera S, Pujol O, Mauri J, et al. Intravascular ultrasound tissue characterization with sub-class error-correcting output codes. J Signal Process Syst. 2009;55(1):35–47.
5. Taki A, Hetterich H, Roodaki A, et al. A new approach for improving coronary plaque component analysis based on intravascular ultrasound images. J Ultrasound Med. 2010;36(8):1245–58.
6. Katouzian A, Laine AF. Methods in atherosclerotic plaque characterization using intravascular ultrasound (IVUS) images and backscattered signals. Atheroscler Dis Manage. 2010; p. 121–52.
7. Glocker B, Komodakis N, Tziritas G, et al. Dense image registration through MRFs and efficient linear programming. Med Image Anal. 2008;12(6):731–41.
8. Katouzian A, Baseri B, Konofagou EE, et al. Texture-driven coronary artery plaque characterization using wavelet packet signatures. Proc IEEE ISBI. 2008; p. 197–200.
9. Katouzian A, Carlier S. Development and performance of a new unsupervised classifier for IVUS-based tissue characterization. In: Proc 31st Belgian Soc Cardiol; 2012. p. accepted.
10. Tanaka K, Carlier S, Katouzian A, et al. Characterization of the intravascular ultrasound radiofrequency signal within regions of acoustic shadowing behind calcium. J Am Coll Cardiol. 2007;49(9 Suppl B).

Improved Image Segmentation with Prospective Motion Correction in MRI

Daniel Stucht[1], Shan Yang[1], Peter Schulze[1], Appu Danishad[1],
Ilja Kadashevich[1], Johannes Bernarding[2], Julian Maclaren[3], Maxim Zaitsev[3],
Oliver Speck[1]

[1]Biomedical Magnetic Resonance, IEP, Otto-von-Guericke University Magdeburg
[2]Institute for Biometry and Medical Informatics, University Hospital of Magdeburg
[3]Medical Physics, Department of Radiology, University Medical Center Freiburg
daniel.stucht@ovgu.de

Abstract. Artifacts caused by patient motion during a magnetic resonance imaging (MRI) scan can corrupt the image data, reduce the effective resolution and make further processing difficult or impossible. Long measurements, as required for high resolution imaging, are particularly prone to motion artifacts, as motion is more likely to occur over longer scan periods. These artifacts can lead to problems in the further image processing of the data. Prospective motion correction offers a possibility to correct for patient motion during the measurement and avoid motion artifacts. Image data from comparative brain scans with and without motion correction are presented and analyzed. Segmentation of gray matter (GM) and white matter (WM) was performed on both datasets using the software packages SPM and Freesurfer, which are widely used in neuroscience studies. The results show that motion correction significantly improves the segmentation quality and suggest that it is also useful for other image processing applications performed on MRI data.

1 Introduction

Artifacts caused by patient motion are often observed in MRI and make examination and further processing of the data difficult if not impossible. Strong motion of subjects unable to co-operate causes pronounced artifacts, which render the MRI data useless. Even for co-operative subjects it is difficult to stay motionless for 10-30 minutes, which is a typical duration for a high resolution brain scan. Involuntary motion induced by respiration, heartbeat and muscle tone changes causes motion artifacts like blurring and ringing, which reduce the effective resolution of the MRI data. For neuroscientists, MRI is an essential method to retrieve information about the brain anatomy. Functional MRI (fMRI) provides insight into even the neural activity of the brain. Often image processing is used to reveal the anatomical or physiological information in the MRI data. Motion artifacts, blurring and reduced contrast can lead to false results when the post processing steps assume uncorrupted data. The clarity of image features like edges is decreased by motion, thus the performance of algorithms relying on those features is decreased. As an example, this study shows the influence of motion artifacts on segmentation with two different software packages.

Several systems to correct for subject motion have been proposed with differences in the methods for motion detection and motion correction. The correction can be accomplished after the measurement (retrospectively) or by recalculating the logical orientation of the gradients and frequencies according to the current position and orientation of the subject during the measurement (prospectively). Some sources of artifacts like spin history effects caused by through-plane motion changing the slice plane or the volume of interest moving out of the imaging volume can only be corrected by prospective correction, which makes it the method of choice for high resolution brain imaging. A variety of motion detection systems have been used: navigator techniques [1] or methods such as PROPELLER [2] need additional scan time and have sequence-specific limitations. This is in contrast to external motion tracking systems (optical tracking systems like infrared based tracking on retro reflective markers [3, 4] or single camera systems using retrograde markers [5], or tracking using features like facial features or 2D patterns [6, 7]), which deliver pose information in real time independent from the scanner and the sequence used. For high resolution imaging, a tracking system with high accuracy and a low noise level is important, since poor motion tracking leads to faulty correction and can introduce new artifacts [8], which decrease the possibilities for image processing.

2   Materials and methods

This section describes the acquisition, analysis and processing of the image data. The software used to process the data was Matlab 2008a (The MathWorks, Natick, MA, USA). The segmentation was performed using a Matlab implementation of statistical parametric mapping (SPM8, Wellcome Trust Centre for Neuroimaging, UCL, London, UK) and the software package Freesurfer (Athinoula A. Martinos Center for Biomedical Imaging, Massachusetts General Hospital, Boston, MA, USA).

2.1   Image acquisition

MRI Measurements were performed on a 7 T whole body MRI (Siemens Medical Solutions, Erlangen, Germany) using a 32-channel coil (Nova Medical, Wilmington, MA, USA) and the following sequence parameters: imaging matrix = $384 \times 384 \times 256$, field of view (FoV) = $230 \times 230 \times 153.6$ mm^3, voxel size = $0.6 \times 0.6 \times 0.6$ mm^3, repetition time and echo time (TR/TE)=2500 ms/2.69 ms, flip angle $\alpha = 5°$. To remove the artifacts that result from RF inhomogeneity, which is dominant at high field MRI systems, a division of the original dataset by a second dataset that was acquired without inversion and short TR was performed. This correction also ensures a purely T1 weighted image contrast [9]. Both datasets were acquired with and without motion correction.

2.2 Prospective motion correction

In a previous study three different optical tracking systems were compared [10].
A single-camera in-bore system based on retrograte reflective (RGR) markers
(University of Wisconsin-Milwaukee, Milwaukee, WI, USA) [5] showed best accuracy and was used to accomplish the motion tracking in the study presented
here. The standard deviation of position-data of the X, Y- and Z- axes are
0.0002, 0.0003 and 0.004 mm, which is sufficiently accurate for resolutions up
to at least 0.1mm voxel size [8]. The tracking marker was attached to a small
retainer with dental impressions, which is tightly fixed to the subject's upper
jaw. The coordinate systems of the tracking system and the MRI scanner were
carefully co-registered prior to the MR session by using a non-iterative cross-
calibration [11].

2.3 Segmentation

The preprocessing was performed in Freesurfer and included intensity normalization and spatial normalization using a Talairach-transformation. Two segmentations were performed on the preprocessed data. The first segmentation was
carried out by SPM, which is capable of processing the dataset in the original
resolution. The segmentation results in three probability maps for GM, WM
and CSF. These maps were thresholded at 0.75 for GM and 0.25 for WM and
CSF. Freesurfer was used to perform the second segmentation. It does not segment CSF. Since Freesurfer uses an atlas-based algorithm, the data had to be
resampled to a voxel size of $1.0 \times 1.0 \times 1.0$ mm^3 to match the atlas datasets.

3 Results

Fig. 1 shows one slice of the datasets acquired with and without motion correction after the post processing described above. Edges are much more distinct
when motion correction is enabled. Small structures like vessels are hardly visible when motion correction is disabled but show up bright and clear in the
corrected data. In the line profile a small (sub-pixel) shift between corrected
and uncorrected data is visible. During the correction, the head position at the
beginning of the measurement of the uncorrected dataset was taken as a reference. The shift is caused by motion during the acquisition of the uncorrected
data. The profile shows mainly three gray levels for WM, GM and CSF in the
image from the corrected data set. In the uncorrected data, the CSF intensity
is not as low as in the corrected data, because it is overlaid by blurring and
ringing artifacts caused by the motion. Both segmentations (Fig. 2 and Fig. 3)
show differences between corrected and uncorrected data. In the SPM segmentation, the edges are frayed. Because of the reduced resolution, this effect is not
as dominant in the Freesurfer segmentation. The elongated segments of WM
and CF often appear interrupted and unconnected in the image without motion
correction. In the Freesurfer segmentation, the border regions of GM to CSF
are not segmented as GM, which results in large regions that might be mistaken
for CSF.

4 Discussion

The results show a significant influence of motion artifacts on the performance of the segmentations. The superior quality of the segmentation based on the corrected data set suggests that other segmentation tasks, vessel segmentation on Time of Flight (ToF) MRI data, would also benefit from prospective motion correction. Differences in the segmentation of corrected and uncorrected MRI data are visible even if that data was down-sampled as it was for the Freesurfer segmentation. Motion correction allows a higher effective resolution, which makes new applications for image processing possible, in high resolution fMRI or in the detection of very small structures. It would also allow the processing of MRI data from patients suffering from neurodegenerative diseases like Parkinson's, who are often unable to remain still during scanning. This would allow neurological studies and the use of established scientific tools like SPM and Freesurfer on MRI data of these patients, which would be very difficult if not impossible without motion correction.

A better quantification of the differences is desirable. A measurement of the effective resolution using a structured phantom might help to accomplish this.

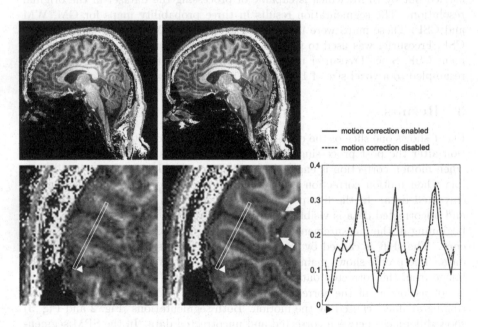

Fig. 1. MRI data acquired without (left) and with (middle) motion correction. The images in the lower row show a magnification of the area marked in the upper row. Two arrows mark vessels that are clearly visible in the corrected data but are hardly visible in the uncorrected images. In the diagram on the right a gray value profile over the line marked in the zoomed images is shown

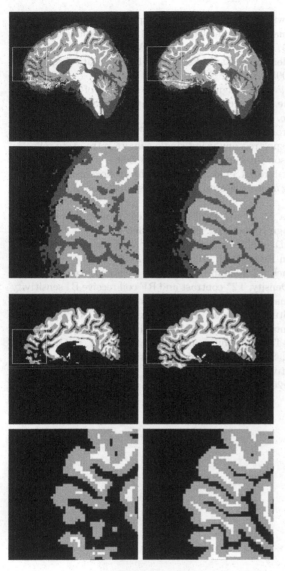

Fig. 2. Results of segmentation using the software package SPM on the uncorrected data (left column) and on the corrected data (right column). The lower row shows a close up of the area marked in the images of the upper row

Fig. 3. Results of segmentation using the software package Freesurfer on the uncorrected data (left column) and on the corrected data (right column). The lower row shows a close up of the area marked in the images of the upper row

Acknowledgement. This project is supported by the BMBF INUMAC project (01EQ0605) and NIDA (1R01DA021146).

References

1. Welch EB, Manduca A, Grimm RC, et al. Spherical navigator echoes for full 3D rigid body motion measurement in MRI. Magn Reson Med. 2002;47(1):32–41.

2. Pipe JG. Motion correction with PROPELLER MRI: Application to head motion and free-breathing cardiac imaging. Magn Reson Med. 1999;42(5):963–9.
3. Dold C, Zaitsev M, Speck O, et al. Prospective Head Motion Compensation for MRI by Updating the Gradients and Radio Frequency During Data Acquisition. Lect Notes Computer Sci. 2005;3749:482–9.
4. Zaitsev M, Dold C, Sakas G, et al. Magnetic resonance imaging of freely moving objects: prospective real-time motion correction using an external optical motion tracking system. Neuroimage. 2006;31(3):1038–50.
5. Andrews-Shigaki BC, Armstrong BSR, Zaitsev M, et al. Prospective motion correction for magnetic resonance spectroscopy using single camera retro-grate reflector optical tracking. J Magn Reson Imaging. 2011;33(2):498–504.
6. Qin L, van Gelderen P, Derbyshire JA, et al. Prospective head-movement correction for high-resolution MRI using an in-bore optical tracking system. Magn Reson Med. 2009;62(4):924–34.
7. Aksoy M, Forman C, Straka M, et al. Real-time optical motion correction for diffusion tensor imaging. Magn Reson Med. 2011;66(2):366–78.
8. Maclaren J, Speck O, Stucht D, et al. Navigator accuracy requirements for prospective motion correction. Magn Reson Med. 2010;63(1):162–70.
9. van de Moortele PF, Auerbach EJ, Olman C, et al. T1 weighted brain images at 7 Tesla unbiased for Proton Density, T2* contrast and RF coil receive B1 sensitivity with simultaneous vessel visualization. NeuroImage. 2009;46(2):432–46.
10. Schulze P, Kadashevich I, Stucht D, et al. Prospective Motion Correction at 7 Tesla Magnetic Resonance Imaging using Optical Tracking Systems. In: Proc 10. Magdeburger Maschinenbau-Tage Forschung und Innovation; 2011. p. C1–3.
11. Kadashevich I, Danishad A, Speck O. Automatic motion selection in one step cross-calibration for prospective MR motion correction. Proc Magn Reson Mater Phy. 2011;24(Supplement 1):266–7/#371.

Diaphragm Tracking in Cardiac C-Arm Projection Data

Marco Bögel[1], Andreas Maier[1], Hannes G. Hofmann[1], Joachim Hornegger[1],
Rebecca Fahrig[2]

[1]Pattern Recognition Lab, Universität Erlangen-Nürnberg, Germany
[2]Department of Radiology, Lucas MRS Center, Stanford University, Palo Alto, CA,
USA
marco.boegel@informatik.stud.uni-erlangen.de

Abstract. Long acquisition times of several seconds lead to image artifacts in cardiac C-arm CT. These artifacts are mostly caused by respiratory motion. In order to improve image quality, it is important to accurately estimate the breathing motion that occurred during image acquisition. It has been shown that diaphragm motion is correlated to the respiration-induced motion of the heart. We describe the development of a method that is able to accurately track the contour of the diaphragm in projection space using a 2D quadratic curve model of the diaphragm to simplify the process. In order to provide robust and stable tracking, additional constraints based on prior knowledge of the projection geometry and human anatomy are introduced. Results show that the tracking is very accurate. A mean model error per pixel of 0.93 ± 0.44 pixels for the left and 0.79 ± 0.19 pixels for the right hemidiaphragm was observed. The diaphragm top is tracked with an even lower error of only 0.75 ± 0.84 pixels for the left and 0.45 ± 056 pixels for the right hemidiaphragm respectively.

1 Introduction

Cardiac C-arm CT makes it possible to reconstruct 3-D images during medical procedures. However, the long acquisition time of several seconds, during which the heart is beating and the patient might breathe, may lead to artifacts, such as blurring or streaks. A commonly used technique to reduce breathing motion is the single breath-hold scan. The physician instructs the patient to hold his breath after exhalation. The data is then acquired during the breath-hold. Although this approach is widely used, several studies have shown that breath-holding does not eliminate breathing motion entirely. Monitoring the position of the right hemidiaphragm during breath-hold, Jahnke et al. observed residual breathing motion to a certain extent for almost half their test group [1]. Therefore, it is necessary to develop better methods to estimate and compensate for respiratory motion in cardiac C-Arm CT.

There are many ways to acquire respiratory signals. Most are based on additional equipment, e.g. Time of Flight- or Stereovision-cameras. Other techniques

Fig. 1. User selected start point and initial rectangular ROI

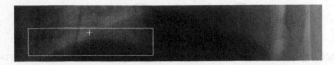

aim to extract the respiratory signal directly from the projection images. Using this approach the extracted breathing signal is perfectly synchronized with the projection images. Image-based respiratory motion extraction often relies on tracking of fiducial markers in the projection images [2, 3]. Wang et al. have shown that the motion of the diaphragm is highly correlated to respiration-induced motion of the heart [4]. Sonke et al. propose to extract a one-dimensional breathing signal by projecting diaphragm-like features on the cranio-caudal axis and selecting the features with the highest temporal change [5]. However, the downside to this approach is that the extracted signal is not the real respiration signal. Due to perspective projection, the projected amplitude depends on the C-arm rotation angle. In this work, we propose to track the diaphragm in a set of rotational projection images.

2   Materials and methods

We propose a method that aims to model the 2-D projection of a hemidiaphragm as a 2-D quadratic function. Most approaches for motion estimation based on tracking of features, assume that the features are unique objects, e.g. spherical fiducial markers. Unlike those methods, the object to be tracked here is not unique. The diaphragm appears as two similar parabolic shapes – the left and right hemidiaphragm.

2.1   Preprocessing

The proposed method works automatically, with the exception of the manual selection of a start point in the first image. The point has to be placed in the rough perimeter of the top of one hemidiaphragm. Next, a Region of Interest (ROI) is defined symmetrically around this point. A rectangular ROI is built such that it includes, ideally, only the contour of the selected hemidiaphragm. We propose an ROI of size 250×55 for projection images of size 640×480. Fig. 1 shows an inaccurately selected start point and the ROI created around it. Even this rough estimate of the initial position is sufficient for our algorithm. In order to reduce noise, the images are then smoothed with a gaussian kernel. The Canny Edge Detector [6] is then applied to extract the diaphragm contour. Hysteresis thresholding is done using percentiles of the edge magnitudes greater than zero. The low threshold was set to the 20th percentile, the high threshold to the 70th percentile.

2.2   Model Estimation

The result is a set of edge points that can now be used to estimate a quadratic model of the hemidiaphragm. However, due to the moderately chosen thresholds in the previous step, this set of points includes many false-positives which are not part of the diaphragm contour. To deal with this, the quadratic model is fit using the Random Sample Consensus (RANSAC) proposed by Fischler and Bolles [7]. RANSAC can deal with datasets with large percentages of gross errors, and is thus the ideal choice to fit a model to our very noisy set of points. The diaphragm is of approximately parabolic shape, and is therefore estimated as a quadratic function $y = ax^2 + bx + c$. Thus, RANSAC has to estimate the three parameters a, b, and c. In the first step, three random points are selected. The model estimation can then be formulated as the following optimization problem

$$\sum_{i=1}^{3} a \cdot x_i^2 + b \cdot x_i + c - y_i \to \min \qquad (1)$$

This way N different models are fit to the data, which are then evaluated to determine the one that fits the data best. The model's quality is determined by the number of inliers. An inlier is a point that lies within a predefined distance to the model. Since an accurate model is desired, we only consider points with a one pixel distance to the model inliers.

Up to this point, the presented method will find a contour, but it is not able to distinguish between the two different hemidiaphragms in cases where they are both visible in the ROI. Hence, we chose additional constraints, based on prior knowledge, that were enforced to obtain the correct models. First of all, the diaphragm's opening is always facing down. Furthermore, assuming small motion between two subsequent frames, the curve's horizontal translation m_x can be limited by a multiple of the average translation $\overline{m}_x$. Also, the contour should deform slowly over time, which can be enforced by limiting the change in the parabola's opening to $\frac{|a_{i-1}-a_i|}{a_{i-1}} < 0.05$, where a_i is the parameter a in the i-th image.

While the previous constraints are sufficient most of the time, the algorithm still fails if the two hemidiaphragms are located close to one another and the models resembling their contours are similar. For this purpose, prior knowledge of the patient's position and the C-arm rotation geometry can be utilized. Suppose acquisition starts from the right lateral view. Rotating towards the frontal view, the contour of the right hemidiaphragm will move to the left, whereas the contour of the left hemidiaphragm moves to the right. From the frontal position to the left lateral position this motion is reversed. We can now enforce the model to move in one direction until the turning point, and then move in the opposite direction. However, since the diaphragm is deforming during respiration, it is better to loosen this constraint, by allowing free-motion around the turning point. Each valid model must therefore fulfill four constraints:

1. Diaphragm opening downwards: $a_i > 0$

Fig. 2. Parabolic ROI used during tracking

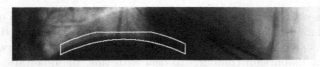

2. Small motion assumption (deformation): $\frac{|a_{i-1}-a_i|}{a_{i-1}} < 0.05$
3. Small motion assumption (translation): $m_x < 3 \cdot \overline{m}_x$
4. Motion based on C-arm trajectory: $\text{dir} = \begin{cases} \text{dir}_A \text{ , if start} \leq \text{angle} \leq 45° \\ \text{dir}_B \text{ , if } 135° \leq \text{angle} \leq \text{end} \end{cases}$

Models that do not fulfill all of the above are discarded immediately. This is done before the more costly determination of the number of inliers, saving computation time.

2.3   Tracking

In order to track the contour throughout the entire image sequence, the ROI has to be moved. This is done by setting the seed point of the ROI to the vertex of the newly estimated model.

Finally, one last optimization is done. After a model was computed for the first image, we know approximately how the contour has to look in the next image, due to the small motion assumption. The ROI is reshaped based on the last estimated model. The new parabolic ROI is then defined as the intersection of the rectangular ROI and the points $\mathbf{p} = (x, y \pm r)^T$, where x and y must satisfy the equation $y = a_{i-1}x^2 + b_{i-1}x + c_{i-1}$, with a_{i-1}, b_{i-1}, and c_{i-1} being the estimated model parameters of the previous image, and the variable $r \in [0, N_r]$ describing the radius of the parabolic ROI. The height of this parabolic ROI is typically much smaller than the height of the rectangular ROI. Therefore, we are able to greatly reduce the number of considered false-positives, further improving the performance of the RANSAC algorithm. Fig. 2 shows an example of a parabolic ROI with $N_r = 10$.

3   Results

The accuracy of the proposed approach was evaluated on XCAT [8] projections of a breathing thorax. We simulated an acquisition time of four seconds with a full respiration cycle with 2.2 cm amplitude. Our algorithm was used to track both the right and the left hemidiaphragm. Projections of only the respective hemidiaphragm were used as gold standard. The projection images were 640 pixels wide and 480 pixels high. An ROI of 250 × 55 pixels was used. Table 1 provides detailed information about the data that was used for the evaluation. The clinical data was acquired on a Siemens AXIOM-Artis system.

Table 1. Properties of the data used for evaluation

	XCAT	Clinical 1	Clinical 2
Frames	200	191	247
Avg. angular increment	1.0°	1.0°	0.8°
Total rotation angle	199°	190°	197.6°
Detector size	640 × 480 px	620 × 480 px	620 × 480 px
Pixel dimension	0.616 mm	0.616 mm	0.616 mm
SID	1200	1199	1199
Source to rotation axis dist.	800	785	785

Table 2. Model error (in pixels) for left and right hemidiaphragm evaluated on windows with different widths around the vertex

	Left full	Left top	Left top euclid.	Right full	Right top	Right top euclid.
Mean	0.93	0.62	0.75	0.79	0.42	0.45
Std. Dev.	0.44	0.60	0.84	0.19	0.52	0.56
Max	5	2	5	2	3	3

First, we evaluate how well the model fits the reference contour. Therefore, the absolute difference of the model's and the contour's y-coordinates is computed. This error is computed over a specified window with the model's vertex as its center and is then normalized by the width. Table 2 shows the normalized error evaluated for the entire model and only at the model's vertex.

In order to further evaluate the accuracy of the model's vertex in x and y direction, we computed the Euclidean distance between the vertex and the true maximum of the contour in the image. The true maximum is often wider than a single pixel. In these cases we evaluated the Euclidean distance for all maximum pixels and then selected the minimum distance. The results show that the model's vertex closely represents the actual top of the diaphragm contour.

Fig. 3 shows the estimated model of the diaphragm in clinical projection data at four projection angles.

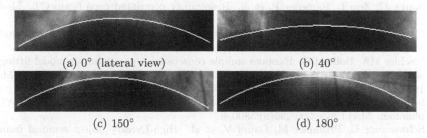

(a) 0° (lateral view)	(b) 40°
(c) 150°	(d) 180°

Fig. 3. Diaphragm tracking on data set clinical 2. Images (a)-(d) show projection images acquired from different angles

4 Discussion

As results show, the proposed method allows us to track the diaphragm in projection data with very high accuracy. The model error is slightly higher when considering larger regions of the diaphragm. This is expected because of the diaphragm's asymmetry. A parabolic model is not a perfect fit for every perspective. Nevertheless, the diaphragm top can still be tracked very accurately, even if the real contour is asymmetric. This method will improve compensation of respiratory motion. Previous studies have shown that diaphragm motion is highly correlated to the respiratory motion of the heart [4]. A very low Euclidean distance of 0.46 ± 0.56 pixels and 0.75 ± 0.84 pixels respectively proves that the vertex of the parabolic model is an excellent estimate of the diaphragm top. Visual inspection of tracking results in clinical projection data suggests that tracking accuracy is comparable to that of the phantom data.

The presented method works well even if parts of the diaphragm are occluded due to bad contrast or overlap with other organs, e.g. the heart. However, high density objects, e.g. catheters, that are located close to the diaphragm contour have to be removed using interpolation [9] to ensure that the parabola is not pulled towards them.

Future work will deal with the extraction of a 1-D respiratory signal based on the tracked position of the diaphragm top. The respiratory signal can then be used to compensate for respiratory motion in cardiac reconstruction.

References

1. Jahnke C, Paetsch I, Achenbach S, et al. Coronary MR imaging: breath-hold capability and patterns, coronary artery rest periods, and beta-blocker use. Radiology. 2006;239:71–8.
2. Wiesner S, Yaniv Z. Respiratory signal generation for retrospective gating of cone-beam CT images. Proc SPIE. 2008;6918:71.
3. Marchant TE, Price GJ, Matuszewiski BJ, et al. Reduction of motion artefacts in on-board cone beam CT by warping of projection images. Br J Radiol. 2011;84:251–64.
4. Wang Y, Riederer S, Ehman R. Respiratory motion of the heart: kinematics and the implications for spatial resolution in coronary imaging. Magn Reson Med. 1995;33:716–19.
5. Sonke JJ, Zijp L, Remeijer P, et al. Respiratory correlated cone beam CT. Med Phys. 2005;32:1176–86.
6. Canny FJ. A computational approach to edge detection. IEEE Trans Pattern Anal Mach Intell. 1986;8(6):679–98.
7. Fischler MA, Bolles RC. Random sample consensus: a paradigm for model fitting with applications to image analysis and automated cartography. Commun ACM. 1981;24:381–95.
8. Segars WP, Mahesh M, Beck TJ, et al. Realistic CT simulation using the 4D XCAT phantom. Med Phys. 2008;35(8):3800–8.
9. Schwemmer C, Prümmer M, Daum V, et al. High-Density object removal from projection images using low-frequency-based object masking. Proc BVM. 2010; p. 365–9.

Optimierte endoskopische Time-of-Flight Oberflächenrekonstruktion durch Integration eines Struktur-durch-Bewegung-Ansatzes

A. Groch[1], S. Haase[2], M. Wagner[3], T. Kilgus[1], H. Kenngott[3], H.-P. Schlemmer[4], J. Hornegger[2], H.-P. Meinzer[1], L. Maier-Hein[1]

[1]Abteilung Medizinische und Biologische Informatik, DKFZ Heidelberg
[2]Lehrstuhl für Mustererkennung, Universität Erlangen-Nürnberg
[3]Allgemein-, Viszeral- u. Transplantationschirurgie, Universitätsklinikum Heidelberg
[4]Abteilung Radiologie, DKFZ Heidelberg
a.groch@dkfz-heidelberg.de

Kurzfassung. Eine der größten Herausforderungen computergestützter Assistenzsysteme für laparoskopische Eingriffe ist die intraoperative akkurate und schnelle Rekonstruktion der Organoberfläche. Während Rekonstruktionstechniken basierend auf Multiple View Methoden, beispielsweise Stereo-Rekonstruktion, schon länger Gegenstand der Forschung sind, wurde erst kürzlich das weltweit erste Time-of-Flight (ToF) Endoskop vorgestellt. Die Vorteile gegenüber Stereo liegen in der hohen Aktualisierungsrate und dem dichten Tiefenbild unabhängig von der betrachteten Szene. Demgegenüber stehen allerdings Nachteile wie schlechte Genauigkeit bedingt durch hohes Rauschen und systematische Fehler. Um die Vorteile beider Verfahren zu vereinen, wird ein Konzept entwickelt, die ToF-Endoskopie-Technik mit einem stereoähnlichen Multiple-View-Ansatz (Struktur durch Bewegung) zu fusionieren. Der Ansatz benötigt keine zusätzliche Bildgebungsmodalität wie z.B. ein Stereoskop, sondern nutzt die ohnehin akquirierten (Mono-) Farbdaten des ToF-Endoskops. Erste Ergebnisse zeigen, dass die Genauigkeit der Oberflächenrekonstruktion mit diesem Ansatz verbessert werden kann.

1 Einleitung

Während der letzten Jahre erfahren computergestützte Assistenzsysteme für laparoskopische Eingriffe zunehmend Aufmerksamkeit in der Wissenschaft. Solche Assistenzsysteme arbeiten in der Regel mit einem präoperativ erstellten Patientenmodell, welches während der Operation auf die aktuell vorliegende Patientenanatomie übertragen wird [1]. Endoskopische Oberflächenrekonstruktion ist in diesem Kontext eine Schlüsseltechnik, da sie markerlos und ohne zusätzliche Bildgebungsmodalität und eventuelle Strahlenbelastung die Registrierung der präoperativ akquirierten Daten in Echtzeit ermöglicht. Häufig angewandte Verfahren zur Oberflächenrekonstruktion basieren auf sogenannten Multiple View Methoden. Dabei wird eine Korrespondenzanalyse auf zwei oder mehreren

40   Groch et al.

Bildern aus verschiedenen Kamerapositionen durchgeführt, was mittels Triangulation eine 3D-Rekonstruktion der abgebildeten Szene erlaubt. Werden zwei fest zueinander definierte Kameras benutzt, spricht man von Stereo-Rekonstruktion. Im Kontext der Endoskopie wird dies mit Stereoskopen als Bildgebungsmodalität realisiert [2]. Bei der Korrespondenzanalyse auf mehr als zwei Bildern werden die Bilder häufig sequentiell über die Bewegung der Kamera akquiriert (Struktur-durch-Bewegung, engl. Structure-from-Motion (SfM)) [3]. Im endoskopischen Kontext werden hierfür gewöhnliche (Mono-) Endoskope benutzt. Andere Ansätze zur Oberflächenrekonstruktion nutzen z.B. Strukturiertes Licht [4], welches auf einer aktiven Triangulation beruht.

Erst kürzlich wurde das erste Endoskop, das auf der neuen Time-of-Flight (ToF) Technik basiert, vorgestellt [5]. Das Prinzip von ToF-Sensoren besteht darin, dass die Flugdauer eines intensitätsmodulierten Lichtsignals gemessen wird. Wegen der Möglichkeit, dichte Tiefendaten mit einer Video ähnlichen Aktualisierungsrate unabhängig von der betrachteten Szene zu generieren, gewinnt die ToF-Technik immer mehr Aufmerksamkeit als Alternative zu konventionellen Distanzmessungen. Nicht zu vernachlässigende Nachteile der ToF-Endoskopie sind dagegen eine schlechte Genauigkeit der rekonstruierten Oberflächen. Dies ist vor allem auf den starken Signalverlust und das damit einhergehende niedrige Signal-zu-Rausch-Verhältnis zurückzuführen, aber auch auf die fehlenden Forschungserfahrungen im Bereich der Kalibrierung von systematischen Fehlern, sowie die endoskopischen Anforderungen an die Genauigkeit im Submillimeterbereich.

Eine Möglichkeit, die niedrige Genauigkeit der rekonstruierten Oberfläche zu kompensieren, besteht darin, weitere Oberflächenrekonstruktionsverfahren in den Rekonstruktionsprozess einzubinden. Es liegt nahe, dies mit einem SfM-Ansatz zu realisieren, da in der ToF-Endoskopie normale (Mono-) Endoskop-Farbbilder ohnehin zusätzlich zu den ToF-Tiefendaten akquiriert werden. Des weiteren sind die Eigenschaften von ToF und SfM komplementär. Während ToF ein dichtes, aber ungenaues Tiefenbild erzeugt, ist SfM an wenigen stabilen Merkmalen sehr genau. Zusätzlich erzielt ToF durch intensitätsbasierte Fehler die besten Ergebnisse bei homogenen Objekten, SfM wegen der Korrespondenzsuche hingegen bei texturierten Objekten. Forschungsarbeiten zur Fusion von ToF mit Multiple-View-Methoden gibt es bereits für herkömmliche, nicht-endoskopische Kameras, hauptsächlich für die Fusion von ToF- mit Stereodaten [6, 7]. Die meisten Arbeiten basieren auf probabilistischen Ansätzen, in denen die unterschiedlichen Fehlerwahrscheinlichkeiten der Bildgebungsmodalitäten modelliert und dann fusioniert werden.

In diesem Beitrag stellen wir ein Konzept zur Verbesserung von ToF-Oberflächen durch Integration eines SfM-Ansatzes im Kontext der Endoskopie vor.

2 Material und Methoden

In diesem Abschnitt werden die benutzte Hardware, das Fusionskonzept von ToF und SfM und die Evaluation des Konzepts näher erläutert.

2.1 Hardware

In dieser Arbeit wurde ein erster ToF-Endoskop-Prototyp (Firma Richard Wolf GmbH) benutzt. Er erzeugt ca 30 Distanzbilder pro Sekunde sowie dazu synchronisierte gewöhnliche endoskopische Farbdaten (Standard Definition (SD)). Die Aufnahme der Farbdaten durch dieselbe Optik ist eine Erweiterung zu dem von Penne vorgestellten ToF-Endoskop [5]. Für die vorliegende Arbeit wurde das Endoskop optisch getrackt, um seine Lage bestimmen zu können. Die intrinsischen Parameter der Farb- und ToF-Kamera wurden mit gängigen Kalibrierungsroutinen bestimmt, die Transformation des Trackingtools zu den Kameras mit einer gewöhnlichen Hand-Auge-Kalibrierung und die Transformation von den Kameras zueinander (ToF- zu Farbkamera) durch eine Stereo-Kalibrierung.

2.2 Fusionsansatz

In jedem Zeit schritt soll mit Hilfe der hier vorgestellten Fusionsmethode eine Oberfläche rekonstruiert werden. Dazu dienen als Input in jedem Zeitschritt (1) eine aus den ToF-Tiefendaten, unter Nutzung der intrinsischen Kameraparameter generierte, dichte Oberfläche sowie (2) eine 3D-Punktwolke aus dem SfM-Ansatz. Die 3D-Punktwolke wird auf Basis der vorangegangen Bildersequenz berechnet. Der Ansatz berücksichtigt nur die „besten" Merkmale in den Farbbildern. Gute Merkmale zeichnen sich dadurch aus, dass sie in jedem Bild der Sequenz eindeutig detektiert und ihren korrespondierenden Merkmalen in allen Vorgängerbildern eindeutig zugeordnet werden können. Von diesen guten Merkmalen werden nur diejenigen n mit der kleinsten Deskriptordifferenz zu ihren korrespondierenden Vorgänger-Merkmalen berücksichtigt. Die Deskriptordifferenz ist ein Maß dafür, wie ähnlich sich die Merkmale sind.

Da für die ToF-Endoskopie noch keine etablierte Distanzkalibrierung existiert und die ToF-Distanzdaten deswegen mit einem Offset in Richtung des Sehstrahls vorliegen können, wird eine rigide Vorregistrierung mit Hilfe des kürzlich vorgestellten anisotropen ICP [8], eine Variante des Iterative Closest Point (ICP) Algorithmus, durchgeführt. Dieser eignet sich besonders gut für rigide Registrierungen von ToF-Oberflächen, da anistrope Fehlerwahrscheinlichkeitsverteilungen, wie sie bei ToF vorliegen, berücksichtigt werden können.

Ein probabilistischer Ansatz, ähnlich wie unter anderem in [6] für die Fusion mit Stereo beschrieben, wird nun für die weitere Fehlerminimierung der Oberflächen realisiert, indem ToF-Endoskop- und SfM-Daten fusioniert werden. Hierfür wird wie z.B. in [9] ein dreidimensionales Belegungsnetz (engl. occupancy grid) aufgestellt, welches das Volumen der zu fusionierenden Oberfläche bzw. Punktwolke umschließt und mit gitterförmig angeordneten Knoten hoher Auflösung (höher als die ToF-Oberfläche) gefüllt ist. Innerhalb dieses quaderförmigen Netzes liegt die gesuchte Oberfläche und setzt sich aus einer Teilmenge der Knoten des Belegungsnetzes zusammen. Jeder Knoten besitzt einen Wert abhängig davon, wie hoch die Wahrscheinlichkeit ist, dass genau dieser Knoten zur gesuchten Oberfläche gehört. Die Wahrscheinlichkeit jedes Knotens v setzt sich zusammen aus $p(v|O_{\text{ToF}}, \Sigma_{\text{ToF}}, O_{\text{SfM}}, \Sigma_{\text{SfM}})$. O_{ToF} ist die Menge aller Knoten des Belegungsnetzes, welche zur ToF-Oberfläche gehören, und O_{SfM} die Menge derjeniger, die zur SfM-Punktwolke gehören. Σ_{ToF} bzw. Σ_{SfM} beschreiben die Fehlerwahrscheinlichkeitsverteilung in alle drei Dimensionen für jeden Knoten $o_{\mathrm{ToF}} \in O_{\mathrm{ToF}}$ bzw. $o_{\mathrm{SfM}} \in O_{\mathrm{SfM}}$. In der jetzigen Implementierung sind die Unsicherheitsverteilungen so gewählt, dass sie für ToF wesentlich höher als für SfM sind und generell in Sehstrahl-Richtung höher als in die Richtungen orthogonal dazu (anisotrope Gaussverteilung mit Erwartungswert 0). Der Ansatz lässt sich leicht erweitern, so dass auch die einzelnen Knoten unterschiedliche Verteilungen erhalten können (Abschnitt 4).

Nach Aufstellung des Belegungsnetzes wird eine Oberfläche in dem dreidimensionalen Netz gesucht, die (1) sowohl durch die Knoten mit möglichst hohen Wahrscheinlichkeiten geht, als auch (2) möglichst glatt ist. Außerdem muss berücksichtigt werden, dass es (3) nur jeweils einen Oberflächenpunkt in Richtung des Sehstrahls geben kann. Dies wird mit einem Graph-Cut basierten Verfahren [10] umgesetzt, welches mit dem Min-Cut-Max-Flow-Theorem einen Schnitt mit minimalen Kosten (= maximaler Wahrscheinlichkeit) bei maximaler Glattheit sucht. Dieses Verfahren gewährleistet zusätzlich, dass der Schnitt das Netz senkrecht zur Sehstrahlrichtung in zwei Teile zerschneidet und somit jeweils genau ein Oberflächenknoten in Sehstrahlrichtung existiert.

2.3   Machbarkeitsstudie

Um die Machbarkeit des vorgestellten Fusionsansatzes zu überprüfen, wurde eine erste Evaluation an in-vitro an Schweineorganen durchgeführt. Hierfür wurden verschiedene Organformen (Abb. 1) und verschiedene Organtexturen aufgenommen. Die Genauigkeit der Oberfläche aus dem Fusionsansatz wurde mit der nur aus den ToF-Endoskopdaten erstellten Oberfläche verglichen. Als Goldstandard dienten CT Aufnahmen aller Objekte. Über Marker, die außerhalb der zu evaluierenden Oberfläche angebracht waren, wurden die rekonstruierten Oberflächen und die Goldstandard-Daten zueinander registriert. Damit konnte die mittlere Distanz aller Knoten der rekonstruierten Oberfläche zu den Goldstandard-Oberflächen berechnet werden. Außerdem wurde verglichen, wie sich die Genauigkeit abhängig von der Anzahl der benutzten SfM-Punkte verbessert.

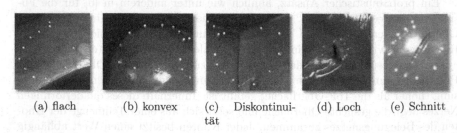

(a) flach   (b) konvex   (c) Diskontinui-   (d) Loch   (e) Schnitt
                                        tät

Abb. 1. Verschiedene Organformen

3   Ergebnisse

Um einen ersten quantitativen Eindruck des Fusionskonzept vor der Gesamtimplementierung zu erhalten, konzentrierte man sich bei dieser Evaluierung auf den probabilistischen Ansatz durch das Belegungsnetz. Dazu wurden ToF-Oberfläche und SfM-Punktwolke mit Hilfe der angebrachten Marker auf die CT-Referenz-Oberfläche registriert und dann fusioniert. Dies verschafft einen Eindruck, wie sehr die relative Genauigkeit der Oberfläche erhöht werden kann, nachdem die Vorpositionierung schon stattgefunden hat.

Ergebnisse an endoskopischen Bilddaten von Leber und Lunge mit verschiedenen Oberflächenformen und -texturen zeigen, dass sich die mittlere Genauigkeit aller akquirierten Organoberflächen bei einer Berücksichtigung schon von ca. 20 SfM-Punkte verdoppelt (Abb. 2).

4   Diskussion

In dieser Arbeit haben wir ein Konzept zur Fusion von endoskopischer, ToF-basierter Oberflächenrekonstruktion mit einem SfM-Ansatz vorgestellt. Dieses kombiniert die Vorteile beider Verfahren, so dass nach ersten Ergebnissen Fehler der noch sehr neuen ToF-Endoskopie reduziert werden. Es ist noch abzuwarten, wie gut die Ergebnisse nach Einsatz des A-ICP sein werden. Außerdem sollen bei der Aufstellung der Unsicherheiten im Belegungsnetz weitere Annahmen getroffen werden, wie z.B. dass Knoten, die aus ToF-Pixeln mit hoher Intensität entstanden sind, eine höhere Wahrscheinlichkeit zugeordnet werden, da helle Objektpixel bei ToF weniger rauschbehaftet sind als dunkle. Ähnliches kann für SfM angenommen werden. Hier sind die Knoten aus Merkmalen mit kleiner Deskriptordifferenz zuverlässiger und könnten deswegen eine höhere Wahrscheinlichkeit erhalten. Trotz des im Moment noch einfachen Ansatzes konnte in diesem Beitrag gezeigt werden, dass eine Fusionierung von ToF mit Stucture from Motion die Genauigkeit der Oberflächenrekonstruktion erhöht.

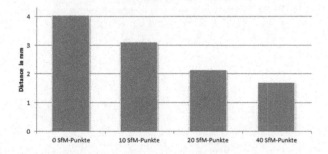

Abb. 2. Mittlerer Fehler aller rekonstruierten Knoten aller akquirierten Oberflächen zur Goldstandard-Oberfläche abhängig von der Anzahl der benutzten SfM-Punkte. Null SfM-Punkte entspricht der nur ToF-basierten Rekonstruktion

Danksagung. Die vorliegende Arbeit wurde im Rahmen des von der Deutschen Forschungsgemeinschaft unterstützten Graduiertenkollegs 1126: „Intelligente Chirurgie" durchgeführt. Vielen Dank an die Firma Richard Wolf GmbH für die Leihgabe des ToF-Endoskop-Prototypen.

Literaturverzeichnis

1. Baumhauer M, et al. Navigation in endoscopic soft tissue surgery: perspectives and limitations. J Endourol. 2008;22(4):751–66.
2. Stoyanov D, Scarzanella MV, Pratt P, et al. Real-time stereo reconstruction in robotically assisted minimally invasive surgery. Proc MICCAI. 2010; p. 275–82.
3. Wengert C, et al. Markerless endoscopic registration and referencing. Lect Notes Computer Sci. 2006;4190:816–23.
4. Clancy NT, Stoyanov D, Yang GZ, et al. An endoscopic structured lighting probe using spectral encoding. Proc SPIE. 2011;8090.
5. Penne J, et al. Time-of-Flight 3-D endoscopy. Lect Notes Computer Sci. 2009;5761:467–74.
6. Zhu J, Wang L, Yang R, et al. Reliability fusion of Time-of-Flight depth and stereo geometry for high quality depth maps. IEEE Trans Pattern Anal Mach Intell. 2011;33:1400–14.
7. Mutto CD, Zanuttigh P, Cortelazzo GM. A probabilistic approach to ToF and stereo data fusion. In: Proc 3DPVT; 2010.
8. Maier-Hein L, Franz AM, dos Santos TR, et al. Convergent iterative closest point algorithm to account for anisotropic inhomogenous localization error. IEEE Trans Pattern Anal Mach Intell. 2012 (in press).
9. Guan L, Franco JS, Pollefeys M. 3D object reconstruction with heterogeneous sensor data. In: Proc 3DPVT; 2008.
10. Li K, Wu X, Chen DZ, et al. Optimal surface segmentation in volumetric images: a graph-theoretic approach. IEEE Trans Pattern Anal Mach Intell. 2006;28(1):119–34.

Motion Compensation for Bronchoscope Navigation Using Electromagnetic Tracking, Airway Segmentation, and Image Similarity

Tobias Reichl[1], Ingmar Gergel[2], Manuela Menzel[3], Hubert Hautmann[3],
Ingmar Wegner[2], Hans-Peter Meinzer[2], Nassir Navab[1]

[1]Computer Aided Medical Procedures (CAMP), Technische Universität München
[2]Div. Med. and Bio. Informatics, German Cancer Research Center, Heidelberg
[3]Medizinische Klinik I, Klinikum rechts der Isar, TUM, München, Germany
reichl@tum.de

Abstract. We present a novel approach to motion compensation for
bronchoscope navigation where the bronchoscope trajectory is modeled
using a spline curve. Initial position and orientation measurements from
electromagnetic tracking are refined using the distance of the trajectory
from airways segmented in preoperative CT data, and similarity between
real and virtual bronchoscopic images. We present an evaluation on a
dynamic motion phantom and on a moving ex-vivo porcine lung. Ground
truth data is provided by human experts.

1 Introduction

Tracking systems are increasingly used for navigated bronchoscopy. While expert
bronchoscopists are commonly well aware of the bronchoscope's current position
and orientation with respect to patient anatomy, the transfer and visualisation
of information from preoperative imaging to the OR may help in targeting small
regions of interest, e.g. lesions or lymph nodes for transbronchial needle aspiration.

However, patients are breathing, maybe even freely, occasionally coughing
and choking, and the insertion of the bronchoscope may cause additional deformation of the lung. Thus, motion correction for tracking is necessary, and
different approaches have been presented during the last decade, including hybrid electromagnetic and image-based tracking [1], particle filtering [2], novel
optical sensors [3], and ex-vivo [4] and in-vivo [5] evaluation of hybrid systems.

2 Materials and methods

For each frame in the video sequence we have a (noisy and erroneous) pose
measurement from electromagnetic (EM) tracking, i.e. position and orientation.
This pose may then be refined using other sources of information.

For image-based tracking virtual bronchoscopy images are generated close to
this initial pose using well-known volume rendering techniques. The similarity

between virtual and real bronchoscopy images can then be maximized. Additional knowledge can be inferred from a prior segmentation of the airways and the fact that the bronchoscope never leaves these.

Thus, when optimizing each frame's position p and orientation q, we evaluate the following

$$E(p,q) = \underbrace{S(p,q)}_{\text{similarity}} - \underbrace{\lambda_1 \cdot R_T(p,q)}_{\text{tension}} - \underbrace{\lambda_2 \cdot R_B(p)}_{\text{bending}} - \underbrace{\lambda_3 \cdot R_S(p)}_{\text{structure}} \qquad (1)$$

where λ_1 through λ_3 are weighting parameters. The image similarity $S(p,q)$ between real and virtual images is computed via Local Normalized Cross Correlation (LNCC), i.e. the Normalized Cross Correlation is computed for a window around each pixel.

R_T, R_B, R_S are regularizers incorporating prior knowledge about EMT measurements, smoothness of motion, and segmentation of anatomical structures, respectively. According to Hooke's law, spring force is proportional to displacement, so we model tension, the cost of distance from the EM tracking measurements, as

$$R_T(p,q) = \sum_k \|p_k - \hat{p}_k\| + \alpha \cdot \theta(q_k, \hat{q}_k) \qquad (2)$$

where $\hat{p}_k$ and $\hat{q}_k$ are the original position and orientation measured by EM tracking at time t_k, and $\theta(\cdot)$ denotes orientation difference. α is the ratio between rotational and translational spring constants and was set to $3.10°/mm$, since this was the ratio of errors observed with the human experts when recording ground truth data (see below). According to Euler–Bernoulli beam theory, the bending moment of the trajectory p_k is proportional to its curvature, so we choose analogously

$$R_B(p) = \sum_k \|\nabla_k^2 p_k\| \qquad (3)$$

$R_S(p)$ is the Euclidean distance from each position p to the nearest airway voxel. Segmentation of airways was performed using an iterative region growing approach [2] and the distance map was computed.

2.1 Spline modeling

Instead of optimizing each frame separately, we interpolate the true trajectory of the bronchoscope using Catmull-Rom-splines [6] for position and SLERP [7] for orientation. Movement of a control point does not influence frames outside its support and gradient computation can be decoupled between control points. In addition, since the total number of frames is constant, the total computational effort does not depend on the number of control points. This spline modeling implies inherent smoothness of the spline curve, in addition to $R_B(p)$ penalizing large translations between control points.

For optimization we employed our existing gradient descent framework [8], where for generality the gradient is approximated via finite differences.

2.2 Setup

We used 3D Guidance (Ascension, Burlington, USA) and Aurora (Northern Digital, Radolfzell, Germany) EM tracking systems, and and BF-P260F (Olympus, Tokyo, Japan) and model 7268 (Richard Wolf, Knittlingen, Germany) flexible fiberoptic bronchoscopes. One 6 DOF (Olympus) or 5 DOF (Wolf) EMT sensor was fixed at each bronchoscope's tip.

Point-based registration was used to determine the spatial relation between CT and EMT coordinate systems, and camera intrinsics and distortion were determined as proposed by Wengert et al. [9].

Prior to a bronchoscopic intervention a visual inspection of all accessible branches is commonly recommended, and after applying our method to the recorded trajectory, we can again employ point-based registration between the corrected and uncorrected point sets, in order to have a refined registration for subsequent use.

Video sequences and CT data were stored in graphics processing unit (GPU) memory, and virtual bronchoscopic image rendering as well as similarity were computed on GPU using OpenGL. Experiments were conducted on a standard workstation (Intel Core Duo 6600, NVidia GeForce 8800 GTS).

2.3 Evaluation

For the dynamic motion phantom a CLA 9 (CLA, Coburg, Germany) was chosen due to its closely human-mimicking surface. Motion was induced through a motor (Lego, Billund, Denmark) via nylon threads (Fig. 1). Four data sets consisting of video sequences and EMT data recordings were acquired with different amplitudes of simulated breathing motion between 7.48 and 23.65 mm.

For the ex-vivo trial an "ArtiChest" thorax phantom (PROdesign, Heiligkreuzsteinach, Germany, Fig. 2), was chosen, where a porcine heart lung explant is placed inside the phantom, and cyclic motion is induced by inflation and deflation of an artificial diaphragm.

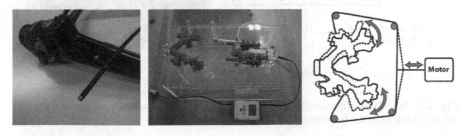

Fig. 1. Bronchoscope with embedded EMT sensor (left), dynamic motion phantom (center), and schematic of phantom operation (right)

48	Reichl et al.

2.4 Expert data

We evaluated the results of our approach using expert-selected positions and orientations, since this enables assessment of the agreement among those experts and a comparison to expert performance. For frames selected in regular intervals across the video sequences, position and orientation of the virtual camera were optimized manually, until virtual and real bronchoscope image matched as closely as possible. This procedure was repeated for two experts and multiple times per expert. For each frame, position and orientation were average per expert, and from both experts those averages were averaged again.

For the phantom trials, intra-expert agreement (mean standard deviation) was 1.66 mm and 5.80° (A) and 1.44 mm and 3.94° (B). Inter-expert agreement was 1.26 mm and 4.78°. Due to the time-consuming process of manual annotation, for the ex-vivo trial data from only one expert was available. Intra-expert agreement here was 2.32 ± 1.76 mm and $5.34 \pm 2.71°$. This agreement might indicate a limit for any approach based on registration of real and virtual bronchoscopy images.

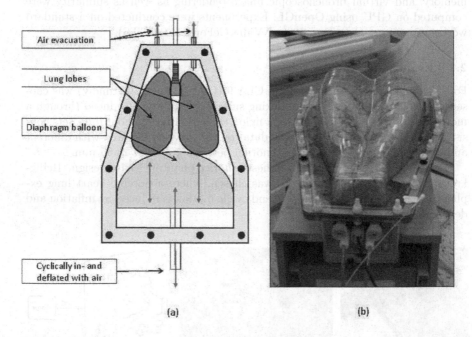

(a)   (b)

Fig. 2. "ArtiChest" thorax phantom: a) schematic of operation, and b) setup with inflated lung and the bronchoscope inserted through trachea

Table 1. Dynamic motion phantom. Accuracy comparison of approaches, in terms of translation and rotation, and smoothness comparison in terms of mean inter-frame distance. Smoothness is significantly improved by the proposed method

Method	Accuracy		Smoothness	
Solomon et al. [10]	5.87 mm	10.55°	3.20 mm	3.40°
Mori et al. [1]	5.59 mm	10.55°	3.72 mm	4.98°
Luo et al. [11]	5.17 mm	10.75°	3.24 mm	4.57°
Proposed method [8]	4.91 mm	11.48°	**1.24 mm**	3.00°
Expert agreement	1.26 mm	4.68°	–	–

3 Results

We compare the proposed method to our own implementations of four previously published approaches, which have already been applied to similar trajectories: bronchoscope tracking by EMT only [10], intensity-based registration (IBR) with direct initialization from EMT [1], and IBR with dynamic initialization from EMT [11].

For the dynamic motion phantom trial, quantitative results for accuracy and smoothness in terms of inter-frame distance are given in Table 1. For the ex-vivo trial, the accuracy including different sources of prior knowledge is given in Table 2.

Method	Accuracy
Uncorrected	10.82 mm
Corrected using spline model (SP)	10.79 mm
Corrected using SP and refined registration	10.70 mm
Corrected using SP and segmentation	9.57 mm
Corrected using SP and image similarity	9.52 mm
Expert agreement	2.32 mm

Table 2. Ex-vivo trial. Accuracy comparison of uncorrected data and data corrected with different approaches [4]. The greatest improvement is due to inclusion of segmentation information

4 Discussion

In the ex-vivo trial, improvement after inclusion of image similarity was limited, since here only a 5 DOF EMT sensor had been used and the arbitrary rotation around the sensor axis was difficult to correct within a limited number of optimization steps. Work is in progress to record ground truth data from more experts, but the process of manual annotation is very time consuming when working diligently, and expert time is a precious routine in clinical practice.

Our contribution is three-fold: First, we present a novel, continuous formulation of the tracking problem by modeling the resulting trajectory as a spline curve. Second, we show that this approach leads to an easily extensible framework for registration to preoperative CT images. Third, we provide a thorough evaluation of our approach using expert-provided ground truth data, including quantitative measurements for these experts' performance.

Acknowledgement. This work was supported by Deutsche Forschungsgemeinschaft under grants NA 620/2-1 and 446 JAP 113/348/0-1, European Union FP7 under grant n°256984, and the TUM Graduate School of Information Science in Health (GSISH).

References

1. Mori K, Deguchi D, Akiyama K, et al. Hybrid bronchoscope tracking using a magnetic tracking sensor and image registration. Proc MICCAI. 2005; p. 543–50.
2. Gergel I, dos Santos TR, Tetzlaff R, et al. Particle filtering for respiratory motion compensation during navigated bronchoscopy. Proc SPIE. 2010; p. 76250W.
3. Luo X, Kitasaka T, Mori K. Bronchoscopy navigation beyond electromagnetic tracking systems: a novel bronchoscope tracking prototype. Proc MICCAI. 2011; p. 194–202.
4. Reichl T, andManuela Menzel IG, Hautmann H, et al. Real-time motion compensation for EM bronchoscope tracking with smooth output: ex-vivo validation. Proc SPIE. 2012.
5. Soper TD, Haynor DR, Glenny RW, et al. In vivo validation of a hybrid tracking system for navigation of an ultrathin bronchoscope within peripheral airways. IEEE Trans Biomed Eng. 2010;57:736–45.
6. Catmull E, Rom R. A class of interpolating splines. Computer Aided Geometric Design. 1974; p. 317–26.
7. Shoemake K. Animating rotation with quaternion curves. Proc SIGGRAPH. 1985.
8. Reichl T, Luo X, Menzel M, et al. Deformable registration of bronchoscopic video sequences to CT volumes with guaranteed smooth output. Proc MICCAI. 2011; p. 17–24.
9. Wengert C, Reeff M, Cattin P, et al. Fully automatic endoscope calibration for intraoperative use. Proc BVM. 2006; p. 419–23.
10. Solomon SB, White Jr P, Wiener CM, et al. Three-dimensional CT-guided bronchoscopy with a real-time electromagnetic position sensor: a comparison of two image registration methods. Chest. 2000;118:1783–7.
11. Luo X, Feuerstein M, Sugiura T, et al. Towards hybrid bronchoscope tracking under respiratory motion: evaluation on a dynamic motion phantom. Proc SPIE. 2010; p. 76251B.

A Simplified Pipeline for Motion Correction in Dual Gated Cardiac PET

Lars Ruthotto[1], Fabian Gigengack[2,3], Martin Burger[4], Carsten H. Wolters[5],
Xiaoyi Jiang[3], Klaus P. Schäfers[2], Jan Modersitzki[1]

[1] Institute of Mathematics and Image Computing, University of Lübeck
[2] European Insitute for Molecular Imaging, University of Münster
[3] Department of Mathematics and Computer Science, University of Münster
[4] Institute for Computational and Applied Mathematics, University of Münster
[5] Institute of Biomagnetism and Biosignalanalysis, University of Münster
lars.ruthotto@mic.uni-luebeck.de

Abstract. Positron Emission Tomography (PET) is a nuclear imaging technique of increasing importance e.g. in cardiovascular investigations. However, cardiac and respiratory motion of the patient degrade the image quality due to acquisition times in the order of minutes. Reconstructions without motion compensation are prone to spatial blurring and affected attenuation correction. These effects can be reduced by gating, motion correction and finally summation of the transformed images. This paper describes a new and systematic approach for the correction of both cardiac and respiratory motion. Key contribution is the splitting of the motion into respiratory and cardiac components, which are then corrected individually. For the considered gating scheme the number of registration problems is reduced by a factor of 3, which considerably simplifies the motion correction pipeline compared to previous approaches. The subproblems are stabilized by averaging cardiac gates for respiratory motion estimation and vice versa. The potential of the novel pipeline is evaluated in a group study on data of 21 human patients.

1 Introduction

Positron Emission Tomography (PET) is a nuclear imaging technique that provides insight into functional processes in the body. Its fields of applications range from oncology via neuroimaging to cardiology. Due to acquisition times in the order of minutes, motion is a well-known problem in PET. In thoracic PET two different types of motion degrade the image quality: respiratory and cardiac motion. Neglecting the resulting spatial mislocalization of emission events during the reconstruction leads to blurred images and affects attenuation correction.

Gating, i.e. grouping the entire list of emission events by breathing and/or cardiac phases reduces the extent of motion contained in each single gate [1, 2]. A downside is the higher noise level in each gate since only a small fraction of the available events is considered. This is a severe problem in dual gating schemes, which demand a very fine division into both respiratory and cardiac gates.

Different strategies for motion correction were proposed in the literature and for a detailed overview [3]. This paper follows the idea of first eliminating the motion in the dual gated data by image registration and finally summation of the gated images to consider all measured emission events and thereby lower the noise level. This strategy has proven successful for respiratory motion correction [4, 5] and cardiac motion correction [6]. Recently, both types of motion were eliminated after dual gating using nonlinear mass-preserving registration [7]. Mass-preservation is a key idea in order to cope with intensity modulations owing to partial volume effects. Another key contribution is the discretization of a hyperelastic regularization energy [8]. This sophisticated regularizer is mandatory as it achieves meaningful motion estimates and guarantees diffeomorphic transformations even for data with high noise level and large deformations. The algorithm was embedded into the registration toolbox FAIR that is freely available (http://www.siam.org/books/fa06/) and documented in [9].

However, the scheme in [7] is computationally very expensive since all gated images are treated individually. This yields a total number of $m \cdot n - 1$ challenging registration problems for a gating into m cardiac and n respiratory gates.

In this paper the nature of the gating scheme is exploited to provide a systematic approach to motion correction and to simplify the registration pipeline. The motion between a template gate and the reference gate is modeled as a simple concatenation of a respiratory and a cardiac transformation under the assumption that cardiac and respiratory motion are approximately independent. This scheme reduces the number of registration tasks to $m + n - 2$ and thus saves computation times which allows finer gating schemes. In the considered 5×5 gating this yields a reduction from 24 to 8 registration subproblems. Furthermore each sub-problem is stabilized by averaging over cardiac phases in the respiratory motion estimation and vice versa. Results for a group of 21 patients indicate the effectiveness of the simplified approach and its positive impact on image quality.

2   Materials and methods

2.1   Data acquisition

Data of 21 patients (19 male, 2 female; 37–76 years old) with known coronary artery disease was acquired in a 20 minute list mode scan on a Siemens Biograph Sensation 16 PET/CT scanner. The data was cropped to the first three minutes to resemble a clinically feasible protocol and dual gating into 5 respiratory and 5 cardiac gates was performed, [2]. The 3D EM software EMRECON was used for reconstruction of all data [10]. The images are sampled with $128 \times 100 \times 44$.

2.2   Mass-preserving hyperelastic registration

A key contribution in [7] is the incorporation of the mass-preserving property of PET into motion correction. The idea is that the total amount of intensity of the template image $\mathcal{T}$ should remain unchanged after registration to the reference $\mathcal{R}$, which is not guaranteed for standard registration approaches. This is realized by an intensity modulation accounting for volumetric changes given by the Jacobian determinant of the transformation [7]. The natural distance term for density images is the sum of squared differences yielding the image registration functional

$$\mathcal{J}[y] := \frac{1}{2} \|(\mathcal{T} \circ y) \cdot \det(\nabla y) - \mathcal{R}\|^2 + \mathcal{S}^{\mathrm{hyper}}(y) \tag{1}$$

where $\mathcal{S}^{\mathrm{hyper}}$ is the hyperelastic energy [8], which was recently integrated into FAIR: $\mathcal{S}^{\mathrm{hyper}}(y) = \alpha_l \mathcal{S}^{\mathrm{length}}(y) + \alpha_a \mathcal{S}^{\mathrm{area}}(y) + \alpha_v \mathcal{S}^{\mathrm{volume}}(y)$. It controls the changes in length, area and volume induced by the transformation y. Since infinite energy is required to annihilate or enlarge a volume $\mathcal{S}^{\mathrm{hyper}}$ guarantees the invertibility of the transformation even for large displacements and noisy data. While this regularizer is a desirable feature in many registration tasks, it is mandatory in this application to guarantee the preservation of mass.

2.3 Simplified registration pipeline

The used gating protocol provides 25 images denoted by $\mathcal{I}_c^r$ which are related to 5 respiratory phases $r = 1, ..., 5$ and 5 cardiac phases $c = 1, ..., 5$. The assumption is that for each fixed respiratory phase r geometric differences in $I_1^r, ..., I_5^r$ are only due to cardiac motion. Hence, all these cardiac phases are displaced by the same respiratory motion y^r. Respiratory motion is eliminated first from the gated dataset as this motion shows less nonlinearities. To this end, cardiac averages $\mathcal{I}^1, ..., \mathcal{I}^5$ are computed, where $\mathcal{I}^r = (\sum_{c=1}^{5} \mathcal{I}_c^r)/5$, and used to estimate the respiratory displacements $y^1, ..., y^5$ based on the above mass-preserving hyperelastic registration. Next, respiratory motion is compensated in all 25 images.

Subsequently, $\mathcal{I}_1, ..., \mathcal{I}_5$ are computed, where $\mathcal{I}_c$ is the average of the transformed respiratory gates. These images are then used to estimate the cardiac displacements $y_1, ..., y_5$. Note that even after removing the respiratory motion each such gate relates to different realization of (stochastic) radioactive decay. Hence averaging reduces the noise level even for perfect spatial alignment.

After these 4 respiratory and 4 cardiac motion estimations both types of motion are eliminated from all 25 images. To this end y^r and y_c are concatenated and the mass-preserving transformation model is applied. Finally, the motion compensated image is obtained by summation over all gates.

3   Results

The proposed motion correction scheme is applied to the image data of 21 human patients. To minimize the geometric mismatch the mid-expiration diastole gate is chosen as reference image denoted by $\mathcal{I}_{\mathrm{Ref}}$. The images are cropped to a rectangular region of $128 \times 100 \times 44$ voxels around the torso. Regularization parameters are set to $\alpha_l = 5$, $\alpha_a = 1$ for length and area term as in [7]. Control of volumetric change is tightened for respiratory by choosing $\alpha_v = 100$ and kept at the same level, $\alpha_v = 10$, for cardiac motion correction. Registration is performed on a coarse-to-fine hierarchy of levels and stopped at the second finest discretization level ($64 \times 50 \times 22$) to improve stability against noise and speed the correction up. The total computation time is about 8 minutes per patient on a Linux PC with a 6 core Intel Xeon X5670@2,93 GHz using Matlab 2010b.

The volumetric change induced by the transformations serves as an indicator to validate the injectivity of the transformation. The minimum and maximum of the Jacobian determinant over all patients and all transformations is between 0.81 and 1.19 for respiratory and 0.55 and 1.31 for cardiac motions. Thus all transformations including their concatenations are diffeomorphic.

Exemplarily, the registration result is illustrated for an arbitrary chosen patient in Fig. 1 using three orthogonal slice views. Presentation is restricted to the most challenging sub-problem of registration between the end-expiration systolic gate and the mid-expiration diastolic reference gate. The difference images before and after registration clearly show the considerably improved image similarity. Furthermore the transformation y_2^5 – obtained by concatenating the respiratory motion y^5 and the cardiac component y_2 is smooth and regular. The positive impact of the new strategy on image quality is illustrated for the same dataset in Fig. 2 in a coronal view. The effect of gating – minimal motion blur, but high noise level – is visible in the reference gate (left). The not motion-corrected reconstruction (center) shows acceptable noise level, but the hearts contour is motion-blurred. Both advantages – minimal motion blur and acceptable noise level – are combined by the resulting image of the new method.

The improvement of image similarity after motion correction is presented in Fig. 3 for the whole group of 21 patients. Normalized cross-correlations (NCC)

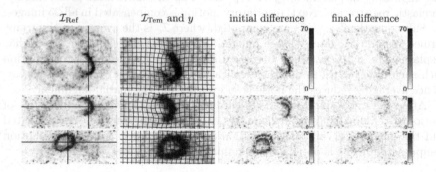

$\mathcal{I}_{\text{Ref}}$ $\mathcal{I}_{\text{Tem}}$ and y initial difference   final difference

Fig. 1. Results of the 3D registration for an arbitrary chosen patient out of the 21 patients. Three orthogonal cross-sections sharing the point marked by a white crosshair are shown. A visualization of the mid-expiration diastolic gate $\mathcal{I}_{\text{Ref}}$ (first col.) is compared to the furthest apart end-expiratory systolic gate $\mathcal{I}_{\text{Tem}}$ that is visualized with superimposed deformation y (second col.) in a small region around the heart. The decline in absolute difference (third and fourth col.) images and the increase of normalized cross correlation from 0.522 to 0.681 before and after nonlinear mass-preserving registration show the positive impact of the proposed method on image similarity

between $\mathcal{I}_{Ref}$ and the 24 template gates computed in a rectangular region around the heart for all patients are illustrated in a box plot. A considerable increase of NCC can be seen by comparing the gray (before registration) and black (after registration) boxes and whiskers.

4   Discussion

This paper presents an systematic approach to cardiac and respiratory motion correction in dual gated thoracic PET. The main contribution is the simplification of the processing pipeline achieved by a splitting of the displacement into a respiration and cardiology component and individually correction of both effects in the dual gated dataset. A considerably lower number of registration problems need to be solved, which are stabilized by averaging cardiac gates for respiratory correction and vice versa. The correction results for a group of 21 patients suggest that the underlying assumption that cardiac and respiratory motion are independent is approximately fulfilled for our data.

The presented pipeline is in principle compatible with existing approaches to cardiac and respiratory motion correction techniques [6, 4, 5, 7]. Here, a nonlinear mass-preserving approach is chosen as it is well-suited for the registration of density images such as PET, [7]. The preservation of mass can be ensured under certain assumptions including the invertibility of the transformation. Therefore an implementation of a hyperelastic regularizer [8], which is integrated in the freely available toolbox FAIR [9], is used. This regularizer guarantees diffeomorphic solutions of the problem, but still allows large and flexible transformations.

Individual treatment of respiratory and cardiac motion seems reasonable as both types of motion are very different in nature. While the further is almost locally rigid, the hearts contraction tends to be more flexible. In the proposed pipeline this can be addressed by e.g. the choice of different regularization parameters for both types as done in this work. This enforces a smaller range of the volumetric changes due to respiratory motion for our data.

Despite the considerably reduced distance, the heart structure is still visible in the final difference images (Fig. 1). The registration could be improved by performing a number of outer loops over respiratory and cardiac motion correction to be investigated in future work. The promising results presented in

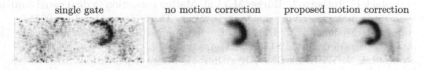

single gate   no motion correction   proposed motion correction

Fig. 2. Reconstruction results for an arbitrary chosen patient out of the group of 21 patients. Coronal views of the mid-expiration diastolic gate $\mathcal{I}_{Ref}$ (left, minimal motion blur, high noise level), reconstruction without motion correction (center, motion blurred, acceptable noise level) and the result using the novel motion correction scheme (right, considerably reduced motion, acceptable noise level) are visualized

Fig. 3. Motion correction results for our group study of 21 patients. Normalized cross-correlations between the 24 template gates and the reference gate are shown before (gray) and after (black) motion correction in a box plot. The considerable increase of NCC shows the effectiveness and robustness of the new method

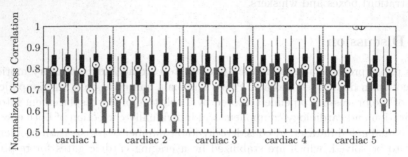

this paper mark a next step towards clinical applicability of motion correction in thoracic PET. With the simplified registration pipeline the quality of motion correction can be further improved as finer subdivision schemes become feasible.

Acknowledgement. The authors thank Otmar Schober, Department of Nuclear Medicine, University of Münster, for providing the interesting data.

References

1. Lucignani G. Respiratory and cardiac motion correction with 4D PET imaging: shooting at moving targets. Eur J Nucl Med Mol I. 2009.
2. Büther F, Dawood M, L LS, et al. List mode-driven cardiac and respiratory gating in PET. J Nucl Med. 2009.
3. Bai W, Brady M. Motion correction and attenuation correction for respiratory gated PET images. IEEE Trans Med Imag. 2011.
4. Dawood M, Büther F, Jiang X, et al. Respiratory motion correction in 3-D PET data with advanced optical flow algorithms. IEEE Trans Med Imag. 2008.
5. Bai W, Brady M. Respiratory motion correction in PET images. Phys Med Biol. 2009.
6. Klein JK, Huesman RH. Four dimensional processing of deformable cardiacd PET data. Med Image Anal. 2002.
7. Gigengack F, Ruthotto L, Burger M, et al. Motion correction in dual gated cardiac PET using mass-preserving image registration. IEEE Trans Med Img. 2011.
8. Burger M, Modersitzki J, Ruthotto L. A hyperelastic regularization energy for image registration. SIAM SISC. 2011; p. submitted.
9. Modersitzki J. FAIR: Flexible Algorithms for Image Registration. SIAM; 2009.
10. Kösters T, Schäfers KP, Wübbeling F. EMrecon: an expectation maximization based image reconstruction framework for emission tomography data. Proc IEEE NSS/MIC. 2011.

FluidTracks

Combining Nonlinear Image Registration and Active Contours for Cell Tracking

Nico Scherf[1,2], Christian Ludborzs[1,2], Konstantin Thierbach[1],
Jens-Peer Kuska[2†], Ulf-Dietrich Braumann[2], Patrick Scheibe[2,3], Tilo Pompe[4],
Ingmar Glauche[1], Ingo Roeder[1]

[1]Institute for Medical Informatics and Biometry, Dresden University of Technology
[2]Interdisciplinary Centre for Bioinformatics, University of Leipzig
[3]Translational Centre for Regenerative Medicine, University of Leipzig
[4]Institute for Biochemistry, University of Leipzig
nico.scherf@tu-dresden.de

Abstract. Continuous analysis of multi-cellular systems at the single cell level in space and time is one of the fundamental tools in cell biology and experimental medicine to study the mechanisms underlying tissue formation, regeneration and disease progression. We present an approach to cell tracking using nonlinear image registration and level set segmentation that can handle different cell densities, occlusions and cell divisions.

1 Introduction

Comprehensive analysis of single cell behavior is an important tool in cell biology to study a variety of fundamental questions. New experimental methods and imaging technologies facilitate continuous spatio-temporal monitoring of single cells over long time periods and in high resolution [1, 2]. One serious limitation is the large amount of data that needs to be analyzed, which obviously calls for computerized tracking and cell detection [2]. Particularly, the accurate detection of cell shapes is manually not feasible for more than just a few images. However, studying the developmental patterns of cells requires the observation over long time periods. On the other hand, automated methods often lack the robustness to reliably follow the cells over the whole course of the experiment. Consequently, these experiments were mainly analyzed in a manual fashion [2].

A number of different techniques for cell tracking have previously been developed [3, 4]. Most of the existing methods can be roughly divided into two classes: detection with subsequent object association [5] or tracking by active contour evolution [3]. Methods of the former class are particular sensitive to the number and duration of occlusions, which introduce a lot of ambiguous assignments that

---

† We are deeply indebted to Jens-Peer Kuska, whose ideas and contributions incomparably influenced our research in image processing and visualization. To our greatest regret, he passed away on July 1, 2009 at the age of 45.

have to be resolved. Active contour based methods aim at segmenting the cells in one image and using the final result to initialize the method for the subsequent image. However, if the initialized contour overlaps with several objects it is hard to ensure convergence to the desired solution. Furthermore, the topology of the contours is either fixed and cell divisions become a problem, or it is flexible and false merging of cell masks can occur. An alternative approach to cell tracking is based on nonparametric image registration [6, 7]. An initial segmentation of the cells is advanced by iteratively applying the obtained displacement fields that map consecutive images onto each other. This approach can in principle overcome some of the above-mentioned problems. Firstly, it takes the movement of surrounding objects into account by virtue of the smoothness constraint of the displacement field. Thus, it provides a rather holistic perspective on changes of groups of pixels as opposed to the sparsity of object assignment or the local perspective of the active contour tracking. Secondly, it provides a prediction for cell movement between frames based on an underlying physical model (viscoelasticity as a reasonable assumption for cell deformation). Since the registration does not care about the regularity of the cell masks, they tend to get smeared out and may become heavily distorted eventually [6]. A combination of segmentation and registration can overcome this problem in principle. However, if both methods are uncoupled as in [7], errors in cell detection and particularly occlusions cannot be resolved. The presented work addresses this issue by coupling registration tracking with a level set segmentation as described in the following section.

2   Materials and methods

2.1   Fast fluid extension for image registration

Given a source image $S(\boldsymbol{x})$ and a template image $T(\boldsymbol{x})$, registration aims at finding a transformation $\boldsymbol{u}(\boldsymbol{x})$ from $S(\boldsymbol{x})$ onto $T(\boldsymbol{x})$ such that $T(\boldsymbol{x}) = S(\boldsymbol{x} - \boldsymbol{u}(\boldsymbol{x}))$. This problem is ill-posed, thus requiring additional constraints on the smoothness of the transformation. These are either derived from physical principles [8], or from a variational formulation [9] of the problem. For our purposes we use the curvature-based regularization introduced by Fischer et al. [9] in a fluid-like formulation as proposed by Kuska et al. [10]. Briefly: A displacement field u is sought that minimizes the sum of squared differences between the source and template (i.e. constant intensity of objects is assumed)

$$\underset{\boldsymbol{u}}{\arg\min} \left(\mathcal{V}[\boldsymbol{u}] = \frac{1}{2} \int_{\Omega} \left(T(\boldsymbol{x}) - S(\boldsymbol{x} - \boldsymbol{u}(\boldsymbol{x}), t) \right)^2 \, \mathrm{d}\boldsymbol{x} \right) \qquad (1)$$

For a fluid formulation, the regularizer $\mathcal{T}$ proposed by Fischer et al. [9] is imposed on the velocity field $\dot{\boldsymbol{u}}$ underlying the displacement

$$\mathcal{T}[\dot{\boldsymbol{u}}] = \frac{\rho}{2} \int_{\Omega} \sum_{i=1}^{2} \left(\Delta \dot{u}_i(\boldsymbol{x}, t) \right)^2 \, \mathrm{d}\boldsymbol{x} \qquad (2)$$

Since the Euler-Lagrange equation for $\mathcal{L}(\dot{u}, u) = \mathcal{T}[\dot{u}] - \mathcal{V}[u]$ is free of dissipation, artificial damping has to be introduced yielding the final formulation

$$\rho \frac{\mathrm{d}^2}{\mathrm{d}t^2} \left(\Delta^2 u \right) - F = -\gamma \dot{u} - \nu \Delta^2 \dot{u} \tag{3}$$

with $F = [T(\boldsymbol{x}) - S(\boldsymbol{x} - u(\boldsymbol{x}, t))] \nabla S(\boldsymbol{x} - u(\boldsymbol{x}, t))$. For a detailed derivation and numerical aspects, we refer to [10]. The resulting registration is considerably faster than the classical fluid model of [8] and allows for an integration of further constraints (vorticity structure).

2.2   Active contours segmentation

Segmentation amounts to dissecting the domain of the image Ω into a number of non-overlapping regions Ω_i, i.e. objects of interest and background. An elegant formulation of the problem is the active contours without edges method introduced by [11]. The level set formulation allows for a segmentation of multiple objects at once with control over the regularity of the solution. Furthermore, a suitable initialization can guide the algorithm to the desired local optimum. These aspects render this method particularly useful to handle the drift of the masks during registration tracking.

2.3   Combined registration-based tracking and segmentation

The principal idea of our method is the following: Cell masks are provided by an initial segmentation. In each step of the algorithm, we first calculate the displacement field $u(\boldsymbol{x})$ between the current and subsequent image of the sequence by using the fluid registration. The cell masks are then propagated to the next frame by applying $u(\boldsymbol{x})$. This provides a prediction of the new position for all cells. The estimate is used to initialize the active contour segmentation, that provides a correction for the prediction step by explicitly taking the actual image data into account. For each segmented cell mask the consistency of the predicted labeling is checked by considering the following cases:

- if the propagated label in the cell mask is unique, the segmentation result is adopted for the labeling
- if contradicting labels are found in a cell mask, an overlap has occurred and only the predicted mask is kept instead
- if two separate masks received the same labeling, a division is detected, the new masks are adopted and a unique label is given to each daughter

It is the basic rationale behind this approach that in case of overlapping objects the segmentation provides ambiguous information. Thus, it is more reliable to revert only to the results of the transformation step until the objects separate again and consistent masks are available from the segmentation. Thus, even under occlusion for several frames, individual masks are kept for each cell. The principal scheme is depicted in Fig. 1.

2.4   Experiments

We tested our method on four different datasets (in vitro and artificial, Fig. 2). Firstly, we used a sequence of unlabeled human primary hematopoietic progenitor cells obtained by usual transmitted-light microscopy (image size 400×300 px). Secondly, a synthetic test data set (256×256 px) was created to simulate a rapidly dividing cell culture with high local cell density to assess the behavior of the algorithm in the presence of multiple occlusions and cell divisions. The last two experiments were conducted on sequences of a murine FDCPmix cell line. These images (554×394 px and 548×390 px, respectively) are characterized by higher local cell densities and a heterogeneity of the cells with respect to shape and migration. Furthermore, the images of the last sequences exhibit weak contrast and imperfect focusing. Manual reference tracking were available for each dataset.

3   Results

Tracking performance was evaluated by counting (i) the number of valid cell tracks and (ii) the number of correctly detected divisions. A cell track is considered valid, if the initialized cell has been correctly detected and tracked for all available time points, and the fate of the cell is correctly determined (cell division, cell death). If the cell has been successfully tracked, but a false cell splitting has been detected the whole track is considered as wrong. Table 1 gives an overview of the tracking results. The number of cells, correct tracks, detected cell divisions, the number of lost cell tracks, the number of lost cells due to false splittings, and the total number of images are given for each sequence.

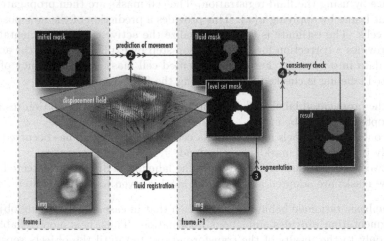

Fig. 1. Principal scheme of proposed algorithm

Table 1. Overview of tracking results

Experiment	cells	correct tracks	divisions	lost tracks	false splittings	frames
HSC	6	6(100%)	0/0	0	0	279
Synthetic	63	63 (100%)	29/29(100%)	0	0	100
FDCPmix1	35	30/35 (86%)	2/2 (100%)	3	2	100
FDCPmix2	34	28/34 (82%)	1/1 (100%)	6	0	44

4 Discussion

All cells of the HSC sequence were successfully tracked and partial occlusions could be resolved. It should be noted, that simple methods as nearest neighbor tracking already fail to handle these rather simple data. The synthetic sequence demands flexible mask handling abilities due to occlusions and divisions. All cells and corresponding offspring were correctly tracked by the algorithm. Even regions with severe overlapping, lasting for a number of frames could be resolved (Fig. 2b). The last two experiments include several difficulties: cells are more similar to background structures and the outlines are blurred, occlusions are frequently occurring, and characteristics of cell motion are quite heterogeneous. Consequently, the algorithm is not able to correctly follow all initialized cells as shown in Table 1. Most of the lost cell tracks result from large jumps of the cell from one image to the next, which is not resolvable by the registration method (Table 1). However, five tracks were lost in the last experiment due to an aggregation of cells that could not even be resolved by manual tracking (lower right region in Fig. 3d). The consistent combination of mask propagation by fluid registration and subsequent level set segmentation yields a robust and flexible method to track cells that undergo divisions even in areas of high local cell density. The main drawbacks of the proposed approach are its vulnerability to large displacements and the the occurrence of newly appearing objects. The first problem can be reduced by including multi-resolution methods in the registration while the latter problem can be handled by keeping a second label image of detected objects that have not yet been labeled. Future work will include the incorporation of these aspects in the existing framework. From a theoretical point of view, a combination of registration and segmentation in a single variational formulation is an attractive aspect for future work.

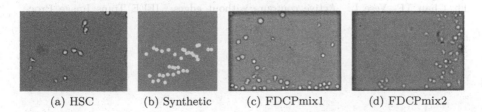

(a) HSC   (b) Synthetic   (c) FDCPmix1   (d) FDCPmix2

Fig. 2. Samples of image data used for experiments

62   Scherf et al.

Fig. 3. Tracking results as space-time trajectories

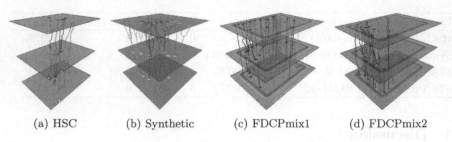

(a) HSC   (b) Synthetic   (c) FDCPmix1   (d) FDCPmix2

Acknowledgement. This research was supported by the European Commission project EuroSyStem (200270) and by the German Ministry for Education and Research, BMBF-grant on Medical Systems Biology HaematoSys (BMBF-FKZ 0315452).

References

1. Megason SG, Fraser SE. Imaging in systems biology. Cell. 2007;130(5):784–95.
2. Schroeder T. Long-term single-cell imaging of mammalian stem cells. Nat Methods. 2011;8:S30–5.
3. Acton ST, Ray N. Biomedical image analysis: tracking. Synthesis Lectures on Image, Video, and Multimedia Processing. 2006;2(1):1–152.
4. Meijering E, Dzyubachyk O, Smal I, et al. Tracking in cell and developmental biology. Semin Cell Dev Biol. 2009;20(8):894–902.
5. Kanade T, Yin Z, Bise R, et al. Cell image analysis: algorithms, system and applications. In: Proc IEEE WACV; 2011. p. 374–81.
6. Hand AJ, Sun T, Barber DC, et al. Automated tracking of migrating cells in phase-contrast video microscopy sequences using image registration. J Microsc. 2009;234(1):62–79.
7. Tokuhisa S, Kaneko K. The time series image snalysis of the HeLa cell using viscous fluid registration. In: Proc ICCSA. Springer; 2010. p. 189–200.
8. Bro-Nielsen M, Gramkow C. Fast fluid registration of medical images. In: Proc VBC; 1996. p. 267–76.
9. Fischer B. A unified approach to fast image registration and a new curvature based registration technique. Linear Algebra Appl. 2004;380:107–24.
10. Kuska JP, Scheibe P, Braumann UD. Fast fluid extensions for image registration algorithms. In: Proc IEEE ICIP; 2008. p. 2408–11.
11. Chan TF, Vese L. Active contours without edges. IEEE Trans Image Proc. 2001;10(2):266–77.

Eine effiziente Parallel-Implementierung eines stabilen Euler-Cauchy-Verfahrens für die Modellierung von Tumorwachstum

A. Mang[1], A. Toma[1,2], T. A. Schütz[1,3], S. Becker[1,2], T. M. Buzug[1]

[1]Institut für Medizintechnik, Universität zu Lübeck (UL)
[2]Centre of Excellence for Technology and Engineering in Medicine (TANDEM)
[3]Graduiertenschule für Informatik in Medizin und Lebenswissenschaften, UL
mang@imt.uni-luebeck.de

Kurzfassung. Die vorliegende Arbeit befasst sich mit der Überführung eines, kürzlich auf dem Gebiet der Bildverarbeitung vorgeschlagenen, beschleunigten Euler-Cauchy Verfahrens (ECV*) in die Modellierung der Progression primärer Hirntumoren auf Gewebeebene in einer parallelen Implementierung. Das biophysikalische Modell ist über ein Anfangsrandwertproblem erklärt. In der vorliegenden Arbeit wird eine Stabilitätsbedingung für das Standard-ECV in der $\ell^{h,2}$-Norm hergeleitet, welche nicht nur eine adaptive Schrittweitensteuerung ermöglicht, sondern auch als Kontrollparameter für das beschleunigte Verfahren dient. Eine vergleichende Gegenüberstellung zu (semi-)impliziten Verfahren demonstriert nicht nur, dass der numerische Fehler für die vorliegende Anwendung dem impliziter Verfahren entspricht, sondern auch die Effizienz der vorgestellten Parallel-Implementierung. Die Rechenzeit ist im Maximum, im Vergleich zu impliziten Verfahren, um ca. einen Faktor 20 reduziert.

1 Einleitung

Die mathematische Modellierung von Erkrankungen des Zentralnervensystems ist ein mächtiges Werkzeug aus der angewandten Mathematik, um Hypothesen über einen Krankheitsverlauf zu prüfen. Mit der vorliegenden Arbeit liefern wir einen Beitrag zur Modellierung der raum-zeitlichen Dynamik kanzeröser Zellen in zerebralem Gewebe. Die betrachtete Tumorentität ist das Gliom – ein hirneigener Tumor, dessen hochgradige Ausprägung eine fatale Prognose aufweist. Ein verbreiteter Ansatz zur bildbasierten Modellierung, ist die Ausbreitung der Krebszellen in zerebralem Gewebe als Anfangsrandwertproblem (ARWP) zu formulieren (§2, Prb. 1). Eine etablierte Grundannahme ist hierbei, dass die Progression des Tumors auf Gewebeebene hinreichend gut durch die Prozesse der Proliferation und der Migration von Zellen in gesundes, umliegendes Gewebe abgebildet werden kann [1, S. 536 ff]. Dieses Modell findet nicht nur Einsatz in der Modellierung patientenindividueller Pathologieverläufe [2, 3] sondern auch als biophysikalischer Prior für hybride Ansätze in der modellbasierten Bildverarbeitung [4, 5, 6, 7, 8]. Sowohl die Integration in rechenintensive Ansätze zur

Schätzung von Modellparametern [3] als auch in Verfahren der modellbasierten Bildverarbeitung [4, 5, 6, 7, 8] geht direkt einher mit der Forderung, effiziente Lösungsstrategien für das zugrundeliegende ARWP bereitzustellen. Eine gängige Strategie [4, 5, 6, 7] ist die Verwendung eines Euler-Cauchy-Verfahrens (ECVs). Dieses besitzt den namhaften Nachteil, dass Stabilität nur dann garantiert werden kann, wenn eine obere Schranke für die zeitliche Schrittweite eingehalten wird ('CFL Bedingung'). Damit wird dieses Verfahren für große Simulationszeiträume ineffizient. (Semi-)Implizite Verfahren sind hingegen stabil, erfordern allerdings die Lösung eines (nicht-/semi-)linearen Gleichungssystems und damit einhergehend einen höheren Implementationsaufwand. Eine sehr viel elegantere Strategie ist die Verwendung eines beschleunigten ECVs (ECV*) [9, 10].

Der wesentliche Beitrag der vorliegenden Arbeit liegt (*i*) in der Überführung des in [9] vorgestellten Verfahrens – in einer *parallelen* Implementierung (pECV*) – in die Modellierung der raum-zeitlichen Dynamik primärer Hirntumoren, (*ii*) der Beschreibung und der Gegenüberstellung zu impliziten Verfahren und (*iii*) einer Verfeinerung des Diffusionsmodells durch die Verwendung unscharfer Gewebekarten. Darüber hinaus liefern wir eine Abschätzung der Stabilitätsgrenze für das ECV, die nicht nur eine adaptive Schrittweitensteuerung erlaubt, sondern zudem als Kontrollparameter für das beschleunigte ECV dient. Es ist hervorzuheben, dass wir uns in dieser Arbeit ausschließlich der numerischen Lösung des ARWP widmen. Wir gehen – mit dem Verweis auf Vorarbeiten [2, 3] – davon aus, dass die Validität des Modells als gesichert gilt.

2   Material und Methoden

2.1   Mathematisches Modell

Die Modellierung der raum-zeitlichen Dynamik einer Populationsdichte u an kanzerösen Zellen innerhalb des zerebralen Gewebes Ω_B basiert auf einem Reaktions-Diffusions-Formalismus [1, S. 536 ff]. Es gilt folgendes ARWP zu lösen:

Problem 1 *Sei* $\Omega := (\omega_1^1, \omega_1^2) \times \cdots \times (\omega_d^1, \omega_d^2) \subset \mathbb{R}^d$, $d \in \{2,3\}$ *und das Gebiet* $\Omega_B \subset \Omega$ *mit Rand* $\partial\Omega_B$ *und Abschluss* $\bar{\Omega}_B$ *gegeben. Weiter seien* $\Omega_B^c := \Omega \backslash \bar{\Omega}_B$, $u_S > 0$, $\sigma > 0$, $\mathcal{P} := \{A \in \mathbb{R}^{d \times d} : A \text{ ist symmetrisch positiv semi-definit}\}$, *das Funktional* $y : C^2(\Omega_B \times \mathbb{R}_0^+, \mathbb{R}_0^+) \cap C^1(\bar{\Omega}_B \times \mathbb{R}_0^+) =: \mathcal{U} \to \mathbb{R}_0^+$ *und die Funktion* $D \in C^1(\Omega, \mathcal{P}) =: \mathcal{D}$ *gegeben. Finde ein* $u \in \mathcal{U}$, *so dass*

$$\partial_t u(\boldsymbol{x}, t) = \nabla \cdot (\boldsymbol{D}(\boldsymbol{x}) \nabla u(\boldsymbol{x}, t)) + y(u(\boldsymbol{x}, t)), \qquad in \; \Omega_B \times \mathbb{R}_0^+, \qquad (1a)$$

$$\partial_{\boldsymbol{n}} u(\boldsymbol{x}, t) = 0, \qquad\qquad\qquad auf \; \partial\Omega_B \times \mathbb{R}_0^+, \qquad (1b)$$

$$u(\boldsymbol{x}, 0) = u_S \exp(-\|\boldsymbol{x} - \boldsymbol{x}_S\|_2^2 / 2\sigma^2), \qquad für \; alle \; \boldsymbol{x} \in \Omega_B, \qquad (1c)$$

erfüllt ist. Hierbei ist $\boldsymbol{x}_S \in \Omega_B$ *und* $\partial_{\boldsymbol{n}}$ *mit* $\|\boldsymbol{n}\|_2 = 1$ *stellt die von* Ω_B *in* Ω_B^c *zeigende Normalenableitung von* u *dar.*

In Prb. 1 markiert $\boldsymbol{D}$ ein Tensorfeld und $\boldsymbol{x}_S$ den Saatpunkt für die Initialbedingung. Das Diffusionsmodell in (1a) basiert auf der anerkannten Annahme einer unterschiedlichen mittleren Diffusivität von Krebszellen innerhalb der weißen ($\Omega_W \subset \Omega_B$) und grauen ($\Omega_G \subset \Omega_B$) Masse. Entsprechend verwenden wir $D(x) = \alpha(x)\hat{D}_l(x)$, $\hat{D}_l \in \mathbb{R}^{d\times d}$ für $x \in \Omega_l$, $l \in \{W, G, C\}$, wobei $\Omega_C := \Omega_B^c \equiv (\Omega_G \cup \Omega_W)^c$, $\hat{D}_G \equiv \hat{D}_C \equiv E = \mathrm{diag}(1, \ldots, 1) \in \mathbb{R}^{d\times d}$, $\hat{D}_W = \psi(\tilde{D}(x))$. Das Funktional $\psi : \mathcal{D} \to \mathcal{D}$ erlaubt eine Skalierung der Anisotropie des Tensorfeldes $\tilde{D} \in \mathcal{D}$ ([11], illustriert in Abb. 1 (rechts)). Wir schlagen eine lokaladaptive Wichtung $\alpha : \Omega \to \mathbb{R}_0^+$ anhand von unscharfen Gewebekarten für die Skalierung der mittleren Diffusivität des Tensorfeldes D vor. Es gilt $\alpha(x) = \alpha_W(x)\kappa_W + \alpha_G(x)\kappa_G$ mit den Wichtungsparametern $\kappa_l > 0$, $l \in \{W, G, C\}$ und den Gewebekarten $\alpha_l : \Omega \to [0, 1]$ für die graue und weiße Masse (Abb. 1 (links)). Für das Proliferations-Modell y gibt es unterschiedliche Möglichkeiten. Wir betrachten exponentielles, $y^{\exp} = \gamma u(x, t)$, und logistisches, $y^{\log} = \gamma u(x, t)(u_L - u(x, t))$, $u_L > 0$, Wachstum mit der Rate $\gamma > 0$.

2.2 Numerische Lösungsverfahren

Die in der vorliegenden Arbeit diskutierten Lösungsschemata lassen sich kompakt über das θ-Verfahren darstellen. Wir führen zunächst die Gitterfunktionen $\tilde{u} \colon \Omega^h \times Q \to \mathbb{R}_0^+$ und $\tilde{y} \colon \{\tilde{u} \colon \Omega^h \times Q \to \mathbb{R}_0^+\} =: \mathcal{U}^h \to \mathbb{R}_0^+$ und $\tilde{D} \colon \Omega^h \to \mathcal{P}$ mit $\Omega^h \in \mathbb{R}^{dm_1 \times \cdots \times m_d}$, $m_i \in \mathbb{N}$, $d \in \{2, 3\}$ (zellzentrierte Diskretisierung des Gebietes Ω) und $Q := \{t^j \in \mathbb{R}_0^+ : t^j = jq, q \in \mathbb{R}^+, j = 0, 1, 2, \ldots\}$ (Diskretisierung der Zeitachse) ein. Überführen wir die Gitterfunktionen in eine lexikographische Anordnung $u^{j,h} \in \mathbb{R}^n$ und $y^{j,h} = \gamma u^{j,h} \in \mathbb{R}^n$ mit $n = \prod_{i=1}^{d} m_i$, lässt sich die numerische Lösung von Prb. 1 in die Lösung eines linearen Gleichungssystems

$$(E - q\theta\mathcal{A})u^{j+1,h} - \gamma\theta y^{j+1,h} = (E + q(1-\theta)\mathcal{A})u^{j,h} + q(1-\theta)y^{j,h}, \quad (2)$$

$j = 0, \ldots, w - 1$, überführen. Hierbei markiert $\mathcal{A} \in \mathbb{R}^{n\times n}$ die Diskretisierung des linearen Diffusionsoperators ((1a)). Für die Approximation der auftretenden Ableitungen verwenden wir finite Differenzen. Der Parameter $\theta \in [0, 1]$ in (2) steuert die konkrete Ausprägung des Lösungsschemas: Für $\theta = 0$ ergibt sich das ECV, für $\theta = 1$ das implizite Euler-Verfahren (iEV), für $\theta = 0.5$ das Crank-Nicholson (CN) Verfahren und für $\theta \in (0, 1) \setminus \{0.5\}$ ein Mischverfahren. Die numerische Lösung $u^{h,j+1}$ bestimmen wir für die impliziten Schemata mittels eines vorkonditionierten, konjugierten Gradientenverfahrens (PCG).

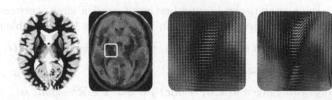

Abb. 1. unscharfe Koeffizientenkarte (invertierte Grauwertkarte) für die mittlere Diffusivität der unterschiedlichen Gewebetypen (links) und Illustration der Skalierung des Tensorfeldes (rechts) für Skalierungsfaktoren $\alpha = 1$ (linker Ausschnitt) und $\alpha = 4$ (rechter Ausschnitt)

Das in [9] vorgestellte Verfahren gehört zur Klasse der ECV. Das Standard-ECV ist, wie aus (2) bereits ersichtlich, durch

$$\boldsymbol{u}^{j+1,\mathsf{h}} = (\boldsymbol{E} + q\mathcal{A})\boldsymbol{u}^{j,\mathsf{h}} + q\boldsymbol{y}^{j,\mathsf{h}} = \mathcal{M}\boldsymbol{u}^{j,\mathsf{h}} + q\boldsymbol{y}^{j,\mathsf{h}} \tag{3}$$

gegeben. Eine namhafte Bedingung für eine stabile Lösung ist die Beschränkung der maximalen, zeitlichen Schrittweite bzgl. der Spektraleigenschaften der Koeffizientenmatrix $\mathcal{A}$. Es gilt $\rho(\mathcal{M}) < 1 \Rightarrow q \leq 2/\rho(\mathcal{A})$. Eine weitere Abschätzung für eine obere Schranke $s > 0$ für die zeitliche Schrittweite q, die nicht die Spektraleigenschaften von $\mathcal{A}$ betrachtet, ergibt sich aus der Fourier-Stabilitätsanalyse. Hiermit ergibt sich

$$s = \left(2\sum_{i=1}^{d} h_i^2 \max_{\boldsymbol{k}\in\mathcal{K}_B} D_{ii,\boldsymbol{k}}\right)^{-1} \tag{4}$$

mit $\mathcal{K}_B := \{\boldsymbol{k} \in \mathbb{Z}^d : \boldsymbol{x_k} \in \Omega_B \cap \Omega^\mathsf{h}\}$. Das in [9] vorgestellte Verfahren umgeht die oben ausgewiesene Stabilitätsbedingung durch eine geschickte Unterteilung des Zeitschrittes $q > 0$ in Unterschritte $q_l^\star > 0$, $0 \leq l < w^\star - 1$. Hervorzuheben ist, dass wir in dem vorliegenden Manuskript eine parallelisierte C++-Implementierung vorstellen. Es gilt die Rechenvorschrift

$$\boldsymbol{u}^{j+1,\mathsf{h}} = \left(\prod_{l=0}^{w^\star-1}(\boldsymbol{E} + q_l^\star\mathcal{A})\right)\boldsymbol{u}^{j,\mathsf{h}} + q\boldsymbol{y}^{j,\mathsf{h}}(\boldsymbol{u}^{j,\mathsf{h}}) \tag{5}$$

Damit relaxiert sich die ursprüngliche Stabilitätsbedingung – ähnlich zu dem in [10] vorgeschlagenen Verfahren – zu einer Forderung nach Stabilität zum Ende eines Rechenzykluss: $\rho\left(\prod_{l=0}^{w^\star-1}(\boldsymbol{E} + q_l^\star\mathcal{A})\right) < 1$. Bemerkenswert ist hierbei, dass $\lceil \frac{1}{2}(w^\star - 1)\rceil$ der Zeitschritte $q_l^\star$ die ursprüngliche Stabilitätsbedingung verletzen [9]. Die Berechnung der Schrittweite ist durch

$$q_l^\star = \nu\left(2\cos^2(\pi(2l+1)/(4w^\star + 2))\right)^{-1} \tag{6}$$

$\nu > 0$ $l = 0, \ldots, w^\star - 1$, mit der resultierenden Zykluszeit $\tau_Z = \sum_{l=0}^{w^\star-1} q_l^\star = \frac{\nu}{3}\binom{w^\star+1}{2}$ erklärt. Um dieses Verfahren auf ein gegebenes Problem übertragen zu können, ist es notwendig, den Skalierungsparameter ν anhand der vorliegenden Koeffizientenmatrix $\mathcal{M}$ zu bestimmen. Hierfür verwenden wir im vorliegenden Manuskript die obige Fourier-Stabilitätsanalyse. Es gilt $\nu = s$ ((4)).

2.3   Numerischer Fehler

Da für Prb. 1 keine analytische Lösung bestimmt werden kann, verwenden wir für die Analyse des numerischen Fehlers ein vereinfachtes Modellproblem:

Problem 2 *Sei $\beta > 0$ und $g \in L^2(\mathbb{R}^3, [0, u_S])$ gegeben. Finde ein $u \in \mathcal{U}$, so dass*

$$\partial_t u(\boldsymbol{x}, t) = \beta \Delta u(\boldsymbol{x}, t) \quad in\ \mathbb{R}^3 \times \mathbb{R}_0^+$$

mit den Anfangsbedingungen $u(\boldsymbol{x}, 0) = g(\boldsymbol{x})$ für alle $\boldsymbol{x} \in \mathbb{R}^3$ erfüllt ist.

Legen wir g mit $g(\boldsymbol{x}) = u_S$, falls $\|\boldsymbol{x} - \boldsymbol{x_S}\|_2 \leq \mu$, $\mu > 0$, und $g(\boldsymbol{x}) = 0$, sonst, fest, lässt sich für Prb. 2 eine Fundamentallösung $\hat{u}$ bestimmen. Der numerische Fehler wird über die $\ell^{\mathsf{h},2}$-Norm des Abstandes zwischen numerischer und analytischer Lösung bestimmt.

3 Ergebnisse

Das erste Experiment analysiert den Trend des numerischen Fehlers für unterschiedliche Schrittweiten $q \in \{\tilde{q} \in (0,4] : \tau \mod \tilde{q} = 0\}$ (Abb. 2, links) basierend auf Prb. 2. Die Parameter sind: $u_S = 1.0$, $\mu = 10\,\text{mm}$; die Konvergenz-Toleranz für das PCG-Verfahren ist $\epsilon_{tol} = 10^{-20}$; die maximale Anzahl an Iterationen ist $\sqrt{n}$, wobei n die Ordnung des linearen Systems (2) bezeichnet. Weiter ist $\beta = 0.5\,\text{mm}^2/\text{d}$. Zudem stellen wir (Abb. 2, rechts) die Rechenzeit δ_{CPU} in Abhängigkeit von der Schrittweite $q \in \{\tilde{q} \in (0,3] : \tau \mod \tilde{q} = 0\}$ für die numerische Lösung von Prb. 1 mittels der diskutierten numerischen Verfahren gegenüber. Für die Berechnungen verwenden wir einen Standard-Desktop-PC (Intel Core i5 760, 2.8 GHz, 8GB DDR3 RAM). Das Wachstumsmodell ist exponentiell mit $\gamma = 0.015/\text{d}$, $\kappa_G = 0.005\,\text{mm}^2/\text{d}$, $\kappa_W = 10\kappa_G$ und $t = 365\,\text{d}$. Abb. 3 zeigt Simulationsergebnisse für ein logistisches Wachstumsmodell ($t = 730\,\text{d} \equiv 2\,\text{a}$).

4 Diskussion

In der vorliegenden Arbeit wurde die Überführung eines kürzlich auf dem Gebiet der Bildverarbeitung vorgestellten, expliziten Lösungsschematas [9] – in einer parallelisierten Implementierung – in die Modellierung der raum-zeitlichen Dynamik kanzeröser Zellen auf Gewebeebene diskutiert. Neben der hierfür notwendigen Bestimmung eines Skalierungsparameters ν wurde der Vergleich zu

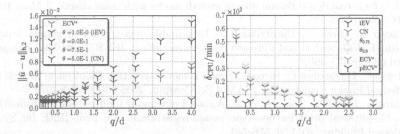

Abb. 2. $\ell^{h,2}$-Norm des Abstandes zwischen der numerischen und der analytischen Lösung des vereinfachten Modellproblems (Prb. 2; links) und Rechenzeiten δ_{CPU} für die Lösung von Prb. 1 (rechts) für unterschiedliche zeitliche Schrittweiten q

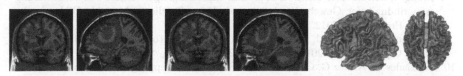

Abb. 3. Simulationsergebnisse für variierende Tensorfeldskalierungen α (links: $\alpha = 1$; zentral: $\alpha = 4$). Dargestellt ist, neben orthogonalen Schnittansichten, eine zu den mittleren Schichtbildern korrespondierende Oberflächensynthese (lateral und superior)

impliziten Verfahren gezogen. Darüber hinaus wurde eine Erweiterung des anisotropen Diffusions-Modells durch eine Wichtung basierend auf einer unscharfen Logik für die verwendeten Gewebekarten vorgestellt. Zusammenfassend wurde gezeigt, dass das diskutierte, beschleunigte ECV nicht nur für die Bildverarbeitung, sondern auch für eine biophysikalische Modellierung eine hinreichende Genauigkeit liefert. Die algorithmische Komplexität entspricht dem Standard-ECV. Die Laufzeit und Speicherauslastung ist gegenüber impliziten Verfahren deutlich reduziert. Hierbei ist zu vermerken, dass der Vergleich zu Mehrgitterverfahren und einer matrixfreien, impliziten und parallelisierten Implementierung noch aussteht. Abschließend ist festzuhalten, dass sich das ECV* im Speziellen für eine Integration in rechenintensive Ansätze zur Parameterschätzung aus Bilddaten [3] bzw. der modellbasierten Bildverarbeitung [4, 5, 6, 7, 8] eignet.

Danksagung. Diese Arbeit wird gefördert durch die Europäische Union und das Land Schleswig-Holstein (AT, SB) [Fördernummer 122-09-024] und die Exzellenzinitiative des Bundes (TAS) [Fördernummer DFG GSC 235/1].

Literaturverzeichnis

1. Murray JD. Mathematical Biology. Springer Heidelberg; 2003.
2. Konukoglu E, Clatz O, Menze BH, et al. Image guided personalization of reaction-diffusion type tumor growth models using modified anisotropic eikonal equations. IEEE Trans Med Imaging. 2010;29(1):77–95.
3. Hogea C, Davatzikos C, Biros G. An image-driven parameter estimation problem for a reaction-diffusion glioma growth model with mass effects. J Math Biol. 2008;56(6):793–825.
4. Gooya A, Biros G, Davatzikos C. Deformable registration of glioma images using EM algorithm and diffusion reaction modeling. IEEE Trans Med Imaging. 2011;30(2):375–390.
5. Hogea C, Davatzikos C, Biros G. Brain-Tumor Interaction Biophysical Models for Medical Image Registration. SIAM J Sci Comput. 2008;30(6):3050–3072.
6. Mang A, Becker S, Toma A, et al. A model of tumour induced brain deformation as bio-physical prior for non-rigid image registration. In: Proc IEEE Int Symp Biomed Imaging; 2011. p. 578–581.
7. Mang A, Becker S, Toma A, et al. Modellierung tumorinduzierter Gewebedeformation als Optimierungsproblem mit weicher Nebenbedingung. Proc BVM. 2011; p. 294–298.
8. Mang A, Schütz TA, Toma A, et al. Ein dämonenartiger Ansatz zur Modellierung tumorinduzierter Gewebedeformation als Prior für die nicht-rigide Bildregistrierung. Proc BVM. 2012.
9. Grewenig S, Weickert J, Bruhn A. From box filtering to fast explicit diffusion. Lect Notes Computer Sci. 2010;6376:533–542.
10. Alexiades V, Amiez G, Geremaud PA. Super-time-stepping acceleration of explicit schemes for parabolic problems. Com Num Meth Eng. 1996;12:31–42.
11. Jbabdi S, Mandonnet E, Duffau H, et al. Simulation of anisotropic growth of low-grade gliomas using diffusion tensor imaging. Magn Reson Med. 2005;54(3):616–634.

Symbolic Coupling Traces for Coupling Analyses of Medical Time Series

Niels Wessel[1], Maik Riedl[1], Hagen Malberg[2], Thomas Penzel[3],
Jürgen Kurths[1,4,5]

[1]Department of Physics, Humboldt-Universität zu Berlin
[2]Institute of Biomedical Engineering, Dresden University of Technology
[3]Sleep Center, Charité Universitätsmedizin Berlin
[4]Potsdam Institute for Climate Impact Research
[5]Institute for Complex Systems and Mathematical Biology, University of Aberdeen
wessel@physik.hu-berlin.de

Abstract. Directional coupling analysis of bivariate time series is an
important subject of current research. In this contribution, a method
based on symbolic dynamics for the detection of time-delayed coupling
is reviewed. The symbolic coupling traces, defined as the symmetric
and diametric traces of the bivariate word distribution, are applied to
model systems and cardiological data as well as sleep data showing its
advantages especially for nonstationary data.

1 Introduction

The cardiovascular systems consist of several subsystems which are interrelated
by feedback loops with time delay. Revealing such time delayed coupling directions is a basic task in understanding the system. Different methods, starting from cross correlation via mutual predictability to information-theoretic approaches are proposed for this purpose, but, due to the non-stationarity, non-
linearity, and the noise, the conclusions are not homogeneous. In this paper,
applications of an enhanced method based on symbolic dynamics [1] for the detection of time-delayed coupling is reviewed. The symbolic coupling traces allow
for a more robust analysis of delayed coupling directions between heart rate and
blood pressure [2, 3, 4].

2 Materials and methods

For bivariate coupling analysis we used the method of symbolic coupling traces
(SCT) [2]. First step of this approach is the transformation of the time series of
beat-to-beat intervals B_i and systolic blood pressure S_i, into symbol sequences
$s_B(t)$ and $s_S(t)$ according to the rule

$$s_z(t) = \begin{cases} 1, z(t) \le z(t + \theta) \\ 0, z(t) > z(t + \theta) \end{cases} \tag{1}$$

where z represents B and S. For analysis of short-term couplings in B_i and S_i the value $\theta = 1$ has been used [2]. Next, words of length l are constructed $w_z(t) = s(t), s(t+1), ..., s(t+l-1)$ which can form $d = 2^l$ different patterns. For short-term dynamics in B_i and S_i, $l = 3$ is used to reliably estimate the bivariate word distribution [2]. $w_x(t)$ and $w_y(t)$ are used to calculate the bivariate word distribution $(p_{ij})_{i=1,...,d,j=1,...,d}(\tau)$

$$p_{ij}(\tau) = P(w_x(t) = W_i, w_y(t+\tau) = W_j) \qquad (2)$$

with the d patterns W_1 to W_d. The parameter τ is included in order to consider delayed interrelationships between the signals. From the bivariate word distribution, the parameters

$$T = \sum_{i=j} p_{ij}(\tau) \qquad (3)$$

$$\overline{T} = \sum_{i=1,...,d;j=d+1-i} p_{ij}(\tau) \qquad (4)$$

$$\Delta T = T - \overline{T} \qquad (5)$$

are calculated. On the one hand, T only captures influences which preserve the structure of the transmitted pattern of dynamics (symmetrical influences). On the other hand, $\overline{T}$ only quantifies influences which inverts the dynamical structure of the driver (diametrical influence). To answer the question if the parameter ΔT is significant or not, a critical value ΔT_{crit} is estimated respectively. Therefore, these parameters are calculated for 1000 realizations of bivariate white noise $N_i(0, \sigma^2)$ with sample length N. We look for the 99th percentile where 99% of the 1000 observation are smaller than that critical value. It represents the critical value of the significance level $\alpha = 0.01$ in an one-side significance test. The nonlinear regression leads to $\Delta T_{\text{crit}}(N) \approx \pm 2.7 \cdot N^{-0.51}$.

3   Results

The SCT-method was applied to real cardiological data to analyze the coupling between B_i and S_i of 20 healthy volunteers (age: 53.0 ± 8.0 years). For all subjects, we measured continuous blood pressure signals (30 min, Portapres Mod. 2, 100 Hz sampling frequency, under standardized supine resting conditions, recorded at the Charité Berlin). A representative example of the coupling analysis is shown in Fig. 1. Parameters based on SCT are not influenced by instationarities of the time series. The parameter ΔT detects significant lags at $\tau = -2$ and $\tau = 0$ for all subjects. This confirms the prevailing opinion about the cardiovascular short term regulation. The symmetric lag at $\tau = 0$ reflects the mechanically induced arterial pressure fluctuations, whereas the diametric lag at $\tau = -2$ represents the vagal feedback from the B_i to the S_i.

Further on, we considered polysomnographical measurements of 18 normotensive (NT, age: 44.6 ± 7.6 years, BMI: 30.2 ± 2.9 kg/m^2 , all male) and 10 hypertensive patients (HT, age: 44.1±8.1 years, BMI: 34.1±4.9 kg/m², all male) suffering from obstructive sleep apnea syndrome (OSAS: repetitive obstruction of the upper airway for more then 10 seconds during sleep) during a diagnostic night (DD, differential diagnosis) and during treatment by means of continuous positive airway pressure (CPAP, positive pressure via mask avoids obstructions of the upper airway during apneas). The first 5 minutes of the largest undisturbed period of light sleep (LS), deep sleep (DS), rapid eye movement (REM) and the awake state (W) for each subject was analyzed. Additionally, a control group of 10 healthy controls (C, age: 44.8 ± 6.7 years, BMI: 25.3 ± 2.7 kg/m², all male) was examined. The results are presented in Fig. 2.

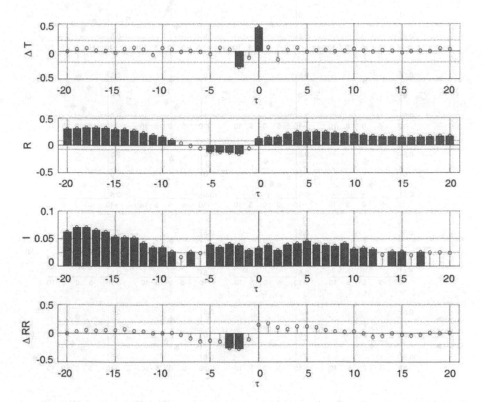

Fig. 1. Comparison of the calculated SCT parameter $\Delta T = T - \overline{T}$, the cross correlation function R, the mutual information I and the recurrence rate difference $\Delta RR = RR_+ - RR_-$ (based on order pattern) for experimental data of a healthy volunteer at different lags τ. Significant lags are drawn as boxes, insignificant as stems. The most significant lags are revealed by ΔT at $\tau = 0$ and $\tau = -2$, i.e. B_i corresponds diametrically ($\tau = -2$) and symmetrically ($\tau = 0$) with S_i. The parameters R, I and ΔRR do not show these lags as clearly as ΔT resp. show false significant lags. This figure is adapted from Wessel et al. 2009 [2]

72   Wessel et al.

Finally, the subjects described in the last paragraph were tested awake with quiet relaxed and regular breathing in a separate room. The duration of the test period was 20 minutes. The test period was conducted at the same time of day in all subjects. The quantification of the dynamics by means of standard parameter of heart rate and blood pressure variability showed neither significant differences between the groups nor significant treatment effects. The SCT during this relaxed breathing are shown in Fig. 3 (Test) and compared to the sleep stages

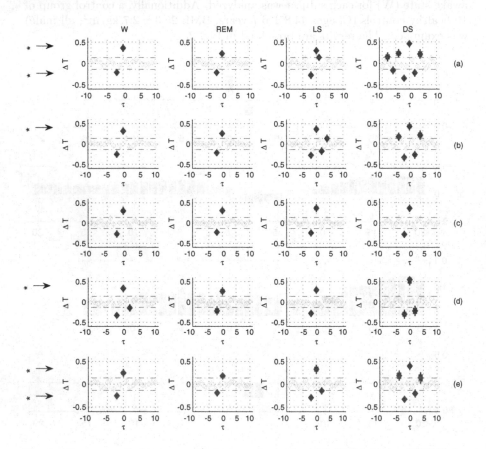

Fig. 2. The comparison between the sleep stages (wake = W, REM-sleep = REM, light sleep = LS, deep sleep = DS) and the different patient groups: (a) healthy controls; (b) NT DD; (c) NT CPAP; (d) HT DD; (e) HT CPAP, clearly shows the short term asymmetry in the coupling during wake and REM characterized by lags $\tau = -2$ and $\tau = 0$. This asymmetry becomes less in light sleep and is lost in deep sleep when periodic breathing leads to a modulation of B_i and S_i. Significant differences in the coupling strength at $\tau = 0$ and $\tau = -2$ between the sleep stages are marked by $\star$ ($p < 0.05$, Kruskal-Wallis test). Differences exist at both lags in the control patients group as well as HT CPAP. In NT DD and HT DD only the lag $\tau = 0$ is significantly different between the sleep stages. This figure is adapted from Suhrbier et al. 2010 [3]

(Fig. 3, REM, light sleep, and deep sleep). At time lag $\tau = 0$ we always observe a significant coupling. In addition to this we do note significant time lags at $\tau = -2$ between heart rate and systolic blood pressure and at $\tau = 1$ between systolic blood pressure and heart rate. The latter time lag can be interpreted as an effect of the baroreflex function.

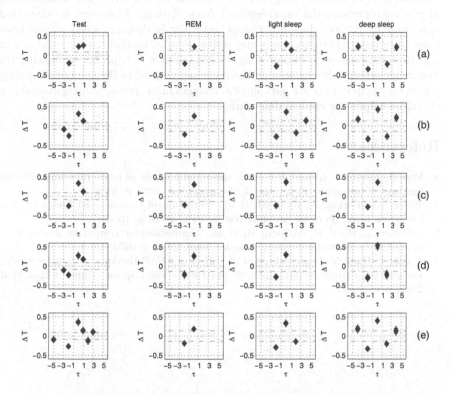

Fig. 3. Symbolic coupling traces of heart rate and systolic blood pressure during daily measurements (Test) for the five different groups. From top to bottom (a) healthy control subjects, (b) normotensive subjects before therapy, (c) normotensive subjects after therapy, (d) hypertensive subjects before therapy, (e) hypertensive subjects after therapy. Negative lags τ indicate the influence of the heart rate on the systolic blood pressure and positive ones vice versa. The thin lines are the significance limits of ΔT(significance level 5%) which depends on the length of time series (awake ≈ 1000 data points, sleep ≈ 300 data points). All significant couplings are marked by purple dots in this plot. For comparison, the symbolic coupling traces during night (REM-sleep=REM, light sleep=LS, deep sleep=DS) are plotted in the three right columns. This figure is adapted from Penzel et al. 2012 [4]

4   Discussion

We confirm the results of [2] where SCT detects significant lags at $\tau = -2$ and $\tau = 0$ for all subjects. This strengthens the prevailing opinion about the cardiovascular short term regulation which is based on antagonistic nervous control via vagus and sympathicus. The symmetric lag at $\tau = 0$ reflects the respiratory induced arterial pressure and heart rate fluctuations, whereas the diametric lag at $\tau = -2$ represents the vagal feedback from B_i to S_i. Moreover, we show that this coupling pattern does not change generally in different sleep stages; however, the strength of interactions may differ. Finally, we find the same pattern at day time measurements except a significant lag at $\tau = 1$, probably showing the baroreflex activity. Summarizing, the proposed method of the symbolic coupling traces may help to indicate pathological changes in cardiovascular regulation and therefore helpful for clinical diagnostics.

References

1. Voss A, Kurths J, Kleiner HJ, et al. improved analysis of heart rate variability by methods of non-linear dynamics. J Electrocardiol. 1995; p. 81–8.
2. Wessel N, Suhrbier A, Riedl M, et al. Detection of time-delayed interactions in biosignals using symbolic coupling traces. EPL. 2009; p. 10004.
3. Suhrbier A, Riedl M, Malberg H, et al. Cardiovascular regulation during sleep quantified by symbolic coupling traces. Chaos. 2010; p. 045124.
4. Penzel T, Riedl M, Gapelyuk A, et al. Effect of CPAP therapy on daytime cardiovascular regulations in patients with obstructive sleep apnea. Comput Biol Med. 2012; p. in press.

Hybride Multi-Resolutions k-Raum Nachbearbeitung für Gadofosveset-verstärkte hochaufgelöste arterielle periphere MR-Angiographie

Egbert Gedat[1], Mojgan Mohajer[1], Ellen Foert[2], Bernhard Meyer[2],
Rainer Kirsch[3], Bernd Frericks[2]

[1]Institut für Medizinische Informatik
[2]Klinik und Hochschulambulanz für Radiologie und Nuklearmedizin
Charité – Universitätsmedizin Berlin
[3]Siemens, Healthcare Sector, Erlangen, Deutschland
egbert.gedat@charite.de

Kurzfassung. Periphere MR-Angiographien mit hoher örtlicher Auflösung und arteriellem Kontrast wurden mit einer vor kurzem vorgestellten Computer-Methode erzeugt. Steady-State und First-Pass MR-Angiographien der Unterschenkel von 10 Patienten wurden zu hoch aufgelösten arteriellen MR-Angiographien kombiniert. Die Bildqualität wurde sehr gut bewertet. Die Ergebnisse einer Befundung von Stenosen waren sehr nah an denen der Steady-State MR Angiographien, die den Standard darstellten.

1 Einleitung

Periphere Angiographie erfordert hohe örtliche Auflösung und arteriellen Kontrast. Bei kontrastmittelverstärkter MR-Angiographie (MRA) kann beides nicht gleichzeitig erreicht werden, da die arterielle Phase des Kontrastmittels zu kurz für eine hoch aufgelöste Akquisition ist. Verschiedene Protokolle wurden entwickelt um die Aufnahme über die arterielle Phase hinaus durchführen zu können. Das sind Keyhole-Imaging [1], weitere Verfeinerungen des k-Raum Samplings [2] und Zeit aufgelöste Sequenzen [3]. Diesen Techniken ist gemeinsam, dass sie den zeitlich veränderten Kontrast mit niedriger Auflösung aufnehmen und in die vorher oder nachher aufgenommene hohe Auflösung substituieren. Dadurch kann aber keine Information, hier die hohe Auflösung der Arterien, gewonnen werden.

Mit Blood-Pool Kontrastmitteln, die bis zu einer Stunde im Gefäßsystem bleiben, lassen sich sehr hoch aufgelöste Steady-State MR-Angiographien aufnehmen [4]. Diese haben allerdings arteriellen und venösen Kontrast. Die Autoren haben ein Schema vorgestellt, das die Hochauflösung aus der Steady-State Phase des Kontrastmittels bewahrt und die venösen Anteile mittels einer niedriger aufgelösten Schablone abzieht [5]. Die Schablone wird aus der arteriellen Phase des Kontrastmittels gewonnen.

Hier wird zusätzlich der klinische Einsatz der Methode in einer Qualitätsstudie an zunächst 12 Patienten vorgestellt und bewertet.

2 Material und Methoden

Zwölf konsekutive Patienten mit Verdacht auf oder bekannter peripherer arterieller Verschlusskrankheit (pAVK) wurden untersucht (6 w./6 m., 65±10 Jahre alt). Die Studie wurde mit Zustimmung der Ethikkommission und der Patienten durchgeführt. Kontrastmittel-verstärkte MR-Angiographie wurde auf einem 1,5 T 32-Kanal MR-Tomographen (Avanto, Siemens Healthcare) durchgeführt. Nach Gabe des Blood-Pool-Kontrastmittels Gadofosveset Trisodium (Vasovist, Bayer Schering Pharma, Berlin, Deutschland) mit einer Dosierung von 0.03 mmol/kg wurde zunächst eine arterielle First-Pass MR-Angiographie (FLASH3D, FOV 500 × 375 × 104 mm^3, Matrix 384 × 288 × 80, aufgenommene Auflösung 1,3 × 1,3 × 1,3 mm^3, SENSE-Faktor 2, Mittelungen 1, TR 3,2 ms, TE 2,1 ms, Flipwinkel 25°, Aufnahmezeit 16 Sekunden) und im Anschluss eine Steady-State MR-Angiographie (FLASH3D, FOV 500 × 375 × 104 mm^3, Matrix 768 × 576 × 160, aufgenommene Auflösung 0,65 × 0,65 × 0,65 mm^3, SENSE-Faktor 1, Mittelungen 2, TR 4,3 ms, TE 1,6 ms, Flipwinkel 18°, Aufnahmezeit 5:15 Minuten) aufgenommen. Zusätzlich wurde vor Beginn der Kontrastmittelgabe eine native Aufnahme (wie First-Pass) gemacht.

Für die Nachbearbeitung wurden die Daten auf einen PC (3.2 GHz, 4 GB RAM) transferiert und entsprechend dem Schema in Abb. 1 prozessiert. Das Ergebnis war ein hoch aufgelöster Datensatz mit arteriellem Kontrast (h.a. arteriell).

Zusätzlich wurden zur Kontrolle zero-fill Datensätze [6] aus den First-Pass Aufnahmen erzeugt. Durch Auffüllen der fehlenden hohen k-Raum Frequenzen mit Nullen und Rücktransformation erhält man Bilder mit pseudo-Hochauflösung mit vielen Pixeln aber nicht der entsprechenden Information.

Zur Darstellung der 3D Daten als maximum intensity projection (MIP) wurden Knochen, Fett und andere Gewebe durch Subtraktion der nativen Bilder entfernt. Für die hoch aufgelösten Datensätze wurden die nativen Daten trilinear interpoliert. Alle Berechnungen wurden mit Matlab R14 (Mathworks, Natick, MA, USA) durchgeführt.

Die MR-Angiographien wurden anonymisiert von zwei Radiologen im Konsens bezüglich Artefakten, Abgrenzung der Gefäße und venöser Überlagerung bewertet. Dazu diente eine Mehrpunktskala (Tab. 1). Eine Befundung stenöser Verengungen wurde durchgeführt. Die für die Befundung benötigte Zeit wurde notiert. Zur statistischen Auswertung wurden die Arterien der Unterschenkel in 13 Segmente eingeteilt und je Segment nur der schwerwiegendste Befund gewertet. Als Standard dienten die Steady-State Aufnahmen [7].

Tabelle 1. Ergebnisse der Qualitätsbeurteilung: Mittelwerte (Standardabweichung)

(n=20)	Abgrenzung der Gefäße[1]	Artefakte[2]	Venöse Überlagerung[2]	Dauer / min.
Steady-State	1,1 (0,31)	0,6 (0,49)	1,5 (0,47)	8,0 (4,6)
h.a. arteriell	1,3 (0,47)	0,4 (0,49)	0,7 (0,59)	4,3 (2,2)
First-Pass	2,0 (0,30)	0,4 (0,56)	0,7 (0,67)	5,1 (2,4)
Zero-Filling	1,7 (0,62)	0,4 (0,56)	0,8 (0,68)	4,6 (2,2)

[1] 1=ausgezeichnet, 2=gut, 3=mäßig, 4=ungenügend

[2] 0=keine, 1=wenig, ohne diagnostische Relevanz, 2=stark, behindert die Befundung

3 Ergebnisse

Für 10 Patienten wurden hoch aufgelöste arterielle Bilder in 90,4±0,1 s berechnet. Zwei Patienten mussten wegen Bewegung ausgeschlossen werden. Die First-Pass Angiographien zeigten in geringerer Auflösung die Unterschenkelarterien der Patienten. Die Steady-State Angiographien zeigten in hoher Auflösung sowohl die Arterien als auch die Venen der Unterschenkel der Patienten. Die h.a. arteriellen Bilder wie auch die zero-fill Bilder zeigten nur die Arterien der Patienten. Insgesamt gab es wenig Artefakte. Die Abgrenzung der Gefäße konnte in h.a. arteriellen Bildern dem Niveau der Steady-State Bilder angenähert werden, während dies bei den zero-fill Bildern nicht der Fall war. Die Ergebnisse der Qualitätskontrolle sind in Tab. 1 gelistet. Die Ergebnisse der Befundung sind in

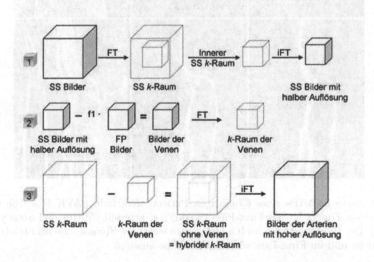

Abb. 1. Schematische Darstellung der Methode zur Erzeugung der hoch aufgelösten arteriellen Angiographien. Der Faktor f1 minimiert die Summe der quadrierten Intensitäten nach Subtraktion [5]

Tab. 2 gelistet. Es wurden in den Steady-State Bildern insgesamt 78 Stenosen
und Verschlüsse gefunden, davon 23 kleinere Stenosen, 34 gravierende Stenosen
und 29 Arterienverschlüsse. In den h.a. arteriellen Bildern gab es insgesamt nur 3
abweichende Befundungen. Bei den first-Pass Bildern gab es 36 abweichende Befundungen und bei den zero-fill Bildern 49. Für die h.a. arteriellen Bilder ergaben
sich eine Sensitivität von 100 % und eine Spezifität von 99,5 %, für die First-Pass
Bilder von 85,7 % und 96,9 %, für die zero-fill Bilder 75,8 % und 94,4 %. Die für
die Befundung benötigte Zeit wurde im Vergleich zum Steady-State für die h.a.
arteriellen Bilder nahezu halbiert.

Beispiele sind in Abb. 2 und 3 gezeigt. In Abb. 2 sieht man deutlich die
Abwesenheit der Venen und die bessere Auflösung in den h.a. arteriellen Bildern.
In Abb. 3 ist die Artefakt-freie Wiedergabe der Information aus den Steady-State
Bildern klar erkennbar, sowie die deutlich bessere Auflösung im Vergleich mit
dem First-Pass Bild und die Abwesenheit der Venen in dem h.a. arteriellen Bild.

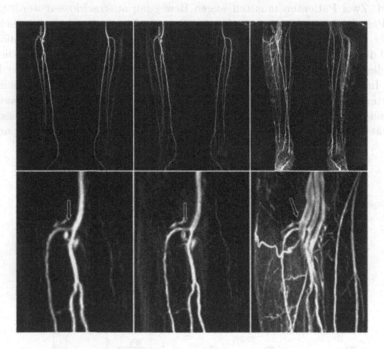

Abb. 2. Sagittale MIPs eines 63-jährigen Patient, männlich, pAVK II a. Die untere
Reihe ist ein Zoom. Jeweils First-Pass (links), h.a. arteriell (Mitte) und Steady-State
(rechts). Der Pfeil zeigt eine im h.a. arteriellen sichtbare Stenose, die im Steady-State
verdeckt ist und im First-Pass wie ein Verschluss aussieht

Tabelle 2. Ergebnisse der Befundung. Für First-Pass und Zero-Filling war ein Segment nicht diagnostisch

(n=260)		Referenz-Standard = Steady-State				
		Keine Stenose	1-50% Stenose	51-99% Stenose	Verschluss	Gesamt
Referenz Standard	Gesamt	174	23	34	29	260
Hoch aufgelöst arteriell	Keine Stenose	174	1	0	0	175
	1-50% Stenose	0	21	0	0	21
	50-99% Stenose	0	1	33	0	34
	Verschluss	0	0	1	29	30
First-Pass	Keine Stenose	162	10	3	0	175
	1-50% Stenose	8	10	5	1	24
	50-99% Stenose	2	3	23	0	28
	Verschluss	1	0	3	28	32
Zero-Filling	Keine Stenose	160	12	11	1	184
	1-50% Stenose	8	6	3	0	17
	50-99% Stenose	5	5	17	0	27
	Verschluss	1	0	3	27	31

4 Diskussion

Die hier vorgestellte Methode zur Gewinnung von hoch aufgelösten arteriellen peripheren MR-Angiographien lieferte für 10 Patienten nahezu Artefakt-freie Bilder in hoher Qualität. Die Venen wurden klar entfernt und die hohe Abgrenzbarkeit der Arterien erhalten. Wie der Vergleich mit den zero-fill Bildern zeigt ist das nicht nur ein Ergebnis der nominell höheren Auflösung sondern der Übernahme der hoch aufgelösten Information aus den Steady-State Bildern.

Bisherige Ansätze Bild-basierter Arterien-Venen-Separation nutzen störanfällige Kriterien wie level-set [8] oder interaktive Verfahren mit seed points in

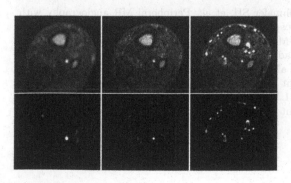

Abb. 3. Axiale Schicht eines 72-jährigen Patienten, männlich, pAVK IV. Oben sind die MR-Angiographien gezeigt, unten die Angiographien nach Subtraktion der nativen Bilder

Fuzzy-Logik [9]. Das Ersetzen des inneren k-Raum des Steady-State mit dem First-Pass k-Raum führt zu Artefakten [5].

Die hohe Sensitivität und Spezifität und die schnellere Befundung mit h.a. arteriellen Bildern macht diese zu aussichtsreichen Kandidaten für einen klinischen Einsatz. Allerdings mangelt es dieser Studie an einem echten Goldstandard, der in der Angiographie die Digitale Subtraktionsangiographie (DSA) ist. Aber es konnte gezeigt werden, dass die Steady-State MRA nahezu gleichwertig mit der DSA ist [7] und damit ein vergleichbarer Standard. Eine Studie mit nur 12 Patienten ist als vorläufig zu betrachten. Ein erster Hinweis ist sie aber dennoch.

Ein Problem ist mögliche Bewegung der Patienten zwischen der First-Pass und der Steady-State Aufnahme, die dann nicht mehr Artefakt-frei kombiniert werden können. Die einzelnen Aufnahmen wären aber für die Befundung nutzbar.

Insgesamt sind die Qualität und die Eignung der hoch aufgelösten arteriellen Bilder zur Befundung eine Weiterentwicklung der peripheren MR-Angiographie mit potentiellem Nutzen für Patienten mit peripherer arterieller Verschlusskrankheit.

Literaturverzeichnis

1. van Vaals JJ, Brummer ME, Dixon WT, et al. Keyhole method for accelerating imaging of contrast agent uptake. J Magn Reson Imaging. 1993;3(4):671–5.
2. Wu Y, Korosec FR, Mistretta CA, et al. CE-MRA of the lower extremities using HYPR stack-of-stars. J Magn Reson Imaging. 2009;29(4):917–23.
3. Fink C, Ley S, Kroeker R, et al. Time-resolved contrast-enhanced three-dimensional magnetic resonance angiography of the chest Combination of parallel imaging with view sharing (TREAT). Invest Radiol. 2005;40(1):40–8.
4. Nikolaou K, Kramer H, Clevert CGD, et al. High-spatial-resolution multistation MR angiography with parallel imaging and blood pool contrast agent: Initial experience. Radiology. 2006;241(3):861–72.
5. Gedat E, Mohajer M, Kirsch R, et al. Post-processing central k-space subtraction for high-resolution arterial peripheral MR angiography. Magn Reson Imaging. 2011;29(6):835–43.
6. Bernstein MA, Fain SB, Riederer SJ. Effect of windowing and zero-filled reconstruction of MRI data on spatial resolution and acquisition strategy. J Magn Reson Imaging. 2001;14(3):270–80.
7. Hadizadeh DR, Gieseke J, Lohmaier SH, et al. Peripheral MR angiography with blood pool contrast agent: Prospective intra-individual comparative study of high spatial-resolution steady-state MR angiography versus standard-resolution first-pass MR angiography and DSA. Radiology. 2008;249(2):701–11.
8. Lei T, Udupa JK, Saha PK, et al. 3D MRA visualization and artery-vein separation using blood-pool contrast agent MS-325. Acad Radiol. 2012;9(Suppl1):127–33.
9. van Bemmel CM, Spreeuwers LJ, Viergever MA, et al. Level-set-based artery-vein separation in blood pool agent CE-MR angiograms. IEEE Trans Med Imaging. 2012;22(10):1224–34.

Surface-Based Seeding for Blood Flow Exploration

Benjamin Köhler[1], Mathias Neugebauer[1], Rocco Gasteiger[1], Gábor Janiga[2],
Oliver Speck[3], Bernhard Preim[1]

[1]Department of Simulation and Graphics, University of Magdeburg
[2]Department of Fluid Dynamics and Thermodynamics, University of Magdeburg
[3]Department of Biomedical Magnetic Resonance, University of Magdeburg
benjamin.koehler@st.ovgu.de

Abstract. Qualitative visual analysis of flow patterns in cerebral aneurysms is important for assessing the risk of rupture. According to current research, the flow patterns close to the aneurysm surface (e.g. impingement zone) provide a good insight. Streamlines can be easily interpreted and are commonly used for visualizing and exploring blood flow. However, standard ways of seeding these streamlines, e.g. manually oriented planes, are not suitable for explicit exploration of local near-wall flow. In this work, we introduce a novel surface-based seeding strategy. Our approach is flexibly applicable to measured as well as simulated data, so we present results for both. Informal domain expert feedback confirmed the suitability of our method to explore near-wall blood flow. The intuitive interaction scheme and the ease of use were appreciated.

1 Introduction

Cerebral aneurysms are a serious health risk for patients. A rupture can cause a subarachnoid hemorrhage with a high fatality rate [1]. Thus, a reliable risk assessment is of major interest. Since experiences have shown that small aneurysms rupture as well, risk assessment by considering only their size or shape is not sufficient. Recent researches [2] pointed out that hemodynamics play an important role for the risk assessment of aneurysms and vascular diseases in general. Since a relation between risk of rupture and complex flow patterns close to the surface is indicated, not only the velocity but also the characteristic of the blood flow is important. Thus, a local, visual analysis of the flow, e.g. at the aneurysm dome, is essential.

In order to qualitatively estimate the flow complexity, adequate flow visualization is necessary. Streamlines can be easily interpreted and are commonly used for visualizing and exploring blood flow [3]. In this work, we want to focus on the seeding of these streamlines. Existing approaches often use centerlines and let the user move an orthogonal plane along the direction of the centerlines [4]. Different seeding patterns are provided by specific probability distributions on the plane. The centerline extraction works well for vessels but often is error-prone in aneurysms due to their shape. Hence, free plane placement correction without assistance is provided. This includes the tedious task of repeated rotation and translation of the plane as well as the necessity for frequent viewport changes. More sophisticated approaches [5] additionally guide the interaction using the aneurysms ostium and provide elaborate exploration widgets, but demand a complex anatomical analysis as prerequisite.

In this work, we introduce a surface-based seeding strategy for streamlines with an intuitive interaction scheme that allows a qualitative analysis of the blood flow especially near vessel boundaries.

2   Material and methods

2.1   Data

There are basically two ways to obtain flow data: direct measurement using 4D PC-MRI or computational fluid dynamics (CDF) simulations [1]. Measured data can be obtained relatively fast and represent the in-vivo flow situation, but can contain image artifacts and noise. Also it is not available in every case. CFD provides a detailed, smooth and noise-free flow representation. Simulating the flow before and after treatment (stenting/coiling) is also possible. However, the accuracy of the flow directly depends on the choice of model assumptions and boundary conditions.

Our first dataset contains three saccular aneurysms and was directly measured using a 4D PC-MRI. Our second dataset contains a basilar aneurysm with distinct satellites and was simulated using CFD. Our approach requires a mesh representation of the surface. This can be obtained by segmenting the vessels using a threshold-based method, removing artifacts by applying a connected component analysis and finally using marching cubes to reconstruct the triangles. Remeshing is applied to gain a mesh quality sufficient for CFD. Given this surface mesh and a vector field of the flow, our approach is generally applicable on simulated and measured data.

2.2   Seeding positions

The principal idea is to select an area directly on the triangular surface, extrude every vertex along a certain vector, connect each triangle to its extruded version (Fig. 1a) and then generate random positions within these prisms. Assuming that a prism with the vertices $p_i, i = 0..5$ is convex, random positions p_{random} within can easily be generated using barycentric coordinates with random weights $w_i \in [0,1]$

$$p_{\mathrm{random}} = \sum_{i=0}^{5} w_i \cdot p_i \quad \text{with} \quad \sum_{i=0}^{5} w_i = 1 \qquad (1)$$

So, the question is how to choose the extrusion vectors. Using the negated normals does not provide a limitation for the maximally allowed translation. If

Fig. 1. Triangle extrusion (left) and extrusion along x (right)

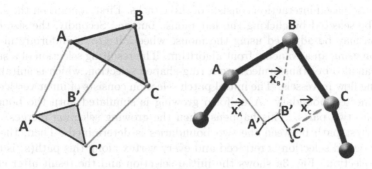

the vertices are moved too far, the prisms degenerate and this causes errors in the barycentric interpolation due to the concavity.

Shrinking of the mesh is usually an unwanted side effect of standard laplacian smoothing. However, we take advantage of this effect and repeatedly apply it until the surface has only about 5% of its original area left. Fig. 2 shows the mesh of our simulated dataset before (a) and after (b) laplacian smoothing. Our (not normalized) extrusion vector x is the difference $p_\Delta - p_{\mathrm{orig}}$ with p_{orig} as the original vertex and p_Δ as the same vertex after shrinking the mesh. An extruded vertex p_x is only allowed to lie between p_{orig} and p_Δ:

$$p_x = p_{\mathrm{orig}} + t \cdot x \quad \text{with } t \in [0,1] \tag{2}$$

Since laplacian smoothing repeatedly replaces every vertex with the average of its direct neighborhood, the problem of degenerating prisms will not occur, illustrated by Fig. 1b.

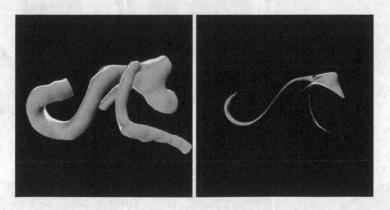

Fig. 2. Full-size (left) and shrunken (right) meshes

2.3   Interaction scheme

The mouse-based interaction consists of three tasks. First, a point on the surface has to be selected by clicking the left mouse button. Secondly, the size of the selection may be adjusted using the mouse wheel. It grows uniformly in every direction using an advancing front algorithm. The resulting selection of a surface patch can also be transformed into a ring-shaped selection, which is suitable for exploring flow in vessels. The initial patch selection consists of inner vertices and one connected boundary. A uniform growing is simulated until the boundary splits into two parts. This happens when the growing selection merges. Now, the shortest path between the two boundaries is determined. Then, the path to the original selection is retraced and every vertex along this path(s) is added to the selection. Fig. 3a shows the initial selection and the result after closing the ring. Finally, the selection has to be extruded. This is achieved by holding the right mouse button and then moving the mouse up or down which changes $t \in [0,1]$ (Chpt. 2.2). Fig. 3b and c illustrate a ring and a cap selection for different t-values.

3   Results and discussion

We proposed a surface-based seeding strategy with an intuitive interaction scheme that improves the exploration of the blood flow and helps to understand its characteristic. Given a surface mesh and a vector field of the flow, our method is generally applicable on simulated as well as measured data.

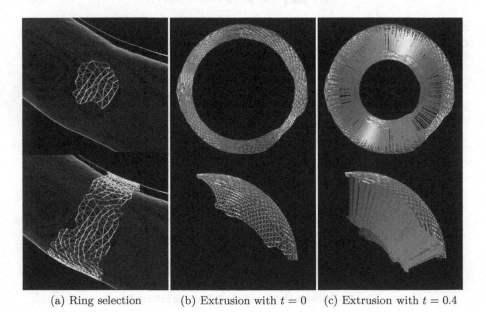

(a) Ring selection   (b) Extrusion with $t = 0$ (c) Extrusion with $t = 0.4$

Fig. 3. Visualization of a vessel

We applied our method to the two datasets described in Sect. 2.1. Fig. 4 and 5 show several selections in the upper and resulting streamlines in the lower rows for the simulated and the measured dataset. Fig. 4a illustrates a cap selection on a basilar aneurysm with distinct satellites and Fig. 4b shows a ring selection on a vessel (Chpt. 2.3). The resulting streamlines are vortex-structured and indicate a complex blood flow characteristic. Parallel to this, Fig. 5a and b show flow behavior in/near saccular aneurysms using a cap selection on an aneurysm (a) and a ring selection on a vessel (b). The streamlines in Fig. 5b visualize the blood flowing partially into the aneurysm showing a swirling behavior and partially following the vessels course. The t-parameter for the extrusion was set to 0.2 in all cases.

A domain expert, who is familiar with Ensight, was asked to interact with the datasets. He seeded only a few streamlines at once with a short integration time, which allowed him to understand the flow characteristics near the boundaries

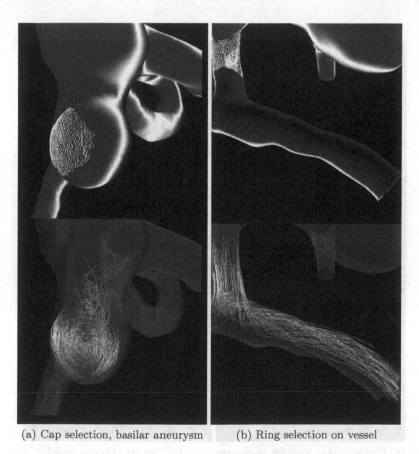

(a) Cap selection, basilar aneurysm   (b) Ring selection on vessel

Fig. 4. Simulated dataset

easily. The suitability of our approach was confirmed and the ease of use was appreciated.

References

1. Gasteiger R, Janiga G, Stucht D, et al. Vergleich zwischen 7 Tesla 4D PC-MRI-Flussmessung und CFD-Simulation. In: Proc BVM; 2011. p. 304–8.
2. Cebral JR, Mut F, Weir J, et al. Association of hemodynamic characteristics and cerebral aneurysm rupture. AJNR Am J Neuroradiol. 2011;32(2):264–70.
3. Salzbrunn T, Jänicke H, Wischgoll T, et al. The state of the art in flow visualization: partition-based techniques. In: SimVis; 2008. p. 75–92.
4. van Pelt R, Olivan Bescos J, Breeuwer M, et al. Exploration of 4D MRI blood flow using stylistic visualization. IEEE Trans Vis Comput Graph. 2010;16:1339–47.
5. Neugebauer M, Janiga G, Beuing O, et al. Anatomy-guided multi-level exploration of blood flow in cerebral aneurysms. Comput Graph Forum. 2011;30(3):1041–50.

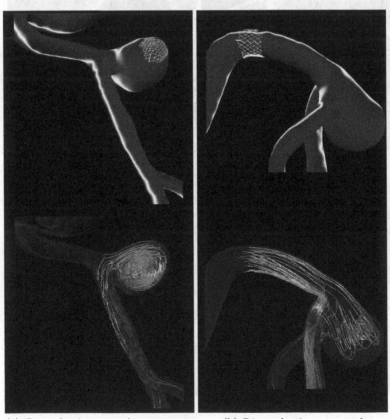

(a) Cap selection, saccular aneurysm   (b) Ring selection on vessel

Fig. 5. Measured dataset

Determination of Heart Valve Fluttering by Analyzing Pixel Frequency

Sven Friedl[1,2], Eugen Herdt[1], Stefan König[1], Michael Weyand[2],
Markus Kondruweit[2], Thomas Wittenberg[1]

[1]Fraunhofer Institute for Integrated Circuits IIS, Erlangen
[2]University Hospital Erlangen
sven.friedl@iis.fraunhofer.de

Abstract. The fluttering of heart valve leaflets is an important aspect regarding the hemodynamics of biological artificial heart valves. Endoscopic high speed recordings allow capturing, visualization and analysis of heart valve movements with significant temporal resolution. In this contribution, a method is presented to determine the fluttering of the leaflets by analyzing the pixel frequency. The intensity value of each image pixel is observed over time and analyzed using Fourier transform. With synthetic sequences the reliability of the method has been proven. First results with ex-vivo recordings show the feasibility to determine fluttering of heart valve leaflets.

1 Introduction

Biological artificial heart valves are preferred as grafts for transplantations because of their more physiological hemodynamics compared to mechanical ones. Depending on the model and the transplantation technique, the movement of the valve leaflets and the hemodynamics are of different quality. One important aspect regarding the hemodynamics is the bending and the fluttering of the leaflets during the systolic period. To capture, visualize and analyze movements of heart valves, different modalities are available. Echocardiography is widely used to determine movements in-vivo, while high speed video recordings are mostly used to analyze artifical grafts in-vitro. With endoscopic high speed recordings in explanted pig hearts [1], the movements of artificial and native heart valves can be recorded under identical physiological conditions. Determination of the bending and fluttering of leaflets has been done based on those modalities with different approaches. E.g., Rishniw [2] has interpreted echocardiographic images, while Erasmi et al. [3] determined the bending in single images of high speed video recordings. An automatic approach for analyzing the fluttering over time in video recordings using image segmentation of the orifice has been presented by Condurache et al. [4]. Due to the large amount of image data in high speed recordings, an automatic approach is desired for motion analysis. Approaches like the orifice-based analysis are depending on the results of the segmentation methods and thus not always stable for all recordings. With this contribution, an alternative method to determine and to describe fluttering of heart valve leaflets, based on a frequency analysis in the spatio-temporal domain will be introduced.

2   Materials and methods

2.1   Pixel frequency analysis

Under constant illumination, intensity changes of pixels can be related to motion depicted in an image sequence. Specifically, for oscillating objects, Granqvist and Lindestad [5] introduced an approach for an intensity based Fourier analysis to determine occurring motion-caused frequencies under the assumption, that no affine motion of the heart valves took place. At each position of an image, the intensity value is extracted over time, generating an intensity signal for each pixel, (Fig. 1(a)) for one example position. These intensity signals are obtained from multiple oscillating periods and the analyzed using a Fourier transform. Thus, for each image position, the frequency spectrum is determined. The fundamental pixel frequency at a given pixel position in the image is defined by the maximum amplitude of the corresponding spectrum. The spectrum is then color-coded and each pixel is colorized using the color, depending on its fundamental frequency. The result is a frequency image (Fig. 1(b)) which visualizes the occurring fundamental pixel frequencies within the image sequence. To improve the visualization, it is possible to eliminate a specific range by filtering the intensity signal or by visualizing only selected frequencies. An overlay of the color-coded image onto the the original sequence indicates the anatomy-based location of the movements.

2.2   Endoscopic high speed recordings

The objective of the proposed approach is to determine the frequencies caused by fluttering of the leaflets. To compare occurring fluttering in native valves with those in biological artificial ones, endoscopic high speed video recordings of native and artificial aortic heart valves are used. The videos have been recorded in explanted and reanimated pig hearts. Regarding blood pressure and heart rate, physiological conditions were achieved. The valves are observed using an endoscopic camera with a recording frame rate of 2000 frames per second. Fig. 2(a)

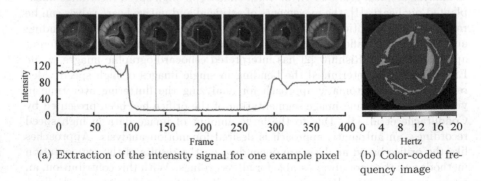

(a) Extraction of the intensity signal for one example pixel   (b) Color-coded frequency image

Fig. 1. Determination of the pixel frequency

shows an example sequence of a biological artificial aortic graft as used for this work. The heart rate for the recordings varies around 80-120 beats per minute, which corresponds to a frequency of approx. 0.75-2 Hz. The fluttering is expected to generate higher frequencies.

2.3 Synthetic image sequences

To prove the reliability of the method, a synthetic image sequence (Fig. 2(b)) was created with exactly defined movements. To emulate the opening and closing of the heart valves, a circle is drawn with increasing and decreasing radius using a frequency of 20 Hz. In the open state with maximum radius, the circle begins to vibrate with 500 Hz to simulate fluttering. To consider lightning conditions, a gradient is moving with 100 Hz in the background. For a second synthetic image sequence, relative movements between the camera and the object are simulated by shifting the complete image with 250 Hz during the complete period.

3   Results

The pixel frequency analysis as described above has been tested with the synthetic image sequences as well as with the endoscopic high speed video recordings. For the first synthetic sequence without simulated relative movement, the defined frequencies of the opening and closing, the fluttering, and the gradient background can be seen clearly in the color-coded frequency image. To improve the visual result, only the significant fluttering frequencies are visualized in Fig. 3(a). It can be seen, that the occurring frequencies can be identified and located precisely in the image. In the resulting frequency image for the synthetic sequence with simulated relative movement (Fig. 3(b)), the defined frequencies can still be identified. However, the regions, where defined frequencies occur, are enlarged and the relative shift is leading to false frequencies by superimposing different movements.

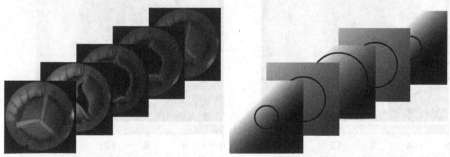

    (a) Artificial aortic heart valve   (b) Synthetic image sequence

Fig. 2. Example image sequences for the evaluation of the method

The same experiments have been made with the real endoscopic recordings. Two different example results are shown in Fig. 3(c) and Fig. 3(d). For the artificial aortic graft, frequencies of 3-20 Hz are identified and visualized. Minor frequencies of approx. 1-2 Hz, corresponding to the heart rate, are recognized but not visualized here. The regions of potential fluttering frequencies are precisely located within the leaflet positions during the open phase. For the native heart valve, similar frequencies can be recognized. In contrast to the artificial graft, the potential fluttering frequencies are not precisely located. Since the relative movement between the camera and the valve is much larger in the recording of

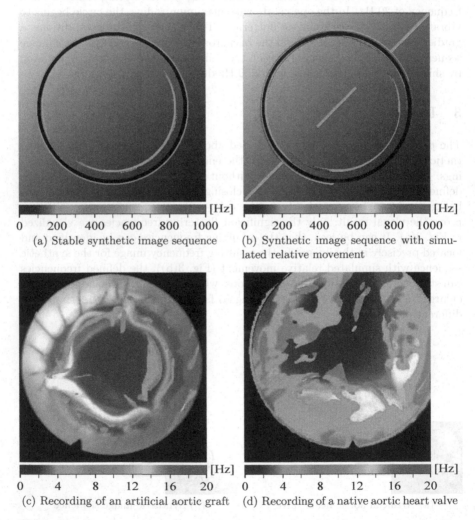

[Hz]

0   200   400   600   800   1000
(a) Stable synthetic image sequence

[Hz]

0   200   400   600   800   1000
(b) Synthetic image sequence with simulated relative movement

[Hz]

0   4   8   12   16   20
(c) Recording of an artificial aortic graft

[Hz]

0   4   8   12   16   20
(d) Recording of a native aortic heart valve

Fig. 3. Resulting frequency images as overlays onto the original sequence images. For an improved visualization only relevant fluttering frequencies are visualized

the native valve, those movements are probably causing the wider distribution of the occurring frequencies.

4 Discussion

The results stated above are indicating that the method presented is able to determine and to visualize the fluttering of heart valve leaflets in endoscopic heart valve recordings. The experiments with synthetic image sequences prove the reliability of the approach. The resulting frequency images show exactly those frequencies, that have been defined in the sequences. In the stable sequence, the appearing frequencies are determined in narrow areas within the image. For the sequence with simulated relative movement, the area of frequency determination is wider and not located as exactly as in stable settings. This can be confirmed by interpreting the results of the endoscopic recordings. In those sequences with large relative movements, the frequency areas are wider as well and the determination of appearing frequencies is slightly imprecise. Aside from the location of the fluttering, the occurring frequencies can be determined and compared in different valves. To obtain best results, a stable recording setup preventing relative movements is desired. Alternatively and since a complete absence of relative movement is unlikely, methods of motion compensation can be considered to deal with this issue.

References

1. Kondruweit M, Wittenberg T, Friedl S, et al. Description of a novel ex-vivo imaging and investigation technique to record, analyze and visualize heart valve motion under physiological conditions. In: 39. Jahrestagung der DGTHG; 2010.
2. Rishniw M. Systolic aortic valve flutter in 6 dogs. Vet Radiol Ultrasound. 2001;42(5):446–7.
3. Erasmi A, Sievers HH, Scharfschwerdt M, et al. In vitro hydrodynamics, cusp-bending deformation, and root distensibility for different types of aortic valve-sparing operations: Remodeling, sinus prosthesis, and reimplantation. J Thorac Cardiovasc Surg. 2005;130(4):1044–9.
4. Condurache AP, Hahn T, Scharfschwerdt M, et al. Video-based measuring of quality parameters for tricuspid xenograft heart valve implants. IEEE Trans Biomed Eng. 2009;56(12):2868–78.
5. Granqvist S, Lindestad P. A method of applying Fourier analysis to high-speed laryngoscopy. J Acoust Soc Am. 2001;110(6):3193–7.

Automatische Detektion des Herzzyklus und des Mitralannulus Durchmessers mittels 3D Ultraschall

Bastian Graser[1], Maximilian Hien[2], Helmut Rauch[2], Hans-Peter Meinzer[1],
Tobias Heimann[1]

[1]Abteilung für Medizinische und Biologische Informatik, DKFZ Heidelberg
[2]Klinik für Anästhesiologie, Universitätsklinikum Heidelberg
b.graser@dkfz.de

Kurzfassung. Mitralklappeninsuffizienz (MI) ist eine weit verbreitete Erkrankung. Für eine erfolgreiche und nachhaltige chirurgische Therapie ist die Ausmessung des Mitralannulus (MA) notwendig. Wir stellen eine Methode zur automatischen Bestimmung des MA Durchmessers auf Basis von Live-3D Ultraschall Daten vor, die zusätzlich für jeden Zeitschritt den Herzzyklus detektiert. Dies erreichen wir hauptsächlich durch die Verwendung von Graph Cut Segmentierung und morphologischen Operationen. Die Evaluation anhand von 13 Patienten zeigt, dass der Herzzyklus in 78% aller Zeitschritte korrekt erkannt wurde, während der MA Durchmesser im Mittel 3.08 mm von der Expertenmessung abweicht. Durch die Nutzung des vorgestellten Verfahrens lässt sich die intraoperative Messzeit des MA reduzieren, da die Messung automatisch und präoperativ erfolgen kann.

1 Einleitung

Die Mitralklappeninsuffizienz (MI) beschreibt eine Undichtigkeit der Mitralklappe (MK). Studien aus den USA [1, 2] besagen, dass 19% der erwachsenen Bevölkerung und 2% der gesamten Bevölkerung von MI betroffen sind. In schweren Fällen ist ein chirurgischer Eingriff notwendig, bei dem eine rigide Ringform, der Annuloplasty Ring, auf dem Mitralannulus (MA) implantiert wird. Die Chancen für eine erfolgreiche Operation sind bei frühzeitiger Erkennung gut. Jedoch kommt es bei 73% aller erfolgreichen Operationen innerhalb von sieben Jahren zu einem erneuten Auftreten von MI und eine weitere Operation ist notwendig[3]. Es gibt Hinweise, dass die Nachhaltigkeit der Operation durch die gewählte Größe des implantierten Annuloplasty Rings beeinflusst wird[4, 5]. Gewöhnlich wird diese Größe während des Eingriffs bestimmt, indem verschiedene Annuloplasty Ringe auf den MA platziert werden und eine möglichst ähnliche Größe gewählt wird. Eine automatische Bestimmung der MA Größe vor dem Eingriff ist erstrebenswert, um OP Zeit bei der Wahl des Annuloplasty Rings einzusparen. Als Grundlage hierfür bieten sich die Bilder des Live-3D Transösophageal Ultraschall an (3D TEE), das vor Herzoperationen meist standardmäßig durchgeführt wird. Allerdings ist für die computergestützte Verarbeitung dieser Daten auch eine automatische Erkennung des Herzzyklus für jeden Zeitschritt notwendig. In Kachenoura et al [6] werden verschiedene Methoden zur Herzzyklus Detektion vorgestellt. Diese benötigen jedoch manuelle Interaktion oder eine Zwei-Kammer oder Vier-Kammer-Ansicht, welche nicht vorliegt wenn der Fokus auf der MK liegt. Interessante Ansätze zur Segmentierung des MA, die letztendlich auch zu dessen Größenbestimmung genutzt werden kann, werden in Schneider et al [7], Ionasec et al [8] und Voigt et al [9] vorgestellt. Allerdings wird bei Schneiders Methode manuelle Interaktion vorausgesetzt, während bei Ionasecs und Voigts Ansatz große Mengen an Trainingsdaten benötigt werden.

2 Material und Methoden

Die Methode lässt sich in drei Schritte unterteilen: (1) Segmentierung von Blut und Gewebe, (2) Detektion des Herzzyklus und (3) Detektion des Mitralannulus

2.1 Segmentierung von Blut und Gewebe

Die einzelnen 3D Bilder der Ultraschallsequenz werden separat verarbeitet. Als erstes wird ein Total Variation Filter [10] ausgeführt. Dadurch wird das Rauschen im Bild verringert, ohne Kanten zu zerstören. Anschließend findet eine grundlegende Einteilung in Blut und Gewebe mittels Graph Cut Segmentierung [11] statt. Dabei wird ein mathematischer Graph erstellt dessen Knoten die Pixel im Bild darstellen, welche durch gewichtete Kanten mit den entsprechenden Nachbarknoten verbunden sind. Einige Knoten werden als Hintergrund- und Objektsaatpunkte deklariert. In diesem Graph wird nun ein Schnitt gesucht, der alle Hintergrund- von den Objektsaatpunkten abtrennt, wobei die Summe der Gewichte aller durchtrennten Kanten minimal ist. Das Ergebnis kann als Segmentierung verstanden werden. Die ausschlaggebenden Faktoren hierbei sind die Saatpunkte und die Kostenfunktion. Bei der vorgestellten Methode werden sehr hohe Intensitäten im Bild als Objekt Saatpunkte deklariert und sehr niedrige Intensitäten als Hintergrund Saatpunkte, da dieser mit hoher Sicherheit als Blut bzw. Gewebe bezeichnet werden können. Um dazwischenliegende Grauwerte korrekt zu deklarieren wird die folgende Kostenfunktion für die Erstellung des Graphen verwendet

$$C(a, b) = f_i C_i(a, b) + f_g C_g(a, b) + f_{gm} C_{gm}(a, b) \tag{1}$$

Die Kostenfunktion beinhaltet drei Terme, die jeweils für zwei benachbarte Pixel a und b den Intensitätsunterschied C_i, den Gradienten C_g und die Größe des Gradienten $C_g m$ beschreiben. Dadurch werden Helligkeitsunterschiede, Kantenpositionen, sowie die Stärke der Kanten bei der Segmentierung berücksichtigt. Das resultierende Binärbild zeigt nun lediglich Gewebe (Abb. 1).

94   Graser et al.

2.2   Detektion des Herzzyklus

Als nächstes werden anatomische Regionen erkannt und der Herzzyklus festgestellt. Hierfür wird zu der vorangegangenen Blut-Gewebe Segmentierung ein
Bildrand hinzugefügt und kleinere Lücken im Gewebe mit morphologischem Closing geschlossen (Abb. 1). Anschließend werden Saatpunkte im Atrium und im
Ventrikel detektiert, indem nach größeren Blutmengen im oberen und unteren
Bereich des Bildes gesucht wird. Beginnend von diesen Punkten wird ein binäres
3D Region Growing ausgeführt. Verbinden sich die Punkte dadurch, war die MK
offen und der Zeitschritt kann zur Diastole gezählt werden. Bei einer Systole besteht keine Verbindung zwischen den Punkten und es entstehen zwei getrennte
Areale (Abb. 2).

2.3   Detektion des Mitralannulus

Wurde ein Zeitschritt als Systole deklariert, wird mit der Suche nach dem MA
fortgefahren. Die in diesem Fall vorliegenden Areale im oberen und unteren Bildbereich stellen Ausschnitte des linken Ventrikels (LV) und des linken Atriums
(LA) dar. Es wird nun der dazwischenliegende Bereich detektiert, der die MK
darstellt. Dazu werden zunächst verbundene Regionen der beiden Areale abgeschnitten, also die am LV anhängende Aorta und die am LA anhängenden
Lungenarterien. Dies wird erreicht in dem die Areale jeweils stark morphologisch erodiert werden, so dass sich anhängende Volumina abtrennen. Anschließend wird das größte Volumen extrahiert und wieder auf die ursprüngliche Größe
morphologisch dilatiert (Abb. 2). Von den resultierenden LV und LA Volumen
wird nun jeweils der Mittelpunkt berechnet. Die beiden Punkte definieren den
Normalenvektor der MA Ebene, der später genutzt wird. Des Weiteren wird
eine Strecke zwischen diesen gebildet, die Gewebepixel in der anfänglichen Blut-
Gewebe Segmentierung schneidet. Diese Pixel liegen nahe der Mitte der MK.

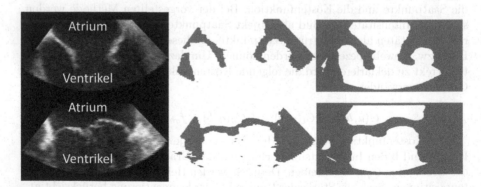

Abb. 1. Zwischenergebnisse für den Fall einer Diastole (oben) und einer Systole (unten). Von links nach rechts: Ausgangsbild, Blut-Gewebe Segmentierung, Basisbild für
die Herzzyklus Detektion

Von hier aus wird wieder ein binärer 3D Region Grower gestartet, der jedoch auf das MK Volumen beschränkt wird. Dies wird erreicht, indem für jedes Pixel überprüft wird, ob beim Folgen des MA Normalvektors ein LA Pixel oberhalb und ein LV Pixel unterhalb des untersuchten Pixels liegt. Das resultierende MK Volumen wird nun auf eine Dicke von einem Pixel verdünnt, so dass eine Oberfläche entsteht. Die Kontur dieser Oberfläche wird anschließend (in Form von einem Satz aus 3D Punkten) extrahiert (Abb. 2 und Abb. 3).

3 Ergebnisse

Die Methode liefert den Herzzyklus zu jeden Zeitschritt (Systole oder Diastole) und zu jeder Systole den Mitralannulus. Um die Methode zu evaluieren, standen klinische 3D TEE Daten verschiedener Patienten zur Verfügung. Dabei wurden

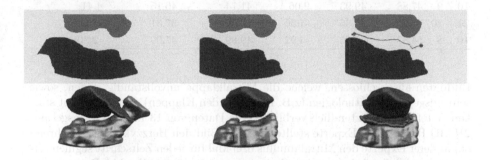

Abb. 2. Zwischenschritte bei der Detektion des Mitralannulus, oben als 2D Darstellung unten als 3D Modell. Links sind an Atrium und Ventrikel noch mit Aorta und Arterien verbunden. Im mittleren Bild wurden diese abgeschnitten. Rechts ist die ermittelte Mitralklappenoberfläche inkl. Mitralannulusring zu sehen

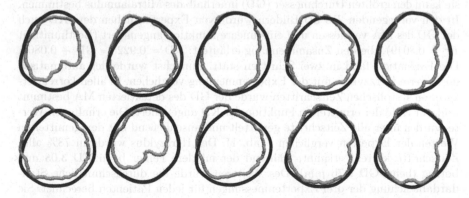

Abb. 3. Der automatische detektierte Mitralannulus (dunkelgrau) im Vergleich zur manuellen Segmentierung (schwarz) für alle Systolen im Datensatz eines Patienten

Tabelle 1. Ergebnisse der Evaluation aller 13 Patienten

Zeitsch./ erkannt	Größter Ø Experte	Größter Ø Methode	Größter Ø Differenz	Kommissur Ø Experte	Kommissur Ø Methode	Kommissur Ø Differenz
12 / 6	47,99	47,89	-0,11	43,80	44,26	0,46
17 / 10	51,87	52,36	0,49	50,27	48,39	-1,88
14 / 7	41,22	47,30	6,08	39,04	43,72	4,67
22 / 16	46,60	46,30	-0,30	42,30	42,80	0,50
16 / 15	50,47	53,79	3,32	44,87	49,71	4,83
17 / 13	42,61	42,40	-0,21	39,88	39,20	-0,69
20 / 17	41,54	48,59	7,05	38,27	44,91	6,64
15 / 12	51,83	49,40	-2,47	49,30	45,65	-3,64
23 / 18	44,07	39,28	-4,78	40,00	36,32	-3,68
21 / 19	48,47	47,65	-0,82	46,65	44,04	-2,61
10 / 9	47,88	49,93	2,06	41,74	46,15	4,41
21 / 20	44,72	40,36	-4,36	40,55	37,31	-3,24
10 / 8	54,87	50,95	-3,92	49,89	47,09	-2,80

Bilddaten ausgeschlossen, welche die Mitralklappe unvollständig zeigen, sowie sehr ausgeprägte Pathologien (z.B. Löcher in den Klappen) und Daten mit starken Artefakten. Letztendlich verblieben die Daten von 13 Patienten (insgesamt 219 3D Bilder). Ein Experte stellte für jedes Bild den Herzzyklus fest, während ein anderer Experte den Mitralannulus drei Mal für jeden Zeitschritt segmentierte, um anschließend eine mittlere Segmentierung zu bilden. Der MA Durchmesser ist ein wichtiger Faktor für die Auswahl des Annuloplasty Rings und sollte das Hauptkriterium der Evaluation sein. Dabei wird für gewöhnlich der Abstand zwischen dem anterior und dem posterior Kommissurpunkt (KD) gemessen. Die automatische Methode kann diese Punkte zwar nicht gesondert detektieren, aber sie kann den größten Durchmesser (GD) innerhalb des Mitralannulus bestimmen. In den vorliegenden 218 3D Bildern wurde von Experten neben dem KD auch der GD des MA vermessen und eine lineare Funktion angenähert (Bestimmtheit $R^2 = 0.8049$), die den Zusammenhang erläutert: KD $= 0.9225 * $ GD $+ 0.0808$. Die Evaluation fand in zwei Schritten statt. Zunächst wurde der automatisch detektierte Herzzyklus mit der Expertenmeinung verglichen. In allen korrekt erkannten systolischen Zeitschritten wurde der GD des detektierten MA bestimmt und mit Hilfe der ermittelten Funktion der KD angenähert. Die erhaltenen Werte wurden über alle Zeitschritte gemittelt und anschließend mit den gemittelten Werten der Experten verglichen (Tab. 1). Der Herzzyklus wurde in 78% aller Zeitschritte korrekt erkannt, während der mittlere Fehler beim KD 3,08 mm betrug (beim GD 2,76 mm). Des Weiteren wurde die durchschnittliche Standardabweichung der drei Expertenmessungen für jeden Patienten berechnet. Sie betrug 2,01 mm.

4   Diskussion

Nach unserem Kenntnisstand handelt es sich hier um die erste Methode, die automatisch den Herzzyklus als auch den MA Durchmesser detektiert. Beim Vergleich der durchschnittlichen Standardabweichung der Expertenmessungen (2,01 mm) zum mittleren Fehler der Methode (3,09 mm), lässt sich die Aussage treffen, dass das Verfahren hinreichend genaue Ergebnisse liefert. Es ist natürlich noch Platz für Verbesserungen: Die Genauigkeit bei der Detektion des Herzzyklus (momentan bei 78%) lässt sich sicherlich verbessern. Die meisten Fehlerkennungen gibt es dabei auf Grund von schwachem Kontrast und Lücken im Ultraschall Bild. Derzeitig werden morphologische Operationen eingesetzt um dies zu kompensieren, was jedoch nicht immer gute Ergebnisse liefert. Stattdessen wäre es besser, anatomisches Wissen in die Methode einfließen zu lassen, z.B. durch statistische Formmodelle. Des Weiteren wäre die zusätzliche Messung des MA während der Diastole hilfreich, um die Dynamik des MA zu quantifizieren. Dennoch kann die vorgestellte Methode bereits genutzt werden, um die Auswahl geeigneter Annuloplasty Ringe für die Operation zu beschleunigen. Da die Nutzung keine Interaktion erfordert, wäre die Integration in die klinische Routine unkompliziert.

Danksagung. Das Projekt wurde vom Graduiertenkolleg 1126 der Deutschen Forschungsgemeinschaft finanziert.

Literaturverzeichnis

1. Singh JP, Evans JC, Levy D, et al. Prevalence and clinical determinants of mitral, tricuspid, and aortic regurgitation (the Framingham Heart Study). Am J Cardiol. 1999; p. 897–902.
2. Nkomo, Gardin, Skelton, et al. Burden of valvular heart diseases: a population-based study. Lancet. 2006; p. 1005–11.
3. Flameng W, Herijgers P, Bogaerts K. Recurrence of mitral valve regurgitation after mitral valve repair in degenerative valve disease. Circulation. 2003; p. 1609–13.
4. Geidel S, Lass M, Schneider C, et al. Downsizing of the mitral valve and coronary revascularization in severe ischemic mitral regurgitation results in reverse left ventricular and left atrial remodeling. Eur J Cardiothorac Surg. 2005; p. 1011–6.
5. Adams DH, Anyanwu AC, Rahmanian PB, et al. Large annuloplasty rings facilitate mitral valve repair in Barlow's disease. Annal Thorac Surg. 2006; p. 2096–101.
6. Kachenoura N, Delouche A, Herment A, et al. Automatic detection of end systole within a sequence of left ventricular echocardiographic images using autocorrelation and mitral valve motion detection. In: Proc IEEE EMBS; 2007. p. 4504–7.
7. Schneider RJ, Perrin DP, Vasilyev NV, et al. Mitral annulus segmentation from 3D ultrasound using graph cuts. IEEE Trans Med Imaging. 2010; p. 1676–87.
8. Ionasec RI, Voigt I, Georgescu B, et al. Patient-specific modeling and quantification of the aortic and mitral valves from 4-D cardiac CT and TEE. IEEE Trans Med Imaging. 2010; p. 1636–51.
9. Voigt I, Ionasec RI, Georgescu B, et al. Model-driven physiological assessment of the mitral valve from 4D TEE. In: Proc SPIE; 2009.

98   Graser et al.

10. Chan TF, Osher S, Shen J. The digital TV filter and nonlinear denoising. IEEE Trans Image Process. 2001; p. 231–41.
11. Boykov Y, Kolmogorov V. An experimental comparison of min-cut/max-flow algorithms for energy minimization in vision. IEEE Trans Pattern Anal Mach Intell. 2004; p. 1124–37.

Automatische Bestimmung von 2D/3D-Korrespondenzen in Mammographie- und Tomosynthese-Bilddaten

Julia Krüger[1], Jan Ehrhardt[1], Arpad Bischof[2], Jörg Barkhausen[2],
Heinz Handels[1]

[1]Institut für Medizinische Informatik, Universität zu Lübeck
[2]Klinik für Radiologie und Nuklearmedizin, Universitätsklinikum Schleswig-Holstein
krueger@imi.uni-luebeck.de

Kurzfassung. Die Tomosynthese verbindet die hohe Auflösung der Mammographie mit den Vorteilen einer überlagerungsfreien Darstellung. In dieser Arbeit wird ein Ansatz zur 2D/3D-Korrespondenzbestimmung zwischen Mammographie- und Tomosynthesebildern beschrieben. Dabei wird das Verfahren unterteilt in eine Punkt-zu-Linien-Korrespondenzbestimmung, die durch ein Mapping zwischen Mammographiebild und dem zentralen Projektionsbild der Tomosynthese bestimmt wird, und eine Punkt-zu-Punkt-Korrespondenzbestimmung, die mithilfe eines Mappings zwischen allen Tomosynthese-Projektionsbildern erfolgt. Die Ergebnisse zeigen, dass mit diesem Verfahren korrespondierende Punkte mit einer Genauigkeit von unter 5 mm bestimmt werden können.

1 Einleitung

Das Mammakarzinom ist ein bösartiger Tumor der Brust und repräsentiert mit 28% die häufigste Krebserkrankung der Frau in Deutschland. Es stellt mit 18% der krebsbedingten Todesfälle die häufigste Krebstodesursache der Frau dar [1]. Die Mammographie ist die primäre Methode in der Brustkrebs-Früherkennung und Diagnostik. Zur genaueren Differenzierung der Diagnose werden weitere bildgebende Verfahren wie MRT, Sonographie oder Tomosynthese eingesetzt. Daher ist eine automatische Gegenüberstellung der Bilder verschiedener Modalitäten von Interesse. Diese Arbeit konzentriert sich dabei auf das Auffinden korrespondierender Strukturen in Mammographie- und Tomosynthesebildern. Die Mammographie hat eine hohe Auflösung, jedoch den Nachteil eines 2D-Projektionsverfahrens, bei dem Strukturen überlagert abgebildet werden. Die Tomosynthese hingegen verbindet die Vorteile der hohen Auflösung innerhalb der Schichten mit einer überlagerungsfreien Darstellung in 3D-Schichtaufnahmen. Bei beiden Verfahren wird die Brust der Patientin bei der Akquisition unter leichtem Druck komprimiert, was bei zweimaligem Einspannen zu Brustlage- und Kompressionsunterschieden in den Bilddaten führen kann. In [2] wurde ein 2D/3D-Ansatz untersucht, um solche Unterschiede mithilfe von Deformationen der 3D-Tomosynthesebilddaten auszugleichen.

Bei bisher veröffentlichten Arbeiten lag das Hauptaugenmerk auf der Entwicklung von CAD-Systemen zur automatischen Lokalisation und Klassifikation von Auffälligkeiten in Mammographie- oder Tomosynthesebildern (z. B. [3]). Weiterhin wurden Verfahren zur Registrierung von Mammographiebildern in Follow-up-Studien entwickelt [4]. Es gibt jedoch nur wenige Arbeiten, die sich mit der Registrierung oder Fusion von Bildern beider Modalitäten beschäftigen. Bakic et al. [5] liefern erste Ansätze zur Fusion von Mammographie- und Tomosynthesebildern, die jedoch auf 2D-Tomosynthesebildern arbeiten und somit auf eine Punkt-zu-Linien-Korrespondenz beschränkt sind.

2   Methoden

Die Tomosynthese liefert überlagerungsfreie 3D-Schichtaufnahmen, die aus 25 2D-Projektionsbildern (Anzahl ist herstellerabhängig) rekonstruiert werden. Die Projektionen werden durch Schwenken der Röntgenröhre aus verschiedenen Blickwinkeln (z.B. -25° bis 25°) aufgenommen. Das „zentrale" Projektionsbild ($\approx$ 0°) unterliegt idealerweise derselben perspektivischen Verzerrung wie das entsprechende Mammographiebild. Aufgrund einer vergleichsweise geringen Auflösung der 3D-Bilder in Projektionsrichtung wird im Rahmen dieser Arbeit ausschließlich auf den Tomosynthese-Projektionsbildern gearbeitet und die 3D-Schichtbilder lediglich zur Anzeige der Ergebnisse genutzt. Das vorgestellte Verfahren unterteilt sich in vier Schritte (Abb. 2).

2.1   Vorverarbeitung

Die Tomosynthese-Projektionsbilder werden mit sehr geringer Strahlendosis akquiriert, sodass es zu einem geringen Signal-Rausch-Verhältnis in den Bilddaten

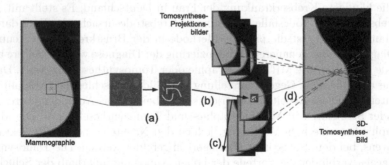

Abb. 1. Ablauf der Korrespondenzbestimmung: Vorverarbeitung der Daten (a), Korrespondenzfindung zwischen Mammographiebild und zentralem Projektionsbild (b), Korrespondenzfindung zwischen den einzelnen Projektionsbildern (c) und Rekonstruktion der 3D-Koordinate aus den detektierten 2D-Punkten/Projektionsstrahlen (d). Dabei kann (b) als Punkt-zu-Linien-Korrespondenzfindung und (c) und (d) als Bestimmung der Punkt-zu-Punkt-Korrespondenz zusammengefasst werden

Abb. 2. Vorverarbeitung der Projektionsbilder: unverarbeitet (a), rauschreduziert (b), Vesselnesswerte (c) und Kombination aus Vesselness- und Grauwerten (d)

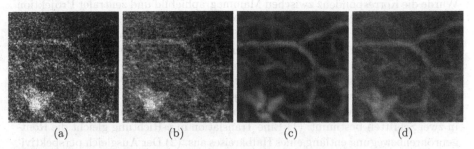

(a)   (b)   (c)   (d)

Abb. 3. Korrespondenzbestimmung zwischen Mammographiebild und zentralem Projektionsbild: Im Mammographiebild (a) werden zwei gesuchte Punkte (weiße Kreuze) markiert. Die Punkte werden in das zentrale Projektionsbild übertragen (schwarze Kreuze (b)) und rigide vorregistriert (rote Kreuze (b)). Nach Verfeinerung durch Template-Matching ergeben sich die korrespondierenden Koordinaten (weiße Kreuze (c))

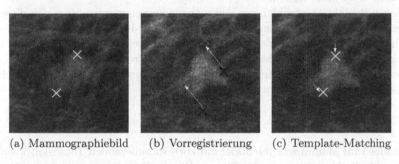

(a) Mammographiebild   (b) Vorregistrierung   (c) Template-Matching

kommt. Um Rauschen zu reduzieren, wird ein morphologischer Ansatz [3] genutzt. Für eine bessere Vergleichbarkeit zweier Aufnahmen werden vorhandene Strukturen (Gefäße) durch einen Vesselnessfilter [6] hervorgehoben (Abb. 2).

2.2 Punkt-zu-Linien-Korrespondenz

Eine Punkt-zu-Linien-Korrespondenz kann hergestellt werden, indem zu einem Punkt im Mammographiebild der korrespondierende Punkt im zentralen Projektionsbild der Tomosynthese, welcher einem Strahl („Linie") im 3D-Tomosynthesebilddatensatz entspricht, bestimmt wird. Hierfür werden beide Bilder grob zueinander ausgerichtet, indem die Außenkonturen der Brust in beiden Bildern per ICP (iterative closest point [7]) rigide registriert werden. Anschließend wird für einen gewählten Mammographie-Punkt mittels Template-Matching der gesuchte korrespondierende Punkt im zentralen Projektionsbild bestimmt (Abb. 3).

2.3   Punkt-zu-Punkt-Korrespondenz

Wurde die Korrespondenz zwischen Mammographiebild und zentraler Projektion korrekt bestimmt, liegt der gesuchte 3D-Punkt entlang des zentralen Projektionsstrahls, der von der Röntgenquelle durch den 3D-Bilddatensatz auf diesen Punkt im zentralen Projektionsbild führt. Um die wahrscheinlichste z-Koordinate zu ermitteln, sind weitere Strahlen nötig, zwischen denen ein „Schnittpunkt" gebildet werden kann (Abb. 4). Dafür wird der gefundene Punkt der zentralen Projektion sukzessiv in alle anderen Projektionen übertragen und weiterverfolgt. Die Korrespondenzen zwischen jeweils adjazenten Projektionen werden hierbei in zwei Schritten bestimmt: (1) Eine Translation in y-Richtung gleicht die Röntgenröhrenbewegung entlang eines Halbkreises aus. (2) Der Ausgleich perspektivischer Unterschiede zwischen den Projektionsbildern wird durch eine nichtlineare Registrierung der Bilder erreicht. Die Güte dieser übertragung wird durch die Kreuzkorrelation zwischen der jeweils lokalen Umgebung der gefundenen Punkte und des Punktes der zentralen Projektion bestimmt. Schlägt die übertragung bei mehr als 75% der Projektionsbilder fehl, kann kein eindeutig korrespondierender 3D-Punkt bestimmt werden.

Liegen Projektionsstrahlen vor, kann angenommen werden, dass sich diese in der gesuchten Tiefe schneiden. Die approximierte z-Koordinate wird durch die Schicht definiert, in der die Verteilung der Punkte, welche die Schnittpunkte von Projektionsstrahl und Schicht beschreiben (Abb. 4 rechts), durch die geringste mittlere quadratische Abweichung zwischen dem zentralen und den restlichen Projektionsstrahlen bestimmt ist.

2.4   Evaluation

Es standen fünf Mammographiebilder mit korrespondierenden Tomosyntheseaufnahmen für die Evaluation zur Verfügung. Für die Bildpaare, wurden zwei Punktepaarmengen manuell bestimmt: Set1: 25 Punktepaare, die eindeutig Struktu-

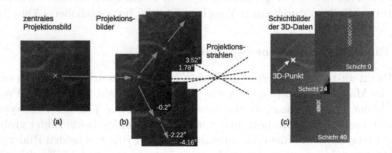

Abb. 4. Punkt-zu-Punkt-Korrespondenzbestimmung: Der im zentralen Projektionsbild ermittelte Punkt (a) wird in die jeweils adjazenten Projektionsbilder übertragen und rekursiv weitergegeben (b). Zwischen den resultierenden Projektionsstrahlen kann anschließend der „Schnittpunkt" bestimmt werden (c), wobei die weißen Kreuze (rechts) die Schnittpunkte dieser Strahlen mit den jeweiligen Schichten markieren

Abb. 5. Zur Evaluation herangezogene Punktepaare (jeweils links Mammographie-, rechts Tomosynthesebild): (a) Set1: Dabei handelt es sich z. B. um Gefäße; (b) Set2: medizinisch relevante Bereiche, die im Mammographiebild nicht eindeutig in Läsion/Auffälligkeit und überlagerung dichteren Gewebes unterschieden werden können

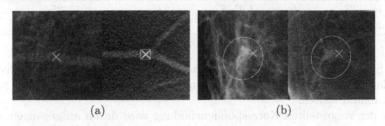

(a)   (b)

ren zugeordnet werden können (z. B. Gefäße) und für die somit eine präzise 3D-Lokalisation möglich ist; Set2: 40 Punktepaare, die in medizinisch relevanten Bereichen in den Mammographiebildern liegen (Abb 5).

Um die Genauigkeit der Punkt-zu-Linien-Korrespondenz zu bestimmen, wurde der Abstand des manuell bestimmten 3D-Tomosynthesepunktes zum automatisch detektierten zentralen Projektionsstrahl errechnet. Dabei wird zwischen einer 2 mm- und einer 5 mm-Abweichung unterschieden. Eine maximale 5 mm-Abweichung innerhalb der Schichten wurde von erfahrenen Radiologen als für die medizinische Untersuchung ausreichend angegeben. Bei der Evaluation der Punkt-zu-Punkt-Korrespondenz muss beachtet werden, dass aufgrund der geringen Rekonstruktionsgüte bei der Tomosynthese die Tiefe des gesuchten Punktes nicht eindeutig festgelegt werden kann. Daher wurde hier lediglich eine visuelle Bewertung durchgeführt und nach „korrekter" und „nicht korrekter" Schichtbestimmung unterschieden.

3 Ergebnisse

Die Tab. 1 zeigt, dass die Ergebnisse den Anforderungen einer maximalen Abweichung von 5 mm entsprechen und lediglich bei 4 der 65 Punktepaare eine Korrektur der Punkt-zu-Linien-Korrespondenz nötig war. Die durchschnittliche Abweichung der Punktepaare liegt für Set1 bei $1,9168$ mm und für Set2 bei $1,7105$ mm. Die Punkt-zu-Punkt-Korrespondenz konnte bei 62 der 65 Punktepaare korrekt bestimmt werden.

4 Diskussion

Die Ergebnisse machen deutlich, dass die mittlere Abweichung der Punktepaare unter einer 2 mm-Abweichung liegt. Bei Punktepaaren, deren Punkt-zu-Linien-Korrespondenz fehlerhaft war, handelt es sich vor allem um kleinere Strukturen wie Kalkablagerungen, die sich nicht ausreichend vom Hintergrund abheben. Außerdem unterliegt die nichtlineare Registrierung, die für die Punkt-zu-Punkt-Korrespondenzbestimmung eingesetzt wird, einer zu starken Regularisierung für

104   Krüger et al.

Tabelle 1. Ergebnisse der beiden Punktepaarmengen

		Punkt-zu-Linie				Punkt-zu-Punkt
	#	< 2 mm	< 5 mm	mittl. Abweich.	manuelle Korrek.	korrekt
Set 1	25	18	24	1.9168	1	25
Set 2	40	33	37	1.7105	3	37

kleine Strukturen. Eine geringere Regularisierung würde jedoch zu einer hypersensiblen Anpassung der Registrierung an Rauschen in den Bilddaten und somit zu Instabilität führen.

Bei der vorgestellten Korrespondenzfindung wird davon ausgegangen, dass die Bilddaten nach standardisierten Einspannrichtlinien (z.B. gegebene Mamillen-Position) akquiriert wurden und die Lageunterschiede daher minimal ausfallen. Kleine Unterschiede können dadurch kompensiert werden, dass bei der Bestimmung der Punkt-zu-Linien-Korrespondenz lediglich lokal die gesuchte Struktur bestimmt wird (Template-Matching). Bei starken Brustlageunterschieden ist eine Korrespondenzfindung mit unserem Verfahrens nicht mehr möglich.

Zusammenfassend hat sich ergeben, dass es mithilfe des vorgestellten Ansatzes möglich ist, zwischen Mammographie- und Tomosyntheseaufnahmen derselben Brust Korrespondenzen automatisch zu bestimmen. Somit kann dem Arzt die Gegenüberstellung und weitere Untersuchung dieser Daten unterschiedlicher Dimensionalität erleichtert werden. Ein weiterer Vorte [6]il der automatischen Korrespondenzfindung ist eine erhöhte Reproduzierbarkeit des Untersuchungsablaufs, da die Diagnostik nicht mehr ausschließlich von der Erfahrung und dem räumlichen Vorstellungsvermögen des untersuchenden Arztes abhängig ist.

Weitergehende Aussagen über die Genauigkeit der Verfahren sind nach einer Analyse einer größeren Anzahl an Datensätzen zu erwarten.

Literaturverzeichnis

1. Zentrums für Krebsregisterdaten am RKI. Verbreitung von Krebserkrankungen in Deutschland – Entwicklung der Prävalenzen zwischen 1990 und 2010. Gesundheitsberichterstattung des Bundes; 2010.
2. Ehrhardt J, Krüger J, Bischof A, et al. Automatic correspondence detection in mammogram and breast tomosynthesis Images. Proc SPIE. 2012 (accepted).
3. Reiser I, Nishikawa RM, Moore RH. Automated detection of microcalcification clusters for digital breast tomosynthesis using projection data only: A preliminary study. Med Phys. 2008;35(4).
4. van Engeland S, Snoeren P, Hendriks J, et al. A comparison of methods for mammogram registration. IEEE Trans Med Imaging. 2003;22(11):1436–4.
5. Bakic P, Richard F, Maidment A. Registration of mammograms and breast tomosynthesis images. In: Digital Mammography. Springer; 2006. p. 498–503.
6. Frangi RF, Niessen WJ, Vincken KL, et al. Multiscale vessel enhancement filtering. Lect Notes Computer Sci. 1998;1469:130–7.
7. Besl PJ, McKay HD. A method for registration of 3-D shapes. IEEE Trans Pattern Anal Mach Intell. 1992;14(2):239–56.

Photometric Estimation of 3D Surface Motion Fields for Respiration Management

Sebastian Bauer[1], Jakob Wasza[1], Joachim Hornegger[1,2]

[1]Pattern Recognition Lab, Department of Computer Science
[2]Erlangen Graduate School in Advanced Optical Technologies (SAOT)
Friedrich-Alexander-Universität Erlangen-Nürnberg
sebastian.bauer@cs.fau.de

Abstract. In radiation therapy, the estimation of torso deformations due to respiratory motion is an essential component for real-time tumor tracking solutions. Using range imaging (RI) sensors for continuous monitoring during the treatment, the 3-D surface motion field is reconstructed by a non-rigid registration of the patient's instantaneous body surface to a reference. Typically, surface registration approaches rely on the pure topology of the target. However, for RI modalities that additionally capture photometric data, we expect the registration to benefit from incorporating this secondary source of information. Hence, in this paper, we propose a method for the estimation of 3-D surface motion fields using an optical flow framework in the 2-D photometric domain. In experiments on real data from healthy volunteers, our photometric method outperformed a geometry-driven surface registration by 6.5% and 22.5% for normal and deep thoracic breathing, respectively. Both the qualitative and quantitative results indicate that the incorporation of photometric information provides a more realistic deformation estimation regarding the human respiratory system.

1 Introduction

Respiratory motion management is an evolving field of research in radiation therapy (RT) and of particular importance for patients with thoracic, abdominal and pelvic tumors. Facing target locations in the upper torso, besides inaccuracies in patient setup and positioning, respiratory motion during treatment delivery induces a fundamental error source. To date, in clinical practice, the tumor is irradiated using RT gating techniques where the linear accelerator is triggered by an external 1-D respiration surrogate [1]. However, gating entails a low duty cycle, increasing the treatment time and hindering an efficient operation of the therapy facility. In contrast, real-time tumor tracking solutions [2, 3, 4] re-position the radiation beam dynamically to follow the tumor's changing position. Under ideal conditions, tracking can eliminate the need for a tumor-motion margin in the dose distribution while maintaining a 100% duty cycle for RT delivery [1].

In particular, methods that infer the internal tumor position from external torso deformations are expected to improve radiation therapy. Based on real-time range imaging (RI), the 3-D surface motion field of the patient's surface with respect to a reference is identified and related to a previously learned model correlating the torso deformation with the target position [2]. Estimating the displacement field using conventional surface registration techniques relies on the pure 3-D topology of the patient. Instead, using modern RI modalities that additionally capture photometric data, we expect the registration to benefit from this secondary information.

Hence, in this paper, we introduce a method for the identification of a dense 3-D surface motion field over non-rigidly moving surfaces observed by RI cameras. Instead of capitalizing on the acquired surface topology, we propose to estimate the optical flow in the 2-D photometric domain. Based on the known relation between the sensor domain and the corresponding surface in world coordinate space, we then deduce the 3-D surface motion field. In experiments on real data from Microsoft Kinect, we have investigated the surface motion fields estimated with our method compared to a purely geometry-driven registration.

2   Materials and methods

The proposed method for estimation of a dense 3-D surface motion field of the patient's respiration state with respect to a reference relies on RI devices that deliver both photometric color and metric depth (RGB-D) information of the scene. Below, let $g(\zeta)$ and $f(\zeta)$ denote the geometric depth and photometric color measurements at a position $\zeta = (\zeta_1, \zeta_2)^T$ in the 2-D sensor domain Ω. Indeed, based on the pinhole camera model, an orthogonal depth measurement $g(\zeta)$ describes a world coordinate position vector $x(\zeta) = (x, y, z)^T \in \mathbb{R}^3$. In homogeneous coordinates, this transformation can be denoted as

$$\begin{pmatrix} x(\zeta) \\ 1 \end{pmatrix} = \begin{pmatrix} \frac{g(\zeta)}{\beta_x} & 0 & 0 \\ 0 & \frac{g(\zeta)}{\beta_y} & 0 \\ 0 & 0 & g(\zeta) \\ 0 & 0 & 1 \end{pmatrix} \begin{pmatrix} \zeta \\ 1 \end{pmatrix} \tag{1}$$

where β_x, β_y denote the focal length. Using triangulation techniques, the point cloud $X = \{x\}$ can be interpreted as a 3-D surface $\mathcal{G}$. Fig. 1 illustrates the torso surface acquired from a male subject, textured with the color-coded orthogonal depth and photometric information, respectively. Below, we introduce our proposed method for photometric estimation of the 3-D deformation. In addition, we oppose a geometry-driven surface registration method. For the purpose of enhanced comparability and in regard to a potential combined formulation in future work, both approaches rely on a variational formulation.

2.1   Photometry-driven surface registration

The proposed method for estimation of a dense 3-D displacement field from 2-D photometric information is based on a two-stage procedure: First, we interpret

Fig. 1. RGB-D data at different respiration states (fully exhale/inhale). On the left, the measured orthogonal depth $g(\zeta)$ is color-coded. On the right, the additionally acquired photometric information $f(\zeta)$ is mapped onto the 3-D surface

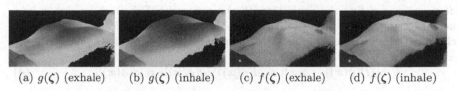

(a) $g(\zeta)$ (exhale)   (b) $g(\zeta)$ (inhale)   (c) $f(\zeta)$ (exhale)   (d) $f(\zeta)$ (inhale)

the acquired photometric information as a conventional planar image and compute a dense optical flow field. Second, we build on this 2-D deformation to extract a dense 3-D surface motion field.

In this work, we have used the combined local-global (CLG) method for optical flow computation proposed by Bruhn et al. [5]. Based on a variational formulation, it combines the advantages of two classical algorithms: the variational approach by Horn and Schunck [6] providing dense flow fields, and the local least-square technique of Lucas and Kanade [7] featuring robustness with respect to noise. The CLG method computes the 2-D photometric optical flow $\tilde{u}_p(\zeta) = (\tilde{u}_p(\zeta), \tilde{v}_p(\zeta), 1)^T$ as the minimizer of the energy functional

$$\mathcal{E}[\tilde{u}_p] = \int_\Omega \left(\tilde{u}_p(\zeta)^T J_\rho(\nabla_3 f)\tilde{u}_p(\zeta) + \alpha_p \|D\tilde{u}_p(\zeta)\|_F^2 \right) d\zeta \qquad (2)$$

where $\tilde{u}_p$ and $\tilde{v}_p$ denote the displacement in direction of ζ_1 and ζ_2, respectively. Further, using the original formulation [5], $\nabla_3 f = (f_x, f_y, f_t)^T$ denotes the spatiotemporal gradient, $J_\rho(\nabla_3 f)$ the structure tensor with some integration scale ρ, $D\tilde{u}_p$ the Jacobian matrix of $\tilde{u}_p$, $\|\cdot\|_F$ the Frobenius norm, and α_p a non-negative regularization weight. In our notation, a tilde placed on top of a variable denotes that it lives in 2-D pixel space, otherwise in 3-D metric real-world space. The numerical minimization of the energy functional $\mathcal{E}[\tilde{u}_p]$ in Eq. 2 is performed by a conjugate gradient solver with a finite difference approximation for spatial discretization [8]. Based on the estimated flow field $\tilde{u}_p$, we are now in the position to infer the 3-D surface motion field $u_p = (u_p, v_p, w_p)^T$ between two respiration states t_1 and t_2

$$u_p(\zeta) = x_{t_2}\left(\zeta + (\tilde{u}_p(\zeta), \tilde{v}_p(\zeta))^T\right) - x_{t_1}(\zeta) \qquad (3)$$

using bilinear interpolation in the sensor domain Ω for computing the position $x_{t_2}\left(\zeta + (\tilde{u}_p(\zeta), \tilde{v}_p(\zeta))^T\right)$ on the surface $\mathcal{G}_{t_2}$.

2.2 Geometry-driven surface registration

For evaluation of the proposed photometric approach, let us compare the estimated surface motion field u_p to a geometry-driven surface registration, based on [9]. Here, we represent the surface $\mathcal{G}_{t_2}$ at time t_2 by its corresponding signed distance function $d(\boldsymbol{x}) := \pm dist(\boldsymbol{x}, \mathcal{G}_{t_2})$, where the sign is positive outside the object domain bounded by $\mathcal{G}$ (outside the body) and negative inside. Furthermore, $\nabla d(\boldsymbol{x})$ is the outward pointing normal on $\mathcal{G}_{t_2}$ and $|\nabla d| = 1$. Based on $d(\boldsymbol{x})$, we can define the projection $P(\boldsymbol{x}) := \boldsymbol{x} - d(\boldsymbol{x})\nabla d(\boldsymbol{x})$ of a point $\boldsymbol{x}$ in a neighborhood of $\mathcal{G}_{t_2}$ onto the closest point on $\mathcal{G}_{t_2}$. Thus, let us quantify the closeness of a displaced template surface point $\phi(\boldsymbol{x}), \boldsymbol{x} \in \mathcal{G}_{t_1}$ to the reference $\mathcal{G}_{t_2}$ using

$$|P(\phi(\boldsymbol{x})) - \phi(\boldsymbol{x})| = |d(\phi(\boldsymbol{x}))\nabla d(\phi(\boldsymbol{x}))| = |d(\phi(\boldsymbol{x}))| \qquad (4)$$

as a pointwise measure. Here, the deformation ϕ is represented by a displacement $\boldsymbol{u}_g = (u_g, v_g, w_g)^T$ defined on Ω, with $\phi(\boldsymbol{x}(\boldsymbol{\zeta})) = \boldsymbol{x}(\boldsymbol{\zeta}) + \boldsymbol{u}_g(\boldsymbol{\zeta})$, minimizing

$$\mathcal{E}[\boldsymbol{u}_g] = \int_{\Omega} \left(d(\boldsymbol{x}(\boldsymbol{\zeta}) + \boldsymbol{u}_g(\boldsymbol{\zeta}))^2 + \alpha_g \|D\boldsymbol{u}_g(\boldsymbol{\zeta})\|_F^2 \right) d\boldsymbol{\zeta} \qquad (5)$$

where $D\boldsymbol{u}_g$ denotes the Jacobian matrix of $\boldsymbol{u}_g$ and α_g the regularization weight. For numerical minimization, we considered a conjugate gradient scheme again.

3   Experiments and results

For experimental evaluation of the proposed method, we have acquired RI data from Microsoft Kinect (640×480 px, 30 Hz) for four healthy subjects S_1-S_4. Reclined on a treatment table, the subjects were asked to perform normal and deep thoracic breathing, respectively. Prior to registration, the range data were preprocessed using edge-preserving denoising. The dataset is available from the authors for non-commercial research purposes.

Qualitative results of the photometry- and geometry-driven 3-D surface motion fields between the respiration states of fully inhale and exhale are illustrated in Fig. 2, using a suitable set of model parameters ($\alpha_p = 0.015, \alpha_g = 10^{-6}$). It can be observed that the photometry-driven surface motion field $\boldsymbol{u}_p$ in superior-inferior (SI) direction is more pronounced than the geometric variant $\boldsymbol{u}_g$. Clinical studies have shown that the SI direction is the prominent direction of human breathing [1]. Thus, let us interpret the results as an indication that even though both motion fields $\boldsymbol{u}_p$ and $\boldsymbol{u}_g$ are meaningful and valuable for application in tumor position correlation, the photometric variant is potentially a better choice for estimating the actual surface motion field regarding the human respiratory system.

Using real data for our experiments, the ground truth 3-D surface motion field is unknown. Hence, for quantitative evaluation, we projected $\boldsymbol{u}_g$ onto the 2-D sensor domain, transferred the deformation from metric real-world to pixel space and applied the resulting displacement $\tilde{\boldsymbol{u}}_g$ to the 2-D photometric data f_{t_1} at time t_1 (fully exhale). For evaluation, we then compared the warped images to the known reference photometric data f_{t_2} at time t_2 (fully inhale) over the patient's torso given by a mask $\mathcal{M}$. In particular, as a scalar distance measure, we computed the root mean square (RMS) photometric distance of the initial

Fig. 2. Glyph visualization of the estimated 3-D surface motion fields u_p (upper row) and u_g (lower row), for subjects S_1 and S_2. The color of the displacement vectors encodes its magnitude in superior-inferior (SI) direction, according to the color bar

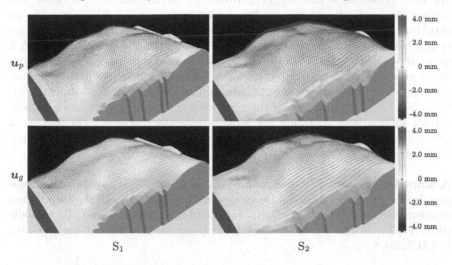

S_1 S_2

Table 1. Photometry-driven vs. geometry-driven estimation of the 3-D surface motion field, for normal and deep thoracic breathing, for four subjects S_1-S_4. Given is the RMS distance before (ϵ_0) and after warping (ϵ_p, ϵ_g)

	Normal breathing					Deep inhale				
	S_1	S_2	S_3	S_4	Mean	S_1	S_2	S_3	S_4	Mean
ϵ_0	0.068	0.078	0.112	0.067	0.082	0.098	0.113	0.127	0.104	0.110
ϵ_p	0.051	0.054	0.081	0.047	0.058	0.061	0.073	0.058	0.060	0.063
ϵ_g	0.056	0.058	0.084	0.051	0.062	0.079	0.086	0.085	0.076	0.081

and warped data w.r.t. the reference f_{t_2}, respectively

$$\epsilon_0 = \sqrt{\frac{1}{|\mathcal{M}|} \sum_{\zeta \in \mathcal{M}} \|f_{t_1}(\zeta) - f_{t_2}(\zeta)\|_2^2} \tag{6}$$

$$\epsilon_{p(g)} = \sqrt{\frac{1}{|\mathcal{M}|} \sum_{\zeta \in \mathcal{M}} \|f_{t_1}(\zeta + (\tilde{u}_{p(g)}(\zeta), \tilde{v}_{p(g)}(\zeta))^T) - f_{t_2}(\zeta)\|_2^2} \tag{7}$$

where ϵ_0 denotes the initial mismatch, $\|\cdot\|_2$ the Euclidean norm. The results on Microsoft Kinect RI data for thoracic respiration of the four subjects is given in Table 1. Note that the individual channels of f (RGB) lie in the range of $[0, 1]$. For normal and deep thoracic breathing, our photometric approach outperformed the geometric variant by $(\epsilon_g - \epsilon_p)/\epsilon_g = 6.5\%$ and $(\epsilon_g - \epsilon_p)/\epsilon_g = 22.5\%$ in average. This underlines the observation that our photometry-driven registration provides a surface motion field that better resembles the actual torso deformation.

4   Discussion

We have presented a method for photometric reconstruction of a dense 3-D surface motion field over non-rigidly moving surfaces using RI sensors. In an experimental study for the application in RT motion management, we have investigated the performance of our photometry-driven method compared to a geometry-driven approach. Both rely on a variational formulation and are capable of providing dense surface motion fields for application in respiratory motion management. However, our results indicate that incorporating photometric information into the estimation of the torso deformation provides a more realistic surface motion field regarding the human respiratory system. Ongoing work investigates the fusion of both photometric and geometric registration within a joint framework.

Acknowledgement. S. Bauer and J. Wasza gratefully acknowledge the support by the European Regional Development Fund (ERDF) and the Bayerisches Staatsministerium für Wirtschaft, Infrastruktur, Verkehr und Technologie (StMWIVT), in the context of the R&D program IuK Bayern under Grant No. IUK338.

References

1. Keall PJ, Mageras GS, Balter JM, et al. The management of respiratory motion in radiation oncology, report of AAPM TG 76. Med Phys. 2006;33(10):3874–3900.
2. Fayad H, Pan T, Roux C, et al. A patient specific respiratory model based on 4D CT data and a time of flight camera. In: Proc IEEE NSS/MIC; 2009. p. 2594–8.
3. Hoogeman M, Prévost JB, Nuyttens J, et al. Clinical accuracy of the respiratory tumor tracking system of the cyberknife: assessment by analysis of log files. Int J Radiat Oncol Biol Phys. 2009;74(1):297–303.
4. McClelland JR, Blackall JM, Tarte S, et al. A continuous 4D motion model from multiple respiratory cycles for use in lung radiotherapy. Med Phys. 2006;33(9):3348–58.
5. Bruhn A, Weickert J, Schnörr C. Lucas/Kanade meets Horn/Schunck: combining local and global optic flow methods. Int J Computer Vis. 2005;61:211–31.
6. Horn BKP, Schunck BG. Determining optical flow. Artiff Intell. 1981;17(1-3):185–203.
7. Lucas BD, Kanade T. An iterative image registration technique with an application to stereo vision. In: Proc IJCAI; 1981. p. 674–9.
8. Liu C. Beyond Pixels: Exploring New Representations and Applications for Motion Analysis. Doctoral Thesis. MIT; 2009.
9. Bauer S, Berkels B, Hornegger J, et al. Joint ToF image denoising and registration with a CT surface in radiation therapy. Lect Notes Computer Sci. 2011;6667:98–109.

ToF/RGB Sensor Fusion for Augmented 3D Endoscopy using a Fully Automatic Calibration Scheme

Sven Haase[1], Christoph Forman[1,2], Thomas Kilgus[3], Roland Bammer[2],
Lena Maier-Hein[3], Joachim Hornegger[1,4]

[1]Pattern Recognition Lab, Dept. of Computer Science, Univ. Erlangen-Nuremberg
[2]Department of Radiology, Stanford University, Stanford, California, USA
[3]Division of Medical and Biological Informatics, DKFZ Heidelberg
[4]Erlangen Graduate School in Advanced Optical Technologies (SAOT)
sven.haase@informatik.uni-erlangen.de

Abstract. Three-dimensional Endoscopy is an evolving field of research and offers great benefits for minimally invasive procedures. Besides the pure topology, color texture is an inevitable feature to provide an optimal visualization. Therefore, in this paper, we propose a sensor fusion of a Time-of-Flight (ToF) and an RGB sensor. This requires an intrinsic and extrinsic calibration of both cameras. In particular, the low resolution of the ToF camera (64×50 px) and inhomogeneous illumination precludes the use of standard calibration techniques. By enhancing the image data the use of self-encoded markers for automatic checkerboard detection, a re-projection error of less than 0.23 px for the ToF camera was achieved. The relative transformation of both sensors for data fusion was calculated in an automatic manner.

1 Introduction

The benefits of three-dimensional (3D) data in medicine to speed up and improve quality of surgeries are described in several publications [1, 2]. In comparison to conventional techniques, Time-of-Flight (ToF) cameras are a popular modality due to their markerless and non-invasive data acquisition. They measure 3D scenes in real-time and hold potential to provide a surgeon with up to date surface data during surgery. Especially 3D endoscopy gained lots of attention recently [3]. It is generally expected that the incorporation of photometric information into geometric data is able to improve segmentation, classification and registration in a significant way. Furthermore, it eases the interpretation of the data for surgeons. As the grayscale information delivered by the ToF sensor is insufficient for texture information due to its low resolution (64×50 px), ToF/RGB data fusion has already been proposed in [4, 5] and for 3D endoscopy in [3]. The 3D endoscope used in this paper is a prototype utilizing a ToF sensor in combination with an RGB chip and is described in Sect. 2.3. Besides an initial calibration of the system, each time the endoscope optics are changed a recalibration needs to be performed. In practice, we experienced that due to in-homogeneous illumination and the low resolution of the ToF sensor, illustrated in Fig. 1, the user has to identify the checkerboard in each acquisition manually, which is a time consuming and tedious procedure. Consequently, data enhance-ment is an inevitable preprocessing step for application of an automatic marker detection framework. For checkerboard detection we propose a method that does not have to recognize the whole checkerboard in each image and that does not have to make sure that both sensors cover all corners during measurement.

In comparison to Penne et al., in this paper, we propose the use of self-encoded markers [6] in order to establish a fully-automatic calibration routine for low-resolution sensor fusion.

2   Materials and methods

The following sections describe our approach to ToF/RGB sensor fusion in detail. This process can be split into two major aspects. First, the camera calibration and the required image enhancement for the ToF amplitude image and second, the fusion of ToF and RGB data.

2.1   Camera calibration

In order to apply a pixel-accurate framework for self-encoded marker detection [6] a bicubic upsampling of the ToF amplitude image data is performed. This technique enables subpixel-accuracy in low-resolution ToF data. In order to compensate for illumination inhomogeneities, we performed the well established technique of unsharp masking for local contrast enhancement [7]. Fig. 1 shows qualitative results of our preprocessing pipeline.

The calibration is split into two major stages. First, the corners of the observed checkerboard are detected and identified. Second, these corners serve as input for intrinsic and extrinsic calibration.

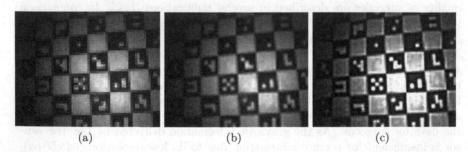

(a)   (b)   (c)

Fig. 1. Illustration of the image enhancement pipeline: (a) shows the original ampli-tude image, (b) the upsampled data using bicubic interpolation and (c) the image after applying an unsharp mask

For automatic detection of the corners, self-encoded markers are utilized. The process is described precisely as follows: The contours of the checkerboard squares are extracted using an adaptive thresholding scheme and are verified using contour shape analysis. Next, the markers are identified according to their unique bar codes using a nearest neighbor classification based on a template database. For eliminating false detection a sanity check of the four diagonal neighbors is performed. Finally, the corners of the verified markers serve as input for subpixel corner detection based on gradient analysis.

Based on the detected corners we apply an established optical calibration method [8] that estimates the intrinsic parameters and the distortion coefficients for both cameras separately. According to [8], the detected corners are re-used to calculate the extrinsic parameters for all image pairs that were acquired for calibration. Next, the poses (position and orientation) of the two cameras w.r.t. each other are calculated by using the extrinsic parameters (rotation and translation) estimated for each view

$$R = R_{\mathrm{RGB}} \left(R_{\mathrm{ToF}}\right)^{\top}, \quad t = t_{\mathrm{RGB}} - R\, t_{\mathrm{ToF}} \tag{1}$$

where $R \in \mathbb{R}^{3 \times 3}$ denotes a rotation matrix and $t \in \mathbb{R}^3$ a translation vector and the index denotes the modality. Due to the fact that for each view a slightly different transformation will be estimated, averaging all results weighted by their certainty is necessary. The certainty of each transformation is calculated depending on the amount of detected corners in the ToF image of this view. Note that the normalized quaternion representation [9] is used for averaging all rotations.

2.2   Sensor Fusion

In order to merge the data of both sensors, the 3D position X_{ToF} is calculated for each rectified ToF pixel $x_{\mathrm{ToF}}^{\mathrm{rect}}$ by utilizing the intrinsic camera matrix K_{ToF} of the ToF camera $X_{\mathrm{ToF}} = K_{\mathrm{ToF}}^{-1} x_{\mathrm{ToF}}^{\mathrm{rect}}$. Next, X_{ToF} is transformed from ToF camera coordinates into RGB camera coordinates, yielding $X_{RGB} = R\, X_{ToF} + t$. Finally, X_{RGB} is projected onto the RGB plane, using the intrinsic camera matrix K_{RGB} of the RGB camera, $x_{RGB} = K_{RGB}\, X_{RGB}$ and eventually distorted. As this usually results in a subpixel coordinate in the sensor domain, the color texture of the ToF pixel is calculated by bilinear interpolating between the surrounding pixels in the RGB image.

2.3   ToF/RGB endoscope prototype

All experiments in this paper are based on a 3D endoscope prototype manufactured by Richard Wolf GmbH, Knittlingen. The prototype utilizes photonic mixer device technology for acquisition of 3D surface data. In comparison to the endoscope used in [3], our device acquires surface and color data through one single endoscope optics by using a beam splitter. The RGB sensor acquires data with a resolution of 640×480 px the low resolution ToF sensor with 64×50 px.

2.4   Experiments

For evaluation of the marker identification, 50 ToF amplitude images of the calibration pattern were acquired considering different angels and distances. The detection rate in Sect. 3.1 is calculated on the total amount of automatically detected markers compared to the total amount of markers detected by a human observer in all 50 images. The identification rate is based on the number of all detected markers compared to the number of correct identified markers.

The experiments for evaluating the camera calibration is only considered for the low resolution ToF camera. The reprojection error is calculated using 50 ToF amplitude images. For evaluation of the robustness of our calibration technique, the intrinsic parameters were estimated based on different number of views of the calibration pattern. For each experiment, the image set was randomly chosen out of 110 views of the calibration pattern. The mean and standard deviation were calculated after 20 repetitions for each number of views.

Finally, for qualitative evaluation of the sensor fusion a red pepper was measured.

3   Results

In the following sections the results of our previously described experiments are presented in detail. Three different outcomes are distinguished. First, the identification of the markers. Second, the calibration results of the ToF camera and third, the camera fusion.

3.1   Marker identification

In terms of the self-encoded marker identification we achieved a detection rate of 93.1 % and an identification rate of 92.0 %. Note that all erroneously identified markers are eliminated due to the sanity check. Furthermore, let us consider the aspect of time as well. As shown in Fig. 2, in practice, at least 50 images need to be acquired in order to achieve a robust estimation of the intrinsics. The expert has to detect and identify all corners of the checkerboard in the ToF amplitude images. Using our approach the automatic identification of these corners was performed within 50 seconds.

3.2   Camera calibration

For the intrinsic calibration, we investigated the reprojection error and achieved a mean error of 0.23 px using 50 images. Besides, Fig. 2 illustrates the mean and the standard deviation of the focal lengths (f_x, f_y) and the principal point (c_x, c_y), given an increasing number N of images considered for calibration. Note that in practice a robust estimation of the camera parameters highly depends on the number of corners that can be detected in each view.

Fig. 2. Plots of the mean and the standard deviation of the focal lengths (f_x, f_y) and the principal point (c_x, c_y) for different number of views N of the checkerboard

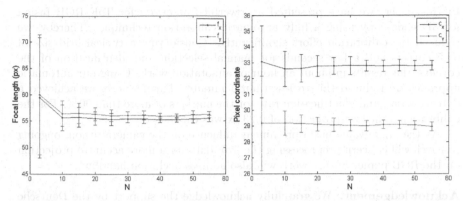

3.3   Sensor fusion

For qualitative evaluation, Fig. 3 shows a checkerboard view of a red pepper, where the texture of the amplitude image of the ToF camera and the merged RGB image are shown in alternating checkerboard patches. Note that at the edges adjacent structures coincide. In order to confirm the qualitative impression, we also computed the normalized mutual information (NMI) [10] as a similarity measure using the RGB image and the amplitude image for both views. Here, we achieved an improvement from 0.84 (0.88) without the alignment to 0.90 (0.93) after mapping the color information using the calculated relative transformation. The value of NMI is located between 0 and 2, where 2 indicates perfect similarity.

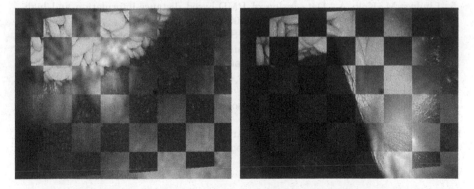

Fig. 3. Two checkerboard views of the ToF/RGB fusion result and the corresponding ToF amplitude image. Please note that at the edges adjacent structure coincide

4 Discussion

In this paper, we have presented a powerful framework for ToF/RGB fusion for 3D endoscopy using a fully automatic calibration technique. Thereby, we reduced the calibration effort significantly. Considering a typical grid size of 6×5 corners and a few seconds for manual selection and identification of the corners, this results in about an hour of annotation work. Using our automatic approach we reduced this to less than a minute. Furthermore, we achieved a detection rate and identification rate for the markers of more than 90 %. For the calibration a mean reprojection of 0.23 px was calculated.

As the range value has a prominent influence on the camera fusion, ongoing research will concern preprocessing the ToF data for a more accurate projection on the RGB plane. Future work will also address occlusion handling.

Acknowledgement. We gratefully acknowledge the support by the Deutsche Forschungsgemeinschaft (DFG) under Grant No. HO 1791/7-1. Furthermore, this research was funded/ supported by the Graduate School of Information Science in Health (GSISH) and the TUM Graduate School.

References

1. Rühl S, Bodenstedt S, Suwelack S, et al. Real-time surface reconstruction from stereo endoscopic images for intraoperative registration. Proc SPIE. 2011;7964:14.
2. Mersmann S, Müller M, Seitel A, et al. Time-of-flight camera technique for augmented reality in computer-assisted interventions. Proc SPIE. 2011;7964:2C.
3. Penne J, Schaller C, Engelbrecht R, et al. Laparoscopic quantitative 3D endoscopy for image guided surgery. Proc BVM. 2010; p. 16–20.
4. Gudmundsson SA, Sveinsson JR. TOF-CCD image fusion using complex wavelets. Proc ICASSP. 2011; p. 1557–60.
5. Lindner M, Kolb A. Data-fusion of PMD-based distance-information and high-resolution RGB-images. Proc ISSCS. 2007;1:121–4.
6. Forman C, Aksoy M, Hornegger J, et al. Self-encoded marker for optical prospective head motion correction in MRI. Med Image Anal. 2011;15(5):708–19.
7. Malin DF. Unsharp masking. AAS Photo-Bulletin. 1977;16:10–3.
8. Zhang Z. A flexible new technique for camera calibration. IEEE Trans Pattern Anal Mach Intell. 1998;22:1330–4.
9. Horn BKP. Closed-form solution of absolute orientation using unit quaternions. J Opt Soc Am A. 1987;4(4):629–42.
10. Studholme C, Hill DLG, Hawkes DJ. An overlap invariant entropy measure of 3D medical image alignment. Pattern Recognit. 1999;32(1):71–86.

GPU-Based Visualization of Deformable Volumetric Soft-Tissue for Real-Time Simulation of Haptic Needle Insertion

Dirk Fortmeier[1,2], Andre Mastmeyer[1], Heinz Handels[1]

[1]Institute of Medical Informatics, University of Lübeck
[2]Graduate School for Computing in Medicine and Life Sciences, University of Lübeck
fortmeier@imi.uni-luebeck.de

Abstract. Virtual reality simulations can be used for training of surgery procedures such as needle insertion. Using a haptic force-feedback device a realistic virtual environment can be provided by computation of forces for specific patient data. This work presents an algorithm to calculate and visualize deformations of volumetric data representing soft-tissue inspired by the relaxation step of the ChainMail algorithm. It uses the coupling of haptic force-feedback computation and the deformation visualization algorithm to enhance the visual experience of our needle insertion training simulation. Real-time performance is achieved by implementing the relaxation on the GPU which outperforms a CPU-based implementation.

1 Introduction

Simulation of needle insertion procedures is an active field of research [1, 2, 3, 4]. For training purposes, a real-time simulation using haptic and visual rendering can create a realistic virtual environment. To augment the realism of such an environment, it is desirable to compute and visualize deformations of tissue caused by interaction between needle and tissue. Interactive flexible needle insertion into soft tissue in 3D has been achieved by [1] using the finite element method. Furthermore, haptic feedback using FEM was incorporated into a training simulation for prostate brachytherapy by [2]. These works are based on tetrahedral meshes to simulate deformation which is considered slow and relies on a segmentation of patient data. An alternative approach for simulation of soft-tissue deformation is the ChainMail algorithm presented in [5] and used for surgery simulation in [6, 7, 8]. Fast and interactive visualization of large deformed volumes using the ChainMail algorithm was done by [9] and adapted for the GPU by [10]. Since deformations in needle insertion procedures mainly occur close to the needle as well as the amount of work needed for creation of a tetrahedral mesh by relying on segmentation is high, it is convenient to use an algorithm which directly deforms parts of the image data. In this work we introduce an approach to calculate soft-tissue deformations in real-time using the relaxation step of the ChainMail algorithm on the inverse of the displacement field similar to diffusive regularization in image registration. The advantages of only using the relaxation step is the small and fixed amount of processing time needed. We use the method developed to visualize the deformation occurring implicitly in a proxy based haptic rendering as presented in [3, 11] by using coupling nodes.

2   Methods

Calculation of haptic force-feedback in general relies on a high haptic rendering rate (1000-2000 Hz) compared to visual rendering (10-30 Hz). We use the haptic algorithms of [3, 11] to calculate force-feedback 2000 times per second. Computing a force is done by the algorithm using a virtual spring which connects the haptic device tip x_{tip} and a proxy x_{proxy}. This proxy-position is computed to simulate effects of surface penetrability, stiffness and viscosity of segmented [3] or partially segmented patient data [11] and implicitly models a deformation process of the soft-tissue surfaces (Fig. 1).

Fig. 1. Deformation of a soft tissue surface implicitly modeled by a proxy based haptic algorithm

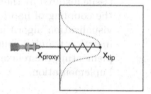

To visualize a deformed volumetric image $J : \mathbb{N}^3 \to \mathbb{R}$ based on the undeformed image of patient data $I : \mathbb{R}^3 \to \mathbb{R}$ we use the information provided by the device tip and the proxy as well as the orientation $r \in \mathbb{R}^3$ of the needle and the orientation $r_{enter} \in \mathbb{R}^3$ at the point where the needle entered the virtual patient. In the following we describe first how deformations are computed in our model. Afterwards, we show how the needle properties calculated by the haptic algorithm is invoking deformations and finally, a rough description of our GPU implementation is given.

2.1   Soft tissue deformation model

Deformation of soft tissue can be expressed using the position of undeformed material $X \in \mathbb{R}^3$, the corresponding deformed position $x \in \mathbb{R}^3$ and the relationship $x = X + u$, where $u : \mathbb{R}^3 \to \mathbb{R}^3$ is a displacement field. In contrast to [9] and [10] we use the inverse of the displacement field $u^{-1} : \mathbb{N}^3 \to \mathbb{R}^3$ to represent and calculate the deformations. This way, we can easily create the deformed image J without having to invert u first. The calculation is done by using trilinear interpolation of the undeformed image so that $J(v) = \text{interp}\left(I, v + u^{-1}(v)\right), v \in \mathbb{N}^3$. For each voxel position v in J, the corresponding value is found by determining the interpolated value at the deformed position of v in I.

For the propagation of deformation in successive time steps of the simulation we choose to use an explicit diffusion process $u_{t+1}^{-1} = u_t^{-1} + \alpha f \Delta u_t^{-1}$ where $\alpha \in [0..1]$ is a constant and f is a material property function describing the stiffness of the material in the deformed image J. In general, this material property function can be constructed from a segmentation of the patient data or the image data directly. In our approach, image data without segmentation is used. Here, we define $f : \mathbb{R} \to [0..1]$ as a simple piecewise-linear transfer function based on the findings presented in [11], for example undeformable (very stiff) material as bone is represented by $f = 0$ and soft-tissue by a range of $0.7 \leq f \leq 1$.

2.2 Tissue deformation induced by the needle

We model the needle as an inflexible 1D rod with a needle tip at $x_0 \in \mathbb{R}^3$ and a direction vector $r \in \mathbb{R}^3$. Interaction of tissue and needle is incorporated into the simulation by $m + 1$ coupling nodes with positions $x_{i=0..m}$ on the needle and corresponding positions in the undeformed tissue $X_{i=0..m}$. In each time step during the computation of the deformations the positions of needle nodes are recalculated.

As shown in Fig. 2, the positions in the undeformed tissue state are calculated accordingly using proxy position x_{proxy} and orientation r_{enter} at the time of entering. The deformation field is adjusted based on the deformed and undeformed positions of needle nodes $u^{-1}(x_i) = X_i - x_i$, $i = 0..m$ and relaxed as described in the previous section.

2.3 GPU accelerated implementation

The deformation and visualization is computed on the GPU (Fig. 3). The deformation algorithm is implemented using nVidia CUDA. In one step of calculating and visualizing deformations, information of the haptic algorithm is transferred to the graphic cards memory where it is used to compute the deformations in the displacement field. The displacement field is stored together with the deformed image as a buffer consisting of four floating point values per voxel (three elements for deformation, one element for the image intensity value). Furthermore, the

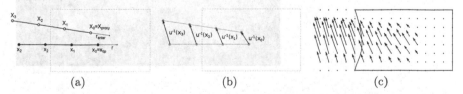

(a)   (b)   (c)

Fig. 2. Calculated needle node positions based on the proxy and haptic device position and orientation (a). Values of u^{-1} are visualized in (b) and the relaxed displacement field and deformed tissue in (c)

buffer is stored two times acting as input and output for one iteration of relaxation. To affect a larger area by deformation and at the same time create a fast response in the vicinity of the needle tip, the relaxation is performed multiple times with different sizes of the affected region (26 times 16^3 voxels, 6 times 48^3 voxels and 2 times 96^3 voxels). The midpoint of the region is the needle tip. After performing the relaxation steps in which the deformed image is resampled as well (needed for the evaluation of the material property function), the deformed image is used to update a pixel buffer object (PBO). Finally, this pixel buffer object is used by a GPU volume renderer provided by the Visualization Toolkit (VTK) to update a 3D texture which it renders to the screen.

Fig. 3. Flow of data in the threaded haptic and visualization architecture

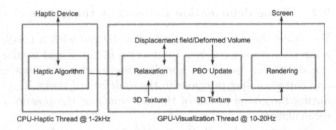

3 Results

Fig. 4 shows a deformed liver object extracted from a CT data set of a human torso ($256 \times 256 \times 326$ voxels). In Fig. 5 (top) the insertion of a needle into the

Fig. 4. Deformed liver object rendered using the VTK volume renderer

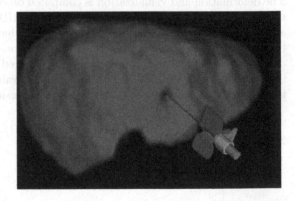

liver on the same CT data set without having removed the surrounding tissue is displayed. The effect of the material stiffness function f is demonstrated in Fig. 5 (bottom) where a virtual phantom of a cubic body is used. In Tab. 1 the processing times of the major components of the visualization algorithm are

Data Set / Voxels	Relaxation	Update	Rendering
Phantom 128^3	24.2 ms	0.3 ms	16.5 ms
Phantom 256^3	25.7 ms	6.8 ms	23.4 ms

Table 1. Median processing times of major components of the visualization thread. For the rendering, the window size was set to 640×480 pixels

shown for the cubic body phantom (measured for $N = 1$ cases). Note that the deformation computation per visualization step consists of multiple relaxations with different sizes of the volume of interest. It can be seen that the amount of time needed for the relaxation (around 25 ms) differs only marginally for different sizes of image data but for the update and rendering process of the 3D texture.

Furthermore, for the relaxation step the GPU implementation has been compared to a single-threaded simplified CPU implementation (without the trilinear interpolation) as shown in Tab. 2. It is noteworthy that for small volume of interests, the CPU implementation is slightly faster but for larger volumes it is easily outperformed by the GPU implementation (for 96^3 voxels the GPU implementation is more than 40 times faster). All results have been obtained on a nVidia Quadro 4000 and an Intel Xeon CPU @ 2.80 GHz.

	16^3 voxels	48^3 voxels	96^3 voxels
GPU	0.47 ms	1.2 ms	6.1 ms
CPU	0.34 ms	14.9 ms	261.8 ms

Table 2. Single Relaxation processing times (median) with different sizes of the VOI

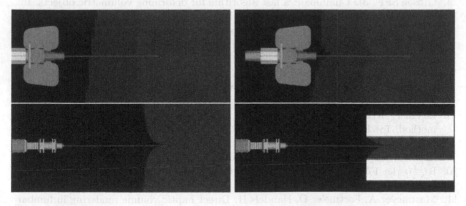

Fig. 5. Sagittal view of a needle on liver surface deforming surrounding tissue (top) and deformed phantom data (bottom) showing the effect of the material stiffness function f

4   Discussion

A fast method for the visual appealing visualization of soft-tissue deformations occurring in a needle insertion training simulation has been presented. Proxy based haptic rendering is used to create deformations on a displacement field which is then used to recalculate the deformed volume. It has been shown that for large volumes of interest, it is very beneficial to use a GPU-based implementation of the relaxation step. Nevertheless, the algorithm is only suitable for small deformations and physical accuracy cannot be claimed.

A future prospect will be the incorporation of the deformations in the calculation of haptic force-feedback. Additional future work will be in the area of bendable needles which are required in most needle insertion scenarios.

Acknowledgement. This work is supported by the German Research Foundation (DFG HA 2355/10-1) and the Graduate School for Computing in Medicine and Life Sciences funded by Germany's Excellence Initiative (DFG GSC 235/1).

References

1. Chentanez N, Alterovitz R, Ritchie D, et al. Interactive simulation of surgical needle insertion and steering. ACM Trans Graph. 2009;28(3):1–10.
2. Goksel O, Sapchuk K, Salcudean SE. Haptic simulator for prostate brachytherapy with simulated needle and probe Interaction. IEEE Trans Haptics. 2011;4(3):188–98.
3. Fï¿½rber M, Hummel F, Gerloff C, et al. Virtual reality simulator for the training of lumbar punctures. Methods Inf Med. 2009;48(5):493–501.
4. Ullrich S, Grottke O, Fried E, et al. An intersubject variable regional anesthesia simulator with a virtual patient architecture. Int J Comput Assist Radiol Surg. 2009;4(6):561–70.
5. Gibson SFF. 3D Chainmail: a fast algorithm for deforming volumetric objects. In: Proc Interactive 3D Graphics; 1997. p. 149.
6. Wang X, Fenster A. A virtual reality based 3D real-time interactive brachytherapy simulation of needle insertion and seed implantation. 2nd IEEE Int Symp Biomed Imaging. 2004; p. 280–3.
7. Gibson SF, Fyock C, Grimson E, et al. Simulating surgery using volumetric object representations, real-time volume rendering and haptic feedback. CVRMed-MRCAS. 1997; p. 367–78.
8. Le Fol T, Acosta-Tamayo O, Lucas A, et al. Angioplasty simulation using chainmail method. In: Proc SPIE. vol. 6509; 2007. p. 65092X–1.
9. Schulze F, Bï¿½hler K, Hadwiger M. Interactive deformation and visualization of large volume datasets. In: Proc Comp Graph Theory and App; 2007. p. 39–46.
10. Rï¿½ï¿½ler FA, Wolff T, Ertl T. Direct GPU-based volume deformation. In: Proc CURAC; 2008. p. 65–8.
11. Mastmeyer A, Fortmeier D, Handels H. Direct haptic volume rendering in lumbar puncture simulation. In: Medicine Meets Virtual Reality; 2012.

In-silico Modellierung der Immunantwort auf Hirntumorwachstum

Alina Toma[1,2], Anne Régnier-Vigouroux[3], Andreas Mang[1], Tina A. Schütz[1,4],
Stefan Becker[1,2], Thorsten M. Buzug[1]

[1]Institut für Medizintechnik, Universität zu Lübeck
[2]Kompetenzzentrum für Medizintechnik (TANDEM)
[3]INSERM U701, Deutsches Krebsforschungszentrum, INF 242, DKFZ Heidelberg
[4]Graduiertenschule für Informatik in Medizin und Lebenswissenschaften
toma@imt.uni-luebeck.de

Kurzfassung. In der vorliegenden Arbeit wird ein neuer mathematischer Ansatz zur Modellierung des Einflusses des Immunsystems, genauer gesagt der Mikrogliazellen (MG) auf die Progression von malignen, primären Hirntumoren vorgestellt. Ein hybrider Ansatz wird zur Modellierung des zellulären Tumorwachstums und der Veränderung lokaler Nährstoffkonzentrationen sowie der Dichte der extrazellulären Matrix genutzt. Die ruhenden MG in Primärtumoren werden mit Hilfe von Tumorsignalen (TS), die durch eine partielle Differentialgleichung beschrieben werden, aktiviert und angelockt. Mit Hilfe eines zusätzlichen Terms für den Abbau der Matrix kann das anschließende Aussenden von degradierenden Enzymen der amöboiden Immunzellen modelliert werden. Dies hilft den Tumorzellen schneller und weiter zu migrieren. Wir stellen erstmalig die Modellierung der MG im Rahmen von Tumorwachstum vor. Der Vergleich mit in-vitro Daten zeigt vielversprechende qualitative Übereinstimmungen. Unser Modell stellt somit einen aussichtsreichen Ansatz zur Modellierung des Hirntumorwachstums auf zellulärer Ebene unter Berücksichtigung des angeborenen Immunsystems dar.

1 Einleitung

Glioblastoma multiforme (GBM) ist der aggressivste und im Erwachsenenalter am häufigsten auftretende primäre Gehirntumor. Mit Hilfe moderner multimodaler Standardtherapie, bestehend aus chirurgischer Entfernung, Strahlentherapie und Chemotherapie, kann häufig nur der Großteil des Tumors beseitigt werden. Aufgrund des infiltrierenden, diffusen Wachstums des Glioblastoms in das umliegende Gehirngewebe und einer effektiven Unterdrückung des Immunsystems, kann lediglich eine mittlere Überlebensdauer von etwas mehr als einem Jahr erreicht werden. Die vorliegende Arbeit befasst sich mit der mathematischen Modellierung der Progression von Tumoren des zentralen Nervensystems, in Wechselwirkung mit dem Immunsystem, präziser, mit der Beschreibung der raum-zeitlichen Interaktionen primärer, hirneigener Tumorzellen mit den Mikrogliazellen/Makrophagen. Ein mächtiges Werkzeug, um beispielsweise Hypothesen über den (patientenindividuellen) Verlauf der Tumorerkrankung zu testen und damit das Verständnis für die Krankheit, insbesondere für das noch nicht vollständig erforschte Verhalten der Immunzellen zu mehren, stellt hierbei die mathematische Modellierung dar. Wir wenden uns hierbei der Beschreibung von Prozessen auf der mikroskopischen Ebene zu. Dies ermöglicht nicht nur eine fein-granularere Beschreibung individueller Zellen, um den infiltrierenden Charakter aufzugreifen, sondern erlaubt es zudem, stochastische Prozesse der Tumorprogression abzubilden.

In der Literatur (z.B. [1, 2]) wird bereits die Modellierung von Interaktionen zwischen Tumor und Immunsystem dargestellt. Hier werden die natürliche Killerzellen (NK) des angeborenen Immunsystems und die cytotoxische T-Lymphozyten (CTL) des adaptiven Immunsystems betrachtet. Beide sind jedoch nur vereinzelt im Hirn vorhanden [3]. Um Tumore des zentralen Nervensystems realitätsnah zu modellieren, muss man zusätzlich zur Tumorprogression die Interaktionen mit den Mikrogliazellen (MG) simulieren. Der wesentliche Beitrag dieser Arbeit liegt in der Neuentwicklung eines Modells, das die Immunantwort auf Tumorwachstum im Hirn beschreibt.

2 Material und Methoden

Das Gewebe wird als ein zwei-dimensionales Gebiet $\Omega = [0,1] \times [0,1]$ mit Abschluss $\overline{\Omega}$ und Dirichlet- und Neumann-Rand $\Gamma_D \cup \Gamma_N = \Gamma = \partial\Omega$ dargestellt und mit einem $M \times M$ Gitter versehen. Da eine Gitterzelle der Größe einer biologischen Tumor- oder Immunzelle (Durchmesser: ca. 10 μm) entsprechen soll und das initiale Tumorwachstum bis zu einer Größe von 4 mm simuliert wird, ergibt sich für M ein Wert von 400.

Da nur MG im Gehirn voll kompetent immunologisch wirken, stellen sie die Makrophagen des Gehirns dar. Sie machen ca. 20% aller Zellen des zentralen Nervensystems aus [4]. Diese tauchen zunächst ausschließlich residenten (ruhend) auf [5]. Erst durch das Auftreten einer Läsion, einer Infektion bzw. eines Tumors werden die MG aktiviert (aMG). Dies geschieht durch Stimulation von Zytokinen (z.B. Interferon-γ, MCP-1, G-CSF), die vom Tumor ausgesendet werden [6] und als Chemoattraktanten für die MG wirken. Im ruhenden Zustand proliferiert eine MG sehr langsam und bewegt sich aufgrund ihres plastischen Charakters viel, legt aber keine weiten Wege zurück. Aus diesem Grund vernachlässigen wir die Proliferation sowie die Bewegung der residenten MG (rMG) für die Modellierung. In den amöboiden Zustand dagegen migrieren die MG in Richtung des höheren Tumor Signalkonzentration. Außerdem exprimieren sie Faktoren, die die Matrix-Metalloproteasen (MMPs) aktivieren. Damit kann die extrazelluläre Matrix (EZM) noch schneller abgebaut werden, was die Tumorzellen invasiver macht [4, 6, 7], d.h. sie helfen dem Tumor schneller und weiter zu migrieren.

Der verwendete mathematische Ansatz für die Progression des Tumors basiert auf einem hybriden Modell zur Beschreibung der Nährstoffverteilung, der Dichte der EZM und der unterschiedlichen zellulären Prozesse. Für die Nährstoffversorgung wird angenommen, dass sich Blutgefäße am Rand des Gebietes befinden. Für die Verteilung von z.B. Glucose und Sauerstoff wird eine

Reaktions-Diffusionsgleichung verwendet, um die Konzentration der diffundie-
renden Nährstoffe u aus nahegelegenen Blutgefäßen über die Zeit zu beschreiben. Die EZM f besteht vorwiegend aus nicht-diffusiblem Collagen, Laminin
und Fibronektin und wird von gesunden und krebsartigen Zellen produziert. Die
EZM kann für die Tumorzellen als ein Trägersubstrat agieren, jedoch auch als
Barriere bei einer höheren Dichte. In letzterem Fall werden von den Gliomazellen
Matrix-degradierende Enzyme wie z.B. MMP freigesetzt. Matrixstrukturprotei-
ne werden dann von MMPs abgebaut. Um das Modell möglichst übersichtlich zu
halten, folgen wir [8] und nehmen an, dass die Tumorzellen selbst die Matrix abbauen können. Die Migration der Zellen c folgt, neben der zufälligen Bewegung
(Diffusion), einem chemotaktischen und einem haptotaktischen Einfluss unter
Berücksichtigung der Umgebung. Die Tumorzellen folgen dem höheren Stoffkon-
zentrationsgradienten, in diesem Fall der Nährstoffkonzentration und bevorzugen
ein Gefälle der Matrix, d.h. eine bereits abgebaute EZM [8]. Für die Bewegung
der aktivierten MG m betrachten wir die Diffusion und die chemotaktische Bewegung aufgrund der vom Tumor ausgesandten Signale s. Es gilt nun folgendes
System partieller Differentialgleichungen

$$\frac{\partial c}{\partial t} = \nabla \cdot (D_c \nabla c) - \chi \nabla \cdot (c \nabla u) - \rho \nabla \cdot (c \nabla f) \qquad \text{in } \Omega \times [0, T] \qquad (1a)$$

$$\frac{\partial u}{\partial t} = \nabla \cdot (D_u \nabla u) - \alpha_u u c \qquad \text{in } \Omega \times [0, T] \qquad (1b)$$

$$\frac{\partial f}{\partial t} = -\alpha_f f(c + m) + \beta_f f(1 - f) \qquad \text{in } \Omega \times [0, T] \qquad (1c)$$

$$\frac{\partial m}{\partial t} = \nabla \cdot (D_m \nabla m) - \lambda \nabla \cdot (m \nabla s) \qquad \text{in } \Omega \times [0, T] \qquad (1d)$$

$$\frac{\partial s}{\partial t} = \nabla \cdot (D_s \nabla s) - \alpha_s s + \beta_s c \qquad \text{in } \Omega \times [0, T] \qquad (1e)$$

mit Randbedingungen

$$\partial c / \partial n = 0, \quad \partial f / \partial n = 0, \quad \partial m / \partial n = 0, \qquad \partial s / \partial n = 0 \quad \text{auf } \Gamma \times [0, T]$$

$$\partial u / \partial n = 0 \quad \text{auf } \Gamma_N \times [0, T], \qquad\qquad u = 1 \quad \text{auf } \Gamma_D \times [0, T]$$

und Anfangswerten $c = c_0$, $u = u_0$, $f = f_0$, $m = m_0$, $s = s_0$, $\forall\, x \in \Omega$, $t = 0$,
wobei D_c, D_u, D_m und D_s Diffusionskoeffizienten sind und χ, λ die chemotaktischen bzw. ρ der haptotaktische Parameter. Als Verbrauchsraten bezeichnen
wir α_u, α_f und α_s und mit β_f die Aufbaurate. Die Produktionsrate der TS wird
mit β_s gekennzeichnet. In jedem Zeitschritt und für jede Tumorzelle berücksichtigen wir die lokale Nährstoffkonzentration und entscheiden dann, wie die Zelle
reagiert. In dem Fall, dass der Sauerstoffwert unter einer kritischen Schwelle
a_{krit} liegt, gehen wir davon aus, dass aufgrund unzureichenden Sauerstoffs mit
einer Wahrscheinlichkeit von 80% die Zelle sterben wird. Diese Zelle wird folglich als nekrotisches Gewebe markiert und nicht für den nächsten Zeitschritt
berücksichtigt. Nach der Überprüfung des Kriteriums für Nekrose, bewegt sich
jede Tumorzelle entsprechend der nachfolgend beschriebenen Regeln. In dem Fall

einer ausreichenden Nährstoffkonzentration wird die Zelle für die Division ausgewählt. Wenn die Signalkonzentration von $s = 0.08$ eine rMG erreicht, so wird diese aktiviert und in den nachfolgenden Zeitschritten als aMG betrachtet. Diese können dann zusätzlich indirekt die Matrix mit abbauen, weswegen wir den Produktionsterm $\alpha_f fm$ in Gleichung (1c) hinzufügen.

Initial wird eine kleine Gruppe von 100 Tumorzellen in der Mitte des Gebietes Ω verteilt. MG sind über das gesamte Gehirn verteilt, deshalb erfolgt die initiale Platzierung zufällig im Gebiet, bis eine Anteil von 10 % der Gitterpunkte belegt ist. Wir skalieren die Variablen und Parameter des Systems (1) und berechnen sie in dimensionslose Größen um, so dass alle berechneten Mengen im Bereich $[0, 1]$ liegen. Die partiellen Differentialgleichungen (1b) sowie (1e) werden für jeden Simulationszeitschritt $t_j = j\Delta t, j = 1, 2, ..., k$; im stationären Zustand (d.h. $\partial u/\partial t = 0$ und $\partial s/\partial t = 0$) mittels der Finite-Elemente-Methode gelöst. Die Tumorgleichung (1a) und die Gleichung für die MG (1d) wird mit Hilfe von finiten Differenzen gelöst. Zentrierte räumliche Ableitungen und für die Zeitableitung eine Vorwärts-Ableitung (FTCS: Forward Time Forward Space) werden verwendet, so dass die resultierenden Koeffizienten proportional zu den Wahrscheinlichkeiten für eine Zelle sind, sich in eine bestimmte Richtung zu bewegen.

3 Ergebnisse

Die Ergebnisse des vorgestellten Modells wurden unter Verwendung der folgenden dimensionslosen Parameter (für die Simulationen) erzielt [8]: $D_c = 10^{-5}$, $D_u = 10$, $\chi = 0.26$, $\rho = 0.26$, $\alpha_u = 6.25 \cdot 10^{-5}$ und $\alpha_f = 0.01$, $\beta_f = 0.001$, $D_m = 10^{-5}$, $\lambda = 0.1$, $D_s = 0.075$, $\alpha_s = 0$, $\beta_s = 1$, $a_{krit} = 0.22$ und $\Delta t = 30$ min.

Abb. 1 zeigt den Tumor nach 40 Iterationsschritten (20 Stunden), wobei eine Nährstoffversorgung durch Blutgefäße am Randbereich Γ des Gebietes Ω angenommen wird 1(d). Rot bzw. hellrot kennzeichnen aktive bzw. in der Ruhephase befindliche Tumorzellen. Gelbe Bereiche entsprechen aufgrund von Nahrungsmangel abgestorbenen Zellen. Die rMG sind in hellblau dargestellt und die aMG in dunkelblau. Für einen späteren Zeitpunkt $t = 230$ h ergeben sich die Resultate in Abb. 2 und für $t = 400$ h sind die Distributionen der Zellen, TS, EZM und Nährstoffe in Abb. 3 zu sehen. Der Vergleich mit in-vitro Daten (Abb. 4) erlaubt uns eine qualitative Gegenüberstellung unsere Ergebnisse.

4 Diskussion

Die Verteilung der Nährstoffe wird in Abhängigkeit von der Tumorzellzahl und deren Position im Gebiet simuliert. In Abb. 3(d) sehen wir einen höheren Nährstoffverbrauch im Vergleich zu vorherigen Zeitpunkten. Hier spielt die Anzahl der Tumorzellen eine wichtige Rolle. Wie in Abb. 3(a) zu sehen, ist der Tumor nach 400 h auf ein Vielfaches seiner ursprünglichen Größe angewachsen und es hat sich ein nekrotischer Kern (gelb) gebildet. Das Absterben in der Mitte des Tumors kann auch in-vitro beobachtet werden (Abb. 4): Die umliegenden Zellen verbrauchen die zur Verfügung stehende Glucose und den Sauerstoff, sodass nur wenige Nährstoffe zum Tumorkern diffundieren können. Die EZM wird von den Tumorzellen abgebaut (Abb. 1(c), 2(c)) und zu einem späteren Zeitpunkt auch von den amöboiden MG (Abb. 3(c)), was anhand der hellroten, im Gebiet verteilten Bereiche zu erkennen ist. Die Tumorzellen (Abb. 1(a), 2(a) und 3(a)) migrieren abgelöst von der Tumorhauptmasse durch die Matrix in das umliegende Gebiet, was man ebenfalls in Abb. 3 beobachten kann. Zum Zeitpunkt 230 h sind aMG zu sehen (Abb. 2(a)), die von den Tumorsignalen 2(b) erreicht wurden.

In diesem Beitrag wurde ein kontinuierliches, stochastisches Modell vorgestellt, das die frühe Wachstumsphase eines Glioblastoms in Wechselwirkung mit Immunzellen in zwei Raumdimensionen betrachtet. Das von uns vorgestellte Modell bildet in der Literatur beschriebene [4] und experimentell bestätigte Verhalten (Abb. 3 und [9]) individueller Tumorzellen ab. Zweifelsfrei unterliegt die raumzeitliche Entwicklung von Hirntumoren komplexen, auf unterschiedlichen Ebenen stattfindenden Mechanismen. Neben der Erweiterung dieses Modells in

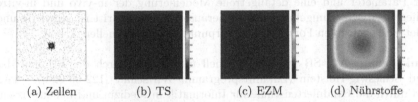

(a) Zellen   (b) TS   (c) EZM   (d) Nährstoffe

Abb. 1. Simulationsergebnisse zum Zeitpunkt $t = 20$ h. Blutgefäße werden an allen Rändern des Gebietes angenommen. Die Farbskala kodiert die Konzentrationen der TS und der Nährstoffe bzw. die Dichte der EZM. Bzgl. der Zellen (1(a)), repräsentiert gelb nekrotisches Gewebe, rot entspricht stillen Tumorzellen und dunkelrot proliferierenden sowie migrierenden Tumorzellen. Die ruhenden MG werden in hellblau dargestellt und die amöboiden MG in dunkelblau

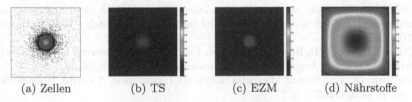

(a) Zellen   (b) TS   (c) EZM   (d) Nährstoffe

Abb. 2. Simulationsergebnisse zum Zeitpunkt $t = 230$ h. Farbkodierung wie in Abb. 1

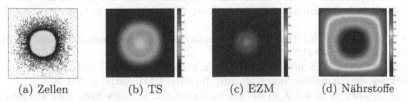

(a) Zellen   (b) TS   (c) EZM   (d) Nährstoffe

Abb. 3. Simulationsergebnisse zum Zeitpunkt $t = 400$ h. Farbkodierung wie in Abb. 1

Abb. 4. In-vitro Ergebnisse: Kokultur von ein Glioma-Sphäroid mit Zusatz von MG in einer Kollagenmatrix ($t = 15$ Tage). MG (in blau) umranden den Glioma-Sphäroid (in grün) oder sammeln sich um abgestorbene Zellen (in rot). Konfokale Aufnahmen nach 3D Modellierung (Amira Software)

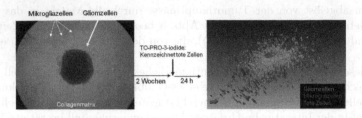

Form eines vaskulären Ansatzes, bestehend aus dem Prozess der Angiogenese, steht eine quantitative Evaluierung gegenüber in-vitro Experimenten aus. Ein derartiger Vergleich erfordert die Integration und Schätzung patientenindividueller Parameter und eine detailgetreue Modellierung der in-vivo und in-vitro vorliegenden Mikroumgebung. Dieser herausfordernde Schritt ist schwierig und bildet einen zentralen Forschungsschwerpunkt unserer aktuellen Arbeit.

Danksagung. AT, SB werden finanziell unterstützt durch die EU und das Land Schleswig-Holstein (Zukunftsprogramm Wirtschaft [122-09-024]). TAS wird durch die Graduiertenschule für Informatik in Medizin und Lebenswissenschaften, Deutsche Exzellenzinitiative [DFG GSC 235/1] unterstützt.

Literaturverzeichnis

1. Mallet DG, Pillis LGD. A cellular automate model of tumor-immune system interactions. J Theo Biol. 2006;239:334–50.
2. Eftimie R, Bramson JL, Earn DJD. Interactions between the immune system and cancer: a brief review of non-spatial mathematical models. Bull Math Biol. 2011;73:2–32.
3. Dix AR, Brooks WH, Roszman TL, et al. Immune defects observed in patients with primary malignant brain tumors. J Neuroimmunol. 1999;100:216–32.
4. Marković D. The Role of Microglia in Glioma Invasiveness. Charité, Universitätsmedizin Berlin; 2007.
5. Roggendorf W, Strupp S, Paulus W. Distribution and characterization of microglia/macrophages in human brain tumors. Acta Neuropathol. 1996;92:288–93.
6. Graeber MB, Scheithauer BW, Kreutzberg GW. Microglia in brain tumors. Glia. 2002;40:252–9.
7. Zhai H, Heppner FL, Tsirka SE. Microglia/Macrophages promote glioma progression. Glia. 2011;59:472–85.
8. Toma A, Mang A, Schütz TA, et al. Is it necessary to model the matrix degrading enzymes for simulating tumor growth? In: Proc VMV; 2011. p. 361–8.
9. Kees T, Lohr J, Noack J, et al. Microglia isolated from patients with glioma gain antitumor activities on poly (I:C) stimulation. Neuro Oncol. 2011.

Pfadbasierte Identifikation von Nanopartikel-Agglomerationen in vitro

Thorsten Wagner[1], Sven Olaf Lüttmann[1], Dominic Swarat[1],
Martin Wiemann[2], Hans-Gerd Lipinski[1]

[1]Biomedical Imaging Group, Fachbereich Informatik, Fachhochschule Dortmund
[2]Institute for Lung Health (IBE R&D gGmbH), Münster
wagner@biomedical-imaging.de

Kurzfassung. Durch eine Laser gestützte Mikroskopietechnik können
Licht streuende Nanopartikel (NP) in Suspensionen anhand ihrer Beu-
gungsmuster sichtbar gemacht und ihre Diffusionspfade durch bildanaly-
tische Methoden erfasst werden. Diese Pfade lassen Rückschlüsse auf den
Diffusionskoeffizienten und damit auf den hydrodynamischen Durchmesser (HD) der NP zu. Eine sprunghafte Änderung der NP-Größe, die im
Beugungsbild keine eindeutigen Veränderungen bewirkt, kann dennoch
als Agglomeration identifiziert werden, da es zu einem nicht-stationären
Verhalten des HD-Zeitreihe kommt. Nicht-agglomerierende Partikel wie
Polystyrol (in H_2O, Durchmesser 100nm) weisen durchweg ein statio-
näres Zeitreihenverhalten auf, während bei „erzwungener"Agglomeration
bestimmter SiO_2 Partikel (Durchmesser 20nm) nach NaCl-Gabe ein statistisch nachweisbares nicht-stationäres HD-Zeitreihenverhalten vorliegt.
Mit diesem indirekten Verfahren lassen sich NP-Agglomerationen aufdecken auch wenn sie nicht direkt mikroskopisch nachweisbar sind.

1 Einleitung

Die Bedeutung von Nanopartikeln (NP) sowohl für die Industrie als auch für
die Medizin nimmt stetig zu. Allerdings weisen Studien darauf hin, dass eine
NP-Exposition beim Menschen möglicherweise zu gesundheitlichen Problemen
führen kann [1, 2]. Unter in vitro-Bedingungen lässt sich u.a. die Wechselwirkung zwischen Immunzellen und NP untersuchen, wobei die NP in ein wässriges
Medium gegeben werden, in dem sich die vitalen Immunzellen befinden. Eine NP Tracking-Analyse (NTA; z.B. die NanoSight^{TM}-Methode) ermöglicht es,
NP in solchen Suspensionen aufgrund ihrer Lichtstreuung bzw. ihrer Beugungsmuster sichtbar zu machen und ihre Größe über zurückgelegte Diffusionspfade
(„Tracks") zu charakterisieren. Offenbar neigen bestimmte Partikelarten zur Agglomeration, wodurch ihre biologische Aktivität oder Toxizität möglicherweise
modifiziert wird. Da die Größenänderung von NP durch Agglomeration unter
dem Mikroskop kaum direkt beobachtet werden kann, wurde eine bildgestützte
Methode entwickelt, mit deren Hilfe Agglomerationen indirekt durch Änderung
des dynamischen Verhaltens detektiert werden können.

2 Material und Methoden

Bei der NTA-Technik wird ein Laserstrahl durch eine Flüssigkeitsschicht geführt, welche die Nanopartikel und ggf. auch die Immunzellen enthält. Trifft der Laserstrahl auf ein NP, wird der Strahl gestreut, wobei ein typisches Beugungsmuster erzeugt wird, das mit einem Mikroskop und einer elektronischen Kamera mit 30 Bildern/s registriert wird. Ein ausgewählter NP kann idealerweise über die gesamte Bildserie hinweg verfolgt werden (Abb. 1). Aufgrund seiner Diffusionsbe-

Abb. 1. Aufnahme einer SiO_2-Suspension mit der Nanosight^{TM}-Technik und exemplarisch eingezeichnetem Pfad eines Nanopartikels

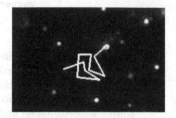

wegung entsteht ein charakteristischer Pfad, den man verfolgen und hinsichtlich seines Verlaufs analysieren kann. Anhand dieses Tracks lässt sich das mittlere Verschiebungsquadrat $\langle r^2 \rangle$ des NP bestimmen, welches die Berechnung des zugehörigen Diffusionskoeffizienten (DC) erlaubt. Die Stokes-Einstein-Beziehung liefert den zum Partikel gehörenden hydrodynamischen Durchmesser (HD) [3]

$$\frac{\langle r^2 \rangle}{4} = D \cdot t = \frac{T K_B}{3\pi\eta d} \tag{1}$$

Unter dem HD d versteht man den Durchmesser einer Kugel, welche die gleichen Diffusionseigenschaften aufweist wie der eigentliche Partikel. Der Parameter T entspricht der absoluten Temperatur der Lösung in Kelvin, η der Viskositäts-Konstante der Lösung und K_B der Boltzmann Konstante. Für die Identifikation von Agglomerationsereignissen ist es notwendig, den zeitlichen Verlauf des HD eines Partikels zu kennen. Dazu werden besonders lange Tracks ($>= 100$ Schritte) ausgewählt und in nicht überlappende Teiltracks mit der Länge Θ (Fensterbreite) unterteilt. Mit der Zeitkomponente $t = n \cdot \Theta$ ergibt sich somit der zeitabhängige Durchmesserschätzer durch folgenden Algorithmus:

1. Bestimmung des mittleren Verschiebungsquadrats

$$\langle r^2 \rangle = \frac{1}{\Theta} \sum_i \left[(x_{i+t} - x_{i-1+t})^2 + (y_{i+t} - y_{i-1+t})^2 \right] \tag{2}$$

2. Berechnung des hydrodynamischen Durchmessers als Zeitfunktion

$$d = d(t) = \frac{T \cdot K_B}{3\pi \cdot \eta} \cdot \frac{4 \cdot \Delta t}{\langle r^2 \rangle} \tag{3}$$

Hierbei sind (x, y) die aktuellen kartesischen Koordinaten des Partikelzentrums und Δt die Zeit zwischen zwei Schritten. Abb. 2 zeigt den zeitlichen Verlauf der Durchmesserkurve für einen Polystyrol-Partikel (100nm) in stabiler Suspension in der keine Agglomeration stattfindet. Der zeitliche Verlauf des Durchmessers weist typische Messschwankungen auf, die größtenteils auf die stochastische Natur der Brownschen Molekularbewegung zurückzuführen ist. Dennoch verhält sich die Zeitreihe der Partikel-Durchmesser stationär (Test nach Kwiatkowski et al./KPSS-Test [4]). Im Fall einer Agglomeration verändern sich allerdings der DC und der damit verbundene HD, so dass ein nicht-stationärer "Trend„ in der HD-Zeitreihe zu erwarten wäre. Um diese Hypothese zu überprüfen, wurde zunächst ein Monte-Carlo-Modell für die Simulation der NP-Bewegungen entwickelt. Die Verteilung der Schrittlänge s in Abhängigkeit vom DC D ist durch folgenden Ausdruck beschrieben [5]

$$p_d(s) = 2s(4D\Delta t)^{-1} exp\left(-s^2(4D\Delta t)^{-1}\right) \qquad (4)$$

Mit Hilfe der Inversionsmethode [6] lassen sich zufällige Schrittlängen dieser Verteilung erzeugen mit denen sich ein Partikelpfad generieren lässt. Ein Agglomerationsereignis wird durch eine schlagartige Verringerung des Diffusions-koeffizienten-Wertes (Halbierung) simuliert, was zu einer Vergrößerung des HD des Partikels führt. Für die Experimenten wurde Partikel aus Polystyrol und SiO_2 eingesetzt. Polystyrol Partikel (NanoSight, Eichstandard 100 nm) lagen in H_2Omonodispers vor. Pegylierte SiO_2-Partikel (BASF, Durchmesser ca. 20-100nm) wurden durch Zugabe von Phosphatpuffer (pH 7,9) und Zugabe von NaCl (Endkonzentration: 0,45% w/v) zur Agglomeration gebracht.

3   Ergebnisse

Auf Basis der Monte-Carlo-Simulation wurde die Leistungsfähigkeit des KPSS-Tests zur Agglomerationsdetektion optimiert und analysiert. Dazu wurden 100

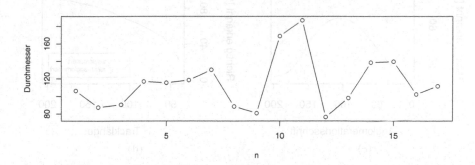

Abb. 2. Zeitlicher Verlauf eines Polystyrol-Partikel-Durchmessers (Tracklänge: 100 Schritte). Der KPSS-Test klassifiziert den Track als stationär

Schritte umfassende Tracks mit und ohne Agglomeration simuliert, wobei die Agglomeration etwas nach Ablauf der halben Zeit (Schritt 50) simuliert wurde. Zur Optimierung des Verfahrens wurden für verschiedene Fensterbreiten und Signifikanzniveaus die Erkennungsraten für agglomerierte Partikel ermittelt. Durch die Ermittlung der Erkennungsraten für nicht agglomerierte Partikel konnte zusätzlich auch eine False-Positive-Rate (1-Erkennungsrate) angegeben werden. Es zeigte sich, dass die Leistungsfähigkeit der Agglomerationsdetektion abhängig war (1.) von dem Zeitpunkt, zu dem die Agglomeration innerhalb des Tracks simuliert wurde und (2.) von der Länge des Partikeltracks. Abb. 3 zeigt, dass die maximale Erkennungsrate bei einer Fensterbreite von sechs Schritten liegt. Die False-Positive-Rate lag dabei praktisch konstant bei ca. 5%. Weitere Untersuchungen ergaben, dass man eine optimierte Fensterbreite erhält, wenn man die Gesamtlänge des Tracks mit 0,06 multipliziert. Für das Signifikanzniveau (Abb. 3b) gilt: Je größer die Erkennungsrate für agglomerierte Partikel sein soll, desto häufiger werden nicht-agglomerierte Partikel fälschlicherweise als agglomerierte Partikel klassifiziert. Daher wurde für die weiteren Analysen ein Signifi-

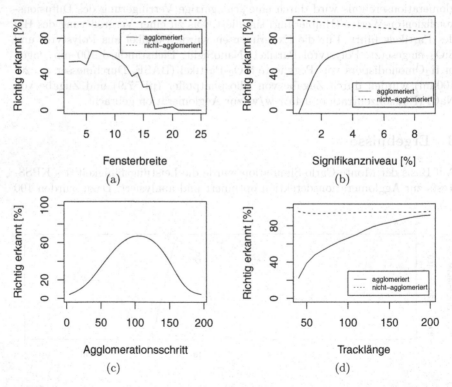

Abb. 3. Analyse Ergebnisse der Optimierungsparameter (a,b) und der Leistungsfähigkeit (c,d). Untersucht wurden die Fensterbreite (a, gemessen in Schritten), das Signifikanzniveau (b), der Agglomerationszeitpunkt (c) und die Länge des Tracks (d)

kanzniveau von 4% gewählt, da hier die False-Positive-Rate von 5% noch relativ niedrig ist. Die Abhängigkeit der Leistungsfähigkeit der Agglomerationsdetektion vom Agglomerationszeitpunkt und von der Tracklänge ist in Abb. 3c bzw. 3d gut zu erkennen. Tritt die Agglomeration in der Mitte des Tracks auf liegt die Erkennungsrate bei ca. 75%. Agglomerationen, die am Anfang und am Ende des Tracks auftreten, werden deutlich seltener erkannt. Die Agglomerationsdetektion wurde abschließend mit in Wasser gelösten pegylierten SiO_2 unter Hinzugabe von NaCl getestet. Dabei wurden 8% der Partikel als mögliche Agglomerate klassifiziert. Abb. 4 zeigt exemplarisch den Zeitverlauf des Durchmessers eines solchen Partikels. Der Trend ist dabei gut erkennbar.

4 Diskussion

Es wurde eine Bild gestützte Trackinganalyse entwickelt, mit der optisch nicht darstellbare NP-Agglomerationen detektiert werden können. Eine Agglomeration lässt sich durch einen nicht-stationären Verlauf der ermittelten Durchmesser-Zeitreihe nachweisen. Dieses Simulationsergebnis wurde mit Messungen an realen NP experimentell überprüft und bestätigt. Während eine Zeitreihenanalyse von nicht-agglomerierbaren Polystyrol-Partikeln zu stationären Partikelgrößen-Zeitreihen führen, können experimentell forcierte Agglomerationen, wie sie etwa bei SiO_2-Partikeln nach NaCl-Gabe auftreten, durch ein nicht-stationäres Verhalten der Partikelgrößen-Zeitreihe nachgewiesen werden. Mit der Methode können schnell verlaufende bzw. induzierte Agglomerationen sowie Deagglomerationen dargestellt und untersucht werden.

Danksagung: Diese Arbeit wurde mit Mitteln des Bundesministeriums für Bildung und Forschung gefördert (NanoGEM; Fördernummer 03X0105G).

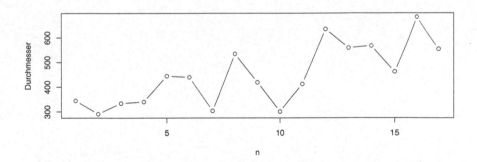

Abb. 4. Zeitlicher Verlauf des hydrodynamischen Durchmessers [nm] eines offenbar agglomerierten SiO_2-Partikels, welcher über ca. 100 Schritte beobachtet werden konnte. Der KPSS-Test klassifiziert den zeitlichen Verlauf des HD als nicht-stationär

Literaturverzeichnis

1. Xia T, Li N, Nel A. Potential health impact of nano particles. Annual Review of Public Health. 2009;30:137–50.
2. Lam C, James JT, McCluskey R, et al. A review of carbon nanotube toxicity and assessment of potential occupational and environmental health risks. Crit Rev Toxicol. 2006;36(3):189–217.
3. Nelson P. Biological Physics. New York: W.H. Freeman and Company; 2008.
4. Kwiatkowski Peter C, et al. Testing the null hypothesis of stationarity against the alternative of a unit root. J Econom. 1992;54(1-3):159–78.
5. Michalet X. Mean square displacement analysis of single-particle trajectories with localization error. Physical Review E. 2010;82(4):041914.
6. Rubinstein RY, Kroese DP. Simulation and the Monte Carlo method. vol. 707. Wiley-interscience; 2008.

Microfluidic Phenotyping of Cilia-Driven Mixing for the Assessment of Respiratory Diseases

Stephan Jonas[1,2], Engin Deniz[3], Mustafa K. Khokha[3,4], Thomas M. Deserno[1], Michael A. Choma[2,3]

[1]Department of Medical Informatics, RWTH Aachen University, Aachen, Germany
[2]Dept. Diagnostic Radiology, Yale University School of Medicine, New Haven, USA
[3]Department of Pediatrics, Yale University School of Medicine, New Haven, USA
[4]Department of Genetics, Yale University School of Medicine, New Haven, USA
stephan.jonas@yale.edu

Abstract. The function of ciliated surfaces to clear mucus from the respiratory system is important for many respiratory diseases and, therefore, has a high impact on public health. In this work, we present a quantitative method to evaluate mixing efficiency of cilia-driven microfluidic flow based on front line deformation as an integrated measurement of cilia function. So far, mixing efficiency has been used mainly for analyzing artificial cilia. Most of this work, however, was either bound to specific imaging modalities or done on simulated data. In this simulations, mixing efficiency has been quantified as the change in length of a virtual dye-strip. We adopt this measure for *in-vivo* data of the Xenopus tropicalis tadpole that is acquired by an innovative low-cost mixing assay (microscopy) and optical coherence tomography (OCT). Mixing is imaged in a water filled well while dye flows into it. The length of front line is extract with the following steps: (i) filtering of the video to reduce compression artifacts, (ii) segmentation of dye based on the hue channel in HSV colorspace, (iii) extracting and converting the front line of segmented dye to curvature scale space, and (iv) smoothing of the front line with a Gaussian filter and calculation of length in curvature scale space. Since dye cannot be used with OCT, we use data from prior work that performs particle tracking to generate a flow vector field and seed virtual dye in this flow field. The following steps extract the vector field: (i) filtering and gray scale thresholding for particle candidate detection, (ii) thresholding size of particle candidates, (iii) pairing of remaining particles from subsequent frames, (iv) estimation of velocity and direction of each particle, and (v) combining these measures into a velocity field. Our *in-vivo* imaging and analysis shows that the front line of dye is actively mixed by the ciliated surface of the Xenopus embryo.

1 Introduction

Motile cilia are organelles that protrude from the surface of cells and generate directional, low Reynolds number fluid flow. Cilia-driven flow is important for human health. For example, the respiratory system is covered with cilia that clear mucus from the respiratory system. Just as artificial cilia can drive microfluidic mixing, we have preliminary data showing that biological cilia can similarly drive microfluidic mixing. Since prior work in artificial cilia has shown that mixing efficiency can be used as a measurement of ciliary function [1, 2, 3], we are interested in translating these measurements to use in biological ciliated surfaces [4]. Since quantification of mixing is bound to the imaging modality, we present a method that can be applied to data of different imaging modalities. We apply our quantitative method to images of cilia-driven fluid flow acquired using optical coherence tomography (OCT) [5] and bright field microscopy.

2   Materials and methods

Since low Reynolds number flow does not have turbulent flow to mixing, other mechanisms are required to drive efficient mixing [6]. Those mechanisms often focus on increasing fluid stirring, thereby facilitating diffusion/mixing. Therefore, the length of front line (LFL) of dye, the length of the interface between dye and water is an important factor that influences the speed of mixing by diffusion. Flow and mixing generated by the ciliated epidermis (skin) of Xenopus embryos (tadpoles) were imaged. We chose Xenopus because (i) it is genetically-manipulable [7] and (ii) it is an emerging animal model in ciliary biology [8].

A measurement similar to the one used by Khatavkar et al. (2007) was implemented to define mixing efficiency in both imaging modalities (Fig. 1). We compare the front (or dye-water interface) length of either virtual dye seeded into vector fields, or of the tracked front of dye the mixing experiments.

2.1   Optical coherence tomography

Two-dimensional two-component vector fields of cilia-driven flow were extracted using a commercially available optical coherence tomography (OCT) system (16kHz swept source OCT, Thorlabs, Inc., Newton, NJ, USA) and particle tracking of tracer particles (Fig. 1(a) and 2(a)) [5]. The particles were micro-beads with a diameter of 5μm. Images of the particles were acquired with a frame rate of 30 fps and filtered with an 3D average filter. Beads were then segmented based on one fixed gray scale threshold chosen manually for all acquisitions. A single fixed threshold is possible due to the consistency of OCT data. The segmented connected components were collected and thresholded with a size-based rejection rule to eliminate false-positives. The centroid of the particles was calculated, thus attaining sub-pixel resolution. Particles were paired based on a maximum-matching algorithm to account for particles leaving the field of view. Tracking results were combined to two-dimensional, two-component flow vector fields. In the resulting field, a line of virtual dye was seeded and the LFL of the virtual dye was calculated as a function of time. We assumed (i) that flow is low Reynolds number (i.e. $Re < 1$), (ii) that dye diffusion is slow compared to flow-mediated transport of dye, and (iii) that flow is 2D. We acknowledge that the last assumption (iii) is violated at certain points in the flow field while highlighting that the method should be readily scaled to three-dimensional flow velocimetry.

2.2 Brightfield microscopy

The mixing assay uses bright field microscopy with a commercially available microscope (SMXZ800, Nikon Instruments, Inc, Melville, NY, USA) and camera (Mark 5 dII, Canon U.S.A., Inc, Lake Success, NY, USA) for acquisition. Dye flow imaging was performed with the ciliated embryo in a round well with inlet for dye or other flow tracers (Fig. 1(b)). Images were acquired in full HD resolution with a frame rate of 30 fps and color-normalized to account for changes in illumination by averaging the RGB channels. The original video is compressed by the camera with the H.264 codec. To reduce compression artifacts, the video is filtered with a moving average filter with kernel size 3 (Fig. 3). The dye was segmented based on the HSV colorspace. Using the hue channel, a piece of the "HSV pie" was cut out corresponding to the observed color of the dye by setting an lower and upper threshold on the hue value. Due to the color normalization, fixed thresholds for hue could be used. The front of the segmented dye was extracted by filtering the segmented image with an edge detector. It was then

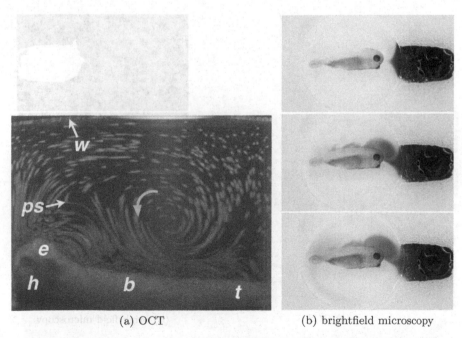

(a) OCT   (b) brightfield microscopy

Fig. 1. Multi-modal source data. The projection over time of OCT images shows a water/air barrier (w), streak lines produced by the particles (ps), and the animal (eye (e), head (h), body (b) and tail (t)). The blue arrow indicates the direction of flow. In video microscopy, the blue dye is clearly visible.

converted into curvature scale space [9], addressing pixels belonging to the dye by coordinates along the front instead of a using binary mask to mark pixels as part of the dye front. The front line is then smoothed by filtering the coordinates with a Gaussian filter before the LFL was calculated.

3 Results

The data acquired by the OCT (Fig. 1(a)) visualizes the tracer particles and can be transferred into a vector field (Fig. 2(a)) by applying particle tracking [5]. Based on this field, the deformation of dye due to flow is simulated. A virtual streak of dye is seeded into the field and deformed according to the velocity field. Movement over time of the simulated dye (Fig. 4(a)) results in a change of LFL (Fig. 4(c)). In contrast for diffusing dye, the LFL is constant over the time as the gradient of the diffusion does not change on the entire front line.

The images acquired by the novel mixing assay (Fig. 1(b)) are segmented based on the hue channel of the HSV colorspace (Fig. 2(b)). The change in LFL during mixing (Fig. 4(b)) is almost linear (Fig. 4(d)), while the LFL of dye moving only by diffusion is almost constant in the observed timespan. This is according to the virtual model and proofs the applicability of this method.

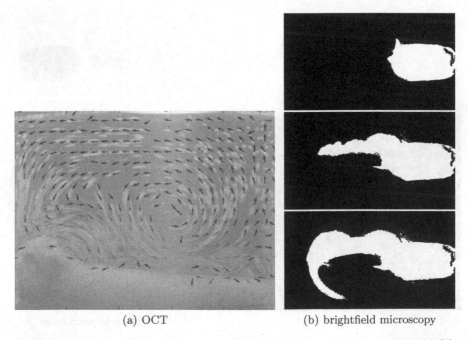

(a) OCT   (b) brightfield microscopy

Fig. 2. Image processing. The velocity vector field is superimposed on Fig. 1(a) [5]. The vectors indicate direction and color indicates velocity. Velocity is scaled from blue (> 0 mm/s) to red (300 mm/s). In video microscopy, dye is segmented by static thresholding in HSV colorspace.

4   Discussion

The results indicate that the front line of dye that is actively being mixed by the ciliated surface of the Xenopus embryo at low Reynolds number flow behaves very differently from undisturbed diffusing dye. While the LFL does not change for simulated undisturbed diffusion, the LFL doubles within three seconds in case of active mixing. Similar observations can be made for the comparison of diffusion and mixing of the real dye in the low cost assay. The length of the diffusing dye only changes a few percent from the initial length, the length of the mixed dye doubles in about two minutes.

We show that by tracking the LFL of dye or simulated dye we can create a readout that can be useful to describe mixing efficiency. After assessing the robustness of our method, the next steps will be testing of gene-manipulated or pharmacologically manipulated animals. We will also investigate our measurement for its suitability for a low-cost screening assay of motile cilia with little available resources.

References

1. Khatavkar VV, Anderson PD, den Toonder JMJ, et al. Active micromixer based on artificial cilia. Phys Fluids. 2007;19:13.
2. Johnson TJ, Ross D, Locascio LE. Rapid microfluidic mixing. Anal Chem. 2002;74(1):45–51.
3. Oh K, Smith B, Devasia S, et al. Characterization of mixing performance for bio-mimetic silicone cilia. Microfluid Nanofluidics. 2010;9:645–55.

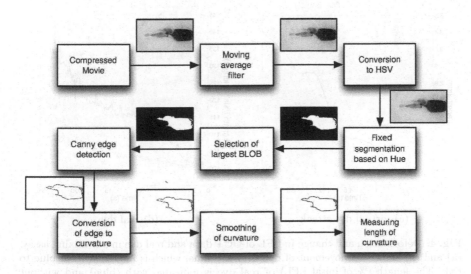

Fig. 3. Processing chain for dye mixing videos of the mixing array

4. Camesasca M, Kaufman M, Manas-Zloczower I. Quantifying fluid mixing with the Shannon entropy. Macromol Theory Simulation. 2006;15(8):595–607.
5. Jonas S, Bhattacharya D, Khokha MK, et al. Microfluidic characterization of cilia-driven fluid flow using optical coherence tomography-based particle tracking velocimetry. Biomed Opt Expr. 2011;2:2022–34.
6. Squires TM, Quake SR. Microfluidics: fluid physics at the nanoliter scale. Rev Mod Phys. 2005;77:977–1026.
7. Khokha MK, Chung C, Bustamante EL, et al. Techniques and probes for the study of Xenopus tropicalis development. Dev Dyn. 2002;225:499–510.
8. Mitchell B, Jacobs R, Li J, et al. A positive feedback mechanism governs the polarity and motion of motile cilia. Nature. 2007;447:97–101.
9. Sadegh Abbasi JK Farzin Mokhtarian. Curvature scale space image in shape similarity retrieval. Multimedia Syst. 1999;7:467–76.

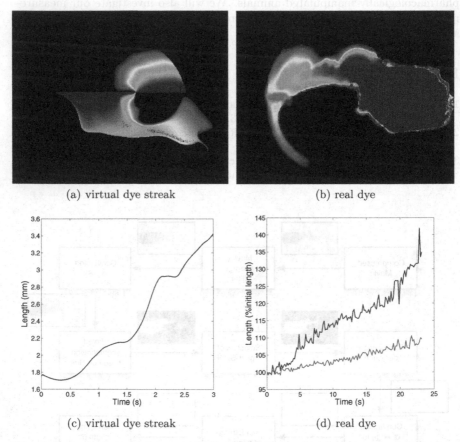

(a) virtual dye streak   (b) real dye

(c) virtual dye streak   (d) real dye

Fig. 4. Deformation and change in LFL of OCT data and real dye in our mixing assay. (a) and (b) show the movement of dye over the time, which is indicated from blue to red. The length (% of inital LFL) of real dye is indicated with (blue) and without active mixing (red)

Sparsity Level Constrained Compressed Sensing for CT Reconstruction

Haibo Wu[1,2], Joachim Hornegger[1,2]

[1]Pattern Recognition Lab (LME), Department of Computer Science
[2]Graduate School in Advanced Optical Technologies (SAOT)
Friedrich-Alexander-University Erlangen-Nuremberg
haibo.wu@informatik.uni-erlangen.de

Abstract. It is a very hot topic to reconstruct images from as few projections as possible in the field of CT reconstruction. Due to the lack of measurements, the reconstruction problem is ill-posed. Thus streaking artifacts are unavoidable in images reconstructed by filtered backprojection algorithm. Recently, compressed sensing [1] takes sparsity as prior knowledge and reconstructs the images with high quality using only few projections. Based on this idea, we propose to further use the sparsity level as a constraint. In the experiments, we reconstructed Shepp-Logan phantom with only 30 views by our method, TVR [2] and stand ART [3] respectively. We also calculated the Euclidean norm of the reconstruction image and the ground truth for each method. The results show that reconstruction results of our method are more accurate than the results of total variation regularization (TVR) [2] and stand ART [3] method.

1 Introduction

In the field of CT reconstruction, it draws a lot of attention to reconstruct the images from few samples (often under the Nyquist sampling rate) to reduce the radiation dose. And in certain applications, it is not possible to sample at Nyquist sampling rate because of motion, cardiac imaging [4]. In these cases, the reconstruction problem is ill-posed. Thus the images reconstructed by FBP (Filtered Backprojection) [2], which is widely used in CT product, contain many streaking artifacts. Recently, compressive sampling (CS) shows that a high quality signal or image can be reconstructed with far fewer measurements than the Nyquist sampling rate. The main idea of CS is to take sparsity as a prior. Based on that, Pan's group developed TVR method [3] and reconstructs high quality images using only few projections. However, the method reduces the contrast of the image [5].

In this paper, we propose to further use the number of the nonzero coefficient (sparsity level) as prior knowledge. This prior knowledge is formulated as an additional constraint in the CS based reconstruction frame work. In practice, the accurate sparsity level is hard to estimate. We suggest to approximate it using the image reconstructed by FBP. From the experiments, even if the sparsity level is 1.4 times as the actual value, the method can still improve the reconstruction accuracy. In the experiments, we used the Shepp-Logan phantom and reconstructed it with our method, TVR [2] and stand ART [3]. The results show that our method reconstruct the images with best accuracy.

2   Materials and methods

A discrete version of the CT scanning process can be described as

$$Ax = b \tag{1}$$

Here $A = (a_{ij})$ is the system matrix representing the projection operator, $x = (x_1,..., x_n)$ represents the object and $b = (b_1, ..., b_m)$ is the corresponding projection data. So to reconstruct the object x is to solve the linear system. In our case, the linear system is underdetermined due to undersampling. There exist infinite solutions. As mentioned above, CS takes sparsity as prior knowledge, which formulates the reconstruction problem as

$$\min_{x} ||\Phi x||_{L1} \ s.t. \ ||Ax - b||_2^2 < \alpha \tag{2}$$

Here, α stands for the variance of the noise. Φ is the sparsifying transform, wavelet transform. The inequality constraint enforces the data fidelity and the L1 norm term promotes the sparsity. For details, we refer to the work [3]. It is well known that the constrained optimization problem (2) can be transformed to an easier unconstrained optimization problem [5].

$$\min_{x} ||\Phi x||_{L1} + \beta ||Ax - b||_2^2 \tag{3}$$

The cost function in the optimization problem is convex. Although there exists a global minimum for a convex function, the minimizer could be non unique (Fig. 1). The function in the picture is convex, but the number of the

Fig. 1.   Convex function with non unique minimizers

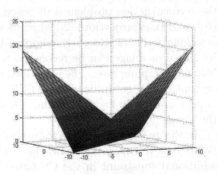

minimizer is infinite. In this case, the initial guess determines the final solution for the iterative reconstruction. The exact reconstruction of CS is guaranteed when there exists only one minimizer [1].

Otherwise the error bound is described by the "size" of the solution set. Sometimes, the "size" of the solution set could be very large. Due to the sampling mechanism, exact reconstruction condition of CS can not be satisfied in the context of CT reconstruction. Is there any way to further select the solution? We propose to use the sparsity level. Then the reconstruction problem can be formulated as

$$\min_{x} ||\varPhi_1 x||_{L1} + \beta ||Ax - b||_2^2 s.t. ||\varPhi_2 x||_{L0} < \chi \qquad (4)$$

where $||\bullet||_{L0}$ is L0 norm, which counts the number of nonzero entries. $||\varPhi_2 x||_{L0} < \chi$ is the sparsity level constraint. χ is a scalar. $\varPhi_1$ and $\varPhi_2$ both are the sparsifying transforms. We use total variation [2] as $\varPhi_1$ and Haar wavelet transform as $\varPhi_2$ in our experiments. These two sparsifying transforms are heavily used in the CS based reconstruction, as the medical images can be expressed sparsely with these two transforms. Some other sparsifying transform can also be used. (3) is a non convex optimization problem. However, all the local minimum should be in the optimal solution set of (3). The sparsity level constraint selects the solutions which satisfies the constraint within the optimal solution set for (3). So this formulation can increase the accuracy of the reconstruction compared to (3). In our experiments, we find that the sparsity level constraint does not have to be very accurate. The most accurate reconstruction is achieved when χ is a little bit bigger than the actual sparsity level. In practice, we can first use FBP to reconstruct the image, then apply the sparsifying transform $\varPhi_2$ to estimate the sparsity level. The optimization problem is hard to solve due to the high dimensions. A splitting method is used to solve (4) [3]. Inspired by this idea, we developed our method based on the splitting method. The algorithm can be summarized as below:

1. Apply the standard ART update [2].
2. Solve the optimization problem $x' = \min ||x-v||_2^2 + \beta ||\varPhi_1 x||_1$ (v is calculated from Step 1 which is the volume estimation from Step 1)
3. Apply the sparsifying transform $\varPhi_2$ on x' (x' is calculated from Step 2)
4. Keep the χ largest coefficients and set others to zero
5. Apply the inverse sparsifying transform $\varPhi_2^{-1}$
6. Repeat Steps 1 to 5 until $||x^{(t)} - x^{(t+1)}||_2^2$ is less than a certain value or the maximum iteration number is reached.

Step 1 and step 2 solve the problem (3) without sparsity level constraint using a splitting method. Step 3 to step 4 force the current estimate to fulfill the sparsity level constraint. We keep the largest coefficients and set others to zero by the assumption that the energy of natural image concentrate on a few basis of an sparsifying transform.

3   Results

In the experiments, we use the Shepp-Logan phantom. We consider image reconstruction of a 128×128 image from projection data containing 30 views and 128 bin on the detector. The projections are equally angular-spaced over 180 degree. We reconstructed the images with standard ART, TVR and our method. The reconstruction results is listed in Fig. 2. In the picture, we can see that the reconstruction from the standard ART contains many streak artifacts. The reconstruction from TVR is better. But the contrast is reduced. The streaks are nearly can not be seen in the reconstruction from our method. Furthermore the contrast is better than the reconstruction of TVR.

The profile of the reconstruction can be found in Fig. 3. The contrast of the reconstruction from our method outperforms the one from TVR.

We also calculated the relative error (RE) over iterations for quantitative evaluation

$$RE = \frac{||x - x^*||_2}{||x^*||_2} \qquad (5)$$

where x is the reconstructed image and x^* is the ground truth. It can be seen from Fig. 4 that the convergence speed of our method is faster than the other two. And the accuracy of our method is the best. In Fig. 5, we set χ to different values. The best reconstruction is achieved when χ is a little bit bigger than the actual sparsity level. Our method still gives more accurate results than the ones from TVR and stand ART, even if we set χ to 1.4 times as the actual sparsity level.(Fig. 4 and Fig. 5). Thus the estimation of sparsity level need not to be very accurate.

4   Discussion

Although CS claims it can reconstruct the image exactly under Nyquist sampling rate, the exact reconstruction condition is hard to be satisfied due to the

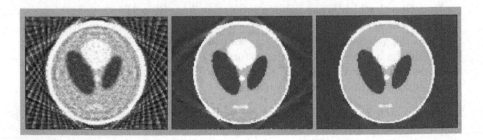

Fig. 2. Reconstruction results. Only 30 projections are used to do the reconstruction. The window level are all [-0.2 0.3]. The reconstruction from the standard ART contains many streak artifacts. The reconstruction from TVR is better. But the contrast is reduced. The streaks are nearly can not be seen in the reconstruction from SLCCS, also the contrast is better than the reconstruction of TVR

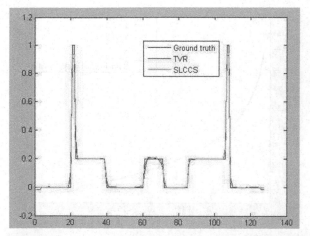

Fig. 3. Profile. The images shows the profile of the center line from the reconstruction of TVR, SLCCS and the ground truth. It can be easily seen that the reconstruction of SLCCS reserves the contrast.

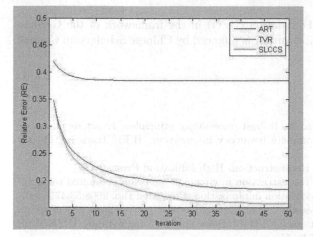

Fig. 4. Converge map. SLCCS converges faster than the other two method and gives best reconstruction quality

sampling mechanism of CT. To further improve the reconstruction quality, we propose to use the sparsity level as prior knowledge as well. The sparsity level constraint shrinks the "size" of the optimal solution set thus increases the reconstruction quality. In the experiment, by taking the sparsity as a prior, TVR which is CS based reconstruction method increase the reconstruction accuracy a lot compared to the classical method (ART). However, the contrast of the TVR reconstruction is reduced. By using the sparsity level constraint, the contrast of our reconstruction is better and relative error of our method is the smallest among the three reconstruction method. We will test the algorithm with vivo data in the future.

Acknowledgement. The first and third authors gratefully acknowledge funding of the Erlangen Graduate School in Advanced Optical Technologies (SAOT)

Fig. 5. Test of χ. We set χ to different values. The most accurate reconstruction is achieved when χ is a little bit bigger than the actual sparsity level. Thus the estimation of sparsity level need not to be very accurate but it should not be less than the actual sparsity level

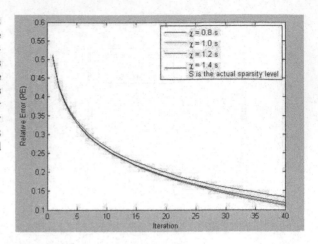

by the German Research Foundation (DFG) in the framework of the German excellence initiative. The first author is financed by Chinese Scholarship Council (CSC).

References

1. Candes E, Romberg J, Tao T. Robust uncertainty principles: Exact signal reconstruction from highly incomplete frequency information. IEEE Trans Inf Theory. 2006;52:489–509.
2. Zeng GL. Medical Image Reconstruction. High Education Press; 2009.
3. Sidky EY, Pan X. Image reconstruction in circular cone-beam computed tomography by constrained, total-variation minimization. Phys Med Bio. 2008;53:4777–807.
4. Hansis E, Schaefer D, Doessel O, et al. Evaluation of iterative sparse object reconstruction from few projections for 3-D rotational coronary angiography. IEEE Trans Med Imag. 2008;27(11):1548–55.
5. Jia X, Lou Y, Li R, et al. GPU-based fast cone beam CT reconstruction from undersampled and noisy projection data via total variation. Med Phy. 2010;37(11):1757–61.

L1-Regularisierung für die Computertomographie mit begrenztem Aufnahmewinkel

Matthias Kleine[1,2], Jan Müller[1], Thorsten M. Buzug[1]

[1]Institut für Medizintechnik
[2]Graduate School for Computing in Medicine and Life Sciences
Universität zu Lübeck
kleine@imt.uni-luebeck.de

Kurzfassung. Das Rekonstruktionsproblem für die Computertomographie (CT) mit begrenztem Aufnahmewinkel ist schlecht gestellt. Mit Standardtechniken wie der gefilterten Rückprojektion oder der Singulärwertzerlegung können nur Kanten rekonstruiert werden, welche tangential zu den aufgenommenen Projektionen liegen. Die Annahme, dass das zu rekonstruierende Objekt dünn besetzt in einer gewählten Wavelet-Basis ist, führt zu einer Regularisierung des Rekonstruktionsproblems mit der L1-Norm. Durch Lösen des sich stellenden Minimierungsproblems lassen sich selbst bei geringem Aufnahmewinkel Kanten im gesamten Winkelbereich rekonstruieren. Für einen Aufnahmewinkel von 90° ist die Rekonstruktion perfekt. Da die Abtastung nicht im Fourier-, sondern im Ortsraum erfolgt, ist keine Interpolation von kartesischen Koordinaten auf Polarkoordinaten erforderlich.

1 Einleitung

Bei tomographischen Aufnahmen mit begrenztem Aufnahmewinkel werden nur wenige Projektionen innerhalb eines begrenzten Winkelbereichs aufgenommen. Dieses Verfahren findet beispielsweise Anwendung bei der digitalen Brust-Tomosynthese oder bei der zerstörungsfreien Prüfung von Gegenständen. Modelliert man die Aufnahme als ein lineares Gleichungssystem $Ax = y$, so ist die Aufgabe, das Bild x aus den gemessenen Daten y zu rekonstruieren, ein schlecht gestelltes inverses Problem [1]. Die Mess- oder Systemmatrix A beschreibt hierbei die Geometrie des Systems, jede Zeile von A entspricht der Röntgenprojektion eines Strahls durch x. Standardverfahren wie die gefilterte Rückprojektion liefern bei der Lösung des Gleichungssystems inakzeptable Ergebnisse (Abb. 1). Bei einem Lösungsansatz mit Singulärwertzerlegung können nur Kanten rekonstruiert werden, welche tangential zu den Richtungen sind, über die im Rahmen der Röntgenprojektion integriert wird [2]. Zusätzliche Annahmen an das zu rekonstruierende Objekt wie beispielsweise Dünnbesetztheit in einer geeigneten Basis können die Rekonstruktion entscheidend verbessern.

Aus der Theorie von Compressed Sensing ist bekannt, dass sich durch die Annahme der Dünnbesetztheit der Lösung auch stark unterbestimmte lineare

148   Kleine, Müller & Buzug

Gleichungssysteme eindeutig lösen lassen. Die Lösung des restringierten Minimierungsproblems

$$\min_x ||x||_1 \text{ so dass } Ax = y \tag{1}$$

liefert die am dünnsten besetzte Lösung x, welche die Messung y erfüllt [3]. Das
in [4] durchgeführte Experiment zeigt beispielsweise, dass die vollständige Rekonstruktion eines dünn besetzten Objekts möglich ist, wenn nur wenige radiale
Linien aus dem Fourier-Spektrum des Objektes bekannt sind. Die Rekonstruktion ist ebenfalls perfekt, wenn nur radiale Linien des Fourier-Spektrums aus
einem begrenzten Winkelbereich bekannt sind.

Ist das zu rekonstruierende Objekt stückweise konstant, so liefert die Minimierung der TV-Norm des Bildes ähnliche Ergebnisse [5]. Dieser Ansatz wird
hier jedoch nicht weiter verfolgt.

Auf Grund des Fourier-Slice-Theorems entsprechen einzelne Projektionen ra-
dialen Linien im Fourier-Raum [6]. Somit entsprechen die in [4] beschriebenen
Experimente einer Messung mit wenigen Projektionen beziehungsweise Aufnahmen aus einem begrenzten Winkelbereich. Im diskreten Fall ist allerdings eine Umrechnung von kartesischen Koordinaten zu Polarkoordinaten erforderlich,
welche in unserem Ansatz vermieden wird.

2 Material und Methoden

Wir fassen die Vorwärtsprojektion als lineares Gleichungssystem $Ax = y$, $A \in
\mathbb{R}^{M \times N}$, $x \in \mathbb{R}^N$, $y \in \mathbb{R}^M$ auf. M ist hierbei das Produkt aus der Anzahl der
Detektorelemente und der Anzahl der Projektionen, während N die Anzahl der
Pixel des Bildes ist. Als zu rekonstruierendes Objekt wählen wir das Shepp-
Logan-Phantom der Größe 256×256 Pixel in MATLAB. Wir rekonstruieren unser Bild in einer vorher bestimmten Wavelet-Basis, da Wavelets besonders gut
die komprimierbare Struktur eines Bildes ausnutzen. Der Vektor w der Wavelet-
Koeffizienten des Bildes ist nicht exakt dünn besetzt, die wichtigen Informatio-
nen des Bildes sind jedoch in wenigen Koeffizienten konzentriert [5]. Das Bild
lässt sich ohne deutliche Verschlechterung der Bildqualität bereits durch diese
Koeffizienten beschreiben.

Um eine dünn besetzte Lösung zu erhalten, lösen wir das restringierte Minimierungsproblem

$$\min_w ||w||_1 \text{ so dass } ||AW^T w - y||_2 \le \epsilon \tag{2}$$

wobei $\epsilon \ge 0$ unsere Fehlertoleranz darstellt. W beziehungsweise W^T beschreiben die Wavelet-Transformation beziehungsweise -Rücktransformation des Bildes x. Hierbei wurden die in MATLAB existierenden Funktionen zur Wavelet-
Zerlegung genutzt.

Sei nun w unser komprimierbares, das heißt annähernd dünn besetztes Bild
(nur wenige Koeffizienten w_j enthalten fast alle Informationen des Bildes) in der
Wavelet-Basis W und $\tilde{w}$ die Lösung des Minimierungsproblems (1). Erfüllt die

Messmatrix A zusätzlich das exakte Rekonstruktionsprinzip ERP [7], so sind die Informationen von $\tilde{w}$ ebenfalls größtenteils in diesen Koeffizienten w_j konzentriert. Allerdings ist bislang nicht bewiesen, ob unsere Messmatrix AW^T diese Eigenschaft erfüllt. Die Ergebnisse in Abb. 1 zeigen zumindest, dass sich die Rekonstruktionsergebnisse durch die Regularisierung im Vergleich zur gefilterten Rückprojektion deutlich verbessern.

Das restringierte Minimierungsproblem (2) lässt sich äquivalent wie folgt formulieren [8]: Wir suchen einen Koeffizientenvektor w, welcher das Funktional

$$J(w) = \frac{1}{2\rho}\|AW^T w - y\|_2^2 + \|w\|_1, \quad \rho > 0 \tag{3}$$

minimiert. Der erste Term ist dabei ein Maß für die Datentreue, während der Regularisierungsterm die L1-Norm von w ist. Für die Lösung von (3) wird der Löser YALL1 verwendet [9]. Als Basis für die Wavelet-Zerlegung wurden Haar-Wavelets bis zum Level $n = 2$ ausgewählt. Der Regularisierungsparameter ρ beträgt 0,001.

Wir simulieren Messungen mit Aufnahmewinkeln von 30°, 60° und 90° in Parallelstrahlgeometrie, wobei die Mittelachse durch die linke obere Bilddecke verläuft. Die Winkelschritte zwischen den einzelnen Projektionen betragen jeweils 1°. Bei angenommenen 500 Detektorelementen ist das lineare Gleichungssystem somit in allen drei Fällen unterbestimmt. Zum Vergleich rekonstruieren wir die Messdaten mit Hilfe der gefilterten Rückprojektion.

3 Ergebnisse

Die Ergebnisse der einzelnen Rekonstruktionen bei konstanter Iterationszahl (3000 Iterationen) sind in Abb. 1 gezeigt. In Abb. 1(a) beziehungsweise Abb. 1(b) ist das Rekonstruktionsergebnis der gefilterten Rückprojektion beziehungsweise die Lösung des Minimierungsproblems (3) bei 30° Aufnahmewinkel dargestellt. In Abb. 1(c) und Abb. 1(d) sind die entsprechenden Ergebnisse bei einem Aufnahmewinkel von 60° abgebildet, während die Ergebnisse der Simulation mit 90° Aufnahmewinkel in Abb. 1(e) und Abb. 1(f) aufgeführt sind.

Betrachten wir die mittlere quadratische Abweichung (MSE) des Original-Phantoms U zu unserer Lösung V,

$$\text{MSE}(U, V) = \frac{1}{MN}\sum_{i,j}(U_{i,j} - V_{i,j})^2, \quad U, V \in \mathbb{R}^{M \times N} \tag{4}$$

so ist der MSE für die Rekonstruktionen der Messungen mit Aufnahmewinkeln von 30° und 60° 0,0236 beziehungsweise 0,0134. Für die Messung mit 90° Aufnahmewinkel beträgt der MSE 1,9038e-05.

Die Rechenzeit beträgt bei gewählten 3000 Iterationen 285 Sekunden im Falle des Aufnahmewinkels von 30°. Für die Aufnahmewinkel von 60° beziehungsweise 90° beträgt die Rechenzeit 536 Sekunden beziehungsweise 730 Sekunden. Die Rechenzeit für die gefilterte Rückprojektion beträgt im Vergleich dazu etwa 1-2 Sekunden.

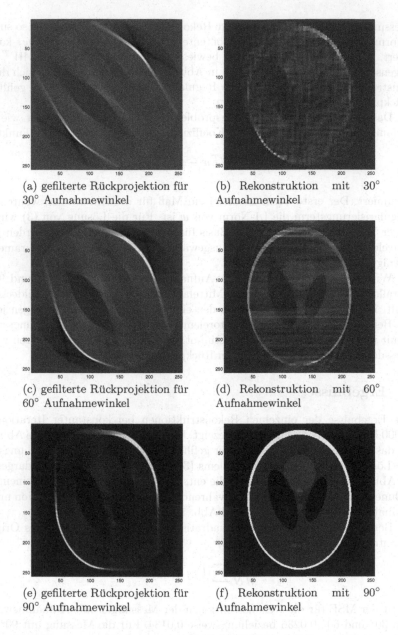

(a) gefilterte Rückprojektion für 30° Aufnahmewinkel

(b) Rekonstruktion mit 30° Aufnahmewinkel

(c) gefilterte Rückprojektion für 60° Aufnahmewinkel

(d) Rekonstruktion mit 60° Aufnahmewinkel

(e) gefilterte Rückprojektion für 90° Aufnahmewinkel

(f) Rekonstruktion mit 90° Aufnahmewinkel

Abb. 1. Rekonstruktionsergebnisse für 3 verschiedene Aufnahmewinkel. Auf der linken Seite ist jeweils das Ergebnis der gefilterten Rückprojektion, während rechts die Lösung des Minimierungsproblems (3) abgebildet ist. Die Winkelschritte zwischen den einzelnen Projektionen betragen jeweils 1°. Die Rekonstruktionen in den oberen beiden Zeilen sind unskaliert. In der unteren Zeile ist der Minimalwert zum besseren Vergleich jeweils auf Null gesetzt

4 Diskussion und Schlussfolgerungen

Mit dem gewählten Ansatz lassen sich nicht nur Strukturen, welche tangential zu den Projektionsrichtungen liegen, sondern Strukturen im gesamten Winkelbereich rekonstruieren. Beispielsweise lassen sich in Abb. 1(b) Kanten im linken oberen Bildbereich erkennen, welche nicht tangential zu den Projektionsrichtungen sind. Die Rekonstruktion mit 90° Aufnahmebereich ist für größere Iterationszahlen perfekt.

Die hier präsentierten Ergebnisse entsprechen im Wesentlichen denen in [4], jedoch wird in unserem Ansatz bei diskret vorliegenden Projektionsdaten eine Umrechnung auf Polarkoordinaten vermieden. Obwohl die Basen des Fourier- und Ortsraums maximal inkohärent sind und sich somit optimal als Basenpaar für die Abtastung beziehungsweise Rekonstruktion eignen [10], erreichen wir ein ähnliches Ergebnis mit der L1-Regularisierung in einer Wavelet-Basis. Somit muss nicht von der Annahme ausgegangen werden, dass radiale Linien des Fourier-Spektrums bekannt seien.

In weiteren Experimenten soll überprüft werden, welche Wavelets sich besonders gut als Basis eignen, eine dünn besetzte Darstellung für medizinische Bilder zu liefern. Des Weiteren soll geprüft werden, inwieweit der Level der Wavelet-Zerlegung Auswirkungen auf die Rekonstruktion hat. Die Rekonstruktionsergebnisse sollen mit der Lösung des Minimierproblems mit TV-Regularisierung verglichen werden.

Danksagung. Diese Arbeit wurde durch die Europäische Union, das Land Schleswig-Holstein (MOIN CC: grant no. 122-09-053) und die „Graduate School for Computing in Medicine and Life Sciences", gegründet durch die Exzellenzinitiative des Bundes und der Länder, unterstützt [DFG GSC 235/1].

Literaturverzeichnis

1. Natterer F, Wübbeling F. Mathematical Methods in Image Reconstruction. Society for Industrial and Applied Mathematics, Philadelphia; 2001.
2. Quinto ET. Tomographic reconstructions from incomplete data-numerical inversion of the exterior Radon transform. Inverse Probl. 1988;4:867–76.
3. Donoho DL. Compressed sensing. IEEE Trans Inform Theory. 2006;52(4):1289–1306.
4. Egiazarian K, Foi A, Katkovnik V. Compressed sensing image reconstruction via recursive spatially adaptive Filtering. In: Proc IEEE ICIP; 2007.
5. Romberg J. Imaging via compressive sampling. IEEE Signal Process Mag. 2008;25(2):14–20.
6. Buzug TM. Computed Tomography. Springer, Berlin Heidelberg; 2008.
7. Candes EJ, Tao T. Near-optimal signal recovery from random projections: universal encoding Strategies? IEEE Trans Inform Theory. 2006;52(12):5406–25.
8. Elad M. Sparse and Redundant Representations: From Theory to Applications in Signal and Image Processing. Springer, New York; 2010.
9. Zhang Y. User's Guide for YALL1: Your Algorithms for L1 Optimization. Rice University, Houston, Texas; 2009.

10. Candes EJ, Wakin MB. An introduction To compressive sampling. IEEE Signal Process Mag. 2008;25(2):21–30.

Advanced Line Visualization for HARDI

Diana Röttger, Christopher Denter, Stefan Müller

Institute for Computational Visualistics, University of Koblenz-Landau
droettger@uni-koblenz.de

Abstract. Diffusion imaging is a non-invasive technique providing information about neuronal connections. Contrary to diffusion tensor imaging (DTI), high angular resolution diffusion imaging (HARDI) is able to model the diffusion pattern in more detail. Tractography approaches reconstruct fiber pathways and result in line representations, approximating the underlying diffusion behavior. However, these line visualizations often suffer from visual clutter and weak depth perception more than reconstructions resulting from DTI, since multiple fibers potentially run within one voxel. In this approach illustrative rendering methods such as depth-dependent halos and ambient occlusion for line data are presented in combination with crucial tract information such as the direction and integrity for HARDI-based fiber representations.

1 Introduction

Brownian motion in white matter architecture is anisotropic since water molecules move with the fiber course in a larger scale than against it. This fact is used in diffusion imaging to reconstruct trajectories, representing major neuronal pathways. DTI is a very common technique, using a second order tensor to describe the direction and scale of diffusion. However, caused by the Gaussian model assumption, it leads to false representations in complex diffusion profiles. High angular resolution diffusion imaging (HARDI) overcomes this limitation and is able to provide more detailed information through a probability density function (PDF).

Illustrative rendering techniques aim to emphasize important features while de-emphasizing less important ones. This leads to a more comprehensible and more recognizable visualization. In medical visualizations illustrative rendering approaches are motivated by anatomical drawings and often include silhouettes, hatching and shading. In terms of diffusion data, representations often suffer from visual clutter caused by the huge amount of dense lines, approximating neuronal pathways. This especially occurs in HARDI fiber results, since more complex configurations are reconstructed. Therefore, understanding the spatial arrangement of lines is very difficult and perception of tubes is considered to be advantageous over simple line representations. However, tube geometry rendering is computationally expensive. Therefore, view-oriented and tube-like textured triangle strips are frequently used to imitate tubes. Merhof et al. [1] proposed a method using triangle strips and point sprites for white matter tract visualization. A further method for dense line data visualization was introduced by Everts et al. [2]. The authors used a shader-based approach to form a view vector oriented triangle strip and depth-dependent halos to emphasize line bundles. A method for illustrative bundles was introduced by Otten et al. [3]. In our approach we use illustrative line rendering methods and add vital color information in terms of tract course and integrity. Additionally, we integrated an ambient occlusion approach to further enhance depth perception.

2   Materials and methods

In this section the used HARDI dataset, tractography algorithms as well as proposed visual enhancements will be introduced.

2.1   Dataset

We used a human brain HARDI dataset of size $128 \times 128 \times 60$ which was acquired with a voxel size of $1.875 \times 1.875 \times 2$ mm [4]. The applied gradient direction scheme included 200 directions and a b-value of 3000 s/mm^2.

2.2   Fiber reconstruction and visualization

Fiber reconstruction was performed using a distance-based tractography approach for HARDI, published by Röttger et al. [5]. In our approach we used a similar rendering method for generating view oriented triangle strips in the manner of Otten et al. [3]. After pathway reconstruction, lines are rendered using the GL_LINE_STRIP_ADJACENCY_EXT primitive. Subsequently, a shader pipeline is designed to form and texture the view vector oriented triangle strip. Using an adjacency primitive, access to neighboring vertices is provided within the geometry shader. Information about the neighbors of each vertex is used in combination with the view vector to generate oriented triangle strips. For a tube-like coloring, fragments far away from the centerline of the triangle strip fade to black.

2.3   Color mapping

Besides directional color coding using the tangent of a point on the line, fiber integrity indices are of great interest in neuroscientific examinations. Therefore, we applied an orientation distribution function (ODF)-based voxel classification index for HARDI, which was proposed by Röttger et al. [6]. The ODF is analyzed and categorized into the following three compartments: isotropic diffusion profiles and anisotropic diffusion into single and multiple fiber populations. A computation pipeline is used which consists of a classification into white and gray matter and a subsequent separation into one and multiple fiber populations. For visualization, we used a heat color map in which black indicates isotropic diffusion, red multiple fiber and yellow single fiber populations.

2.4 Halo rendering

The generated geometry can be additionally used to illustrate line surrounding halos. In the following visual enhancements to the halos, based on the work by Everts et al. [2], are presented. In this case, similar to the tube-like appearance, parts of the triangle strips are colored either according to a color map or white, white parts represent halos. After having generated the triangle strips with white halos surrounding them, on the one hand halos hide the visual clutter, but on the other hand, it also becomes more difficult to understand areas with a high degree of fiber-density. This is due to the fact that halos of fibers located more in the foreground will hide those very close or even almost parallel to them. To remedy this, Everts et al. suggested to shift the halos in depth along the view vector according to a, in our case linear, function. Therefore, fiber-dense areas are recognizable, since they now have significantly less visible halos. Additionally, we can draw more distant fibers with a smaller line width to support depth perception. This depth cueing approach conveys the idea in which fibers closer to the view port are thicker than those far away.

2.5 Ambient occlusion

Furthermore, shadows are an important aspect in depicting depth. One way of incorporating shadowing in OpenGL renderings that is independent from the complexity of the geometry is Screen-Space Ambient Occlusion (SSAO), first introduced by Mittring [7]. By sampling the depth buffer with a kernel in the neighborhood of any given fragment, we can determine how many neighboring fragments are closer to the viewpoint than the currently examined fragment. This number is used in turn to darken the current fragment's color, based on the assumption that fragments with a higher number of potentially occluding fragments will in general be darker.

3 Results

An illustration of lines showing fibers of the corpus callosum, the major white matter tract in the brain, is displayed in Fig. 1. The tube rendering approach is used in combination with a directional color coding.

Fig. 2 shows the same tube visualization method, but with applied tract integrity color encoding. Yellow parts highlight regions comprising single fiber populations, red multiple fiber populations and black isotropic diffusion. Considering the region of the centrum semiovale, one can clearly estimate the crossing regions of the corticospinal tract and the corpus callosum, indicated in red.

An illustration of the halo visualization with directional color coding is shown in Fig. 3. Depth cueing provides hints about the spatial depth of fibers, in this case blue fibers are further away than red fibers. To emphasize fiber-dense areas, a halo depth shift is performed in the right image.

Fig. 4 displays the tube-like geometry in combination with the screen-space ambient occlusion approach. Occluded lines in the bottom of the image appear darker in the right illustration.

4   Discussion

In this paper we have presented illustrative approaches for tractography results, featuring both advanced line rendering and visualization of diffusion characteristics. The presented approaches lead to an improved visualization of spatial depth for line rendering. An advanced rendering approach including tube visualization, halo generation, depth cueing and screen-space ambient occlusion was shown. By adding color encodings to fiber representations such as pathway direction or tract integrity, visualizations become even more comprehensible and meaningful for neurosurgical examinations.

References

1. Merhof D, Sonntag M, Enders F, et al. Hybrid visualization for white matter tracts using triangle strips and point sprites. IEEE Trans Vis Comput Graph. 2006;12:1181–88.
2. Everts M, Bekker H, Roerdink J, et al. Depth-dependent halos: illustrative rendering of dense line data. IEEE Trans Vis Comput Graph. 2009;15:1299–306.

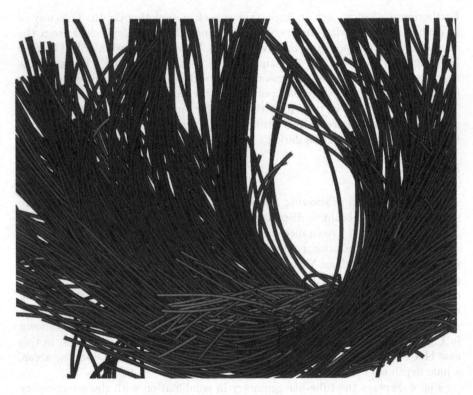

Fig. 1. Tube-like rendering of callosal fibers, represented by view vector oriented triangle strips with applied directional color coding

3. Otten R, Bartroli AV, van de Wetering HMM. Illustrative white matter fiber bundles. Comput Graph Forum. 2010;29(3):1013–22.
4. Poupon C, Poupon F, Allirol L, et al. A database dedicated to anatomo-functional study of human brain connectivity. 12th HBM Neuroimage. 2006;12(646).
5. Röttger D, Seib V, Müller S. Distance-based tractography in high angular resolution diffusion imaging. The Visual Comput. 2011;27:729–39.
6. Röttger D, Dudai D, Merhof D, et al. ISMI: a Classification Index for High Angular Resolution Diffusion Imaging. Proc SPIE. 2012.
7. Mittring M. Finding next gen: CryEngine 2. ACM SIGGRAPH 2007 Courses. 2007; p. 97–121.

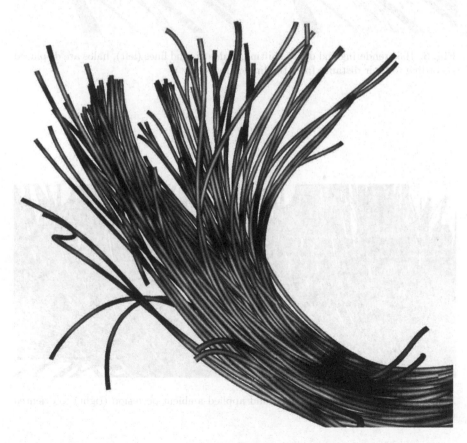

Fig. 2. Tube-like rendering of line representations with applied tract integrity color coding

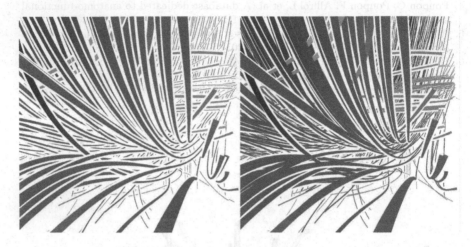

Fig. 3. Halo rendering and depth shifting: halos around lines (left), halos are displaced according to their distance from the line center (right)

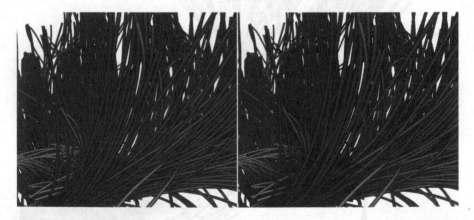

Fig. 4. No ambient occlusion (left) and applied ambient occlusion (right) to oriented color coded line representation

Modellfunktion zur Approximation von Ultraschallkontrastmittelkonzentration zur semi-quantitativen Gewebeperfusionsbestimmung

Kai Ritschel, Claudia Dekomien, Susanne Winter

Institut für Neuroinformatik, Ruhr-Universität Bochum
Kai.Ritschel@ini.ruhr-uni-bochum.de

Kurzfassung. Kontrastmittelultraschall wird zur Diagnose von Tumoren der Leber oder Schlaganfällen eingesetzt. Die Eignung von Kontrastmittelultraschall zur Darstellung von Hirntumoren wurde ebenfalls bereits nachgewiesen. Eine Möglichkeit zur Auswertung ist die Approximation von Modellfunktionen, welche insbesondere den Hauptanstieg der Kontrastmittelkonzentration abbilden. In dieser Arbeit wird ein Modell zur Approximation von Kontrastmittelverläufen in Ultraschalldaten vorgestellt, welches in der Lage ist zusätzlich zu diesem Hauptanstieg weitere Eigenschaften im Zeitverlauf, wie z. B. einen zweiten Anstieg durch Rezirkulation, abzubilden. Das Modell erreichte eine höhere Genauigkeit der Approximation als die zum Vergleich herangezogenen Modelle.

1 Einleitung

Als Ultraschallkontrastmittel werden in der Sonographie hüllenstabilisierte Mikroblasen eingesetzt. Die charakteristischen Eigenschaften des Echos erlauben eine spezifische Abbildung des Kontrastmittels, z. B. durch das $2^{nd} Harmonic-Imaging$. Die nicht gewebegängigen Mikroblasen erlauben es, die Perfusion von Gewebe darzustellen und zu beurteilen.

Bolusinjektionen des Kontrastmittels werden z. B. zur Diagnose von Tumoren der Leber [1] oder Schlaganfällen [2] eingesetzt [3]. Die Veränderung des Gefäßsystems durch das Wachstum von Tumoren führt zu lokalen Veränderungen der Perfusion, welche u. a. bei Neoplasien der Leber erfolgreich identifiziert werden können [1]. Die Eignung von Kontrastmittelultraschall zur Darstellung von Hirntumoren wurde ebenfalls bereits nachgewiesen [4].

Die Interpretation der gewonnenen Bilddaten ist allerdings oft schwierig. Sie erfolgt klinisch zumeist durch visuelle Beurteilung der Bilder. Eine Möglichkeit zur Auswertung ist die Approximation von Modellfunktionen, welche insbesondere den Anstieg der Konzentration abbilden [2, 5, 6]. In dieser Arbeit wird ein neues Modell vorgestellt, welches eine erweiterte Flexibilität aufweist und einen möglichen zweiten Anstieg durch Rezirkulation abbilden kann.

2 Material und Methoden

2.1 Daten

Die in dieser Arbeit verwendeten Video-Datensätze wurden während Tumorresektionsoperationen am offenen Schädel der Patienten aufgenommen. Dabei wurde dem Patienten ein Bolus von 2 ml Ultraschallkontrastmittel in eine Armvene injiziert, um einen möglichst hohen Gradienten der Kontrastmittelkonzentration im Verlauf der Aufnahme zu erzeugen.

Abhängig von den Einstellungen des Ultraschallsystems traten große Unterschiede im Kontrast und damit in der Intensität der Aufnahme auf. Für diese Arbeit wurden drei Datensätze von drei Patienten verwendet. Alle Aufnahmen wurden mit dem Toshiba Aplio XG unter Verwendung der Ultraschallsonde PST-65AT bei einer Mittenfrequenz von 6,5 MHz aufgenommen. Die drei verwendeten Datensätze wurden in einer Auflösung von 340×408 Bildpunkten über einen Zeitraum von ca. 80 sek. aufgezeichnet.

2.2 Modellfunktionen

Da die Messdaten starkes Rauschen aufweisen, werden Modellfunktionen an die Daten angepasst und zur Auswertung und Interpretation verwendet. Drei in der Literatur verwendete Modelle wurden anhand eines idealen Verlaufs der Bolusinjektion entworfen und bilden einen zweiten Anstieg der Konzentration nicht ab. Das *Gamma Variate Function Model* erlaubt es, den Anstieg durch eine exponentielle Wachstumsfunktion zu modellieren [5]. Diese Modellierung führt zu einer direkten Abhängigkeit der Abfallgeschwindigkeit v_{out} von der Anflußgeschwindigkeit v_{in}. Das *Bolus Kinetic Function Model* [7] ermöglicht es hingegen, durch einen anderen Modellansatz die beiden Geschwindigkeiten unabhängig voneinander zu modellieren. Im *Bolus Method Function Model* [6] wurde das *Bolus Kinetic Function Model* um einen Parameter erweitert, welcher unterschiedliche Werte vor und nach dem Anstieg modelliert. Das Modell kann so beispielsweise eine verbleibende Konzentration des Kontrastmittels abbilden.

Das in dieser Arbeit entwickelte Modell $I_{sig}(t)$ verwendet eine Kombination von vier sigmoiden Funktionen, um den Verlauf der Intensität in der Zeit t abzubilden. Mit dieser Funktion kann z. B. auch ein zweiter Anstieg durch Rezirkulation abgebildet werden. Jede einzelne der sigmoiden Funktionen wird durch drei Parameter bestimmt. Die Amplitude der ersten Sigmoiden wird durch a_1 realisiert. Die Geschwindigkeit des Anstiegs wird durch v_1 beschrieben und der Parameter t_1 bezeichnet den mittleren Zeitpunkt des Anstiegs der Funktion. Die Parameter der drei weiteren sigmoiden Funktionen verhalten sich analog. Die Parameter t_1 bis t_4 beschreiben dabei die Verschiebung der Sigmoiden relativ zur vorherigen. Der Parameter b beschreibt die Grundintensität vor dem Anstieg (Formel 1).

Tabelle 1. Durchschnittlicher Fehler der vier Modelle über drei Datensätze je Gewebetyp

Modell	Tumor	Gefäß	Normal	Durchschnitt
Gamma Variate Function Model	3,12	6,50	1,74	3,78
Bolus Kinetic Function Model	3,12	6,48	1,83	3,81
Bolus Method Function Model	2,79	6,35	1,82	3,66
Sigmoide Kombination	2,63	5,81	1,78	3,41

$$
\begin{aligned}
I_{\text{sig}}(t) = b &+ \frac{a_1}{1 + e^{-v_1 \cdot (t - t_1)}} + \frac{-a_2}{1 + e^{-v_2 \cdot (t - t_1 - t_2)}} \\
&+ \frac{a_3}{1 + e^{-v_3 \cdot (t - t_1 - t_2 - t_3)}} + \frac{-a_4}{1 + e^{-v_4 \cdot (t - t_1 - t_2 - t_3 - t_4)}}
\end{aligned}
\tag{1}
$$

2.3 Optimierungsalgorithmen

Zur Approximation der Modellparameter wurden zwei Optimierungsalgorithmen, das gradientenbasierte Rprop-Verfahren [8] und die evolutionäre Strategie CMA-ES [9] eingesetzt und miteinander verglichen. Das Optimierungsproblem bestand dabei in der Minimierung einer Fehlerfunktion, dem *Mean Squared Error* (MSE). Hierbei wird der Abstand der approximierten Modellkurve zum Intensitätsverlauf als Fehler verwendet.

3 Ergebnisse

In drei Datensätzen wurde je eine Tumor- und Gefäßregion sowie ein gesunder Bereich ausgewählt und mit jedem der vier vorgestellten Modelle approximiert. Die Approximation wurde mit den beiden Algorithmen Rprop und CMA-ES durchgeführt, die Startbedingungen der Algorithmen waren identisch.

Die Laufzeiten und Fehler wurden über die Modelle pro Datensatz gemittelt. Keiner der beiden Algorithmen Rprop und CMA-ES konnte eindeutig als schneller oder präziser identifiziert werden. Die erreichte Qualität der Approximationen durch die Modelle ist in Abb. 1 beispielhaft am Verlauf über eine Tumorregion dargestellt.

Alle vier Modelle bilden den ersten Anstieg der Intensität ab. Unterschiede bestehen vor allem in den Bereichen der Grundintensität und des Abfalls der Konzentration. Die Kombination sigmoider Funktionen approximiert zusätzlich den zweiten Anstieg der Intensität und erreicht auf allen Datensätzen in allen Regionen -bis auf einen Wert- den niedrigsten Fehlerwert bei der Approximation der Messdaten (Tab. 1). Das sigmoide Modell erreichte einen durchschnittlichen Fehler von 3,41, die anderen Modelle erreichten Werte zwischen 3,66 und 3,81.

Zusätzlich zu diesen 72 Approximationen wurde für einen gesamten Datensatz der Verlauf der Intensitätsänderung an jedem Bildpunkt durch die vier

Abb. 1. Intensitätsverlauf von Ultraschallkontrastmittel über einer Tumorregion und die durch CMA-ES approximierten Modellverläufe. Die Kombination der Sigmoiden modelliert zusätzlich den zweiten Anstieg der Intensität

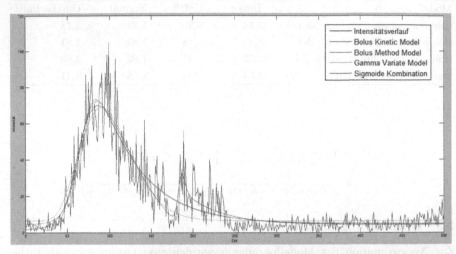

Abb. 2. Einzelbild einer kontrastmittel-spezifischen Ultra-schallaufnahme

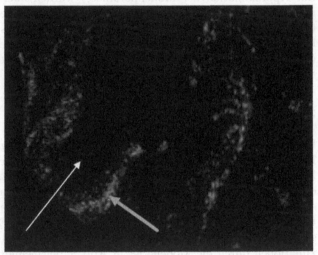

Modelle approximiert. Abb. 3 zeigt ein Einzelbild des hier verwendeten Datensatzes. Es können einige größere Blutgefäße visuell identifiziert werden. Abb. 4 und Abb. 5 zeigen zwei Parameter der sigmoiden Modellfunktion: den erreichten Fitnesswert und den maximalen Wert des Modellkurvenverlaufs.

In beiden Parameterbildern stellen sich die Gefäße gut dar. Im Randbereich des abgebildeten Tumors zeigt sich eine graduelle Abnahme der Intensitäten zum Tumorzentrum hin. Im Gegensatz dazu zeigt sich auf der tumorabgewandten Seite eine scharfe Begrenzung der Gefäße.

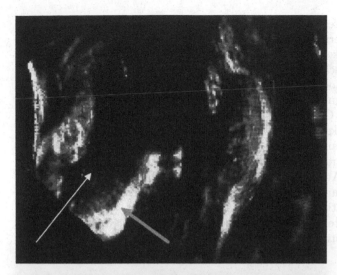

Abb. 3. Darstellung der – durch die CMA-ES erreichten – Fitness des sigmoiden Modells

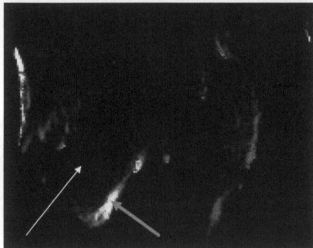

Abb. 4. Darstellung des Maximums des Modellverlaufs des sigmoiden Modells; der dünne Pfeil zeigt die Mitte des Tumors, der dicke Pfeil ein am Tumorrand liegendes Gefäß

4 Diskussion

Es konnte gezeigt werden, dass die hier vorgestellte Modellfunktion die Messdaten mit einem geringeren Fehler approximieren kann als die zum Vergleich herangezogenen exponentiellen Modelle [2, 5, 6].

Die Parameter beeinflussen den Verlauf der Modellkurven auf sehr unterschiedliche Weise, sodass ein direkter Vergleich der entsprechenden Parameter der Modelle nicht möglich war. Die Darstellung des Maximums des Kurvenverlaufs in Abb. 4 erlaubt eine visuelle Beurteilung der Blutgefäße im Bereich der Aufnahme. Eine Interpretation der einzelnen Parameter in Bezug auf die Art des zugrunde liegenden Gewebes ist nur bedingt möglich. Die Abb. 3 und Abb. 4

zeigen einen weichen Verlauf der Parameter in den Randbereichen des abgebildeten Tumors; diese Perfusion des Gewebes ist nicht direkt auf den verwendeten Ultraschalldaten zu erkennen.

Um das starke Rauschen in den Zeitverläufen zu unterdrücken, sollen in einem nächsten Schritt die Modellkurven an geglättete Daten approximiert werden.

Zudem soll die Eignung von modellunabhängigen Parametern zur Bestimmung des abgebildeten Gewebetyps untersucht werden, um die Anwendung einer automatischen Klassifikation zu ermöglichen. Die modellunabhängigen Parameter können je Modell analytisch anhand der Parameter bestimmt werden und bilden so die Modellparameter auf diagnostisch relevante Kenngrößen ab.

Die diagnostische Aussagekraft des in den Daten abgebildeten zweiten Anstiegs ist derzeit unbekannt. In den bisher bekannten Modellen wird nur der erste Anstieg des Konzentrationsverlaufes betrachtet.

Das hier vorgestellte Modell soll unter Verwendung eines Klassifikators zeigen, ob der zweite Anstieg zusätzliche Informationen zur Perfusion des abgebildeten Gewebes liefert.

Danksagung. Wir bedanken uns bei I. Pechlivanis, Universitätsklinik für Neurochirurgie in Mannheim, für die freundliche Bereitstellung der Kontrastmittelaufnahmen.

Literaturverzeichnis

1. Albrecht T, Oldenburg A, Homann J, et al. Imaging of liver metastases with contrast-specific low-MI real-time ultrasound and SonoVue. Eur Radiol. 2003;13(3):79–86.
2. Seidel G, Meairs S. Ultrasound contrast agents in ischemic stroke. Cerebrovasc Dis. 2009;2:25–39.
3. Claudon M, Cosgrove D, Albrecht T, et al. Guidlines and good clinical practice recommendations for contrast enhanced ultrasound (CEUS). Eur J Ultrasound. 2008;29:28–44.
4. Engelhardt M, Hansen C, Schmieder K, et al. Feasibility of contrast-enhanced sonography during resection of cerebral tumours: Initial results of a prospective study. Ultrasound Med Biol. 2007;33(4):571–5.
5. Esaote. Qonstrast-Operator manual; 2006. Technisches Handbuch.
6. Hansen C. Kontrastmittelspezifische Ultraschall-Computertomographie. Ruhr-Universität Bochum. Bochum, Deutschland; 2009.
7. Eyding J, Hölscher T, Postert T. Transkranielle Neurosonologie beim akuten Schlaganfall. Dt Ärzteblatt. 2007;6:340–6.
8. Igel C, Hüsken M. Improving the Rprop learning algorithm. In: Proc 2nd ISBC; 2000. p. 115–121.
9. Suttorp T, Hansen N, Igel C. Efficient covariance matrix update for variable metric evolution strategies. Machine Learning. 2009;75:167–97.

Diameter Measurement of Vascular Structures in Ultrasound Video Sequences

Matthias Bremser[1,2], Uwe Mittag[2], Tobias Weber[2], Jörn Rittweger[2],
Rainer Herpers[1,3,4]

[1]University of Applied Sciences Bonn-Rhine-Sieg, Department of Computer Science
[2]German Aerospace Center, Institute of Aerospace Medicine
[3]Dept. of Computer Science and Engineering, York University,Toronto, Canada
[4]Faculty of Computer Science, University of New Brunswick, Fredericton, Canada
matthias@bremser.eu

Abstract. Diameter measurements of vessel structures are of interest
for a number of cardiovascular examinations. To support manual analysis of duplex ultrasound (US) images of human vessels and to improve the
measurement accuracy and reproducibility, a semi-automatic approach
has been developed which applies image processing techniques to compute reliably the vessel diameter. The proposed approach presents an
interactive tool for measuring vessel diameters from US image sequences.
A first derivative of a Gaussian (DoG) is applied for vessel wall detection
followed up by a skeletonization step, and computation of horizontal line
segments. Within a final classification step those line segments which
show the highest likelihood are selected. The classification score is computed based on length, edge strength and linearity information. The
overall approach has been evaluated at several sample sequences showing results outperforming "manual" measurements. It is currently applied
in physiological studies.

1 Introduction

The function and structure of the human vessel system is a fundamental factor
regarding cardiovascular health. Both elements are highly adaptable to its environmental conditions, for example micro-gravity. Vascular ultrasound scanning
is a proven method to assess human vessel structure and function [1, 2, 3].

US assessments are usually performed on computer aided basis. There are
semi-automatic and complete automatic algorithms. The algorithms cover a
range of different kinds of techniques. Early approaches use image differentiation
to detect the vessel walls [4]. However, most up-to-date approaches are using
an active contours technique [5, 6], also called snake. The snake model defines
a curve based upon prior knowledge, approaching the vessel wall by adjusting
parameters, iteratively. Differentiation methods, however, are straight forward
edge detection techniques, and are therefore less computationally intensive.

Ordinary US devices are capable of analyzing the diameter of vascular structures under certain requirements during acquisition. In general, they are designed for single frame based measurements on current preselected images but

not for systematic analysis of US time series. For some in particular scientific applications however, repeated analysis of very precise measurements are necessary, to determine vascular changes e.g. during exercise conditions. At DLR aerospace center physiological studies are conducted which search for vascular adaptation mechanisms durning special conditions (e.g. exercise, zero-gravity). Therefore, the proposed approach has been developed to extend the basic capabilities of standard video output out of different standard US devices by semi-automatic stand-alone post-acquisition analysis procedures. It does not compete with complex raw data analysis methods. Prior knowledge and edge detection methods are combined to provide a less intensive, but reliable vessel wall detection approach. Additional features like archiving of analysis configurations and synchronous automatic extraction of text information from the video frames by OCR are provided as well.

2   Materials and Methods

During the development process US data of several areas of healthy adult human bodies (male + female; arteria femoralis superficialis, arteria brachialis) at a resolution of 330×290, 8-bit grayscale, have been used. US data are preprocessed by automatic cropping of the central area of interest form the raw image sequence. Fig. 1 shows a sample B-mode US image and a schematic illustration of the notation of near wall, far wall, lumen, and diameter. US images in general

Fig. 1. Sample US image area (enlarged) of a healthy adult human including a schematic illustration of the used notation and setup

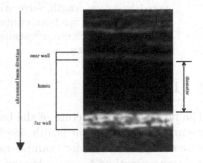

suffer from noise and artifacts and may differ strongly in quality from subject to subject and device to device. Depending on the individual habitus, higher amounts of tissue surrounding the blood vessel usually leads to poor quality of the US images. Most noted kind of noise is the so called speckle noise [5, 6, 7] causing the typical speckle type structures in ultrasound images (Fig. 2a). Also, blood backscattering the US waves may result in a distribution of gray values in the more or less homogeneous vessel lumen (Fig. 2b). Especially the appearance of the far wall is affect by high blood scattering (Fig. 2c). Other sources of disturbances of the US signal are echo shadows [6, 5] (Fig. 2d). Echo shadows may appear behind strong reflecting v essel walls or when tissue is absorbing

Fig. 2. Examples of different noise and artifacts in ultrasound scans. The images have been inverted for better conspicuity. a: Typical speckle noise of US scans. b: Blood backscattering causing artifacts in the lumen. c: Excessive blood backscattering texturing the vessel wall. d: Echo shadow behind strong reflecting vessel wall

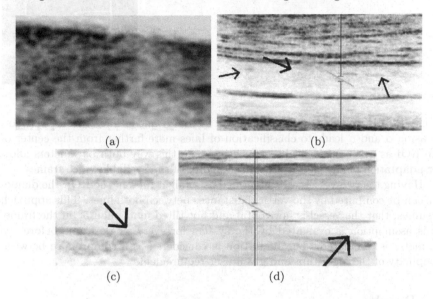

(a)   (b)

(c)   (d)

the US signal. Principle steps of the approach are to first apply edge detection methods, then identify both edges on the vessel walls and finally measure the diameter between the two. A region of interest (ROI) has to be defined where diameter measurement should be executed. This ROI selection has to be done in a way, that it is appropriate for the entire set of frames under investigation. In this step the experience of the operator, where best results can be expected, and his special anatomical interest need to be considered. In the next step the image sequences are subsequently analyzed frame-by-frame. To detect the vessel walls, a longitudinal first derivative of a Gaussian filter is applied. It has been shown, that a DoG parameterization of $\sigma_{xx} \leftarrow 10$ and $\sigma_{yy} \leftarrow 5$ for $(7\sigma_{xx} \times 7\sigma_{yy})$ kernel sizes result in meaningful values for our data sets. In the next process step the edge images are skeletonized and smaller edge segments are excluded. Adjacent edge elements are computed to horizontal "Line"structures (horizontal lines are defined quite generously (Fig. 3)). Each line is considered as a candidate for a vessel wall. During a classification step the most likely line segment pair is determined as near and far vessel wall representatives. Fig. 3 shows typical pattern of computed line candidates (all horizontal lines) and the final selection of the vessel wall representatives (dashed lines). The classification of the line segments as edges of the vessel walls is computed on the basis of length, edge strength, linear regression coefficient, and distance to the vertical center of the ROI, for each line. Length, edge strength and linear regression coefficient are mandatory for the classification process while the distance of the line to the vertical center

Fig. 3. Computed line segments and selected near and far vessel wall candidates (dashed) of arteria femoralis superficialis

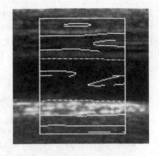

of the ROI is weighted by two tolerance factors α and β have to be given. Increasing α and β leads to classification of lines more farther from the center of the ROI as near and far walls, respectively. In this way both parameters allow for adaptation of the algorithm to the quality of the available video frames.

Having the two vessel walls identified as straight lines in the ROI, the diameter can be computed by the vertical distances between both lines. This approach assumes, that the vessel is horizontal and not tilted more than 5° in the frame. This assumption is evaluated by the system for every single frame before the diameter is calculated. The limitation is considered as a compromise between simplicity of the algorithm and given user requirements.

3   Results

An evaluation of the approach has been conducted at DLR aerospace center. Manual measurements of image sequences of 6 subjects performed by 2 examiners, summing up to 15,608 frames, have been compared to diameter measurements obtained by the approach as well operated by the both raters. All measurements were obtained twice. Manual measurements were obtained on the basis of a reduced set of frames.

The intra-individual deviations were obtained by calculating the absolute differences of frame measurements of both iterations and then averaging all those differences. Table 1 lists the intra-tester and inter-tester deviations in millimeters that were obtained. The chart in Fig. 3 shows the measurement results of one

Table 1. Intra-tester and inter-tester deviation (manually and automatic): For intra-tester absolute difference between 2 measurements; for inter-tester mean of value of 2 measurements per frame and tester respectively; Average deviation over all testers and frames

Deviation	mm	Std.
Intra-tester manual	0.209	0.232
Intra-tester automatic	0.130	0.251
Inter-tester manual	0.173	0.202
Inter-tester automatic	0.014	0.016

sample examined sequence. The measurement results computed by the approach, on average, lie between both results of manual measurement, concluding a lower inter-individual deviation. For the evaluations conducted, the ground truth of the vessel diameter should be considered as rather constant. However due to the current of the blood flow within a living subject the measurements may vary naturally in a range of ± 10%. Variations of this magnitude, however, may not occure within the range of preselected frames as we have seen it during purely manual measurements. Fig. 5 shows results of the sequential frames analysis of one sequence. It can be seen that approach constitutes accuracy and stability by capturing characteristic movement of the blood vessel walls generated by pulse effects. A clear advantage over the manual measurements is obvious, the latter not being able to resolve the pulse shape.

4 Discussion

The evaluation shows, that the results for semi-automatic diameter detection vary less or similar in comparison to the manual results. The measured values, in principle, lie between the results of manual assessment. Comparison to manual measurements have been the basis for evaluation of the results. Not only the coherence of the manual and semi-automatic results, was considered as convincing enough for a practical application.

The approach turned out to be reliable and flexible and has already shown it's main benefit, that lies in it's enormous saving of time. The approach has

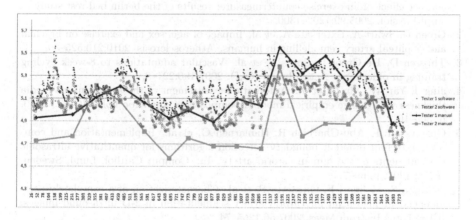

Fig. 4. Measurement results of a sample sequence obtained by both examiners, manually and by the proposed approach. The abscissa shows frame numbers. The ordinate axis shows measured lumen diameter in mm. The values shown, are the mean of both iterations with the support of the approach and manual reference. Offset of start and stop frames were defined by the operators due to the quality of the video sequences. It is clearly visible that the diameter variations of the manual references vary more than the approach supported ones

Fig. 5. Measurement results a sample sequence where 75 sequential frames have been analyzed by both testers, manually and semi-automatically

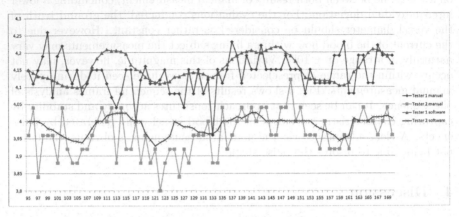

proven its performance in two physiological studies with 28 subjects to assess vascular adaptations to resistive vibration exercises on the one hand and to immobilization on the other, at DLR aerospace center.

References

1. Bleeker M, De Groot P, Rongen G, et al. Vascular adaptation to deconditioning and the effect of an exercise countermeasure: results of the berlin bed rest study. J Appl Physiol. 2005;99:1293–1300.
2. Green D, Swart A, Exterkate A, et al. Impact of age, sex and exercise on brachial and popliteal artery remodelling in humans. Atherosclerosis. 2010;210:525–30.
3. Thijssen D, De Groot P, Smits P, et al. Vascular adaptations to 8-week cycling training in older men. Acta Physiol (Oxf). 2007;190:221–8.
4. Jing J, Yan W, Xin G, et al. Automatic measurement of the artery intima-media thickness with image empirical mode decomposition. In: Proc IEEE ICIST; 2010. p. 306–10.
5. Gustavsson T, Abu-Gharbieh R, Hamarneh G, et al. Implementation and comparison of four different boundary detection algorithms for quantitative ultrasonic measurements of the human carotid artery. In: Comput Cardiol. Lund, Sweden: IEEE; 1997. p. 69–72.
6. Delsanto S, Molinari F, Giustetto P, et al. Characterization of a completely user-independent algorithm for carotid artery segmentation in 2-D ultrasound images. IEEE Trans Instrum Meas. 2007;56:1265–74.
7. Loizou C, Pattichis C, Christodoulou, et al. Comparative evaluation of despeckle filtering in ultrasound imaging of the carotid artery. IEEE Trans Ultrason Ferroelectr Freq Control. 2005;52:1653–69.

Ein Prototyp zur Planung von Bohrpfaden für die minimal-invasive Chirurgie an der Otobasis

Ralf Gutbell, Meike Becker, Stefan Wesarg

Graphisch-Interaktive Systeme, TU Darmstadt
meike.becker@gris.tu-darmstadt.de

Kurzfassung. Bei Operationen an der Otobasis ist es wichtig, umliegende Risikostrukturen wie Gesichtsnerv oder Blutgefäße nicht zu verletzen. Bisher legt der Arzt dazu alle Strukturen frei. Unser Forschungsprojekt untersucht nun einen minimal-invasiven Multi-Port-Ansatz. Im Rahmen dieses Projektes haben wir basierend auf SOFA einen Prototypen zur Planung von Bohrpfaden an der Otobasis entwickelt. Damit kann der Arzt sowohl einen Bohrkanal genauer analysieren als auch sich die Menge aller zulässigen Pfade anzeigen lassen, aus der er schließlich die besten Bohrpfade für die Operation auswählt. Dies ist ein erster Schritt, den Arzt bei der Planung von mehreren Bohrkanälen zu unterstützen.

1 Einleitung

Im Rahmen des Forschungsprojektes MUKNO (DFG Forschergruppe FOR 1585, http://www.mukno.de) soll die Durchführung minimal-invasiver Operationsverfahren an der Otobasis (z.B. Kochleaimplantate, Tumorentfernungen) untersucht werden. Bisher legt der Chirurg bei diesen Eingriffen alle Strukturen frei. Um das Risiko für den Patienten zu minimieren und die Reproduzierbarkeit zu erhöhen, soll in Zukunft nur mittels mehrerer linearer Bohrkänale gearbeitet werden. Je nach Anwendung sind bis zu drei Bohrkanäle sinnvoll, um mit Endoskop sowie ein bis zwei Instrumenten am Ziel des Eingriffs zu operieren. Dabei ist es wichtig, dass bestimmte Strukturen, wie z. B. der Gesichtsnerv oder die innere Halsschlagader beim Bohrvorgang nicht verletzt werden. Daher ist eine genaue Planung der Bohrkanäle unumgänglich.

Zur Planung von Trajektorien wurden in der Neurochirurgie und Abdominalchirurgie verschiedene Ansätze entwickelt [1, 2, 3, 4, 5]. In der Hals-Nasen-Ohren-Chirurgie gibt es nur wenige Arbeiten zu diesem Thema [6, 7]. Außer Riechmann et al. betrachten diese Arbeiten nur eine einzelne Trajektorie. Riechmann et al. ermöglichen das manuelle Platzieren mehrerer einzelner Bohrkanäle, jedoch findet keine automatische Bestimmung einer Kombination mehrerer Bohrkanäle statt.

Im Folgenden stellen wir unseren Prototypen zur Planung von Bohrpfadkombinationen an der Otobasis für einen Multi-Port-Ansatz vor. Dabei wird sowohl der Sicherheitsabstand zu den Risikostrukturen als auch die Unsicherheit in der Bohrbewegung berücksichtigt.

2   Material und Methoden

Unser Planungstool basiert auf dem Simulationsframework Simulation Open Framework Architecture (SOFA) [8], welches auf medizinische Anwendungen zugeschnitten ist. Ein großer Vorteil von SOFA ist, dass wir jede anatomische Struktur durch mehrere Modelle (visuelles Modell, Kollisionsmodell, physikalisches Modell) darstellen können und so z. B. Zusatzinformationen, wie der minimale Sicherheitsabstand zu den Risikostrukturen und die Unsicherheit in der Bohrbewegung, bei der Kollisionsberechnung und der Visualisierung unterschiedlich behandelt werden können. Des Weiteren sind verschiedene Algorithmen für Kollisionsdetektion und Zeitintegration implementiert.

Unser Prototyp besteht aus zwei Komponenten, die im Folgenden näher erläutert werden: der manuellen Suche, bei der ein bestimmter Bohrkanal genauer analysiert werden kann und der automatischen Suche, bei der alle zulässigen Bohrkanäle berechnet werden.

2.1   Analyse eines Bohrkanals

Zunächst werden die aus den Computertomographiedaten des Patienten rekonstruierten 3D-Modelle als Szene in SOFA geladen. In Abb. 1 ist eine solche SOFA-Szene abgebildet. In dieser Szene gibt der Arzt den Start- und Endpunkt des Bohrkanals vor. Dann wird der Bohrvorschub mit der zeitabhängigen Simulation von SOFA visualisiert. Für jeden Zeitschritt prüfen wir auf Kollision des Bohrers mit den Risikostrukturen. Als Kollisionsmodell für den Bohrer verwenden wir eine Kugel, deren Radius r_{Kugel} von der Größe des Bohrkopfes r_{Bohrer}

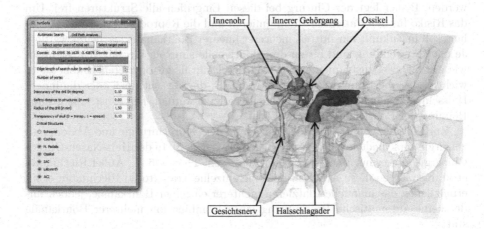

Abb. 1. SOFA-Szene. Auf der linken Seite ist unser Graphisches User-Interface zur Parametereingabe und Steuerung des Planungstools abgebildet. Auf der rechten Seite sehen wir den Schädel (transparent) mit den kritischen Strukturen

sowie den folgenden zwei Parametern abhängt: dem vorgegebenen minimalen Sicherheitsabstand d_{min} zu den Risikostrukturen sowie der Bewegungsungenauigkeit des Bohrers α_{Bohrer}. Sei d_{curr} die Distanz vom Startpunkt zur aktuellen Position auf dem Bohrkanal. Dann ist der Radius der Kugel wie folgt definiert

$$r_{Kugel} = r_{Bohrer} + d_{min} + \tan(\alpha_{Bohrer})d_{curr} \tag{1}$$

Für die Risikostrukturen verwenden wir das Dreiecksnetz des visuellen Modells auch als Kollisionsmodell.

Visualisiert wird eine Kollision mit einer Risikostruktur, indem die entsprechenden Dreiecke auf der Risikostruktur rot hervorgehoben werden (Abb. 2(b)). Die Bewegungsungenauigkeit des Bohrers wird durch einen semi-transparenten, wachsenden Bohrkopf visualisiert, damit der Betrachter ein Gefühl für diesen Faktor bekommt (Abb. 2(a)). Für diese Visualisierungen haben wir die Module von SOFA entsprechend erweitert.

Ein weiteres Feature ist, dass der Arzt die Perspektive wählen kann, aus der er die Szene betrachtet: entweder kann der Arzt wie üblich von außen auf die Szene schauen, oder die Kamera wird kurz hinter dem Bohrkopf positioniert. Im zweiten Fall hat der Arzt die Möglichkeit, entlang des Bohrkanals zu „fliegen", um ein räumliches Gefühl für die Abstände zu bekommen.

2.2   Bestimmung aller zulässigen Bohrkanäle

Bei der zweiten Komponente bestimmen wir alle zulässigen Bohrkanäle für die gegebenen Patientendaten. Dazu markiert der Arzt zunächst den Zielpunkt des Bohrkanals in der Szene, sowie einen Punkt auf dem Schädel. Um diesen Punkt

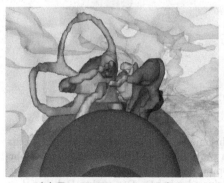 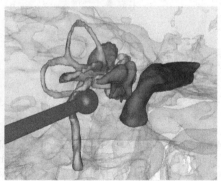

(a) Bewegungsungenauigkeit   (b) Kollision mit dem Gesichtsnerv

Abb. 2. Simulation des Bohrvorschubs für einen Bohrkanal. Die Bewegungsungenauigkeit des Bohrers wird durch eine semi-transparente Kugel um den Bohrkopf visualisiert (links). Kollidiert ein Bohrkanal mit den kritischen Strukturen, so werden die Dreiecke rot eingefärbt (rechts). Links wurde die Kamera auf dem Bohrkopf fixiert, während rechts die übliche Ansicht mit fixem Beobachter gewählt wurde

werden durch Nachbarschaftssuche auf dem Kollisionsmodell alle Dreiecke in einem bestimmten Bereich extrahiert. Die Mittelpunkte dieser Dreiecke bilden die Startmenge, von der aus Bohrpfade zum Zielpunkt getestet werden.

Zwischen jedem Mittelpunkt der Startmenge und dem Endpunkt wird nun ein Kegelstumpf aufgespannt. Seine Größe hängt von dem Mindestabstand zu den Risikostrukturen und der Bewegungsungenauigkeit des Bohrers ab. Den Kegelstumpf haben wir als neues Kollisionsmodell zu SOFA hinzugefügt. Für jeden Kegelstumpf wird geprüft, ob er mit einer Risikostruktur kollidiert. Dadurch erhalten wir die Menge der zulässigen Bohrkanäle (Abb. 3(a)). Anschließend kann der Arzt aus dieser Menge der zulässigen Bohrkanäle die drei auswählen, die er als am geeignetsten erachtet. Als ein mögliches Kriterium haben wir in Rücksprache mit den Ärzten den Winkel zwischen den Bohrpfaden ausgewählt und bieten die Möglichkeit, die drei Bohrpfade mit dem stumpfesten Winkel zueinander anzeigen zu lassen (Abb. 3(b)). Gleichzeitg achten wir dabei darauf, dass die Winkel möglichst gleichgroß sind.

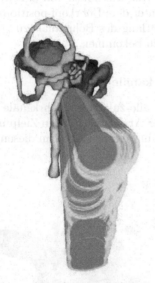 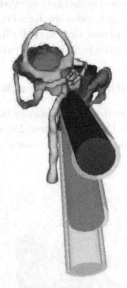

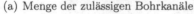

(a) Menge der zulässigen Bohrkanäle   (b) Bohrkanalkombination

Abb. 3. Automatische Bestimmung der Bohrkanäle. Zunächst wird die Menge der zulässigen Bohrkanäle berechnet (links). Dann werden daraus Kombinationen von Bohrkanälen bestimmt (rechts). Hier ist eine Kombinationen abgebildet, bei der die Bohrkanäle einen möglichst stumpfen Winkel zueinander haben. Der exakte Bohrkanal ist opak dargestellt, während der Mindestabstand und die Bohrungenauigkeit transparent gezeichnet werden. Für eine bessere Sicht wurde der Schädel ausgeblendet

3   Experimente

Wir haben unseren Prototypen mit jeweils der rechten Otobasis aus drei Computertomographiedatensätzen getestet. Dazu wurden die Risikostrukturen Gesichtsnerv, innere Halsschlagader, Ossikel und Innenohr zunächst manuell segmentiert und der Schädel durch ein einfaches Schwellwertverfahren extrahiert. In Zukunft wollen wir semi-automatisch segmentieren. Die 3D-Modelle wurden als Szene in SOFA geladen. Anschließend haben wir die zulässige Menge an Bohrpfaden für jeden Patienten bestimmt und uns die nach den in Abschnitt 2.2 beschriebenen Kriterien beste Bohrpfadkombination anzeigen lassen. Des Weiteren haben wir einzelne Bohrpfade mit der manuellen Suche genauer analysiert und konnten uns so für jeden Punkt des Bohrkanals ansehen, wieviel Abstand zu den umliegenden Risikostrukturen bleibt.

Die Parameter wurden wie folgt gewählt: der Radius des Bohrer betrug $1.5\,mm$ und die Bohrungenauigkeit haben wir auf 0.1 Grad festgesetzt. Der Mindestabstand zu den Risikostrukturen betrug für den ersten Patienten $0.5\,mm$ und wurde für den zweiten und dritten Patienten nicht berücksichtigt. Für diese Parameter haben wir in allen drei Fällen zulässige Bohrkanäle gefunden. Eine Bohrkanalkombination, die basierend auf diesen Parametern am besten ist, haben wir für den ersten Patient in Abb. 3(b) abgebildet und für den zweiten und dritten Patienten in Abb. 4 dargestellt.

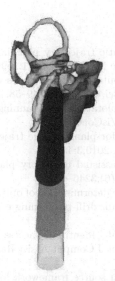 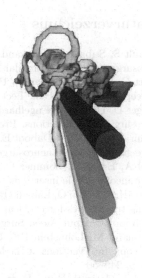

(a) Bohrkombination zweiter Patient   (b) Bohrkombination dritter Patient

Abb. 4. Ergebnisse der Experimente. Hier ist jeweils die Bohrkombination abgebildet, bei der die Bohrkanäle gleichzeitig einen möglichst gleichgroßen und möglichst stumpfen Winkel zueinander haben. Für eine bessere Sicht wurde der Schädel ausgeblendet

4   Diskussion

In dieser Arbeit haben wir unseren Prototypen zur Planung von Bohrpfaden an der Otobasis vorgestellt. Dabei haben wir SOFA um spezifische Komponenten für die Simulation in der Schädelbasischirurgie erweitert.

Zur Zeit verwenden wir für die Bestimmung der zulässigen Bohrkanäle die Brute-Force-Methode. Obwohl diese relativ schnell ist, wollen wir eine effizientere Methode implementieren. Des Weiteren kann durch eine verbesserte Visualisierung (wie z. B. von Röttger et al. [3] vorgestellt) der Arzt noch besser bei der Analyse der Bohrkanäle unterstützt werden.

Unser Prototyp ist ein erster Schritt in Richtung Multi-Port-Knochenchirurgie. Der nächste Schritt ist nun eine Evaluation durch die Ärzte. Der Arzt bestimmt mit Hilfe unseres Planungstools geeignete Bohrpfade für eine Reihe von Patienten. Anhand dieser Daten können wir statistisch lernen, was eine sinnvolle Kombination von Bohrkanälen ist und in einem weiteren Schritt diese Bohrkanäle automatisch bestimmen.

Danksagung

Diese Arbeit wurde von der Deutschen Forschungsgesellschaft (DFG) gefördert: FOR 1585; FE 431/13-1.

Literaturverzeichnis

1. Bériault S, Subaie FA, Mokand K, et al. Automatic trajectory planning of DBS neurosurgery from multi-modal MRI datasets. Proc MICCAI. 2011;1:259–66.
2. Essert C, Haegelen C, Jannin P. Automatic computation of electrodes trajectory for deep brain stimulation. Lect Notes Computer Sci. 2010;6326:149–58.
3. Röttger D, Denter C, Engelhardt S, et al. An Exploration and Planning Tool for Neurosurgical Interventions. Proc IEEE VisWeek VisContest. 2010.
4. Shamir RR, Tamir I, Dabool E, et al. A method for planning safe trajectories in image-guided keyhole neurosurgery. Proc MICCAI. 2010;3:457–64.
5. Seitel A, Engel M, Sommer C, et al. Computer-assisted trajectory planning for percutaneous needle insertions. Med Phys. 2011;38(6):3246–60.
6. Noble JH, Majdani O, Labadie RF, et al. Automatic determination of optimal linear drilling trajectories for cochlear access accounting for drill-positioning error. Int J Med Robot Comput Assist Surg. 2010;6(3):281–90.
7. Riechmann M, Lohnstein PU, Raczkowsky J, et al. Identifying access paths for endoscopic interventions at the lateral skull base. Int J Comput Assist Radiol Surg. 2008; p. 249–50.
8. Allard J, Cotin S, Faure F, et al. SOFA: an open source framework for medical simulation. In: Medicine Meets Virtual Reality; 2007. p. 13–8.

Integration eines globalen Traktographieverfahrens in das Medical Imaging Interaction Toolkit

Peter F. Neher[1], Bram Stieltjes[2], Marco Reisert[3], Ignaz Reicht[1],
Hans-Peter Meinzer[1], Klaus H. Fritzsche[1,2]

[1]Abteilung Medizinische und Biologische Informatik, DKFZ Heidelberg
[2]Quantitative bildgebungsbasierte Krankheitscharakterisierung, DKFZ Heidelberg
[3]Medizin Physik, Universitätsklinikum Freiburg
k.fritzsche@dkfz-heidelberg.de

Kurzfassung. Traktographiealgorithmen liefern potentiell wertvolle Informationen für die Neurochirurgie sowie für automatisierte Diagnoseansätze. Dennoch werden sie im klinischen Umfeld bisher kaum oder gar nicht eingesetzt. In diesem Paper präsentieren wir eine open-source Integration des von Reisert et al. vorgestellten globalen Tracking-Algorithmus in das open-source Medical Imaging Interaction Toolkit (MITK) welches von der Abteilung für Medizinische und Biologische Informatik am Deutschen Krebsforschungszentrum (DKFZ) entwickelt wird. Die Integration dieses Algorithmus in eine standardisierte und offene Entwicklungsumgebung wie MITK erleichtert die Zugänglichkeit von Traktographiealgorithmen für die Wissenschaftsgemeinschaft und ist ein wichtiger Schritt in Richtung klinischer Anwendungen. Die MITK Diffusion Anwendung, verfügbar auf www.mitk.org, beinhaltet alle Schritte die für eine erfolgreiche Traktographie notwendig sind: Vorverarbeitung, Rekonstruktion der Bilder, das eigentliche Tracking, live Beobachtung von Zwischenergebnissen, Nachbearbeitung und Visualisierung der Tracking-Ergebnisse. Dieses Paper beschreibt typische Tracking-Ergebnisse und demonstriert die Schritte die zur Vor- und Nachbearbeitung der Bilder und Ergebnisse durchgeführt werden.

1 Einleitung

Bis heute ist die diffusionsgewichtete Bildgebung die einzige Technik um nichtinvasiv Einblicke in die Architektur der Faserstruktur des menschlichen Gehirns zu bekommen. Tracking-Algorithmen versuchen aus der gegebenen voxelweisen Information explizite Aussagen über die zugrundeliegende Struktur der Faserstränge zu rekonstruieren. In den letzten Jahren wurde eine große Bandbreite verschiedener Tracking-Ansätze entwickelt die grob in die beiden Unterkategorien lokal und global eingeteilt werden können. Lokale Methoden versuchen eine Faser Schritt für Schritt aus der lokalen Bildinformation zu rekonstruieren indem sie sukzessive neue Segmente an die Faser anfügen. Während lokale Methoden

178   Neher et. al.

vor allem für ihre hohe Performanz bezüglich Rechenzeit bekannt sind, scheitern sie doch häufig an Bildartefakten oder komplexen Faserkonfigurationen wie Kreuzungen oder sog. Kissings. Globale Methoden rekonstruieren alle Fasern des Bildvolumens simultan, indem sie nach einem globalen Optimum suchen. Diese Methoden sind wesentlich rechenaufwändiger als lokale Methoden, allerdings versprechen sie auch deutlich robustere Ergebnisse.

Diese Arbeit stellt die Integration des erfolgreichen [1] und performanten globalen Ansatzes, genannt Gibbs Tracking [2, 3], sowie Komponenten für die Vor- und Nachbearbeitung der Daten in das Medical Imaging Interaction Toolkit (MITK), genauer gesagt in die Diffusion Imaging Komponente MITK-DI [4], vor. MITK ist ein open-source Software System für die Entwicklung von Interaktiver Software zur Verarbeitung medizinischer Bilddaten [5]. Die open-source Anwendung MITK Diffusion ist auf www.mitk.org verfügbar.

2   Material und Methoden

Um die Wiederverwendbarkeit und Kompatibilität mit anderen Applikationen zu garantieren ist der Algorithmus selbst (itk::GibbsTrackingFilter) als ein Insight Toolkit (ITK, www.ITK.org) Filter Objekt realisiert welches die bekannten ITK Mechanismen wie Smart-Pointer und Pipeline Processing aufgreift. Neue MITK Datenstrukturen (z.B. mitk::FiberBundle) erweitern MITK-DI und garantieren die nahtlose Integration in MITK Basierte Anwendungen. Dies schließt Erweiterungen des MITK Factory Mechanismus zur Unterstützung von Laden, Speichern und Drag and Drop von Fiber Bundle Dateien mit ein. Zum speichern der Daten kann entweder das xml-basierten *.fib Dateiformat oder das weit verbreiteten vtkPolyData Format (ASCII) mit der Dateiendung *.vfib verwendet werden.

Die folgenden Abschnitte beschreiben die Pipeline von der Vorverarbeitung der Rohdaten über das eigentliche Tracking bis zur Nachbearbeitung der Tracking-Ergebnisse (Abb. 1).

2.1   Vorverarbeitung

Der Tracking-Algorithmus benötigt Orientation Distribution Functions (ODF) als Eingabedaten. Falls die Bilder mittels High Angular Resolution Imaging (HARDI) Sequenzen aufgenommen wurden kann eine Q-Ball Rekonstruktion zur Generierung der ODFs direkt durchgeführt werden. Wenn keine HARDI Daten zur Verfügung stehen wird eine standard Tensor Rekonstruktion benutzt. Aus diesen Tensordaten kann MITK-DI entweder HARDI Daten schätzen um eine Q-Ball Rekonstruktion zu ermöglichen oder direkt ODFs aus den Tensoren berechnen. Zur Q-Ball Rekonstruktion stellt MITK-DI mehrere Methoden zur Verfügung: eine numerische Rekonstruktion (Tuch et.al. [6]), eine Spherical Harmonics (SH) Rekonstruktion (Descoteaux et.al. [7]) und eine SH Rekonstruktion mit Solid Angle Consideration (Aganj et.al. [8]). Um den Tracking-Prozess zu beschleunigen kann der Suchraum des Algorithmus mittels einer binären Maske eingeschränkt werden.

2.2 Traktographie

Die grundsätzliche Idee des Algorithmus ist es ein Modell M, bestehend aus gerichteten Punkten (Partikeln) und Verbindungen zwischen diesen Partikeln, an die Bilddaten D anzupassen indem zwei Energieterme minimiert werden. Diese Minimierung ist als iterativer Prozess gestaltet, der zufällige Änderungen in M einführt die mit einer gewissen Wahrscheinlichkeit, die aus den beiden Energietermen berechnet wird, akzeptiert werden. Die Energien beschreiben zum einen wie gut M die Daten D erklärt (externe Energie) und zum anderen wie wohlgeformt, im Sinne gewisser biologischer Einschränkungen, die einzelnen Fasern sind (interne Energie). Die Gibbs Tracking View erlaubt die Konfiguration der wichtigsten Parameter:

– Anzahl der Iterationen
– Partikel Länge/Breite/Gewicht, die den Beitrag jedes Partikels zu M kontrollieren
– Start und Endtemperatur, die kontrollieren wie schnell der Algorithmus einen stabilen Zustand erreicht
– Gewichtung zwischen den beiden Energien
– Minimale akzeptierte Faserlänge

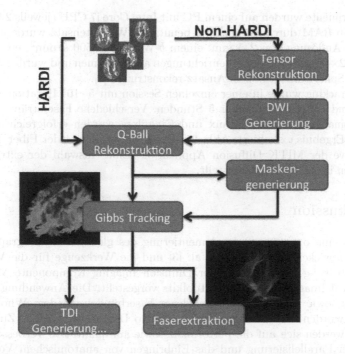

Abb. 1. Flowchart der Verarbeitungsschritte von den Rohdaten zur Nachbearbeitung der Ergebnisse

Der Tracking-Prozess wird, um die Anwendungs-GUI nicht zu blockieren, in einem Separaten Worker-Thread gestartet was mittels Mechanismen aus QTs QThread Klasse realisiert ist. Zusätzlich zu einer Textanzeige, die Informationen über den Fortschritt des Trackings zeigt, kann der gesamte Prozess auch durch eine kontinuierliche Visualisierung der Zwischenergebnisse beobachtet werden. Um die Anzahl der resultierenden Fasern zu erhöhen und um die statistische Natur des Verfahrens zu berücksichtigen, kann der Tracking-Prozess mehrfach wiederholt werden. Die so gewonnenen Ergebnisse können dann im Nachhinein zu einem Gesamtergebnis kombiniert werden.

2.3 Nachbearbeitung

MITK-DI stellt die Fiber Bundle Operations View zur Verfügung um die Tracking-Ergebnisse nachzubearbeiten. Diese View integriert alle Mechanismen die notwendig sind um mit Fiber Bundles zu arbeiten, wie Tract Density Image, Envelope und Oberflächenmesh Generierung, Visualisierung der Faserenden und die Extraktion von Faser-Untermengen durch manuelle ROI Platzierung.

3   Ergebnisse

Die Experimente wurden auf einem PC mit Intel Core i7 CPU (jeweils 2,93 GHz) und 16 Gb RAM durchgeführt. Der benutzte DWI Datensatz wurde mit einer isotropen Auflösung von $2,5$ mm, einem b-Wert von 3500 s/mm^2, einer Größe von $96 \times 82 \times 40$ und 65 Gradientenrichtungen aufgenommen und wurde mit einem standard Spherical Harmonics Ansatz rekonstruiert [7].

Das Tracking wurde in einer einzelnen Session mit $5 \cdot 10^8$ Iterationen durchgeführt und benötigte ungefähr 5 Stunden. Verschiedene Faserstränge wie der Corticospinaltrakt (CST), Fornix und Cingulum wurden erfolgreich aus dem Tracking-Ergebnis extrahiert. Abb. 2 zeigt einen Screenshot der Fiber Tracking Perspektive der MITK Diffusion Applikation. Eine Auswahl der extrahierten Strukturen ist in Abb. 3 dargestellt.

4   Diskussion

Es wurde eine open-source Implementierung des globalen Traktographiealgorithmus entwickelt von Reisert et al. [3] und die Werkzeuge für die Vor- und Nachbearbeitung der Daten in der Diffusion Imaging Komponente MITK-DI des Medical Imaging Interaction Toolkits vorgestellt. Die Anwendung des Algorithmus sowie Extraktion verschiedener Faserbündel aus dem Whole Brain Ergebnis wurden erfolgreich auf einem in-vivo Datensatz getestet. Zukünftige Arbeiten werden sich auf die Performanz sowie auf qualitative Verbesserungen, z.B. durch Parallelisierung und das Einbringen von anatomischem Vorwissen, des Tracking-Ansatzes konzentrieren.

Literaturverzeichnis

1. Fillard P, Descoteaux M, Goh A, et al. Quantitative evaluation of 10 tractography algorithms on a realistic diffusion MR phantom. Neuroimage. 2011;56(1):220–34. Available from: http://dx.doi.org/10.1016/j.neuroimage.2011.01.032.
2. Krcher BW, Mader I, Kiselev VG. Gibbs tracking: a novel approach for the reconstruction of neuronal pathways. Magn Reson Med. 2008;60(4):953–63. Available from: http://dx.doi.org/10.1002/mrm.21749.
3. Reisert M, Mader I, Anastasopoulos C, et al. Global fiber reconstruction becomes practical. Neuroimage. 2011;54:955–62.
4. Fritzsche K, Meinzer HP. MITK-DI A new diffusion imaging component for MITK. Proc BVM. 2010.
5. Wolf I, Vetter M, Wegner I, et al. The medical imaging interaction toolkit. Med Image Anal. 2005;9(6):594–604.
6. Tuch DS. Q-ball imaging. Magn Reson Med. 2004;52:1358–72.
7. Descoteaux M, Angelino E, Fitzgibbons S, et al. Regularized, fast, and robust analytical Q-ball imaging. Magn Reson Med. 2007;58:497–510.
8. Aganj I, Lenglet C, Sapiro G. ODF reconstruction in q-ball imaging with solid angle consideration. Proc IEEE ISBI. 2009.

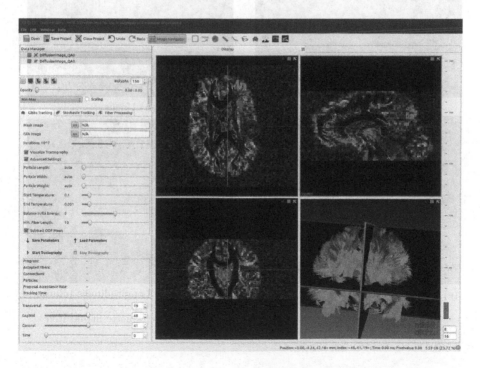

Abb. 2. Screenshot der Fiber Tracking Perspektive sowie Q-Ball und Faservisualisierung, eingebettet in die MITK Diffusion Applikation

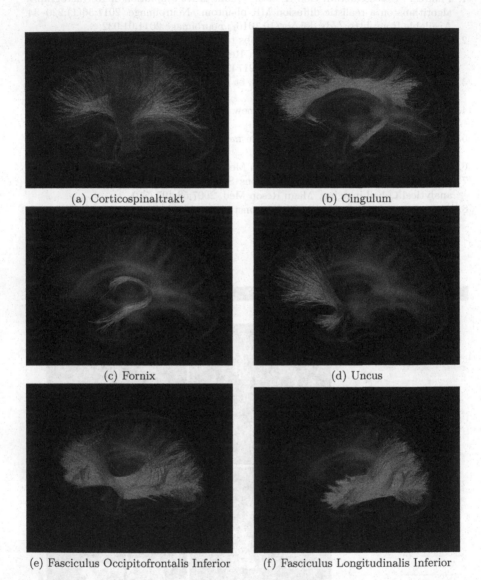

(a) Corticospinaltrakt

(b) Cingulum

(c) Fornix

(d) Uncus

(e) Fasciculus Occipitofrontalis Inferior

(f) Fasciculus Longitudinalis Inferior

Abb. 3. Auswahl der aus dem Whole Brain Tracking extrahierte Strukturen

Interaktive 3D Segmentierung auf Basis einer optimierten Oberflächeninterpolation mittels radialer Basisfunktionen

Andreas Fetzer, Hans-Peter Meinzer, Tobias Heimann

Abteilung für Medizinische und Biologische Informatik, DKFZ Heidelberg
a.fetzer@dkfz-heidelberg.de

Kurzfassung. In dieser Arbeit wird ein Verfahren zur effizienten und interaktiven Erstellung einer 3D Segmentierung vorgestellt. Dafür wird die Oberfläche des zu segmentierenden Bereiches auf Basis manuell gezeichneter Konturen mittels radialer Basisfunktionen interpoliert. Um die Auswirkung zusätzlicher Konturen auf die interpolierten Oberfläche in wenigen Sekunden visualisieren zu können, wurden gezielte Maßnahmen getroffen, um den Algorithmus auf Geschwindigkeit zu optimieren. Eine Evaluation auf Basis von Expertensegmentierungen ergab, dass sich der Aufwand für die Erstellung einer manuellen Segmentierung deutlich reduzieren ließ, wobei gleichzeitig eine hohe Genauigkeit erzielt werden konnte.

1 Einleitung

Die Segmentierung anatomischer Strukturen ist eine zentrale Aufgabe in der medizinischen Bildverarbeitung. Da eine rein manuelle Segmentierung sehr Zeit intensiv ist, wurden in der Vergangenheit eine Vielzahl halb- und vollautomatischer Segmentierungsalgorithmen entwickelt. Qualitativ schlechte Bilder oder pathologische Strukturen erfordern dennoch häufig eine Segmentierung von Hand. Das Ziel dieser Arbeit ist es daher, die manuelle Segmentierung durch eine effiziente Interpolation zu unterstützen und dabei gleichzeitig eine hohe Güte bzgl. der Referenz zu erzielen.

Ein Verfahren dafür stellten Wolf et al. [1] vor, bei dem die Oberfläche des segmentierten Bereiches auf Basis weniger Konturen anhand sog. Coons-Patches interpoliert wird. Ein Nachteil dieser Methode ist, dass die Kanten eines Coons-Patches durch maximal vier Konturen definiert werden können, was zu Einschränkungen bzgl. der Lage der eingezeichneten Konturen führt. Dagegen unabhängig von der Position der Konturen ist der Ansatz von Wimmer et al. [2], bei dem mittels radialer Basisfunktionen (RBF) aus existierenden Konturen eine initiale Oberfläche interpoliert und anschließend unter Einbindung von Bildinformationen verfeinert wird. Eine Einschränkung bei diesem Verfahren ist, dass die Konturen nur durch Interpolation zwischen vom Benutzer gesetzten Kontrollpunkten erzeugt werden. Des Weiteren ist die initiale Interpolation mit einer

Dauer von ca. 2 Min. bei 6 - 8 Konturen relativ zeitaufwändig. Hinzu kommt die anschließende Level-Set-Verfeinerung mit ca. 5 Min.

In dieser Arbeit wird ein optimierter Algorithmus zur Oberflächeninterpolation mit RBF vorgestellt. Eine interaktive Nachbesserung der eingezeichneten Konturen resultiert in einer schnellen Aktualisierung der Oberfläche. Sowohl bzgl. der eingesetzten manuellen Segmentierungswerkzeuge als auch bzgl. der Lage der eingezeichneten Konturen bestehen keinerlei Einschränkungen. Selbst Verästelungen und Löcher sind modellierbar.

2 Material und Methoden

In unserer Arbeit verwenden wir für die mathematische Beschreibung der Oberfläche eine Distanzfunktion. Sie ist eine implizite Funktion und hat die Form

$$d(p) = d(x, y, z) = c \tag{1}$$

p ist ein Punkt des R^3 und c ein Maß für den Abstand von p zur gesuchten Oberfläche. Die Interpolation der Distanzfunktion erfolgt, ähnlich zu Wimmer et al., mittels RBF. Die Distanzfunktion erhält dadurch das Aussehen

$$d(p) = \sum_{i=1}^{n} \lambda_i \cdot \Phi(\|p - p_i\|_2) = c \tag{2}$$

Φ ist dabei die biharmonische RBF mit $\Phi(x) = x$. Für diese ist das resultierende Interpolationsproblem immer lösbar [3]. $\|.\|_2$ steht für die euklidische Distanz, die Punkte p_i sind die Stützstellen der Interpolation und c ist der Distanzwert des Punktes p. λ_i sind die Interpolationsgewichte. Sie werden durch Lösen des folgenden Gleichungssystems berechnet

$$\begin{pmatrix} \Phi(\|p_1 - p_1\|_2) & \Phi(\|p_1 - p_2\|_2) & \dots & \Phi(\|p_1 - p_n\|_2) \\ \vdots & \vdots & \ddots & \vdots \\ \Phi(\|p_n - p_1\|_2) & \Phi(\|p_n - p_2\|_2) & \dots & \Phi(\|p_n - p_n\|_2) \end{pmatrix} \cdot \begin{pmatrix} \lambda_1 \\ \vdots \\ \lambda_n \end{pmatrix} = \begin{pmatrix} c_1 \\ \vdots \\ c_n \end{pmatrix} \tag{3}$$

Da die Randpunkte $p_{1..n}$ der eingezeichneten Konturen per Definition auf der gesuchten Oberfläche liegen, gilt $c_{1..n} = 0$ und deshalb auch $\lambda_{1..n} = 0$. Um das zu verhindern, müssen zusätzlich Punkte mit einer Distanz $\neq 0$ definiert werden, sog. Offsurface-Points. Dazu werden die Normalvektoren der gesuchten Oberfläche an jedem Randpunkt approximiert. Die Normalen werden anschließend zu jedem Punkt addiert bzw. subtrahiert, um zusätzlich Punkte mit einer Distanz von -1 bzw. $+1$ zu erhalten. Aus n Konturrandpunkten ergeben sich somit $3n$ Punkte für die Interpolation. Die Anzahl der Randpunkte und somit die der Summanden der Distanzfunktion verdreifacht sich dadurch, die Größe des zu lösenden Gleichungssystems verneunfacht sich sogar. Aus diesem Grund ist das Lösen des Gleichungssystems und die Berechnung der Distanzwerte sehr rechenintensiv. Um eine möglichst schnelle Interpolation und Auswertung der

Distanzfunktion zu erreichen, werden in dem Algorithmus die folgenden Schritte und Optimierungen durchgeführt:

Da der Algorithmus unabhängig von den eingesetzten Segmentierungswerkzeugen ist, arbeitet dieser ausschließlich auf dem Segmentierungsbild. Dieses liegt als Binärbild vor, aus dem im ersten Schritt die Randpunkte der eingezeichneten Konturen extrahiert werden müssen. Das Ergebnis ist für jede Kontur eine dichte Rand-Punktwolke. Da die Anzahl der Punkte die Geschwindigkeit der Oberflächeninterpolation maßgeblich beeinflusst, wird als erster Optimierungsschritt eine Reduzierung der Randpunkte durchgeführt. Dazu wurden mehrere Verfahren implementiert und miteinander verglichen. Für die Interpolation hat sich eine abgewandelte Form des von Douglas et al. [4] vorgestellten Algorithmus als am geeignetsten erwiesen. Dabei wird zusätzlich darauf geachtet, dass die Abstände zwischen den resultierenden Randpunkten p_i nicht zu groß werden und diese gleichmäßig verteilt sind.

Anschließend erfolgt die Erzeugung der Offsurface-Points. Bei der Berechnung der Oberflächennormalen muss darauf geachtet werden, dass diese nicht in das Innere der Oberfläche zeigen. Besonders relevant wird dies, wenn aus einer bestehenden Kontur eine Weitere herausgeschnitten wird, was bei röhrenförmigen Strukturen der Fall sein kann. Abb. 1 verdeutlicht diese Problematik.

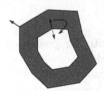

Abb. 1. Die Invertierung des Normalenvektors bei Konturen, die innerhalb einer Anderen liegen. Bei ihnen müssen die approximierten Normalenvektoren negiert werden, damit den Offsurface-Points die richtigen Distanzwerte zugewiesen werden. Dadurch können selbst röhrenförmige Strukturen interpoliert werden

Aus den so erhaltenen Punkten wird das Gleichungssystem entsprechend (3) für die Interpolation aufgestellt und die Gewichte λ_i für die Distanzfunktion berechnet. Mit diesen kann letztendlich die Distanzfunktion angegeben und damit auch die Distanz eines jeden Pixels zur gesuchten Oberfläche berechnet werden. Die Stellen im Bild, an denen der Distanzwert 0 ist, geben den Verlauf der Oberfläche an. Wie bereits erwähnt ist die Berechnung der Distanzwerte sehr aufwändig, da die Distanzfunktion bei p_n Stützstellen n Summanden hat. Zwei Maßnahmen wurden ergriffen, um diesen Aufwand zu minimieren.

Zum Einen wurde das Volumen des Distanzbildes unabhängig von der Größe des segmentierten Bereiches und der Auflösung des Originalbildes auf eine bestimmte Anzahl Voxel festgelegt. Tests haben ergeben, dass ein Volumen von 50.000 Voxel gute Ergebnisse liefert. Des Weiteren wurde eine Narrowband Distanzwertberechnung durchgeführt. Dabei werden nur die Distanzwerte der Punkte berechnet, die sich in unmittelbarer Nachbarschaft der gesuchten Oberfläche befinden. Beginnend mit einem Punkt der auf der Oberfläche liegt, werden die Distanzen der Punkte in der 6er Nachbarschaft berechnet. Liegt ein Distanzwert innerhalb eines definierten Grenzwertes, so wird für den dazugehörigen Punkt wiederum die 6er Nachbarschaft berechnet. Dies geschieht solange, bis alle Punkte abgearbeitet sind. Das Ergebnis ist ein Distanzband, dass durch das Distanzbild verläuft, an dessen Nullstellen die Oberfläche liegt. Alle Voxel außerhalb des Bandes erhalten den Wert 10 und alle innerhalb den Wert -10. Aus dem Distanzbild wird im letzten Schritt die Oberfläche extrahiert. Abb. 2 zeigt den Verlauf des Distanzbandes.

Abb. 2. Das erzeugte Distanzbild. Die Linien in der Detailansicht beschreiben den Verlauf der Narrowband Distanzwertberechnung. ähnlich eines Bereichswachstums werden nur für die Pixel die Distanzwerte berechnet, deren Wert innerhalb eines Grenzwertes liegt. Alle Pixel innerhalb des vom Band eingeschlossenen Bereiches erhalten den Wert -10, alle Pixel außerhalb den Wert +10. An den Stellen im Bild, an denen die Pixel den Wert 0 annehmen verläuft die gesuchte Oberfläche

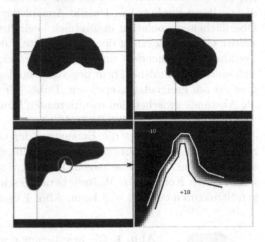

Aus dem resultierenden Distanzbild wird im letzten Schritt die gesuchte Oberfläche mit Hilfe des Marching Cubes Algorithmus [5] extrahiert.

Evaluiert wurde der Algorithmus anhand einer Expertensegmentierung der Leber und eines Rattenfemurs. Aus diesen wurden sukzessive Konturen extrahiert. Für unterschiedliche Anzahlen von Konturen wurde die interpolierte Segmentierung mit der Referenz verglichen. Dazu wurden die von Heimann et al. in [6] vorgestellten Metriken genutzt. Die Evaluation wurde auf einem Apple iMac 3,4 GHz mit 16 GB Arbeitsspeicher durchgeführt.

3   Ergebnisse

Die Abb. 3 und 4 zeigen jeweils für die Leber und den Femur die interpolierte Oberfläche bei unterschiedlicher Konturenzahlen. Die schwarzen Konturen markieren die Positionen, an denen Schichten aus der Expertensegmentierung extrahiert wurden. Tab. 1 und 2 enthalten die Ergebnisse der Evaluation. Neben der Anzahl der Konturen und entsprechend der Anzahl der Randpunkte, wurde die Dauer der Interpolation, die mittlere und maximale Distanz zur Referenzsegmentierung und der volumetrische überlappungsfehler gemessen.

4   Diskussion

Aus Tab. 1 wird ersichtlich, dass sich bei großen und komplexen Strukturen wie der Leber zusätzliche Konturen deutlich auf die Ergebnisqualität auswirken. Bei

Tabelle 1. Evaluierung der 3D Segmentierung für die Leber bei unterschiedlicher Anzahl eingezeichneter Konturen

Anzahl Konturen	Anzahl Punkte	Dauer [s]	Mittl. Dist. [mm]	Max. Dist. [mm]	Überlappungsfehler [%]
3	299	0,73	4,47	22,59	22,73
8	793	5,12	1,09	15,45	6,77
14	1155	19,34	0,62	10,08	4,16

Tabelle 2. Evaluierung der 3D Segmentierung für einen Rattenfemur bei unterschiedlicher Anzahl eingezeichneter Konturen

Anzahl Konturen	Anzahl Punkte	Dauer [s]	Mittl. Dist. [mm]	Max. Dist. [mm]	Überlappungsfehler [%]
3	295	0.49	0,05	1,08	7,20
6	494	1,58	0,04	1,22	6,11
8	539	2,05	0,04	1,20	5,9

einfacheren Formen, wie dem Femur sind hingegen bereits wenige Konturen ausreichend, um ein gutes Ergebnis zu erzielen (Tab. 2). Generell zeigt sich, dass sich die Ergebnisqualität ab einer gewissen Anzahl Konturen, nicht mehr signifikant verbessert, die Dauer der Interpolation sich allerdings stark erhöht. Im Falle der Leber liefern 14 Konturen das genaueste Ergebnis mit einem überlappungsfehler von 4,16 %, allerdings dauerte die Interpolation bereits über 19 Sekunden. Dagegen führen 8 Konturen mit einem überlappungsfehler von 6,77 % ebenfalls zu einer genauen Segmentierung und benötigen lediglich knapp ein Viertel der Zeit.

Abschließend kann gesagt werden, dass das entwickelte Verfahren dank der Optimierungen, wie z.B. der Narrowband Distanzberechnung effizient genug ist, um eine schnelle Nachbesserung zu ermöglichen und dadurch zu einem guten Ergebnis führt. Der Umstand, dass die Positionen der Schnittebenen für die Konturen frei im Raum wählbar sind, erlaubt es, den Femur mit bereits drei Konturen gut zu interpolieren. Selbst röhrenförmige Strukturen können mit dem Verfahren segmentiert werden. Mit deutlich reduziertem Aufwand lässt sich so

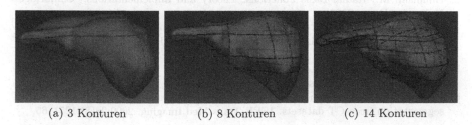

(a) 3 Konturen   (b) 8 Konturen   (c) 14 Konturen

Abb. 3. Lage der eingezeichneten Konturen für die Lebersegmentierung

Abb. 4. Lage der eingezeichneten Konturen für die Femursegmentierung

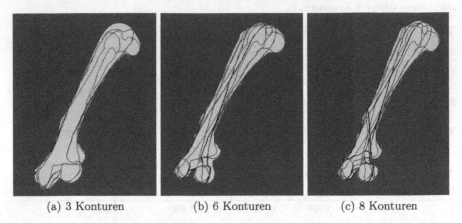

(a) 3 Konturen   (b) 6 Konturen   (c) 8 Konturen

eine vollständige 3D Segmentierung erstellen, die z.B. als Trainingsdaten für Formmodelle oder als Ausgangspunkt für die Erstellung einer neuen Referenzsegmentierung verwendet werden kann. Da der Algorithmus ausschließlich auf Binärdaten arbeitet, ist er unabhängig von den eingesetzten Segmentierungswerkzeugen.

Zukünftige Arbeiten könnten das Verfahren bzgl. Qualität und Geschwindigkeit verbessern. Qualitativ wäre die Einbindung von Bildinformationen interessant, um die Oberfläche im letzten Schritt, ähnlich zu Wimmer et al. [2], zu verfeinern. Eine Parallelisierung der Auswertung der Distanzfunktion, ein Schritt der sehr rechenintensiv ist, würde die Interpolation zusätzlich beschleunigen.

Literaturverzeichnis

1. Wolf I, Vetter M, Hassenpflug P, et al. Extension of 2D segmentation methods into 3D by means of Coons-patch interpolation. In: Proc SPIE. vol. 5032; 2003. p. 1413–20.
2. Wimmer A, Soza G, Hornnegger H. Two-Staged Semi-automatic Organ Segmentation Framework using Radial Basis Functions and Level Sets. 3D Segmentation in Clinic. 2007; p. 179 – 88.
3. Buhmann M. Radial Basis Functions: Theory and Implementations. Cambridge University Press; 2003.
4. Douglas DH, Peucker TK. Algorithms for the reduction of the number of points required to represent a digitized line or its caricature. Int J Geogr Inf Geovisualization. 1973;10:112–22.
5. Schroeder W, Martin K, Lorensen B. The Visualization Toolkit An Object Oriented Approach To 3D Graphics. 4th ed. Kitware Inc.; 2006.
6. Heimann T, van Ginneken B, et al. Comparison and evaluation of methods for liver segmentation from CT datasets. IEEE Trans Med Imaging. 2009;28(8):1251–65.

Inkrementelle lokal-adaptive Binarisierung zur Unterdrückung von Artefakten in der Knochenfeinsegmentierung

Patrick Scheibe[1], Philipp Wüstling[2,3], Christian Voigt[4], Thomas Hierl[5], Ulf-Dietrich Braumann[3,6]

[1]Translationszentrum für Regenerative Medizin, Universität Leipzig
[2]Fak. Inform., Math. u. Naturwiss., Hochsch. f. Technik, Wirtsch. u. Kultur Leipzig
[3]Interdisziplinäres Zentrum für Bioinformatik, Universität Leipzig
[4]Klinik und Poliklinik für Orthopädie, Universitätsklinikum Leipzig
[5]Klinik u. Poliklin. f. Mund-, Kiefer- u. Plast. Gesichtschir., Universitätsklin. Leipzig
[6]Institut für Med. Informatik, Statistik und Epidemiologie, Universität Leipzig

pscheibe@trm.uni-leipzig.de

Kurzfassung. Das präzise Segmentieren von Knochen in klinischen CT-Aufnahmen spielt heutzutage eine wichtige Rolle. Vor allem, um operative Eingriffe zu planen oder das maßgeschneiderte Anfertigen von Implantaten zu ermöglichen, ist eine Erkennung auch feiner Knochendetails unabdingbar. Gerade die feinen, lamellenartigen Strukturen im Nasenbereich können bei CT-Aufnahmen, die in der klinischen Routine angefertigt werden, durch ihre zu geringe Signalstärke oft nicht als Knochen identifiziert werden. Um diese, vom sogenannten Partialvolumeneffekt betroffenen Strukturen dennoch automatisch segmentieren zu können, stellen wir hier eine Methode vor, die ausgehend von einer Initial-korrekten, aber unzureichenden Segmentierung, iterativ angrenzende, schwache Strukturen erkennt. Dabei wird für Voxel, die am Rande des segmentierten Knochens als Hintergrund erkannt wurden, lokal die Wahrscheinlichkeit geschätzt, eine knöcherne Struktur zu repräsentieren. Mit dieser Reevaluierung wird die bestehende Segmentierung so lange iterativ erweitert, bis sich eine Konvergenz einstellt. Durch den lokalen Charakter der Randvoxel-Neubewertung kann der vorgestellte Algorithmus ausgezeichnet parallel implementiert werden.

1 Einleitung

Grundlegend für die meisten Bildverarbeitungsaufgaben ist eine initiale Segmentierung der Daten, also eine Abtrennung des interessanten Vordergrundes von dem für die beabsichtigte Analyse uninteressanten Hintergrund (figure-ground separation). In realen Daten wird dieser Vorgang oft erschwert durch Abbildungsfehler, die dem zugrunde liegenden Aufnahmesystem geschuldet sind. Bildrauschen ist dabei eines der bekanntesten Beispiele, aber auch Sensoren-bedingte Abbildungsfehler zählen dazu. Ein Artefakt, das unter anderem bei Computertomografie-Aufnahmen von sehr feinen Knochenstrukturen auftritt, ist der Partialvolumeneffekt. Dabei kommt es etwa im Bereich der Nasennebenhöhlen dazu, dass die feinblättrigen Knochen nicht mehr korrekt durch das CT aufgelöst werden können. Durch Mittelung in den Sensordaten werden diese Bereiche dann mit einem viel zu niedrigen Hounsfieldwert-bezogenen Grauwert dargestellt und sind dadurch mit rein globalem Schwellwertverfahren nicht mehr ohne weiteres als Knochengewebe zu identifizieren.

In einer kürzlich publizierten Arbeit stellten Zhang et al. mit dem Anspruch, gerade Partialvolumeneffekte tolerieren zu können, eine Methode zur Knochensegmentierung vor, die ausgehend von einer Übersegmentierung durch lokale Neubewertung dekrementell ein besseres Segmentierungsergebnis erreicht [1]. Der Nachteil dieses Vorgehens liegt allerdings darin, dass, wenn Gewebe vollständig von Knochen umgeben ist und dieses Gewebe zu Beginn als Vordergrund klassifiziert wird, es niemals als tatsächlicher Hintergrund segmentiert werden kann. Aufgrund der umgebenden Knochen wird das falsch klassifizierte Gewebe niemals als Randpixel erkannt, aber nur an Randpixeln erfolgt eine Reklassifikation.

Lokal arbeitende Schwellwertmethoden sind an sich nicht neu, für eine Übersicht sei auf [2] verwiesen. Gradienten-basierte lokale Schwellwertverfahren etwa sind unter stark vorherrschenden Partialvolumeneffekten von daher nicht geeignet, als dass ja gerade die Gradienten beeinträchtigt sein können. Wasserscheiden-basierte Verfahren als mögliche Alternative zu lokalen Schwellwertverfahren hingegen bringen oftmals einen erheblichen Nachverarbeitungs-Aufwand mit sich, etwa zum Fusionieren von Segmenten. Lokale intensitätsbasierte Statistiken erscheinen demgegenüber also grundsätzlich als durchaus vielversprechend. Zu einfache Statistiken allerdings, etwa der direkte Bezug von lokalen Schwellen auf lokale Mittelwerte und Streuungen, lassen Möglichkeiten zur Differenzierung, etwa anhand mehrerer Histogramm-Moden, ungenutzt. Genau da hatten die Autoren von [1] angesetzt und ein lokales Clusterverfahren vorgeschlagen.

Wir greifen diesen Ansatz grundsätzlich auf und erweitern ihn für die Problemstellung der Knochenfeinsegmentierung. Dabei werden ebenso am Rand der bestehenden Segmentierung lokal die Zufallsverteilungen von Vorder- und Hintergrund geschätzt und mit Hilfe dieser die Wahrscheinlichkeit approximiert, ob – umgekehrt zu [1] – ein Hintergrundpixel richtiger weise doch zum Vordergrund eingeordnet werden muss, oder nicht.

2 Material und Methoden

Die hier vorgestellte Methode besteht aus zwei Schritten, wobei zuerst der Datensatz initial binarisiert wird und danach diese erste Segmentierung an den Rändern iterativ verbessert wird. In diesem letzten Teil des Algorithmus kann die Segmentierung nur wachsen, d.h. es können ausschließlich Hintergrundpixel zum Vordergrund dazu genommen werden, aber nicht umgekehrt.

Dieses Vorgehen impliziert, dass die initiale Segmentierung der Daten, die dann zur iterativen Verbesserung herangezogen wird, möglichst wenige falschpositive Pixel erzeugen sollte. Das wird im einfachsten Fall durch einen globalen Schwellwert bewerkstelligt, der ausreichend hoch gewählt wurde. Aus Konsistenzgründen, die später noch klarer werden, haben wir uns hier für eine Variante des bekannten ISODATA-Algorithmus (Iterative Self-Organizing Data Analysis Technique) entschieden [3]. Damit ergibt sich zusammengefasst folgender Ablauf:

1. Initiale Binarisierung des Datensatzes
2. Für alle Hintergrundpixel p, die in direkter Nachbarschaft zum Vordergrund liegen:
    (a) Berechnen der statistischen Parameter der lokalen Verteilungen
    (b) Bewertung, ob p falsch klassifiziert wurde und somit zum Vordergrund dazu genommen werden muss
3. Falls sich Pixel geändert haben, dann gehe zu 2. mit der erweiterten Binarisierung.

2.1 Binarisierungsmethode

Die Binarisierung hat die Aufgabe, das Bild in zwei Klassen zu unterteilen, jedoch finden sich gerade im Schädel-CT meist mindestens drei Klassen: Knochen, weiches Gewebe und Hintergrund. Bei einer automatischen Bestimmung eines Schwellwertes würde der Hintergrund, der meist einen Großteil des Bildes einnimmt, den gefundenen Schwellwert maßgeblich beeinflussen.

Um trotzdem eine möglichst gute Trennung von Knochen und Weichgewebe zu erreichen, wurde in den ISODATA-Algorithmus ein minimaler Schwellwert $t_{\min}$ eingeführt. Die Berechnung erfolgt somit nicht auf allen Pixeln des Bildes B, sondern nur auf denen, die größer als $t_{\min}$ sind.

Als Startwert für den Algorithmus wird der Mittelwert aller Pixel $p > t_{\min}$ benutzt und dann solange iteriert, bis sich die Schwelle nicht mehr ändert. Dabei besteht eine Iteration daraus, mittels der aktuellen Schwelle die Daten in Vorder- und Hintergrund zu unterteilen, für jeden Teil unter Berücksichtigung der minimalen Schwelle $t_{\min}$ die Mittelwerte μ_V und μ_H zu berechnen, und mit diesen Mittelwerten eine neue Schwelle $t = (\mu_V + \mu_H)/2$ zu bestimmen.

Dabei ändert sich t genau dann nicht mehr, wenn keine Pixel mehr von Vordergrund zu Hintergrund oder vice versa umsortiert werden, und es ergibt sich daraus die Startsegmentierung für die folgende, inkrementelle Erweiterung der Binarisierung.

2.2 Lokal-adaptiver Binarisierungsschritt

In diesem Schritt wird für jeden Hintergrundpixel, der an einen Vordergrundpixel angrenzt (Randpixel), überprüft, ob er lokal falsch klassifiziert wurde, d.h. ob er nicht nachträglich dem Vordergrund zugeordnet werden sollte.

Dazu werden lokal die Wahrscheinlichkeitsverteilungen für Vorder- und Hintergrund approximiert und mit Hilfe des Bayes'schen Theorems entschieden, ob ein Randpixel der Vordergrundverteilung zuzuordnen ist. Dazu werden die bedingten Wahrscheinlichkeiten $P(V|G)$ und $P(H|G)$ verglichen, d.h. unter der Annahme, dass ein bestimmter Grauwert G für einen Randpixel p auftritt, ist es wahrscheinlicher, dass p zum Vordergrund V gehört, oder nicht. Es reicht hier aus, das Verhältnis der beiden bed. Wahrscheinlichkeiten zu betrachten

$$q = \frac{P(V|G)}{P(H|G)} \tag{1}$$

und zu überprüfen, ob $q > 1$. Nach dem Bayes'schen Theorem ergibt sich

$$q = \frac{P(G|V)P(V)}{P(G|H)P(H)} \tag{2}$$

Um die benötigten Wahrscheinlichkeiten lokal zu approximieren, wird eine Umgebung N um jeden Randpixel p betrachtet. Mit Hilfe der in 2.1 beschriebenen Methode wird für N eine lokale Schwelle bestimmt, anhand derer N in Vordergrund V und Hintergrund H unterteilt wird.

Mit Hilfe dieser lokalen Binarisierung kann für den Vordergrund (und äquivalent für den Hintergrund) der Mittelwert μ_V und die Standardabweichung σ_V ermittelt werden.

Somit kann für alle Randpixel des Bildes das Verhältnis q bestimmt und anhand dessen Größe entschieden werden, ob ein Pixel zum Vordergrund klassifiziert werden soll. Nachdem alle Randpixel auf diese Weise behandelt wurden, werden alle neu hinzugekommenen Vordergrundpixel zur bestehenden Segmentierung addiert. Mit der Ermittlung aller neuen Randpixel beginnt nun eine Iteration von vorn. Das Verfahren konvergiert, wenn in einer Iteration keine Randpixel mehr zum Vordergrund hinzukommen.

3 Ergebnisse

Abb. 1 zeigt die CT-Aufnahme eines Schädels und soll ein typisches Anwendungsgebiet der hier vorgestellten Methode demonstrieren. Dabei sollen hier besonders die im Nasenbereich befindlichen, sehr dünnen Knochenwände betrachtet werden. Diese liegen an der Auflösungsgrenze und werden deshalb, anders als der restliche Knochen, viel zu hell dargestellt. Versucht man nun, wie in der klinischen Praxis immer noch üblich, durch einen globalen Schwellwert die Daten zu segmentieren, wird das immer zu suboptimalen Ergebnissen führen.

Dazu erkennt man in Abb. 1 (mitte) das Segmentierungsergebnis mit der kleinstmöglichen Schwelle, die ausschliesslich Knochen und kein Weichgewebe segmentiert. Die feinen Strukturen im Nasenbereich werden nur marginal richtig klassifiziert. Versucht man hingegen die globale Schwelle weiter abzusenken, sodass der Nasenbereich wenigstens partiell richtig segmentiert wird, erhält man eine übersegmentierung im Hirn (Abb. 1, rechts).

Benutzt man dagegen die hier vorgestellte Methode, so erkennt man, dass von der Initialbinarisierung in Abb. 2 (links) ausgehend, der Nasenbereich an vielen Stellen korrekt nachklassifiziert wurde. Zu bemerken ist, dass Abb. 2 (mitte) die exakte numerische Umsetzung der hier gezeigten Methode darstellt, d.h. die Initialbinarisierungsschwelle wurde vollkommen automatisch bestimmt und Pixel wurden positiv klassifiziert, falls $q > 1$ (Gleichung 2). Der Algorithmus stoppte nach 164 Iterationen.

In unserer numerischen Implementierung, auf die hier aus Platzgründen leider nicht näher eingegangen werden kann, besteht die Möglichkeit $q > v$ zu wählen, wobei v ein freier Klassifizierungsparameter ist. Um bei zu niedriger Wahl von v ein Auslaufen der inkrementellen Erweiterung zu verhindern, kann man weiterhin einen Mindestabstand für $|\mu_V - \mu_H|$ setzen. Mit geeigneter Wahl dieser Parameter und einer manuell optimierten Startbinarisierungsschwelle konvergiert der Algorithmus im Abb. 2 (rechts) schon nach 56 Iterationen und liefert ein deutlich besseres Ergebnis.

Die Anwendung muss aber nicht auf klinische Schädel CTs beschränkt bleiben. Abb. 3 zeigt das Blatt einer Pflanze. Die fein verzweigten Blattadern können mit einem globalen Verfahren nicht segmentiert werden. Erschwerend kommt die ungleichmäßige Ausleuchtung des Bildes (schwach zu erkennen in Abb. 3 (mit-

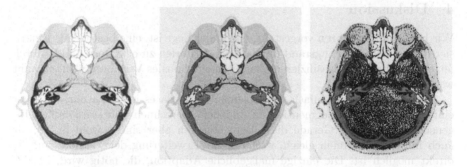

Abb. 1. Die Abbildung zeigt, dass es mit einem globalen Schwellwert nicht möglich ist, eine Binarisierungsschwelle zu finden, die die feinen Knochenstrukturen im Na/sen/-be/-reich segmentiert und dabei im Hirnbereich nicht übersegmentiert. Die CT-Darstellung wurde zur besseren Sichtbarkeit invertiert

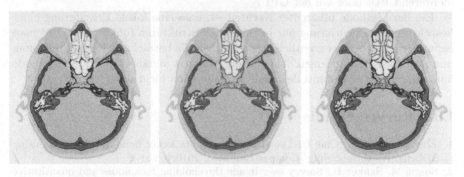

Abb. 2. Die Abbildung zeigt die vorgestellte Methode. Im Hintergrund zu erkennen das zugrunde liegende Grauwertbild, in blau die initiale Binarisierung und in rot die inkrementell erweiterten Bereiche

194   Scheibe et al.

Abb. 3. Die Abbildung zeigt, dass das Verfahren auch unter anderen Bedingungen Verwendung finden kann, bei denen feine Strukturen an der Auflösungsgrenze nicht mehr akkurat vom Hintergrund getrennt werden können. In der Mitte ist das Ergebnis mit globalem Schwellwert und rechts das Ergebnis unserer Methode zu sehen

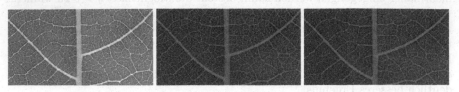

te) in der unteren, rechten Ecke) hinzu. Mit einer starken Untersegmentierung als Ausgangspunkt kann mit 51 Iterationen unserer Methode die Segmentierung stark verbessert werden.

4   Diskussion

Wir haben ein Verfahren vorgestellt, das in der Lage ist, eine bestehende Binarisierung am Binarisierungsrand durch lokale Kriterien zu erweitern und dadurch feine Strukturen zu klassifizieren, die durch ein globales Verfahren nicht erkannt werden können.

Das Verfahren ist einfach zu implementieren, da es im Kern nur aus einer einfachen, iterativen Segmentierung und dem Berechnen von statistischen Eigenschaften besteht. Gerade diese Berechnungen aber sind sowohl in 2D, als auch in 3D vollkommen gleich, weshalb eine Erweiterung der Methode auf 3D direkt möglich ist. Die einzige maßgebliche Adaption, die nötig wird, ist das Extrahieren der Randvoxel und der Voxel in der lokalen Umgebung.

Da der adaptive Schritt des Algorithmus für jeden Randpunkt unabhängig geschieht und dabei nur Lesezugriffe in den Originaldatensatz stattfinden, ist dieser Teil der Methode prädestiniert für eine parallele Architektur, sei es auf mehreren CPUs oder auf der GPU.

Ein der Methode inhärenter Nachteil ist, dass eine lokale Erweiterung einer bestehenden Segmentierung nur bei kleineren Strukturen funktioniert. Hat man bspw. Strukturen, die wesentlich größer sind als die betrachtete lokale Umgebung und sich noch dazu graduell dem Hintergrundwert annähern, wird die Methode fehlschlagen, da eine sinnvolle, lokale Klassifikation nicht mehr möglich ist.

Literaturverzeichnis

1. Zhang J, Yan CH, Chui CK, et al. Fast segmentation of bone in CT images using 3D adaptive thresholding. Comput Biol Med. 2010;40:231–6.
2. Sezgin M, Sankur B. Survey over image thresholding techniques and quantitative performance evaluation. J Electron Imaging. 2004;13:465–73.
3. Ridler TW, Calvard S. Picture thresholding using an iterative selection method. IEEE Trans Syst Man Cybern. 1978;8:630–2.

Farbbasierte Entfernung von Artefakten bei der Blutgefäßsegmentierung auf Dickdarmpolypen

Sebastian Gross[1,2], Cosmin Adrian Morariu[1], Alexander Behrens[1],
Jens J.W. Tischendorf[2], Til Aach[1]

[1]Lehrstuhl für Bildverarbeitung, RWTH Aachen
[2]Medizinische Klinik III, Universitätsklinikum Aachen
sebastian.gross@lfb.rwth-aachen.de

Kurzfassung. Darmkrebs ist in Deutschland die zweithäufigste Tumorerkrankung und wird jährlich bei 32.000 Frauen und 36.000 Männern diagnostiziert. Die Blutgefäßstruktur auf Dickdarmpolypen kann Aufschluss über die potentielle Bösartigkeit des Gewebes geben. Für die automatisierte Analyse von Dickdarmpolypen werden daher die Blutgefäße segmentiert. Artefakte, die bei der Segmentierung durch Rauschen oder Strukturen der Polypenoberfläche entstehen, können zu Fehlern in einer anschließenden Klassifikation führen. Wir schlagen daher vor, eine farbbasierte Unterscheidung zwischen Artefakten und Blutgefäßen nachzuschalten. Diese basiert auf einer Darstellung der Strukturen im HSV-Farbraum, einer Verteilungsschätzung durch eine bivariate Gaußfunktion und einer Berechnung der Mahalanobis-Distanz. Abschließend präsentieren wir Ergebnisse für die Gesamtgenauigkeit eines Polypenklassifikationsalgorithmus mit und ohne Artefaktentfernung.

1 Einleitung

Darmkrebs ist in Deutschland die zweithäufigste Tumorerkrankung und wird jährlich bei 32.000 Frauen und 36.000 Männern diagnostiziert [1]. Die Anzahl der dokumentierten Neuerkrankungen hat in den letzten Jahren stetig zugenommen, was auf neue Diagnoseverfahren und flächendeckendes Screening zurückzuführen ist. Im gleichen Zeitraum nahm allerdings die Sterblichkeit ab, da innovative Therapien und frühzeitige Erkennung die Behandlungsmöglichkeiten verbessert haben. In 2004 veröffentlichten Gono et al. eine Studie zur Nutzung einer speziellen, schmalbandigen Beleuchtung in der Endoskopie [2]. Tischendorf et al. verglichen 2007 diese neue Technik mit der Chromoendoskopie, bei der farbige Markerstoffe eingesetzt werden, um die Oberflächenbeschaffenheit von Dickdarmpolypen diagnostisch auszuwerten [3]. Sie kamen zu dem Ergebnis, dass die Zuverlässigkeit der beiden Verfahren bei der Einschätzung der Bösartigkeit von wucherndem Gewebe (Polypen) ähnlich hoch zu bewerten ist. Hierbei ist die Schmalbandbeleuchtung (NBI) jedoch weniger aufwändig, da lediglich die Lichtquelle vom Untersucher auf Knopfdruck umgestellt werden muss [3]. Stehle et al. veröffentlichten im Jahr 2009 ein Verfahren zur automatisierten Klassifikation von Dickdarmpolypen unter NBI-Beleuchtung [4], welches in [5]

weiterentwickelt wurde. Hierbei werden nach Vorbild des ärztlichen Diagnose-
prozesses die Blutgefäßstrukturen analysiert. Ein Segmentierungsprozess isoliert
die Blutgefäßstrukturen und diese werden anschließend durch Merkmale, die an
die Entscheidungskriterien der Ärzte angelehnt sind, beschrieben. Auf Basis dieser Beschreibung bestimmt dann ein Klassifikationsalgorithmus die wahrschein-
liche Klasse (harmloser Hyperplast oder potentiell bösartiges Adenom) des Polypen. Bei der Segmentierung von Blutgefäßen unter NBI tritt jedoch oftmals das
Problem auf, dass Artefakte entstehen oder Oberflächenstrukturen der Polypen
mitsegmentiert werden. Um diese zu unterdrücken, stellen wir ein Verfahren vor,
das die segmentierten Ergebnisse objektweise farblich klassifiziert.

Der Aufbau des Papers ist wie folgt: Abschnitt 2 schildert die auf der Transformation in den HSV-Farbraum basierende Trennung von Artefakten und Blutgefäßen und stellt die Polypendatenbank sowie das experimentelle Setup vor.
Die Ergebnisse der Polypenklassifikation basierend auf den erstellten Gefäßkarten werden in Abschnitt 3 vorgestellt und in Abschnitt 4 diskutiert.

2 Material und Methoden

Blutgefäßkarten enthalten häufig Übersegmentierungen und andere Segmentie-
rungsfehler. Der Grund hierfür ist, dass viele Verfahren zur Segmentierung von
Blutgefäßen in erster Linie nach tubulären Strukturen im Grünkanal suchen
(z.B. Matched Filter, [4, 6, 7, 8]). Hierbei werden Strukturen, im Folgenden Artefakte genannt, segmentiert, die lediglich von ihrer Form her Ähnlichkeit mit
Blutgefäßen aufweisen. Bei vielen Verfahren jedoch werden die Farbinformatio-
nen nahezu vollständig außer Acht gelassen. Blutgefäße sind für menschliche
Beobachter farblich meist deutlich von fälschlicherweise segmentierten Strukturen wie z.B. Pit-Patterns, Furchen auf der Polypenoberfläche oder Einblutungen
zu unterscheiden. Das für die Analyse von Dickdarmpolypen eingesetzte NBI-
Licht wird stark von Hämoglobin, dem Farbstoff in den roten Blutkörperchen,
absorbiert. So treten Blutgefäße im Bild deutlich hervor und der Kontrast zum
umliegenden Gewebe wird verbessert. Für eine Artefaktentfernung ist daher eine
genaue Betrachtung der Farbinformation hilfreich. Unterschiede in der Helligkeit
sind jedoch meist auf den Abstand des Endoskops zum Polypen und damit auf
eine variierende Beleuchtungsstärke zurück zu führen. Um diese Problematik zu
überwinden, wird das Ausgangsbild des Koloskops in den HSV-Farbraum [9]
überführt. Hier wird die Helligkeit auf der Achse „value" (Helligkeitswert) aufgetragen, die Farbkomponenten sind in den Achsen „hue" (Farbton) und „satu-
ration" (Farbsättigung) repräsentiert. Somit kann durch Vernachlässigung des
Helligkeitswertes Beleuchtungsinvarianz erreicht werden. Für jedes vermutete
Blutgefäß werden der durchschnittliche Farbton und Farbsättigungswert berechnet und in ein 2-dimensionales Histogramm, welches in Abb. 1 abgebildet ist,
eingetragen. Die unimodale Verteilung der Einträge im Histogramm ist deutlich
einer bivariaten Gaußverteilung ähnlich. Das Histogramm umfasst sowohl Blutgefäße als auch Artefakte. Letztere weisen bei näherer Betrachtung häufig höhere
Farbtonwerte sowie niedrige Sättigungswerte auf. Wir schätzen die Verteilungs-

dichtefunktion mit Hilfe einer bivariaten Gaußverteilung. Somit sind Höhenlinien
in der Verteilung durch die quadratische Funktion

$$d(x, m_x) = (x - m_x)^T K_x^{-1} (x - m_x) \tag{1}$$

gegeben, wobei m_x den Mittelwertvektor und K_x die Kovarianzmatrix der Farb-
ton-Sättigungs-Paare präsentiert. Die quadratische Distanz $d(x, m_x)$ nach Maha-
lanobis beschreibt den varianznormierten Abstand des Vektors x vom Mittelwert
m_x und folgt selbst der χ^2-Verteilung mit n Freiheitsgeraden für den Fall, dass die
Ausgangsverteilung eine multivariate Gaußverteilung ist [10]. Die multivariate
χ^2-Verteilungsdichtefunktion wird durch

$$p_n(d(x, m_x)) = \frac{x^{\frac{n}{2}-1} e^{-\frac{d(x,m_x)}{2}}}{2^{\frac{n}{2}} \Gamma(\frac{n}{2})} \tag{2}$$

bestimmt. Für den Fall $n = 2$ (bivariate Gaußverteilung) lässt sich die Vertei-
lungsdichtefunktion mit

$$p_2(d(x, m_x)) = \frac{1}{2} e^{-\frac{d(x,m_x)}{2}} \tag{3}$$

für $d(x, m_x) \geq 0$ leicht angeben, da die Γ-Funktion $\Gamma(u) = (u - 1)! = 1$ ist
für $u = \frac{n}{2}$ mit $n = 2$. Man kann unter Angabe eines Quantils mit der inversen χ^2-Verteilungsfunktion mit $n = 2$ Freiheitgraden einen Cut-Off-Wert für die
Mahalanobis-Distanz bestimmen. So wird die Festlegung der zugelassenen varianznormierten Abweichungen vom Mittelwert der Verteilung bei der Bewertung
von Strukturen möglich. Weiterhin entfernen wir alle gefundenen Strukturen,
deren Größe in Pixeln unter der Schwelle $t_{\text{connected}}$ liegt. Für die Auswertung
nutzen wir den Algorithmus aus [11].

Die Ergebnisse der Blutgefäßsegmentierung werden anschließend mit unseren neuen Verfahren gefiltert. Jedes $p(d(x, m_x))$ ergibt einen neuen Satz von
Blutgefäßsegmentierungen für das Bilderset. Für die Ergebnisse mit verschiedenen $p(d(x, m_x))$ und ohne Artefakterkennung werden im Anschluss mit Hilfe der
in [11] vorgeschlagenen Merkmalselektionsverfahren Sequential Backward Feature Selection (SBFS) und Simulated Annealing (SA) mit SBFS-Initialisierung

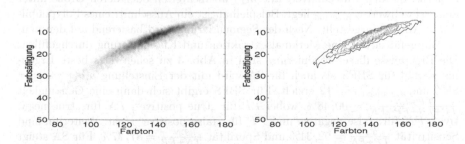

Abb. 1. Histogramm der HS-Wertepaare (links) und Höhenliniendarstellung (rechts)

198   Gross et al.

Tabelle 1. Quantile der χ^2-Verteilungsfunktion und zugehörige Cut-Off-Werte für die Mahalanobis-Distanzen

$p(d(x, m_x))$	60%	70%	80%	85%	90%
$d(x, m_x)$	1,83	2,41	3,22	3,79	4,61

optimale Merkmalskombinationen bestimmt. Hierzu wird eine Leave-one-out-Klassifikation und die 22 Features aus [11] verwendet. Unser Datenset enthält jedoch mit 463 Bildern deutlich mehr Polypen, wobei viele Aufnahmen mit mäßiger Bildqualität inkludiert wurden. Insofern ist anzunehmen, dass unsere Datenbasis größere Anforderungen an die Robustheit der Klassifizierung stellt. Die Bilder von 216 Patienten entstanden am Universitätsklinikum Aachen und zeigen 463 unterschiedliche Polypen aus verschiedensten Winkeln und Beleuchtungssituationen. Die Aufnahmen wurden von verschiedenen Untersuchern mit einem NBI-Zoom-Endoskop vom Typ Olympus Exera II CV-180 gemacht. 274 Aufnahmen zeigen adenomatöse Polypen, die potentiell Krebs entwickeln könnten, und auf 188 Bilder sind harmlose hyperplastische Polypen abgebildet.

3 Ergebnisse

Aus dem Datenset und den dazugehörigen Gefäßkarten ermitteln wir den Mittelwertvektor

$$m_x = \begin{pmatrix} 14,46 \\ 135,63 \end{pmatrix} \tag{4}$$

und die Kovarianzmatrix

$$K_x = \begin{pmatrix} 46,03 & -108,33 \\ -108,33 & 332,65 \end{pmatrix} \tag{5}$$

durch die Schätzung der Gesamtverteilung aller gefundenen Objekte. Es ergibt sich die in Tab. 1 ablesbare Zuordnung von Quantilen $p(d(x, m_x))$ und Cut-Off-Werten $d(x, m_x)$. Aus sämtlichen Blutgefäßkarten werden diejenigen Strukturen entfernt, die den Cut-Off-Wert $d(x, m_x)$ überschreiten oder deren Größe unter dem Schwellwert $t_{connected}$ liegt. Beispielhaft ist ein Ausschnitt eines Polypenbildes in Abb. 2 dargestellt. Nach der Segmentierung wird basierend auf den neuen Blutgefäßkarten eine Merkmalsextraktion und Klassifizierung durchgeführt. Die Ergebnisse dieser Evaluierung sind in Abb. 3 zu sehen. Das beste Ergebnis sowohl für SBFS als auch für SA wird mit der Einstellung $p(d(x, m_x)) = 85\%$ und $t_{connected} = 12$ erzielt. Für SBFS ergibt sich dann eine Genauigkeit $\frac{TP+TN}{TP+TN+FP+FN} = 90,48\%$, wobei TP für „true positive", TN für „true negative", FN für „false negative"und FP für „false positive" steht. Weiterhin sind Sensitivität $\frac{TP}{TP+FN} = 92,34\%$ und Spezifität $\frac{TN}{TN+FP} = 87,77\%$. Für SA steigt der Wert auf $92,21\%$ (Sensitivität von $93,80\%$, Spezifität $89,89\%$). Alternativ, falls eine hohe Sensitivität im Vordergrund steht, kann mit $p(d(x, m_x)) = 86\%$

und $t_{\text{connected}} = 9$ eine Sensitivität von 94,16% erreicht werden (Genauigkeit 90,69%, Spezifität 85,64%). Zum Vergleich wurde das System aus [11] ohne Artefaktentfernung auf dem neuen Datensatz mit 463 Polypen getestet. Es erreichte eine Genauigkeit von 88,10% (Sensitivität 91,24%, Spezifität 83,51%).

4 Diskussion

Die automatisierte Klassifizierung von Dickdarmpolypen auf Basis von Blutgefäßsegmentierungen liefert gute Klassifikationsraten. Artefakte jedoch, die bei der Segmentierung von Blutgefäßen entstehen, beeinträchtigen die Genauigkeit des Gesamtsystems. Mit der vorgeschlagenen Artefaktentfernung wurde auf der neuen Datenbasis ein um 4,2% besseres Ergebnis erzielt als mit dem in [11] beschriebenen System. Insgesamt bestätigt sich auch die Vermutung, dass unsere Datenbasis aufgrund der niedrigeren durchschnittlichen Bildqualität eine größere Herausforderung für die Algorithmen darstellt. Die nächsten Schritte werden von der Entwicklung eines Demonstrators für klinische Studien geprägt sein. Hierzu wird eine Implementierung des Gesamtverfahrens in C++ und die Integration in medizinische Hardware notwendig sein. Weiterhin rückt auch die Detektion der Polypen aus Gründen der einfachen Handhabung wieder in den Fokus.

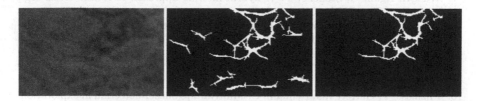

Abb. 2. Beispielhafte Segmentierungsergebnisse für das System: Original Bildausschnitt (links), Segmentierungsergebnis vor der Artefaktentfernung (mitte) und danach (rechts)

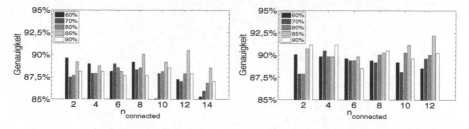

Abb. 3. Klassifikationsgenauigkeit des Gesamtsystems für unterschiedliche Mindestpixelzahlen der Blutgefäße $n_{\text{connected}}$ nach Anwendung der Artefaktunterdrückung mit verschiedenen Quantilen $p(d(x, m_x))$ (Legende) und einer Merkmalsselektion mit SBFS (links) bzw. SA (rechts)

200   Gross et al.

Danksagung. Die Autoren danken den Unterstützern des Projekts: dem Bundesministerium für Bildung und Forschung sowie der Exzellenzinitiative des Bundes und der Länder.

Literaturverzeichnis

1. Robert Koch Institut, editor. Krebs in Deutschland 2005/2006: Häufigkeiten und Trends. Robert Koch Institut und Gesellschaft der epidemologischen Krebsregister in Deutschland e.V.; 2010.
2. Gono K, Obi T, Yamaguchi M, et al. Appearance of enhanced tissue features in narrow-band endoscopic imaging. J Biomed Opt. 2004;9(3):568–77.
3. Tischendorf JJW, Wasmuth HE, Koch A, et al. Value of magnifying chromoendoscopy and narrow band imaging (NBI) in classifying colorectal polyps: A prospective controlled study. Endoscopy. 2007;39(12):1092–6.
4. Stehle T, Auer R, Gross S, et al. Classification of colon polyps in NBI endoscopy using vascularization features. Proc SPIE. 2009;7260.
5. Gross S, Palm S, Behrens A, et al. Segmentierung von Blutgefäßstrukturen in koloskopischen NBI-Bilddaten. Proc BVM. 2011; p. 13–7.
6. Sofka M, Stewart CV. Retinal vessel centerline extraction using multiscale matched filters, confidence and edge measures. IEEE Trans Med Imaging. 2006;25(12):1531–46.
7. Wu CH, Agam G, Stanchev P. A hybrid filtering approach to retinal vessel segmentation. Proc ISBI. 2007; p. 604–7.
8. Chaudhuri S, Chatterjee S, Katz N, et al. Detection of blood vessels in retinal images using two-dimensional matched filters. IEEE Trans Med Imaging. 1989;8(3):263–9.
9. Joblove GH, Greenberg D. Color spaces for computer graphics. Proc SIGGRAPH. 1978;12:20–5.
10. Filzmoser P, Garrett RG, Reimann C. Multivariate outlier detection in exploration geochemistry. Comput Geosci. 2005;31:579–87.
11. Gross S, Palm S, Tischendorf JJW, et al. Automated classification of colon poylps in endoscopic image date. Proc SPIE. 2012;8315.

Evaluation of Algorithms for Lung Fissure Segmentation in CT Images

Alexander Schmidt-Richberg, Jan Ehrhardt, Matthias Wilms, René Werner,
Heinz Handels

Institute of Medical Informatics, University of Lübeck, Lübeck, Germany
schmidt-richberg@imi.uni-luebeck.de

Abstract. Automatic detection of the interlobular lung fissures is a crucial task in computer aided diagnostics and intervention planning, and
required for example for determination of disease spreading or pulmonary
parenchyma quantification. Moreover, it is usually the first step of a subsequent segmentation of the five lung lobes. Due to the clinical relevance,
several approaches for fissure detection have been proposed. They aim at
finding plane-like structures in the images by analyzing the eigenvalues of
the Hessian matrix. Furthermore, these values can be used as features for
supervised fissure detection. In this work, two approaches for supervised
an three for unsupervised fissure detection are evaluated and compared
to each other. The evaluation is based on thoracic CT images acquired
with different radiation doses and different resolutions. The experiments
show that each approach has advantages and the choice should be made
depending on the specific requirements of following algorithm steps.

1 Introduction

The human lungs consist of five separate lobes, three in the right lung and
two in the left. The lobes have individual bronchial and vascular systems and
are functioning relatively independent of each other. A robust segmentation
of the individual lobes is required for many applications in computer aided diagnostics and intervention planning. For example, it is clinically important to
determine if affections in early stages are confined to single lobes, since the interlobular fissures stem the spread of diseases. Moreover, accurate segmentations
are required to characterize and quantify malfunctions like residual pulmonary
parenchyma. First step of lobe segmentation is usually a detection of the interlobular fissures [1, 2, 3, 4]. Fissure detection most commonly aims at finding
planar structures in 3D space by considering the eigenvalues of the Hessian Matrix at each voxel. This approach was first proposed by Wiemker et al. [5].
Lassen et al. later proposed an alternative formulation [1]. Furthermore, Antiga
provided a generalized open source implementation for the Insight Segmentation
and Registration Toolkit (ITK) [6]. Alternatively to these approaches, a supervised fissure detection was proposed by van Rikxoort et al. [7]. Besides gray
value and gradient information, the features considered for classification are also

based on the Hessian matrix. In this work a comparison of the common unsupervised an supervised approaches for fissure segmentation is presented. The goal is to evaluate their performance for images of different quality, i.e. resolution and radiation dose.

2   Material and methods

Most approaches for fissure detection aim at finding two-dimensional, i.e. planar objects in three-dimensional space. This shape information has to be considered to differentiate between vessels and fissures, which have very similar gray values in CT images (around -800 HU). Let $I : \Omega \mapsto \mathbb{R}$ be an image with the domain $\Omega \subset \mathbb{R}^3$. The local shape of a structure at a point $x \in \Omega$ can be assessed by considering the eigenvalues λ_0, λ_1 and λ_2 of the Hessian matrix $\mathcal{H}$ with $|\lambda_0| \geq |\lambda_1| \geq |\lambda_2|$. For plane-like structures, λ_0 is big (across plane) and λ_1 and λ_2 are small (in-plane). For unsupervised fissure segmentation, the eigenvalues are used to formulate a single feature – the fissureness measure F – that is used to separate fissures from background. Approaches for unsupervised segmentation however use several features to train a classifier; its output is then post-processed to obtain the fissure segmentation. Both approaches are detailed in the following.

2.1   Unsupervised fissure segmentation

Wiemker et al. [5] first proposed the fissureness measure

$$F^W := \frac{|\lambda_0| - |\lambda_1|}{|\lambda_0| + |\lambda_1|} \exp \left(\frac{-(I - \mu)^2}{2\sigma^2} \right) \tag{1}$$

The first term is close to one for voxels with $|\lambda_0| \gg |\lambda_1|$. This term is then weighted with a Gaussian function to restrict detection to gray values typical for fissures, with μ and σ being the mean and standard deviation. Moreover, voxels with $\lambda_0 < 0$ are set to zero since fissures are light objects on dark background. Later, Lassen et al. [1] proposed an alternative formulation

$$F^L := \exp \left(\frac{-(|\lambda_0| - \alpha)^6}{\beta^6} \right) \exp \left(\frac{-|\lambda_1|^6}{\gamma^6} \right) \tag{2}$$

While the first term quantifies the strength of a structure by considering the absolute value of λ_0, the second term differentiates between planar structures and vessels or nodules, for example. The parameters α, β and γ are used to weight the terms. Finally, Antiga [6] presented a generalization of the vesselness measure to detect m-dimensional objects in n-dimensional space, originally introduced by Frangi et al. [8]. For $m = 2$ and $n = 3$, this results in

$$F^A := \exp \left(-\frac{|\lambda_1|^2}{2\beta^2|\lambda_0|^2} \right) \left(1 - \exp \left(-\frac{\lambda_0^2 + \lambda_1^2 + \lambda_2^2}{2\gamma^2} \right) \right) \tag{3}$$

The Frobenius norm of the Hessian is included to suppress background noise and β and γ are used as weights. The different functions are visualized in Fig. 1. All terms can be computed on several scales by using images smoothed with varying sigmas to find vessels of different sizes. The maximal value over all considered scales is then used as fissureness measure. The final segmentation S is obtained using a vector-connected-component analysis based on the first eigenvector following [9] and a morphological closing.

2.2 Supervised classification

Alternatively to an unsupervised detection, van Rikxoort et al. propose a supervised approach [7]. A set of 57 features was defined containing the original image value as well as gradient components (3 features), gradient magnitude (1), values of the Hessian (6), eigenvalues (3) and Gray value (1) computed on four different scales with $\sigma = 1, 2, 4, 8$. A subset of these features was used to train a classifier. Moreover, a two-phase strategy was applied. That means, the output of the first run of the classification is used as input for a second run. This procedure significantly reduces background noise. In the original paper four classifiers were tested, whereof the support vector machine (SVM) and k-nearest neighbors (kNN) performed best. These are also considered in this work. To obtain the segmentation S, the output of the classifiers – the number of nearest neighbors classified as fissure F^{kNN} in case of kNN and the probability F^{SVM} of the voxel to belong to a fissure in case of SVM – is thresholded and a connected-component analysis is applied, followed by a morphological closing.

2.3 Image data and validation procedure

First, nine normal dose CT images (120 kVp, $450 - 750$ mAs, $0.79 \times 0.79 \times 0.7$ mm spacing) were used. Moreover, detection was tested for five 4D-CT datasets (120 kVp, 80 mAs, $0.98 \times 0.98 \times 1.5$ mm spacing) supplied by the Washington University in St. Louis. This data set is especially challenging since quality

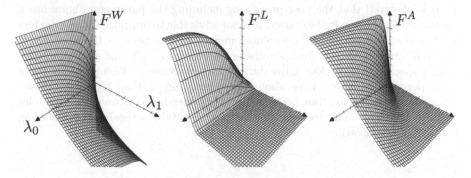

Fig. 1. Comparison of different functions used as fissureness measure

suffers from motion and reconstruction artifacts as well as the low radiation dose per time point. For each dataset manual segmentations were generated as gold standard. All five approaches were used to segment the fissures. Parameters in formulas (2) and (3) and for the post-processing steps were optimized with respect to the Dice coefficient of the manual and the post-processed automatic segmentation. The classifiers were trained using a leave-one-out strategy as described in [7]. First indicator for detection quality is the area under the ROC-Curve (plot of fallout against sensitivity for different thresholds [7]) of each fissureness image F. However, since the volume of the lung is much bigger than the volume of the fissures, the fallout is always very small (i.e. specificity is always close to one) and thus unreliable as a metric. We therefore further analyze additional metrics for the post-processed fissure segmentation S: sensitivity (true positive rate), precision (positive prediction value, PPV) and the Dice coefficient.

3   Results

The results of the evaluation are found in Table 1. In all experiments, segmentations based on F^W show the highest sensitivity for the unsupervised detection, while PPV and Dice coefficient are highest for F^L. This means, most fissures are detected using F^W while F^L features less false positives. This observation can be explained with regard to the graphs in Fig. 1, where only F^L strictly classifies voxels with a high value of λ_1 as background. F^A is outperformed by all other terms. A similar observation can be made for the supervised approaches: While the SVM-based detection has the highest detection rate, it is also more prone to noise than kNN.

Comparing supervised and unsupervised detection, the differences are especially apparent for the ultra-low dose data. Here, the supervised approaches have a significantly higher detection rate than the unsupervised approaches while featuring a comparable amount of noise. The relatively small precision compared to the unsupervised approaches can be explained by the fact that detected fissures are generally thicker due to the higher amount smoothing with a σ of up to 4 (cf. Fig. 2).

It is observed that the post-processing including the parameter choice has a big impact on the result. Moreover, it is not advisable to optimize the parameters for the computation of the fissureness image with respect to the area under the ROC curve. Instead, to optimize sensitivity and PPV one should aim for a high specificity and close gaps during post-processing. Computation times for supervised detection were about four times longer than for unsupervised detection; the exact run time however strongly depends on the number of samples used for training. The training of the SVM can take several hours including parameter optimization.

Evaluation of Algorithms for Lung Fissure Segmentation   205

Table 1. Results for the 3D normal-dose (left) and 4D ultra-low lose data (right). Best results for supervised and unsupervised detection are printed bold for the most meaningful metrics (sensitivity, PPV and Dice coefficient). The segmentation generated using F^i is denoted with S^i

	F^W	F^L	F^A	F^{kNN}	F^{SVM}		F^W	F^L	F^A	F^{kNN}	F^{SVM}
ROC-Area	0.82	0.80	0.80	0.99	0.99	ROC-Area	0.78	0.77	0.80	0.99	0.99
Sensitivity	**0.58**	0.51	0.46	0.82	**0.92**	Sensitivity	**0.55**	0.53	0.52	0.80	**0.91**
Specificity	1.00	1.00	0.98	0.99	0.99	Specificity	1.00	1.00	0.98	0.99	0.99
PPV	0.81	**0.90**	0.16	**0.54**	0.38	PPV	0.51	**0.58**	0.19	**0.52**	0.41
Dice	0.65	**0.76**	0.24	**0.65**	0.58	Dice	0.53	**0.55**	0.28	**0.63**	0.57
	S^W	S^L	S^A	S^{kNN}	S^{SVM}		S^W	S^L	S^A	S^{kNN}	S^{SVM}

4 Conclusion

All examined algorithms were applicable to segment fissures in the normal-dose CT data. For the 4D data, only the supervised approaches supplied reasonably good results. The choice of detection algorithm strongly depends on the application. If computation time is not very crucial or if the images are of very bad quality, supervised detection is advised. To choose between F^W and F^L or f^{kNN} and F^{SVM}, characteristics of following steps should be considered: For example,

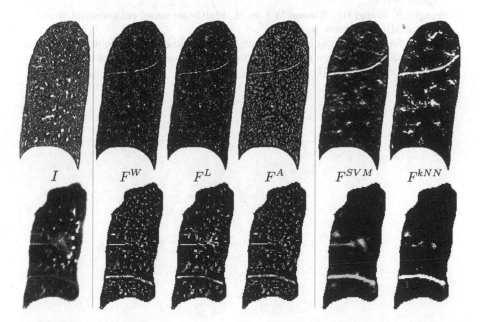

Fig. 2. Comparison of unsupervised fissureness values an the outputs of the supervised classifiers for the normal use (upper row) and ultra-low dose data (lower row)

if a subsequent lobe segmentation is prone to noise [4], F^L or f^{kNN} should be used. If the algorithm requires the fissures to be computed as comprehensively as possible, F^W or F^{SVM} are advised.

References

1. Lassen B, Kuhnigk JM, Friman O, et al. Automatic segmentation of lung lobes in CT images based on fissures, vessels, and bronchi. In: Proc IEEE ISBI; 2010. p. 560–563.
2. Pu J, Zheng B, Leader JK, et al. Pulmonary lobe segmentation in CT examinations using implicit surface fitting. IEEE Trans Med Imag. 2009;28(12):1986–96.
3. van Rikxoort EM, Prokop M, de Hoop BJ, et al. Automatic segmentation of pulmonary lobes robust against incomplete fissures. IEEE Trans Med Imag. 2010;29(6):1286–96.
4. Schmidt-Richberg A, Ehrhardt J, Wilms M, et al. Pulmonary lobe segmentation with level sets. In: Proc SPIE; 2012. (in press).
5. Wiemker R, Bülow T, Blaffert T. Unsupervised extraction of the pulmonary interlobar fissures from high resolution thoracic CT data. In: Proc CARS; 2005. p. 1121–26.
6. Antiga L. Generalizing vesselness with respect to dimensionality and shape. Insight J. 2007.
7. van Rikxoort EM, van Ginneken B, Klik M, et al. Supervised enhancement filters: application to fissure detection in chest CT scans. IEEE Trans Med Imag. 2008;27(1):1–10.
8. Frangi AF, Frangi RF, Niessen WJ, et al. Multiscale vessel enhancement filtering. In: Proc MICCAI; 1998. p. 130–7.
9. Ross JC, San José Estépar R, Kindlmann G, et al. Automatic lung lobe segmentation using particles, thin plate splines, and maximum a posteriori estimation. In: Proc MICCAI; 2010. p. 163–71.

Real-Time Intensity Based 2D/3D Registration for Tumor Motion Tracking During Radiotherapy

Hugo Furtado[1], Christelle Gendrin[1], Christoph Bloch[1], Jakob Spoerk[1],
Suprianto A. Pawiro[1], Christoph Weber[1], Michael Figl[1], Helmar Bergmann[1],
Markus Stock[2], Dietmar Georg[2], Wolfgang Birkfellner[1]

[1]Center for Biomedical Engineering and Physics
[2]University Clinic for Radiotherapy, Division of Medical Physics
Medical University Vienna, Vienna, Austria
hugo.furtado@meduniwien.ac.at

Abstract. Organ motion during radiotherapy is one of the causes of uncertainty in dose delivery creating the need to enlarge the planned target volume (PTV) to guarantee full tumor irradiation. In this work, we investigate the feasibility of using real-time 2D/3D registration for tumor motion tracking during radiotherapy based on purely intensity based image processing, thus avoiding markers or fiducials. X-rays are acquired during treatment at a rate of 5.4 Hz. We iteratively compare each x-ray with a set of digitally reconstructed radiographs (DRR) generated from the planning volume dataset, finding the optimal match between the x-ray and one of the DRRs. The DRRs are generated using a ray-casting algorithm, implemented using general purpose computation on graphics hardware (GPGPU) for best performance. Validation is conducted off-line using a phantom and five clinical patient data sets. The phantom motion is measured with an RMS error of 2.1 mm and mean registration time is 220 ms. For the patient data sets, a sinusoidal movement that clearly correlates to the breathing cycle is seen. Mean registration time is always under 105 ms which is well suited for our purposes. These results demonstrate that real-time organ motion monitoring using image based markerless registration is feasible.

1 Introduction

Organ motion during radiotherapy is one of the main sources of uncertainty in dose application. Periodic movements, correlated with the breathing or cardiac cycle and other aperiodic movements create the need to extend the margins of the planned target volume (PTV) in order to guarantee full tumor irradiation. This can result in organs at risk being irradiated. Attempts at tumor motion tracking include the use of x-ray imaging and implanted fiducial markers [1], the tracking of passive electromagnetic transponders implanted close to the tumor tissue [2], the correlation of surface landmarks with internal motion [3], and the correlation of surface motion with lung motion models [4, 5, 6]. While these efforts present promising results, most of these approaches are stricken with challenges such as the implantation of markers which add an additional burden in clinical routine or, in the case of respiratory models, drift problems, an insufficient correlation of organ movement patterns and external surrogate markers, and aperiodic motion.

The aim of our work is to investigate the feasibility of continuous tumor motion tracking using purely intensity based image registration techniques. Modern radiotherapy devices include the possibility of kiloVoltage high contrast image aquisition during treatment at rates as high as 5Hz. We aim at providing registration with a sufficient update rate to be able to follow tumor motion in real-time thus enabling further reduction of the PTV with the consequent reduction of total dose delivery to the patient. This work extends previous research performed in our group where a similar evaluation has been done but where the performance was still well bellow our goal [7]. The work was extended by reimplementing the ray-casting algorithm in the graphics card using CUDA which increased the performance significantly.

2   Materials and methods

Our approach requires no markers or fiducials and works as follows: X-ray images, acquired during treatment, are compared to digitally rendered radiographs (DRRs) generated from the planning volume dataset. The two images are compared using a intensity based merit funtion. An optimizer searches for the spatial transformation which generates the best match between the DRR and the x-ray. The registration is complete when a maximum of similarity is reached. The DRRs are generated using a ray casting algorithm which is implemented on a general purpose graphics processing unit (GPGPU) and programmed in CUDA (as described in [8]) for best performance. The registration is done on a region of interest (ROI) centered around the PTV. This is the region where we want to follow movement and where the assumption of a rigid transformation is valid. The DRR and the x-ray are compared using normalized mutual information [9] as merit function.

We validated our approach off-line using a respiratory phantom and datasets from five clinical patients undergoing therapy in our center. The data sets consist of x-ray images acquired during tumor irradiation, a planning CT volume and a CBCT volume acquired at the beginning of each fraction. The x-rays were acquired at a rate of 5.4Hz and stored on hard-drive for off-line processing. The alignment of the CBCT to the x-rays is easy since these are generated with the same device. Therefore, we used the CBCT volume for the phantom registration. On the other hand, the planning CT offers better image quality compared to the CBCT and contains also the planning structures for the patients. For this reason, we chose to use the planning CT volume for the patient registration.

The phantom consists of three spheres of the same diameter and several materials embedded in a circular cylinder. The cylinder is fixed to an axle that can translate in one direction to simulate breathing motion. This phantom was set to the respiration mode at 15 cycles per minute during acquisition of the x-ray images. The movement was simultaneously recorded in six degrees-of-freedom by means of an optical tracking system. The accuracy of the tracking system is of 0.5 mm (95% confidence interval) allowing us to use this measurement as ground-truth.

The five patients suffering from non-small cell lung tumor or lung metastases were undergoing treatment in a routine procedure at the department of radiotherapy. For each of them, a planning CT was acquired and treatment specific contours were defined by the medical team (Fig. 1). From these datasets, we extracted the PTV contour, which we used to define our ROI. In all cases, a set (between 105 and 150) of x-rays were acquired during treatment.

3   Results

The movement of the phantom was measured with an RMS error of 2.1 mm in relation to the known displacement (Fig. 2a). On the patient datasets we measure a movement which clearly correlates with the respiratory cycle which was obtained by extracting the diaphragm movement from the treatment x-rays (Fig. 3). Patient four has been omitted from the results because it exhibited almost no movement due to the tumor being situated in the apex of the lung. Table 1 gives the RMS and maximum amplitude of the resulting tumor displacements in each direction, cranial caudal (CC), left right (LR) and anterior posterior (AP). The movement is always more pronounced along the CC direction with the exception of patient 3 exhibiting a movement of higher amplitude along LR than CC direction. The larger motion along the CC direction, especially in patients 1 and 5 (8.5 mm and 19.4 mm respectively) is related to the

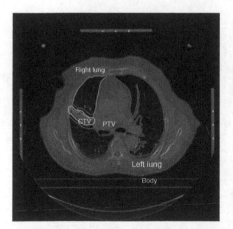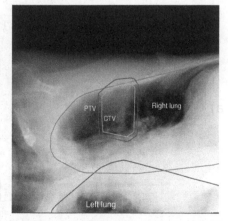

Fig. 1. Example patient data set used for off-line validation of the method. One slice of the 3D dataset, with annotated contours of the lungs, the PTV and the CTV is shown on the left side. On the right, one x-ray with the contours projected is shown

Table 1. RMS and maximum amplitude of the tumor motion along CC, LR and AP directions for the patients. If the extracted displacement did not feature a sinusoidal like signal, the statistics are not relevant and N.A. (non applicable) is written in the table

	RMS (mm)			Amplitude (min-max)			Mean reg. time (ms)
	CC	LR	AP	CC (mm)	LR (mm)	AP (mm)	
Patient 1	2.0	0.9	0.6	8.5	3.0	1.8	69.6
Patient 2	1.3	0.8	0.9	5.0	3.1	2.4	101.4
Patient 3	0.5	0.5	0.2	1.3	2.4	1.2	91.7
Patient 5	6.7	N.A	N.A	19.4	N.A	N.A	67.9

tumors being located close to the diaphragm. In the table, the mean registration time for each of the patients is also shown. Finally, Fig. 4 shows three intra-fractional x-rays in different points in time with the clinical target volume (CTV), the middle contour (green), following the result of our registration.

4   Discussion

We implemented an image based markerless registration framework, able to robustly follow tumor motion during radiotherapy treatment with sufficient update rate to process data in real-time. The registration for all the patients is well bellow our target which was a maximum of 185 ms (5.4Hz update rate) and the extracted movement clearly correlates with the breathing motion. The phantom mean registration time is around 220 ms due to the bigger ROI. Nevertheless,

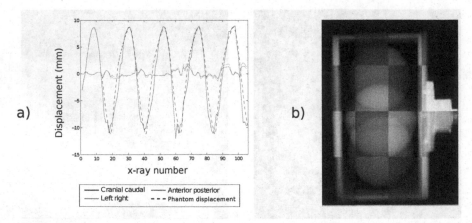

Fig. 2. a) Reconstructed motion of the phantom displacement along SI (blue line), LR (green line) and AP (red line). The dashed line represents the phantom motion measured with an optical tracking system. b) checkerboard image of x-ray and corresponding registered DRR images acquired during phantom motion

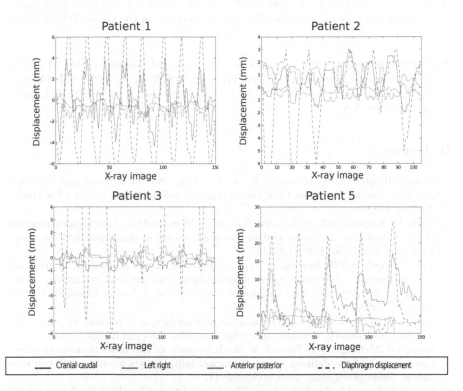

Fig. 3. Reconstructed motion of the centroid of the tumor along CC (blue line), LR (green line), AP (red line) directions for patients 1, 2, 3 and 5. The diaphragm motion of each patient is also shown as a black dotted line

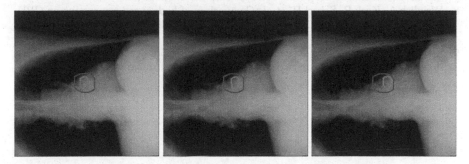

Fig. 4. Tumor motion tracking example. In the images, the planned target volume (PTV) is represented as the outer contour, in red and the clinical target volume (CTV) as the inner contour, in green. The images were taken in different point in time. In each of the images, the CTV was represented in the final position extracted by our registration algorithm

seldom a PTV will be this big for patients in this kind of treatment. Further steps include increasing the update-rate by implementing other components of the registration scheme – such as the merit function – in the GPGPU and online validation.

Acknowledgement. We acknowledge the financial support of the Austrian FWF Translational Research Program (Project P19931 and L503), of the ASEA-Uninet foundation and of the EC Marie Curie Research Action PIIF-GA-2009-252305 ROBOGYN.

References

1. Shirato H, Shimizu S, Kitamura K, et al. Organ motion in image-guided radiotherapy: lessons from real-time tumor-tracking radiotherapy. Int J Clin Oncol. 2007;12(1):8–16.
2. Shah AP, Kupelian PA, Willoughby TR, et al. An evaluation of intrafraction motion of the prostate in the prone and supine positions using electromagnetic tracking. Radiother Oncol. 2011;99(1):37–43.
3. Cho B, Poulsen PR, Sawant A, et al. Real-time target position estimation using stereoscopic kilovoltage/megavoltage imaging and external respiratory monitoring for dynamic multileaf collimator tracking. Int J Radiat Oncol Biol Phys. 2010;79(1):269–78.
4. Ren Q, Nishioka S, Shirato H, et al. Adaptive prediction of respiratory motion for motion compensation radiotherapy. Phys Med Biol. 2007;52(22):6651–61.
5. Hughes S, McClelland J, Tarte S, et al. Assessment of two novel ventilatory surrogates for use in the delivery of gated/tracked radiotherapy for non-small cell lung cancer. Radiother Oncol. 2009;91(3):336–41.
6. Lin T, Cervino LI, Tang X, et al. Fluoroscopic tumor tracking for image-guided lung cancer radiotherapy. Phys Med Biol. 2009;54(4):981.
7. Gendrin C, Furtado H, Weber C, et al. Monitoring tumor motion by real time 2D/3D registration during radiotherapy. Radiother Oncol. 2011.
8. Weinlich A, Keck B, Scherl H, et al. Comparison of high-speed ray casting on GPU using CUDA and OpenGL. In: Buchty R, Weiß JP, editors. Proc HIPHAC. vol. 1. Karlsruh; 2008. p. 25–30.
9. Maes F, Collignon A, Vandermeulen D, et al. Multimodality image registration by maximization of mutual information. IEEE Trans Med Imaging. 1997;2:187–98.

Registration of Lung Surface Proximity for Assessment of Pleural Thickenings

Peter Faltin[1], Kraisorn Chaisaowong[1,2], Thomas Kraus[3], Til Aach[1]

[1]Lehrstuhl für Bildverarbeitung, RWTH Aachen University
[2]King Mongkut's University of Technology North Bangkok
[3]Institut für Arbeitsmedizin und Sozialmedizin, UK Aachen
peter.faltin@lfb.rwth-aachen.de

Abstract. Follow-up assessment of pleural thickenings requires the comparison of information from different points in time. The investigated image regions must be precisely registered to acquire this information. Since the thickenings' growth is the target value, this growth should not be compensated by the registration process. We therefore present a non-rigid registration method, which preserves the shape of the thickenings. The deformation of the volume image is carried out using B-splines. With focus on the image regions located around the lung surface, an efficient way of calculating corresponding points combined with the reuse of information from different scale levels leads to the non-rigid registration, which can be performed within a short computation time.

1 Introduction

Inhaled carcinogenic asbestos fibers can cause pleural thickenings which may evolve to pleural mesothelioma. To reduce the mortality, an early stage diagnosis is essential. Hence high-risk patients undergo a regular medical check-up including CT imaging. Manual analysis of CT data is time consuming and subject to strong inter- and intra-reader variability [1]. The application of a computer assisted diagnosis system reduces the workload and provides objective analysis. Within this framework a non-rigid registration is required to compare information from multiple points in time. The system is designed for the clinical routine. Therefore all algorithms are designed with respect to their computation time.

B-spline registration utilizes different methods to determine the mesh, controlling the deformation. Rueckert et al. [2] use mutual information while Loeckx et al. [3] use conditional mutual information to iteratively optimize the mesh. Faster methods like Chui et al. [4] or Kwon et al. [5] utilize features to calculate the deformation, but are still based on iterative optimization schemes. These methods however are not capable to protect the thickening growth from being undesirably compensated. We explicitly address this problem and additionally calculate the transformed mesh from matched points non-iteratively.

2   Materials and methods

The images $G_t^{(0)}, t \in \{0, 1\}$ from the same patient at two different points in time consist of the voxels $G_t^{(0)}(r)$, with the image coordinates $R^{(0)} = \{(x, y, z)^T : 0 \leq x < X^{(0)}, 0 \leq y < Y^{(0)}, 0 \leq z < Z^{(0)}\}$. The superscripts $^{(0)}$ address the scaling level and can be ignored for the first step. The lung masks $R_{L,t}^{(0)} \subset R^{(0)}$ and the associated surfaces $\partial R_{L,t}^{(0)}$ are extracted using two-step supervised range-constrained Otsu thresholding [6]. The thickenings $R_{T,t=0}^{(0)} \subset R^{(0)}$ for $t = 0$ are segmented by the comparison of the actual lung with a healthy lung model [6]. With the known mask data $R_{L,t}^{(0)}$, the rigid transformation T_r can be determined using e.g. a Gibbs-Markov random field based approach from Faltin et al. [7].

We present here an efficient method for the non-rigid part of the registration. First, the surface of interests (SOI) is extracted. The local registration for each included point is identified and the image is deformed accordingly. Offsets and deformations are determined for each scaling level of an image pyramid.

2.1   Extracting the surface of interest

It is hard to distinguish between the healthy lung boundary and the boundary implied by a pleural thickening (Fig. 1). Therefore the thickening growth can easily been misinterpreted as a deformation. The critical thickening regions $R_{T,t}^{(0)} \subset R^{(0)}$ are first increased by a dilation with a sphere W of radius 5 (voxels) and then masked in the point-set approximating the lung surface $\partial R_{L,t}^{(0)}$. This leads to the discrete SOI

$$R_{\text{SOI},t}^{(0)} = \partial R_{L,t}^{(0)} \setminus (R_{T,t}^{(0)} \oplus W) \tag{1}$$

which contains the voxel coordinates at lung surface excluding regions close to thickenings.

2.2   Applying the image pyramid

The unregistered and downsampled images of the lungs are determined iteratively applying $G_t^{(q)} = \text{B}_{\downarrow 2}\{G_t^{(q-1)}\}$, where q, $0 < q < Q$, denotes the scaling

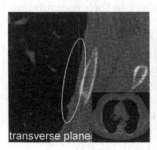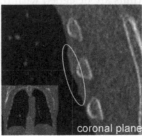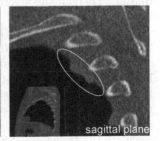

transverse plane   coronal plane   sagittal plane

Fig. 1. A pleural thickening shown in different planes

level and $\boldsymbol{R}^{(q)}$ its image domain for each of the Q scaling levels. $B_{\downarrow 2}$ includes downsampling of factor 2 and a previous smoothing with an appropriate Gaussian kernel. Analogue to the Gaussian kernel which prevents aliasing in the image, a rounding operation is applied, when downsampling the point-set of the SOI, to keep all surface information

$$R_{\text{SOI},t}^{(q)} = \left\{ \left\lfloor \frac{\boldsymbol{r}^{(q-1)}}{2} \right\rfloor : r^{(q-1)} \in R_{\text{SOI},t}^{(q-1)} \right\}, 0 < q < Q \tag{2}$$

2.3 Determining the local displacements

The data obtained from the image pyramid at level q is modified considering the results from the previous level $(q + 1)$, which is denoted by a tilde on top of the identifiers and described in section 2.4. The deformation is determined at each level q in the SOI by 3D block matching. As an error metric the sum of absolute differences is calculated

$$\mathbf{SAD}^{(q)}(\boldsymbol{d}, \boldsymbol{r}) = \sum_{\|\boldsymbol{r}' - \boldsymbol{r}\|_\infty \le b, \boldsymbol{r}' \in \mathbb{Z}^3} \left| \tilde{G}_{t=0}^{(q)}(\boldsymbol{r}' + \boldsymbol{d}) - G_{t=1}^{(q)}(\boldsymbol{r}') \right|, \boldsymbol{r} \in \tilde{R}_{\text{SOI},t=0}^{(q)} \tag{3}$$

for each displacement $\boldsymbol{d}$, with the block size b. For densely sampled surfaces and large block dimensions $(2b + 1)^3$, overlapping of the blocks results in multiple calculation of the absolute differences. An more efficient way is to separately create an error image and summing up the differences. An error image

$$E^{(q)}(\boldsymbol{d}, \boldsymbol{r}) = \left| \tilde{G}_{t=0}^{(q)}(\boldsymbol{r} + \boldsymbol{d}) - G_{t=1}^{(q)}(\boldsymbol{r}) \right|, \boldsymbol{r} \in R^{(q)} \tag{4}$$

is created for each displacement $\boldsymbol{d} \in \{\boldsymbol{s}; \forall \boldsymbol{s} \in \mathbb{Z}^3, \|(0,0,0)^T - \boldsymbol{s}\|_\infty \le 1\}$, which includes all 27 combinations of displacements $\{-1, 0, 1\}$ per dimension. Calculating the error for the full image domain $\boldsymbol{R}^{(q)}$ in parallel can be faster than to determine which voxels are required for the block-wise calculation and individually addressing them. Larger displacements are implicitly considered due to the image pyramid. The computationally intensive summation is only applied for the SOI, resulting in the SAD for each displacement $\boldsymbol{d}$

$$\mathbf{SAD}^{(q)}(\boldsymbol{d}, \boldsymbol{r}) = \sum_{\|\boldsymbol{r}' - \boldsymbol{r}\|_\infty \le b, \boldsymbol{r}' \in \mathbb{Z}^3} E^{(q)}(\boldsymbol{d}, \boldsymbol{r}'), \boldsymbol{r} \in \tilde{R}_{\text{SOI},t=0}^{(q)} \tag{5}$$

Finally for each feature point the displacement $\boldsymbol{D}$ is determined choosing the displacement, which minimizes the SAD

$$D^{(q)}(\boldsymbol{r}) = \arg \min_{\boldsymbol{d}} \mathbf{SAD}^{(q)}(\boldsymbol{d}, \boldsymbol{r}), \boldsymbol{r} \in \tilde{R}_{\text{SOI},t=0}^{(q)} \tag{6}$$

2.4 Deforming the images

The deformed image $G_{t=0}^{(q)}$ can be interpolated using B-splines, which are controlled by a mesh of $N_x \times N_y \times N_z$ points $\tilde{\boldsymbol{\Phi}}_{\mu,\nu,\epsilon}^{(q)}$, with the uniform spacing δ.

The positions of these control points are determined by the B-spline approximation (BA) of Lee et al. [8], which utilizes the SOI $R^{(q)}_{\mathrm{SOI},t=0}$ and the associated displacements $D^{(q)}(r)$. The deformation for each image point is given by

$$
T^{(q)}_{\mathrm{nr}}(r) = \begin{cases} \sum_{l=0}^{3}\sum_{m=0}^{3}\sum_{n=0}^{3} B_l(u)B_m(v)B_n(w)\tilde{\Phi}^{(q)}_{i+l,j+m,k+n} & 0 < q < Q-1 \\ r & q = Q-1 \end{cases} \tag{7}
$$

with $i = \lfloor \frac{x}{N_x} \rfloor + 1$, $j = \lfloor \frac{y}{N_y} \rfloor + 1$, $k = \lfloor \frac{z}{N_z} \rfloor + 1$, $u = \frac{x}{N_x} - \lfloor \frac{x}{N_x} \rfloor$, $v = \frac{y}{N_y} - \lfloor \frac{y}{N_y} \rfloor$, $w = \frac{z}{N_z} - \lfloor \frac{z}{N_z} \rfloor$. $B_c(s)$ is the c-th basis function of the cubic and uniform B-spline [2]. To avoid iterative interpolations for the following scale levels we adapt the control points using

$$
\tilde{\Phi}^{(q)}_{\mu,\nu,\epsilon} = 2 \cdot T^{(q+1)}_{\mathrm{nr}} \left(\frac{\Phi^{(q)}_{\mu,\nu,\epsilon}}{2} \right) \tag{8}
$$

Therefore the transformed image data and SOI from the first point in time ($t = 0$) are given by

$$
\tilde{G}^{(q)}_{t=0}(r) = G^{(q)}_{t=0} \left(2 \cdot T^{(q+1)}_{\mathrm{nr}} \left(\frac{r}{2} \right) \right), r \in R^{(q)} \tag{9}
$$

and

$$
\tilde{R}^{(q)}_{\mathrm{SOI},t=0} = \left\{ \left\lfloor 2 \cdot T^{(q+1)}_{\mathrm{nr}} \left(\frac{r}{2} \right) + (0.5, 0.5, 0.5)^T \right\rfloor : r \in R^{(q)}_{\mathrm{SOI},t=0} \right\} \tag{10}
$$

3   Results

The presented method is applied to CT datasets from 4 different patients. For each patient 2 CT scans from different points in time are non-rigidly registered. The CT scans for the patients I - III consist of 400-700 slices, while the the CT scans from patient IV consist of approx. 60 slices. The SAD within a lung surface proximity $R_{P,t=1}$ is used as an indicator to evaluate the registration quality. After dilation with a sphere W of radius 10 (voxels) on the lungs surface $\partial R_{t=1}$ the proximity $R_{P,t=1} = \partial R_{t=1} \oplus W$ is created. Additionally the average surface distance (ASD), from each point of the lung surface $\tilde{R}^{(0)}_{\mathrm{SOI},t=0}$ to the closest point in $R^{(0)}_{\mathrm{SOI},t=1}$ is determined.

First we investigate the results using varying block size b (fixed $\delta = 8$) then mesh spacing δ (fixed $b = 4$). The resulting SAD are shown in Fig. 2. Finally we compare the performance of our method to the implementation from Kroon (MATLAB central file ID: #20057). SAD and ASD are compared in Fig. 3 for both methods and all patients. We chose for patient I - III $\delta = 8$, $b = 8$ and for patient IV with the low slice count $\delta = 4$, $b = 4$.

Fig. 2. SAD using different parameters

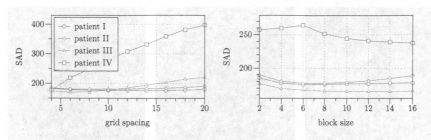

Fig. 3. Comparison of the Kroon implementation and our approach

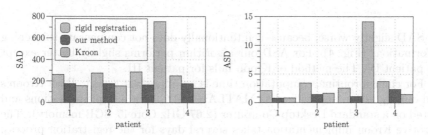

4 Discussion

Fig. 2 shows that our method does not optimally perform for patient IV, which is a consequence of the low slice count. For higher slice count the method shows a stable and low SAD for the parameter $\delta = 8$, $b = 8$. Visual examples of the results are shown as difference images in Fig. 5. The rigid registration (Fig. 5a) performs an overall optimization and is not optimal for each individual part of the lung surface. The visualizations of the non-rigid results (Fig. 5b, Fig. 5c) show good performance in the surface regions. While our approach shows weaknesses in the disregarded image regions (Fig. 5b), the Kroon approach performs well for whole image (Fig. 5c).

Comparing our approach to the Kroon implementation reveals that the SAD values are in a similar range (Fig. 3). As expected our implementation performs

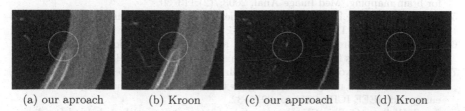

(a) our aproach   (b) Kroon   (c) our approach   (d) Kroon

Fig. 4. Visible thickening growth influenced by non-rigid registration comparing CT image data (a),(b) and difference images (c),(d)

Fig. 5. Visual comparison of registrations by regarding the difference image

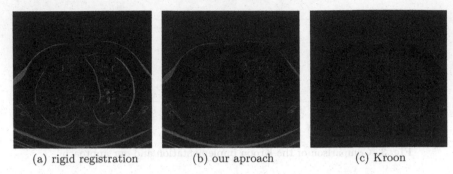

(a) rigid registration   (b) our aproach   (c) Kroon

for SAD slightly worse, because it intentionally does not compensate thickening deformations (Fig. 4). For ASD our algorithm performs slightly better except for patient IV. The method of Kroon fails for patient III.

For clinical routine, computation time is an important aspect. Both Kroon's and our algorithm are realized as MATLAB and C hybrid implementations and tested on a standard Desktop Computer (2.67 GHz Core i5, 8GB memory). The iterative Kroon implementation takes several days for the registration process, while our approach takes at maximum 2.5 minutes.

For future work we plan to use the obtained registration for a consistent segmentation of the thickenings at both points in time.

References

1. Ochsmann E, Carl T, Brand P, et al. Inter-reader variability in chest radiography and HRCT for the early detection of asbestos-related lung and pleural abnormalities in a cohort of 636 asbestos-exposed subjects. Int Arch Occup Environ Health. 2010;83:39–46.
2. Rueckert D, Sonoda LI, Hayes C, et al. Nonrigid registration using free-form deformations: Application to breast MR images. IEEE Trans Med Imaging. 1999;18:712–21.
3. Loeckx D, Slagmolen P, Maes F, et al. Nonrigid image registration using conditional mutual information. IEEE Trans Med Imaging. 2007;29(1):725–37.
4. Chui H, Win L, Schultz R, et al. A unified non-rigid feature registration method for brain mapping. Med Image Anal. 2003;7(2):113–30.
5. Kwon D, Yun ID, Lee KH, et al. Efficient feature-based nonrigid registration of multiphase liver CT volumes. In: BMVC; 2008.
6. Chaisaowong K, Bross B, Knepper A, et al. Detection and follow-up assessment of pleural thickenings from 3D CT data. In: ECTI; 2008. p. 489–92.
7. Faltin P, Chaisaowong K, Kraus T, et al. Markov-Gibbs model based registration of CT lung images using subsampling for the follow-up assessment of pleural thickenings. In: IEEE ICIP; 2011. p. 2229–32.
8. Lee S, Wolberg G, Shin SY. Scattered data interpolation with multilevel B-splines. IEEE Trans Vis Comput Graph. 1997;3:228–244.

Effiziente Verpunktung pulmonaler MR-Bilder zur Evaluierung von Registrierungsergebnissen

Jan Strehlow[1], Jan Rühaak[2,3], Christina Kluck[3], Bernd Fischer[2,3]

[1]Fraunhofer MEVIS - Institut für Bildgestützte Medizin, Bremen
[2]Fraunhofer MEVIS - Projektgruppe Bildregistrierung, Lübeck
[3]Institute of Mathematics and Image Computing, Universität zu Lübeck
jan.strehlow@mevis.fraunhofer.de

Kurzfassung. Die aussagekräftige Validierung von nichtlinearen Registrierungsverfahren gehört nach wie vor zu den großen Herausforderungen der medizinischen Bildverarbeitung. Ein vielversprechender Ansatz besteht in der Generierung vieler Landmarken in den zu registrierenden Objekten, welche dann in einem zweiten Schritt zur Validierung des Deformationsfeldes genutzt werden können. Wir präsentieren ein flexibles Verfahren zur Erstellung solcher Referenzstandards für MR-Scans. In einem ersten Schritt werden in der Referenz (Baseline-Scan) automatisch Landmarken erzeugt. Die entsprechende Zuordnung im Template (Follow-up-Scan) erfolgt nach einer kurzen Benutzerinitialisierung automatisch durch Thin-Plate-Spline-Transformation und lokale, affin-lineare Nachregistrierung. Eine fehleranfällige und zeitaufwändige manuelle Verpunktung entfällt fast vollständig. Wir evaluieren unser Verfahren anhand einer Studie mit drei Experten auf pulmonalen MR-Scans. Die ersten Ergebnisse erwiesen sich als sehr vielversprechend. Es stellte sich heraus, dass die vom System bestimmten Punkte im Bereich der Variabilität der Experten untereinander liegen.

1 Einleitung

Die CT-Aufnahmetechnik repräsentiert den derzeitigen klinischen Standard der Lungenbildgebung. In jüngerer Zeit eröffnen sich durch neue Aufnahmesequenzen und Kontrastmittel jedoch zunehmend vielversprechende Anwendungen der pulmonalen MR-Bildgebung (MRI) [1]. Die MRI erzeugt keine Strahlenbelastung und bietet daher große Vorteile etwa für die Pädiatrie sowie im Therapiemonitoring. Typischerweise werden beim Monitoring von COPD- und Asthmapatienten mehrere funktionelle und morphologische Scans zu verschiedenen Zeitpunkten erstellt [2]. Die morphologischen Scans stellen dabei anatomische Informationen bereit, können aber auch dazu genutzt werden, die funktionellen Aufnahmen zueinander in Beziehung zu setzen. Es entsteht aufgrund der auftretenden Lungendeformationen unmittelbar ein nichtlineares Registrierungsproblem.

Für den klinischen Einsatz solcher Verfahren ist eine umfangreiche Evaluierung insbesondere der nichtlinearen Registrierungen unerlässlich. Hierzu stehen verschiedene Kriterien zur Wahl; es hat sich jedoch unter anderem in der umfangreichen EMPIRE10-Studie über CT-Lungenregistrierung [3, 4]) gezeigt, dass der Target Registration Error, also der durchschnittliche Abstand manuell annotierter Landmarkenpunkte, die gegenwärtig aussagekräftigste Bewertung verschiedener Registrierungsverfahren erlaubt. Die Aussagekraft einer solchen Methodik hängt dabei entscheidend von der Güte der gewählten Landmarken und ihrer zuverlässigen Korrespondenz ab [5]. Die manuelle Erstellung eines solchen Referenzstandards in einem großen 3D-Datensatz ist jedoch außerordentlich mühselig, zeitaufwändig und zudem fehleranfällig.

In [6] wurde ein Verfahren vorgestellt und evaluiert, das automatisch eine große Anzahl Landmarken in Lungen-CT-Aufnahmen generieren kann und einen medizinischen Experten bei der Zuordnung korrespondierender Punkte in einem zweiten Scan unterstützt. Wir präsentieren in dieser Arbeit eine Verallgemeinerung des Ansatzes am Beispiel pulmonaler MR-Scans und zeigen anhand einer ersten Studie an klinischen Datensätzen die Nützlichkeit unserer Neuerungen.

2   Material und Methoden

2.1   Bisherige Arbeiten

Das speziell zur Verpunktung von Lungen-CTs entwickelte Verfahren von Murphy et al. [6] generiert zunächst n Landmarken in der Referenzaufnahme. Die Zuordnung korrespondierender Punkte in einem zweiten CT-Scan verläuft für $n = 100$ in drei Phasen:

1. Manuelle Zuordnung der ersten vier Landmarken
2. Semiautomatische Zuordnung der Landmarken 5 bis ca. 30
3. Vollautomatische Zuordnung der verbleibenden ca. 70 Landmarken

Der Benutzer wird nach den ersten vier manuellen Zuordnungen bei der Auswahl korrespondierender Punkte durch eine Kombination aus einer Thin-Plate-Spline-Transformation (TPS), die aus den bisher bestimmten Korrespondenzen berechnet wird, und einer lokalen Verfeinerung mittels Blockmatching unterstützt. Während dieser Phase wird die TPS-Transformation durch die Korrekturen des Benutzers fortwährend verfeinert. Nach ca. 30 Zuordnungen ist das System dann so gut trainiert, dass die verbleibenden Korrespondenzen vollautomatisch gefunden werden können [6]. Die Autoren stellen zudem eine Übertragung der Methode auf neurologische MR-Daten vor, verzichten jedoch aufgrund der MR-Besonderheiten explizit auf das Sum of Squared Differences (SSD)-Blockmatching und erzielen ungenauere Ergebnisse als auf CT-Daten.

2.2   Erweiterungen für MR-Daten

Murphy et al. [6] realisieren die Verfeinerung der TPS-Vorschläge durch eine vollständige Suche nach dem Minimum der SSD-Distanz in einem lokalen Fenster (Blockmatching). Hierzu werden zwei Suchblöcke fester Größe in Baseline-

und Follow-Up-Bild entlang des Voxelgitters gegeneinander verschoben. Die Verwendung von SSD als Distanzmaß ist jedoch für MR-Daten nicht adäquat, da die Intensitäten korrespondierender Strukturen nicht notwendigerweise übereinstimmen, wie es bei CT-Bildern der Fall ist. Des Weiteren ist die Einschränkung auf Translationen der Suchblöcke bei größeren Deformationen nicht ideal.

Wir ersetzen daher das Blockmatching durch eine affin-lineare, lokal beschränkte Registrierung. Um die Landmarke im Baseline-Bild wird hierfür ein quaderförmiger Suchbereich definiert. Das Follow-Up-Bild wird daraufhin so verschoben, dass der TPS-Vorschlag mit der Landmarke im Baseline-Bild übereinstimmt. Von diesem Startpunkt wird die affin-lineare Registrierung des MERIT-Frameworks [7] gestartet. Als Distanzmaß wurde die normalisierte Kreuzkorrelation (NCC) [8] gewählt, da wir davon ausgehen, dass korrespondierende Strukturen lokal zueinander korrelieren und wir lediglich lokale Ausschnitte ausrichten. Die berechnete Transformation wird dann genutzt, um die vorgeschlagene Landmarkenposition im Follow-Up-Scan zu korrigieren.

2.3   Evaluierung

Das System wurde mit Hinblick auf zwei Fragestellungen evaluiert: Zum einen soll untersucht werden, ob die Abstände zwischen Experten-Landmarke und Systemvorschlag in der selben Größenordnung liegen wie die Abstände zwischen den einzelnen Experten (Inter-Observer-Variabilität). Zum anderen soll überprüft werden, ob eine Nachregistrierung der TPS-Vorschläge mit MERIT zu einer genaueren Verpunktung der Scans führt.

Zu diesem Zweck wurden drei über Jahre hinweg mit Lungenbildgebung vertraute Experten gebeten, in drei morphologischen Scanpaaren jeweils 30 Landmarkenkorrespondenzen manuell zu annotieren. Bei den Scans handelt es sich um aufeinanderfolgende, morphologische MR-Scans der Lunge mit einer Voxelgröße von $0.9766 \times 0.9766 \times 4$ mm^3. Die in der Studie genutzten Bilder wurden von der Abteilung Diagnostische und Interventionelle Radiologie am Universitätsklinikum Heidelberg zur Verfügung gestellt. Abb. 1 zeigt eine koronale Projektion der wie in [6] automatisch generierten Landmarken auf die mittlere Schicht eines der Scans.

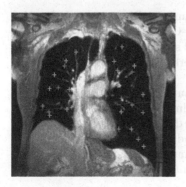

Abb. 1. Koronale Projektion von 30 automatisch generierten Landmarken

222   Strehlow et al.

Tabelle 1. Mittelwert und Standardabweichung der Inter-Observer-Abstände in mm

	Fall 1	Fall 2	Fall 3
Experte 1 ↔ Experte 2	3.73 ± 2.83	3.25 ± 1.87	3.66 ± 2.81
Experte 1 ↔ Experte 3	2.67 ± 2.59	2.33 ± 1.80	4.69 ± 3.90
Experte 2 ↔ Experte 3	4.19 ± 2.91	2.98 ± 2.33	4.66 ± 3.52

Tabelle 2. Mittelwert und Standardabweichung der Abstände zwischen TPS- bzw. MERIT-Vorschlag und Expertenannotation in mm bei automatischer Verpunktung nach Initialisierung mit fünf manuell gesetzten Landmarken

	TPS	MERIT
Fall 1	3.66 ± 1.96	2.88 ± 2.04
Fall 2	3.50 ± 1.69	2.78 ± 1.64
Fall 3	4.30 ± 2.46	3.66 ± 2.44

Nach dem rein manuellen Verpunkten von vier Landmarken wurden vom System Vorschläge für korrespondierende Landmarken generiert. Die Vorschläge blieben dem Annotierenden jedoch verborgen. Um unnötiges Suchen zu ersparen, wurde im Datensatz koronal eine Schicht angezeigt, die zwischen TPS-Vorschlag und MERIT-Nachregistrierung lag. Hierdurch soll vermieden werden, dass der Experte einen der beiden Punkte bevorzugt.

In einer weiteren Untersuchung sollten die Verbesserungen durch die MERIT-Nachkorrektur unter fast vollautomatischen Bedingungen untersucht werden. Um robuste TPS-Schätzungen zu gewährleisten wurden dafür zunächst fünf Landmarken manuell definiert. Zum einen wurde aus diesen Landmarken eine TPS-Transformation berechnet, mit der Vorschläge für die restlichen 25 Landmarken berechnet wurden. Zum anderen wurden die selben Landmarken als Initialisierung für eine TPS-Transformation genutzt, die in jedem Schritt durch die lokal-affine Registrierung verfeinert wurde.

3   Ergebnisse

In Tab. 1 sind Mittelwert und Standardabweichung der Distanzen zwischen den Landmarken der Experten aufgelistet. Die Inter-Observer-Variabilität über alle Landmarken liegt bei 3.57 ± 2.87 mm. In Abb. 2 sind die Abstände der manuell annotierten Landmarken zu den vom System verborgen berechneten Landmarken dargestellt.

Die Ergebnisse der zweiten Studie, der vollautomatischen Verpunktung auf Basis von lediglich fünf manuell gesetzten Landmarken, sind in Abb. 3 dargestellt. Der Box-Whisker-Plot zeigt die Verteilung der Abstände zu den Expertenlandmarken nach der reinen TPS-Schätzung und nach der Verfeinerung durch die lokal-affine Registrierung. Die Abstände konnten durch die lokal-affine Verfeinerung im Mittel um 18.7% verringert werden (Tab. 2).

4 Diskussion

Schon nach fünf manuell gesetzten Landmarken kann das hier vorgestellte Verfahren automatisch die restlichen Landmarken robust generieren (Abb. 3). Im Vergleich zu einer reinen TPS-Transformation, wie sie von Murphy et al. [6] für MR-Bilder vorgeschlagen wurde, konnte mit der lokal-affinen Verfeinerung der TPS-Transformationen eine substantielle Verbesserung der Landmarkenvorschläge erreicht werden. Der Aufwand für die Erstellung eines aussagekräftigen Referenzstandards für pulmonale MR-Bilder ist damit erheblich gesenkt.

Das Verfahren generiert in fast allen Fällen Landmarkenvorschläge, die im Bereich oder sogar unterhalb der Inter-Observer-Abstände liegen (Abb. 2). Eine mögliche Bevorzugung in der Bewertung von Registrierungsverfahren, die sich einer ähnlichen Methodik bedienen, halten wir daher für unwahrscheinlich [6]. In vier Fällen ist der erste Landmarkenvorschlag des Systems unbrauchbar (Abb. 2). In diesen Fällen lagen die ersten rein manuell zuzuordnenden Landmarken sehr dicht beieinander und führten daher zu einer schlechten Schätzung durch die TPS-Transformation. Dies kann vermutlich durch eine einfache Umsortierung der Landmarken behoben werden.

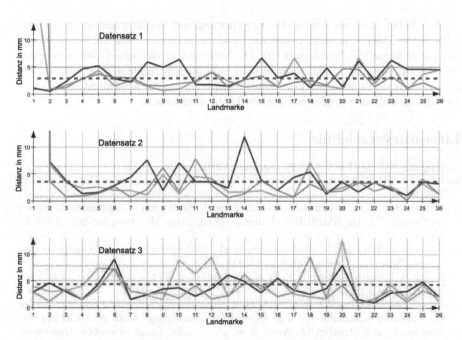

Abb. 2. Distanzen der MERIT-Vorschläge zu den Landmarken der drei Experten (Grüntöne) sowie mittlere Distanz und Standardabweichung zwischen den Experten (rot)

Abb. 3. Abstände der TPS-Vorschläge (jeweils links) und lokaler Nachregistrierung (rechts) zu den von Experten gewählten Punkten

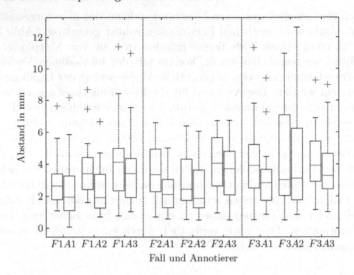

Wir haben in dieser Arbeit eine Erweiterung und Verallgemeinerung des Verfahrens von Murphy et al. [6] präsentiert und dadurch eine effiziente Verpunktung von pulmonalen MR-Scans realisiert. Die hierdurch erleichterte Übertragung auf weitere Organe und Modalitäten soll in zukünftigen Implementierungen erfolgen. Zudem sind umfangreichere Studien geplant, um die Leistungsfähigkeit des Verfahrens auf einer größeren Datenbasis zu untersuchen.

Literaturverzeichnis

1. Kauczor HU. MRI of the Lung. Springer Verlag; 2009.
2. Risse F. MR Perfusion in the lung. In: MRI of the Lung. Springer Verlag; 2009. p. 25–34.
3. Murphy K, van Ginneken B, Reinhardt J, et al. Evaluation of registration methods on thoracic CT: the EMPIRE10 challenge. IEEE Trans Med Imaging. 2011;1(99):1–20.
4. Papenberg N, Lange T, Heldmann S, et al. Bildregistrierung. In: Computerassistierte Chirurgie. Elsevier; 2010. p. 85–118.
5. Kabus S, Klinder T, Murphy K, et al. Evaluation of 4D-CT lung registration. Proc MICCAI. 2009;1:747–54.
6. Murphy K, van Ginneken B, Klein S, et al. Semi-automatic construction of reference standards for evaluation of image registration. Med Image Anal. 2011;15(1):71–84.
7. Boehler T, van Straaten D, Wirtz S, et al. A robust and extendible framework for medical image registration focused on rapid clinical application deployment. Comput Biol Med. 2011;41(6)(41):340–9.
8. Modersitzki J. FAIR: Flexible Algorithms for Image Registration. vol. 6. Society for Industrial and Applied Mathematics (SIAM); 2009.

Automatische atlasbasierte Differenzierung von klassischen und atypischen Parkinsonsyndromen

Nils Daniel Forkert[1], Alexander Schmidt-Richberg[4], Alexander Münchau[2],
Jens Fiehler[3], Heinz Handels[4], Kai Boelmans[2]

[1]Institut für Computational Neuroscience
[2]Klinik für Neurologie
[3]Klinik für Diagnostische und Interventionelle Neuroradiologie
Universitätsklinikum Hamburg-Eppendorf
[4]Institut für Medizinische Informatik, Universität zu Lübeck
n.forkert@uke.uni-hamburg.de

Kurzfassung. In der klinischen Praxis müssen Patienten mit klassischem Parkinsonsyndrom von Patienten mit atypischem Parkinsonsyndrom unterschieden werden um eine optimale Therapie zu gewährleisten. Eine korrekte Diagnose auf Basis von klinischen Kriterien kann jedoch sehr schwierig sein. Im Rahmen dieser Arbeit wird eine automatische Methode zur Differenzierung von Parkinsonsyndromen unter Verwendung von T2'-gewichteten MR-Bildsequenzen präsentiert. Die vorgestellte Methode wurde auf Basis von Datensätzen von 24 gesunden Probanden, 25 Patienten mit klassischem Parkinsonsyndrom und 17 Patienten mit atypischem Parkinsonsyndrom entwickelt und evaluiert. In einem ersten Schritt wurde zunächst ein Atlas basierend auf den Datensätzen der gesunden Probanden generiert und in diesem VOIs definiert, die für eine Klassifikation relevant sein könnten. In einem folgenden Schritt wurden die Patientendaten auf den Atlas registriert und die T2'-Intensitäten in den VOIs analysiert. Hiermit wurde in einem folgenden Schritt ein LAD-Entscheidungsbaum trainiert. Die Evaluation mittels 10-facher Kreuzvalidierung zeigte, dass der Klassifikator klassische von atypische Parkinsonsyndrome mit einer Genauigkeit von 90,5% differenzieren kann. Zusammenfassend zeigen die ersten Ergebnisse, dass sich T2'-Bildsequenzen für eine automatische Differenzierung von Patienten mit klassischen und atypischen Parkinsonsyndromen eignen.

1 Einleitung

Parkinsonsyndrome sind genetisch und pathologisch heterogene neurodegenerative Erkrankungen. Das klassische Parkinsonsyndrom (KPS) ist unter anderem durch eine asymmetrische auftretende Akinese, Rigor und Tremor charakterisiert. Vom klassischen Parkinsonsyndrom abgesehen existieren noch weitere atypische Varianten. Hierzu zählen unter anderem die Multi-System-Atrophie (MSA), Progressive supranukleäre Blickparese (PSP) und Cortikobasale Degeneration (CBD). Atypische Parkinsonsyndrome weisen teilweise eine zum klassischen Parkinsonsyndrom klinisch sehr ähnliche Symptomatik auf, was eine korrekte Diagnose erschwert. Die Differentialdiagnose zwischen den verschiedenen

Parkinsonsyndromen basiert heutzutage in der diagnostischen Routine hauptsächlich auf klinischen Kriterien. Eine definitive gesicherte Diagnose ist derzeit noch ausschließlich anhand von post mortem Untersuchungen möglich [1].
Klinisch-pathologische Studien haben unter anderem gezeigt, dass lediglich 41
bis 88% der pathologisch belegten PSP-Fälle zu Lebzeiten korrekt diagnostiziert wurden [2]. Eine korrekte Diagnose ist jedoch insbesondere wichtig, da
dieses direkte Auswirkungen auf die Behandlungsstrategie und folglich auf den
Therapieerfolg hat. In der Vergangenheit wurden vermehrt verschiedenste Bild-
gebungstechniken verwendet um die Genauigkeit der Diagnose von Parkinsonsyndromen zu steigern. Hierbei hat sich gezeigt, dass sich insbesondere morphologische und metabolische Parameter für die automatische Differenzierung von
klassischen und atypischen Parkinsonsyndromen eignen. So konnte zum Beispiel
gezeigt werden, dass atypische Parkinsonsyndrome häufig zu einer Atrophie des
rostralen Mittelhirns führen. Duchesene et al. [3] haben sich diese Beobachtung
zu Nutzen gemacht und für eine automatische Klassifikation verwendet. Hierbei
wurden T1-gewichtete MR-Sequenzen nicht-linear auf einen Atlas registriert. In
einem folgenden Schritt wurden dann die Deformationen im Bereich des Mittelhirns analysiert und dazu verwendet eine Support Vector Maschine zu trainieren.
Dieser Ansatz wurde auf Basis von 32 Datensätzen evaluiert, wobei eine Klassifikationsgenauigkeit von 91% für PSP- und KPS-patienten nachgewiesen werden
konnte. Der Nachteil dieser Methode ist, dass die Akquisition von hochaufgelösten T1-Datensätzen relativ lange dauert. Insbesondere bei Parkinsonpatienten
mit Tremor ist diese Bildgebung daher schwieriger einzusetzen. Im Gegensatz
dazu wurde von Tang et al. [4] ein Klassifikationsansatz auf Basis von Positron-
Emissions-Tomographie (PET) Datensätzen vorgestellt. Hierbei konnte gezeigt
werden, dass KPS- und PSP-Patienten regional unterschiedliche metabolische
Profile aufweisen. Der vorgestellte Klassifikationsansatz erreichte bei der Evaluation auf Basis von 30 PSP und 96 KPS Patienten eine Spezifizität von >90%. Der
größte Nachteil an dieser Methode ist, dass die PET-Akquisition mit schädlicher
ionisierende Strahlung einhergeht und diese Bildgebungstechnik nicht flächen-
deckend verfügbar ist. Ein möglicher Biomarker, der sich für eine automatische
Klassifikation von Parkinsonsyndromen eignen könnte und in Beziehung zum
Metabolismus steht, ist die regionale Eisenverteilung im Gehirn [5, 6]. So konnte im Rahmen von post mortem Untersuchungen gezeigt werden, dass sich die
Eisenverteilung und -Akkumulation zwischen Parkinsonsyndromen unterscheidet. Paramagnetische Substanzen wie die Depot-Eisen Ferritin und Hämosiderin
erzeugen lokale Feldinhomogenitäten und folglich eine Verkürzung der trans-
versalen Relaxationszeiten bei der MR-Bildgebung. Aus diesem Grund eignen
sich T2-gewichtete und insbesondere T2'-Bildsequenzen dazu den Eisengehalt
im Gewebe abzuschätzen. Das Ziel dieser Arbeit ist es einen Klassifikator auf
Basis dieses Biomarkers zu entwickeln und zu evaluieren.

2 Methoden

2.1 Material

Für die Entwicklung und Evaluation des automatischen Klassifikationsansatzes waren insgesamt 67 Datensätze verfügbar. Hierbei standen 24 Datensätze von gesunden Probanden (mittleres Alter: 62,8), 25 Datensätze von Patienten mit klassischen Parkinsonsyndrom (mittleres Alter: 60,1) und 17 Datensätze von Patienten mit einem atypischen Parkinsonsyndrom (mittleres Alter: 64,2) zur Verfügung. Bei elf Patienten mit atypischen Parkinsonsyndrom wurde eine Progressive supranukleäre Blickparese (PSP), bei vier Patienten eine Multi-System-Atrophie (MSA) und bei zwei Patienten eine Cortikobasale Degeneration (CBD) diagnostiziert. Patienten mit unsicherer Differentialdiagnose wurden nicht in die Datenbasis aufgenommen. Alle MR-Aufnahmen wurden auf einem 1,5T Siemens Sonata Scanner akquiriert. Unter anderem umfasste das MR Protokoll T2- und T2*-Sequenzen. Zur quantitativen T2-Bestimmung wurde eine Triple-Echo Sequenz unter Verwendung von drei TE-Zeiten verwenden (12, 84 und 156 ms). Zur quantitativen T2*-Bestimmung wurde eine echo-planar Bildgebung ebenfalls unter Verwendung von drei TE-Zeiten verwendet (20, 52 und 88 ms). Alle Datensätze wurden mit einer räumlichen Auflösung von $1,9 \times 1,9 \times 5$ mm^3 aufgenommen. Aus den akquirierten T2- und T2*-Triple-Echo Sequenzen wurden dann für jeden Patienten eine quantitative T2- bzw. T2*-Karte berechnet. Hierbei wurde voxelweise die exponentielle Funktion $SI(t) = SI_0 \exp(-t/T2)$ an die Intensitätskurve $SI(t)$ angepasst, die durch die jeweils drei TE-Zeiten gegeben war. Auf Basis der beiden berechneten quantitativen T2- (qT2) und T2*- (qT2*) Karten wurde dann die korrespondierende T2'-Karte mittels $1/T2' = 1/qT2 - 1/qT*$ berechnet (Abb. 1).

2.2 Atlas Generierung

Die so generierten T2'-Datensätze stellen eine Abschätzung der Eisenkonzentration im Gewebe dar. Aufgrund von unterschiedlichen Patientenanatomien und

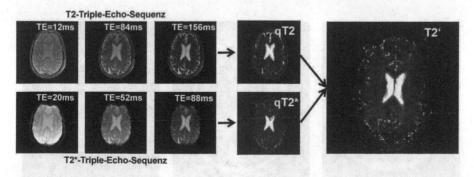

Abb. 1. Triple-Echo T2- und T2*-Bildsequenz und hieraus berechnete quantitative T2-, T2*- und T2'-Karten

Positionen im MR-Scanner ist eine Registrierung der Datensätze auf einen Atlas notwendig um die lokalen T2'-Signale in korrespondierenden Geweben zu analysieren. Die T2'-Datensätze weisen jedoch relativ viel Rauschen auf und beinhalten eher metabolische als morphologische Informationen. Aus diesem Grund wäre eine direkte Registrierung auf Basis dieser Datensätze relativ fehleranfällig und ungenau. Daher wurde die Registrierung auf Basis des Datensatzes aus der T2-Triple-Echo Sequenz mit der längsten TE-Zeit berechnet, da dieser den besten Gewebekontrast aufweist. Die am häufigsten verwendeten neuroanatomischen Atlanten wurden typischerweise auf Basis von hochaufgelösten T1-gewichteten MR-Bildsequenzen erzeugt und eignen sich daher nur bedingt für die vorliegenden Datensätze. Darüber hinaus wurden die meisten Atlanten auf Basis von Bildsequenzen einer Kontrollgruppe von Probanden erzeugt die deutlich jünger sind als typische Parkinson-Patienten. Um eine optimale Atlas-Registrierung zu ermöglichen wurden daher die Datensätze von den gesunden Probanden verwendet um einen speziell für diese Fragestellung optimierten Atlas zu generieren. Insbesondere ist dieses von Vorteil bei der Registrierung da die Datensätze von den Probanden mit denselben MR-Parametern aufgenommen worden sind wie die Patientendaten. Für die Atlasgenerierung wurde in einem ersten Schritt ein Datensatz aus der Kontroll-Datenbasis als Referenz selektiert. Dieser Datensatz wurde ausgewählt da alle wichtigen Gehirnareale abgedeckt waren, keine Bewegungsartefakte vorlagen und der Kopf zentral im Bild abgebildet wurde. In einem weiteren Schritt wurden die übrigen Datensätze von den gesunden Probanden dann auf diesen Datensatz registriert. Durch voxelweise Berechnung des Mittelwertes wurde dann der finale Atlas erzeugt (Abb. 2).

2.3 Klassifikation

In dem so unter Verwendung der Probanden-Datensätze generierten T2-Atlas wurden dann in einem folgenden Schritt manuell VOIs (Volume-of-Interest) in Gehirnarealen definiert von denen angenommen wurde, dass sie unterschiedliche Eisenkonzentrationen bei klassischen und atypischen Parkinsonsyndromen aufweisen. Unter anderem wurde folgende Areale in der linken und rechten

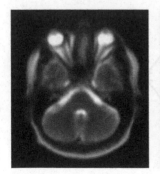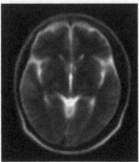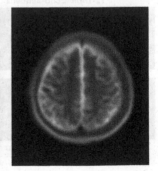

Abb. 2. Drei ausgewählte Schichten vom generierten T2-Atlas

Hemisphäre bestimmt: Pallidum (anterior und posterior), Nucleus Caudatus, Putamen (anterior und posterior), Thalamus, frontale weiße Hirnsubstanz und occipitale weiße Hirnsubstanz. Um die T2'-Signale in diesen VOIs zu analysieren mussten die entsprechenden Patienten-Datensätze auf den Atlas registriert werden. Hierzu wurden für jeden Patienten der T2-Datensatz mit der längsten TE-Zeit unter Verwendung einer affinen Transformation und Minimierung der SSD-Metrik auf den Atlas registriert. Nach der affinen Registrierung wurden die T2-Datensätze dann unter Verwendung einer intensitätsbasierten diffusiven Registrierung [7] an den Atlas angepasst, so dass auch nicht-lineare Unterschiede ausgeglichen werden konnten. Nach der nicht-linearen Registrierung wurden die berechneten Transformationen dann dazu verwendet die korrespondierenden T2'-Datensätze auf den Atlas anzupassen. Nach der Transformation der T2'-Datensätze konnten die T2'-Signale für alle manuell definierten VOIs ausgewertet werden und dazu verwendet werden einen Klassifikator zu trainieren. Als Klassifikator wurde im Rahmen dieser Arbeit ein LAD-Entscheidungsbaum (LogitBoost Alternating Decision Tree) [8] eingesetzt. Dieser Klassifikator hat den Vorteil, dass die Ergebnisse direkt interpretierbar sind, so dass relativ einfach Rückschlüsse gezogen werden können, welche der manuell definierten VOIs wirklich für die Klassifikation wichtig sind.

3 Ergebnisse

Der LAD-Entscheidungsbaum Klassifikator wurde unter Verwendung einer 10-fachen Kreuzvalidierung evaluiert. Hierbei zeigte sich, dass der Klassifikator klassische von atypische Parkinsonsyndrome mit eine Genauigkeit von 90,5% differenzieren kann. Insgesamt wurden 38 der 42 Patienten richtig klassifiziert. Zwei Datensätze von Patienten mit atypischem Parkinsonsyndrom wurden falsch als klassisches Parkinsonsyndrom eingestuft. Gleichermaßen wurden zwei Datensätze von Patienten mit klassischem Parkinsonsyndrom falsch als atypisch eingestuft. Insgesamt ergibt sich so eine Sensitivität von 0.88 und eine Spezifizität von 0.92 für die Klassifikation mittels LAD-Entscheidungsbaum. Die Analyse der für die Klassifikation nach Training verwendeten Parameter zeigte, dass lediglich die T2'-Intensitäten im anterior Pallidum, posterior Pallidum, anterior Putamen und in der occipitalen weißen Hirnsubstanz für die Klassifikation relevant waren.

4 Diskussion

Die ersten Ergebnisse zeigen, dass sich T2'-Bildsequenzen für eine automatische Differenzierung von Patienten mit klassischen und atypischen Parkinsonsyndromen eignen. Die erreichte Genauigkeit von 90,5% bei einer Sensitivität von 0.88 und einer Spezifizität von 0.92 liegt dabei im oberen Bereich von zuvor publizierten Ergebnissen für automatische Klassifikationsansätze [3, 4]. Im Gegensatz zu früheren Methoden hat der vorliegende Ansatz jedoch den Vorteil, dass T2'-Bildgebung relativ schnell ist und keine ionisierende Strahlung verwendet. Obwohl das vorliegende Patientenkollektiv bestmöglich charakterisiert ist und auch geringfügig unsichere Fälle von dieser Studie ausgeschlossen wurden, bleibt eine geringe Unsicherheit bezüglich der Goldstandard-Klassifikation bestehen, was auch einen Grund für die Fehlklassifizierungen darstellen könnte. Dieses lässt sich jedoch nicht verhindern, da zu dem verwendeten Patientenkollektiv keine post mortem Untersuchungen vorliegen. Bisher wurde beim vorgestellten Ansatz nicht zwischen den atypischen Parkinsonsyndromen selbst unterschieden da die einzelnen Subgruppen derzeit noch zu klein sind. Sobald die einzelnen Subgruppen groß genug sind, soll evaluiert werden ob sich die beschriebene Methode auch für eine solche Subgruppen-Klassifikation eignet. Der beschriebene Ansatz bietet noch weitere Möglichkeiten zur Verbesserung. So wurde zum Beispiel die nicht-lineare Transformation bisher noch nicht analysiert und in den Klassifikationsansatz integriert. Zusammenfassend bietet der vorgestellte Klassifikationsansatz auf Basis von T2'-Bildsequenzen Potenzial die Differentialdiagnostik von Parkinsonsyndromen zukünftig zu verbessern.

Literaturverzeichnis

1. Rizzo G, et al. Diffusion-weighted brain imaging study of patients with clinical diagnosis of corticobasal degeneration, progressive supranuclear palsy and Parkinson's disease. Brain. 2008;131(10):2690–700.
2. Hughes A, Daniel S, Ben-Shlomo Y, et al. The accuracy of diagnosis of Parkinsonian syndromes in a specialist movement disorder service. Brain. 2002;125(4):861–70.
3. Duchesne S, Rolland Y, Vérin M. Automated computer differential classification in Parkinsonian syndromes via pattern analysis on MRI. Acad Radiol. 2009;16:61–70.
4. Tang C, et al. Differential diagnosis of Parkinsonism: a metabolic imaging study using pattern analysis. Lancet Neurol. 2010;9:149–58.
5. Graham J, Paley M, Grünewald R, et al. Brain iron deposition in Parkinson's disease imaged using the PRIME magnetic resonance sequence. Brain. 2000;123(12):2423–31.
6. Schenck J, Zimmerman E. High-field magnetic resonance imaging of brain iron: birth of a biomarker? NMR Biomed. 2004;17:433–45.
7. Schmidt-Richberg A, Ehrhardt J, Werner R, et al. Diffeomorphic diffusion registration of lung CT images. Proc MICCAI Grand Challenge Workshop. 2010;7962:55–62.
8. Holmes G, Pfahringer B, Kirkby R, et al. Multiclass alternating decision trees. In: ECML. Springer; 2001. p. 161–72.

Tracking Virus Particles in Microscopy Images Using Multi-Frame Association

Astha Jaiswal[1], William J. Godinez[1], Roland Eils[1], Maik J. Lehmann[2],
Karl Rohr[1]

[1]University of Heidelberg, BIOQUANT, IPMB, and DKFZ Heidelberg
[2]Molecular Parasitology, Humboldt-University Berlin
astha.jaiswal@bioquant.uni-heidelberg.de

Abstract. Automatic tracking of fluorescent particles is an essential task to study the dynamics of a large number of biological structures at a sub-cellular level. We have developed a probabilistic tracking approach based on multi-frame association finding and the Kalman filter. We have successfully applied the approach to synthetic as well as real microscopy image sequences of ALV virus particles and have performed a quantitative comparison with previous approaches.

1 Introduction

Automatic tracking of subcellular structures in fluorescence microscopy images is important to study the behavior of, for example, virus particles under different experimental conditions. Virus particle tracking is challenging due to the similar appearance of different virus particles, the high particle density, the large number of spurious objects, the appearance and disappearance of particles, as well as their hardly predictable motion. Moreover, a high level of noise, a frequent clustering and unclustering of the virus particles, and out-of-focus movement of the virus particles are additional challenges for an automatic tracking algorithm.

Previous work on particle tracking include deterministic and probabilistic approaches. Deterministic approaches consist of particle detection and association finding ([1, 2]). While being computationally efficient, deterministic approaches often have difficulties in dealing with spurious objects and detection errors [3]. In contrast, probabilistic tracking approaches perform spatial-temporal filtering which allows robust estimation of the position of particles under noisy conditions [3, 4]. Thus, probabilistic approaches generally outperform deterministic approaches. For multiple particle tracking, probabilistic approaches typically employ a temporally local association finding algorithm. Two-frame approaches ([3, 4]) do not cope well with difficult tracking tasks (e.g., appearance and disappearance of particles) for which information from multiple frames is important. In contrast, multi-frame approaches ([2, 5]) exploit more temporal information. The deterministic approach in [1] achieves multi-frame association (MFA) by multiple two-frame associations (TFA). Thus, the approach is in fact temporally local (two-frame approach). Deterministic association finding approaches that uncouple particle linking from the detection of clustering and unclustering events ([5]) are prone to yield incorrect associations. In [2], a MFA finding algorithm has been proposed which performs particle linking and detection of clustering and unclustering simultaneously. However, the approach is deterministic and thus does not cope well with high object density and many spurious objects.

In this work, we have developed a probabilistic tracking approach based on MFA finding and the Kalman filter. Key properties of our approach are multi-frame optimization, verification of associations with past as well as subsequent positions of the particles, correction of erroneous associations, and robust estimation of the position of particles. Our approach performs particle linking and detection of clustering and unclustering simultaneously. We have quantitatively evaluated our approach using synthetic as well as real fluorescence microscopy image sequences of avian leukosis virus (ALV) particles and performed a comparison with previous approaches.

2 Materials and methods

2.1 Multi-frame association

We model the association finding problem using a w-partite graph for a temporal window of size w. Vertices of the graph represent particles, and edges of the graph denote possible associations. The edges are assigned weights that correspond to the likelihood of the association. Partite sets of the graph correspond to the set of measurements (or predictions) at time points within the window. For a particle i at time point t, with position p_t^i, and a particle j at time point $t + r$, with position p_{t+r}^j, where $r \epsilon [1, 2, ..., w - 1]$, the likelihood that the two particles correspond to the same object over time is given by a gain function $g(p_t^i, p_{t+r}^j)$. The MFA algorithm initially generates soft associations which can be changed when more information becomes available. The soft associations between the first two frames within a window are changed into hard associations only after processing all frames within the window. The MFA finding problem has been modeled as a split graph of a w-partite graph for a temporal window of size w [2]. The optimal solution corresponds to the maximum matching of the split graph. The optimization objective has been defined as finding a hypothesis $M_{\max}$ with the maximum total gain from the set of all hypotheses C

$$M_{\max} = \arg \max_{M \epsilon C} \sum_{(p_t^i, p_{t+r}^j) \epsilon M} g(p_t^i, p_{t+r}^j) \qquad (1)$$

$$\text{subject to} \sum_{k=1}^{N} M_{k,l} = 1, \sum_{l=1}^{N} M_{k,l} = 1 \qquad (2)$$

where N is the total number of measurements and predictions within a temporal window. A hypothesis M is a feasible solution represented by an association matrix consisting of 0 and 1, where 1 indicates presence of the association and 0 indicates absence of the association in the solution. The constraints ensure a one-to-one association. We solve the optimization problem (1) using the Hungarian algorithm.

2.2 Probabilistic tracking approach using multiple frames

We developed a probabilistic tracking approach that combines a deterministic MFA algorithm with the Kalman filter (KF), and is denoted by MFAKF. A block diagram of the approach is shown in Fig. 1. MFA uses as input the predicted positions of the particles (predictions) at the current time point and the measured positions (measurements) of the particles at all time points within a window. The goal of MFA is to find associations between the predicted and measured positions of the particles. Based on the association results of MFA, the KF determines an estimate of the positions of the particles at the current time point.

3 Results

We have applied the developed tracking approach to synthetic as well as real microscopy image sequences of avian leukosis virus (ALV) particles and have performed a quantitative comparison with previous approaches. In total, we evaluated four different approaches: MFAKF (described above), a deterministic TFA approach [1], a deterministic MFA approach [2], and a KF based multiple particle tracking approach which uses TFA for motion correspondence [4]. We have used the spot enhancing filter for particle detection and the gain function $g(\boldsymbol{p}_t^i, \boldsymbol{p}_{t+r}^j)$ exploits the Euclidean distance between two positions of a particle. The synthetic images have been generated to simulate real fluorescence microscopy images. An advantage is that ground truth is available. The synthetic image sequences show multiple particles with different motion patterns (confined motion, random motion, and directed motion), and a high object density. The image sequences consist of 100 time points with image dimensions 256×256 pixels and include intensity dependent additive Poisson noise (SNR = 4.55). To evaluate the approach under different conditions, we generated image sequences for 7 different levels of object density (number of particles). To quantify the performance of the tracking approaches, we computed the track error

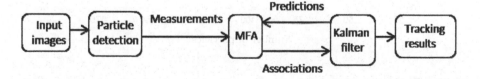

Fig. 1. Overview of the probabilistic tracking approach MFAKF

234   Jaiswal et al.

E_{track} which is defined based on the number of correct trajectories $n_{\text{track,correct}}$ and the number of the true trajectories $n_{\text{track,total}}$ as $E_{\text{track}} = 1 - \frac{n_{\text{track,correct}}}{n_{\text{track,total}}}$. A trajectory is considered to be correct if it contains more than 75% correct positions (positions within a tolerance of 2 pixels).

We generated 20 synthetic image sequences for each of the 7 different numbers of particles (25, 50, 75, 100, 125, 150, 175) and computed the mean track error (Fig. 2). In total, we have used 140 image sequences. It can be seen that MFA yields a better result than TFA. The best result is achieved by MFAKF for all different numbers of particles (object density).

We have also applied all four tracking approaches to 5 real microscopy image sequences displaying fluorescently labeled ALV virus particles. The images were acquired every 15 seconds using a confocal microscope [6]. The image sequences differ in the level of the image noise, the object density, the motion pattern of the particles, and the number of spurious objects. For the image sequences the image dimensions vary between 512×512 pixels and 1024×1024 pixels, the number of time points ranges from 36 to 180, and the number of particles varies from 28 to 380. For the real images the temporal resolution is relatively low and consequently the motion of particles is quite abrupt. Ground truth for the real images has been determined by manual tracking using the ImageJ plugin MTrackJ. The mean track error $\bar{E}_{\text{track}}$ (and standard deviation) over all image

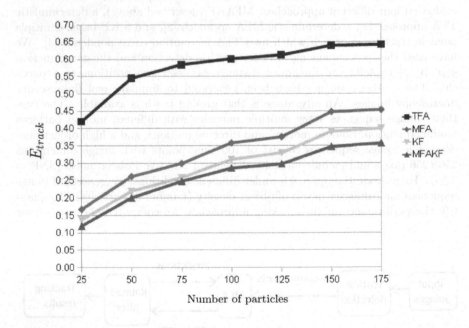

Fig. 2. Tracking results of different approaches for synthetic image sequences as a function of the number of particles (mean track error $\bar{E}_{\text{track}}$, 140 image sequences)

Table 1. Tracking results of different approaches for real microscopy images (mean track error $\bar{E}_{\text{track}}$ and standard deviation)

	TFA	MFA	KF	MFAKF
$\bar{E}_{\text{track}}$	0.345	0.321	0.298	0.284
Std. dev.	0.165	0.210	0.166	0.167

sequences is shown in Table 1. It can be seen that MFA is better than TFA. Consequently, MFAKF is found to be better than KF. Among all approaches, the best result is obtained by MFAKF. As an example, Fig. 3 shows tracking results of MFAKF and a comparison with ground truth and results from a different probabilistic approach (KF). In the enlarged section two particles cluster and uncluster. As can be seen, KF generates a broken trajectory. In contrast, MFAKF generates correct trajectories by effectively dealing with the clustering and unclustering.

4   Discussion

We have presented a probabilistic tracking approach based on MFA finding and the Kalman filter. On the basis of a quantitative performance evaluation and a comparison with previous approaches we found that multi-frame-based approaches outperform two-frame-based approaches. Consequently, our probabilistic approach based on MFA and the Kalman filter yields a better result than the

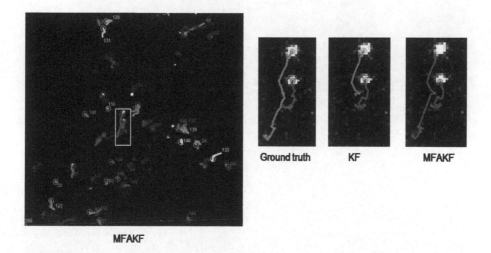

Fig. 3. A real microscopy image with tracking results of MFAKF as well as enlarged sections of ground truth and tracking results of KF and MFAKF. The image contrast has been enhanced for better visualization

Kalman filter approach using TFA. We also found that probabilistic approaches outperform corresponding deterministic approaches.

Acknowledgement. This work has been supported by the BMBF (FORSYS) project VIROQUANT and HGS MathComp, University of Heidelberg.

References

1. Sbalzarini IF, Koumoutsakos P. Feature point tracking and trajectory analysis for video imaging in cell biology. J Struct Biol. 2005;151:182–95.
2. Shafique K, Shah M. A noniterative greedy algorithm for multiframe point correspondence. IEEE Trans Pattern Anal Mach Intell. 2005;27:51–65.
3. Smal I, Draegestein K, Galjart N, et al. Particle filtering for multiple object tracking in dynamic fluorescence microscopy images: application to microtubule growth analysis. IEEE Trans Med Imaging. 2008;27:789–804.
4. Godinez WJ, Lampe M, Wörz S, et al. Deterministic and probabilistic approaches for tracking virus particles in time-lapse fluorescence microscopy image sequences. Med Image Anal. 2009;13:325–42.
5. Jaqaman K, Loerke D, Mettlen M, et al. Robust single-particle tracking in live-cell time-lapse sequences. Nat Methods. 2008;5:695–702.
6. Lehmann MJ, Sherer NM, Marks CB, et al. Actin- and myosin-driven movement of viruses along filopodia precedes their entry into cells. J Cell Biol. 2005;170:317–25.

Parameteroptimierte und GPGPU-basierte Detektion viraler Strukturen innerhalb Plasmonen-unterstützter Mikroskopiedaten

Pascal Libuschewski[1,2], Frank Weichert[1], Constantin Timm[2]

[1]Lehrstuhl für Graphische Systeme, Technische Universität Dortmund
[2]Lehrstuhl für Eingebettete Systeme, Technische Universität Dortmund
pascal.libuschewski@tu-dortmund.de

Kurzfassung. Die lokale Verfügbarkeit von effizienten und leistungs-
fähigen Biosensoren, z.B. an Flughäfen, gewinnt durch die zunehmende
Verbreitung viraler Infektionen zunehmend an Bedeutung. Die zentralen Herausforderungen für entsprechende in situ Virusdetektionssyste-
me sind eine schnelle und sichere Erkennung der Viren respektive die
Adaptivität an unterschiedliche Ausprägungen von Erregern. Optische
Verfahren, wie die neuartige Plasmonen-unterstützte Mikroskopie von
Nanoobjekten erlauben es, diesen Anforderungen zu entsprechen. Aufgrund starker multipler Artefaktbelastung des Signals und hohen Datenmengen (zeitlichen und örtlichen), werden nachhaltige Anforderungen
an die Bildrestauration und -analyse gestellt. Hier setzt die vorliegende
Arbeit an, welche eine GPGPU-basierte Bildrestaurations- und Bildanalysepipeline vorstellt. Über eine Kombination aus lokaler und globaler
Parameteroptimierung mittels Genetischer Algorithmen kann eine höhere Effektivität der einzelnen Stufen der Verarbeitung erzielt werden,
aber auch im übergreifenden Verbund – dies zeigt sich nachhaltig in der
Erkennungsrate des Biosensors für Viren.

1 Einleitung

Insbesondere vor dem Hintergrund eines Anstiegs epidemisch auftretender viraler
Infektionen ist ein großflächiger Einsatz von mobilen Biosensoren zunehmend re-
levant [1] – dies setzt aber eine präzise und schnelle Erkennungsleistung voraus.
Die neuartige Plasmon-assisted Microscopy of Nano-size Objects (PAMONO)
Technik [2] erfüllt, im Gegensatz zu etablierten Verfahren [3], wie z.B. ELISA
oder PCR, die gestellten Anforderungen. Der PAMONO-Sensor basiert auf der
Erkennung von markierungsfreien biomolekularen Bindungsreaktionen an einer
Goldoberfläche, in einer mit einer CCD-Kamera aufgenommenen Bildserie. Zur
Detektion wird der Effekt ausgenutzt, dass polarisierendes Licht (Laser), welches
auf eine Metallschicht trifft, dort Oberflächenplasmonen anregt [2]. Abb. 1 zeigt
einen exemplarischen Bildausschnitt einer Bildserie und verdeutlicht an drei exemplarischen Zeitreihen (Graustufenwerte an einer Bildposition über die Zeit)
die Manifestierung der Ausprägungen Virus, Artefakt (z.B. Staub) und Hintergrund. Da eine (Virus-)Bindung die reflektierte Intensität verändert, prägt sich

dies in einem prägnanten Sprung in der Zeitreihe aus. Zur Analyse entsprechender (Pixel-)Zeitreihen eignen sich Transformations- und Template-basierte Verfahren [4], zur bildbasierten Vorverarbeitung Denoising-Verfahren [5], die auch im Fokus der vorliegenden Arbeit liegen.

Durch die Nutzung von General Purpose Computation on Graphics Processing Units (GPGPU) wird zudem die Echtzeitfähigkeit der Pipeline gewährleistet. GPUs werden zunehmend in der medizinischen Bildverarbeitung angewendet, z.B. bei der echtzeitfähigen Segmentierung histologischer Schnittpräparate [6], da sie im Gegensatz zu Spezialprozessoren [7] einen flexibleren Entwurf von Algorithmen unterstützen. Die eingesetzten Bildverarbeitungsverfahren sind hoch variabel im Hinblick auf ihren Einsatzzweck, allerdings auch bzgl. ihrer Parametrisierung, welche für ein optimales Detektionsergebnis, auch bei variablen Erregern, wichtig ist. Durch eine automatische Parameteroptimierung mittels Genetischen Algorithmen (GA) und der Berücksichtigung Pipelineübergreifender Abhängigkeiten, wird eine global optimierte Parameterauswahl erzielt. Für einen Überblick zur Parameteroptimierung sei auf die Literatur verwiesen [8].

Ausgehend von dieser einleitenden Darstellung thematisiert Abschnitt 2 die mehrstufige und GPGPU-basierte Bildrestaurations- und Bildanalysepipeline und Abschnitt 3 die automatische Parameteroptimierung. Zur Bewertung der Nachhaltigkeit erfolgt eine Bewertung der Erkennungsrate für unterschiedliche Nanostrukturen (Abschn. 3) und leitet über zur Diskussion (Abschn. 4).

2   Material und Methoden

Als Ausgangsbasis der nachfolgend thematisierten GPGPU-basierten Verarbeitungspipeline, sind T Bilder der Auflösung $M \times N$ Pixel zu untersuchen (Abb. 1). Bezogen auf die Analyse der (Pixel-)Zeitreihen ist eine ausgezeichnete Zeitreihe im Folgenden mit $f_i(t)$ mit $i = 0, \ldots, (M-1) \cdot (N-1)$ und $t = 0, \ldots, T-1$ referenziert – $f_i(t) \in \mathbb{R}$ repräsentiert den 12 Bit-Graustufenwert (Intensität I) an der Bildposition i zum Zeitpunkt t.

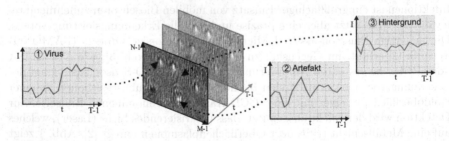

Abb. 1. Darstellung eines exemplarischen Ausschnitts innerhalb der durch den PAMONO-Sensor bereitgestellten Bildfolge und Ableitung repräsentativer (Pixel-)Zeitreihen für die Ausprägungen Virus, Artefakt und Hintergrund

2.1   GPGPU-basierte Bildrestaurations- und Bildanalysepipeline

Die im Folgenden beschriebene echtzeitfähige, hoch-parallele GPGPU-Verarbeitungspipeline (Abb. 2) basiert im Hinblick auf eine hohe Plattformvariabilität auf OpenCL und ist dabei generisch gehalten [9]. In der ersten Pipelinestufe werden die Bilddaten mit einer Fuzzy-Logik gestützten Rauschreduktion aufbereitet, in der zweiten Stufe per Pixel die Kandidaten für eine Anhaftung ermittelt, im nachfolgenden Segmentierungsschritt zu Polygonen aggregiert und anschließend zur Differenzierung klassifiziert. Im Unterschied zu [9] erfolgt auf jeder Stufe eine lokale und übergreifend eine globale Optimierung.

Vorverarbeitung Zielsetzung der Vorverarbeitung (erste Pipelinestufe) ist eine Kompensierung des (Signal-)Rauschens. In Anbetracht der hohen Durchdringung der Bilddaten durch multiple Artefakte, dient dieser Schritt zur Verbesserung der Erkennungsleistung. Zur Anwendung kommt hierbei ein in Anlehnung an [5] entwickelter 3D Denoisingfilter (2D+t), welcher Konzepte der Fuzzy-Logik auf der GPU nutzt. Dabei wurden die einzelnen Regeln durch Zwischenevaluierungen an die speziellen Herausforderungen zur Filterung der PAMONO-Sensordaten angepasst. Diese liegen beispielsweise im Erhalt des marginalen Nutzsignals ($\approx$ 6% vom Mittelwert) im Verhältnis zum konstruktionsbedingten Rauschen ($\approx$ 3% um den Mittelwert). In einer kaskadierten Filterung erfolgt über Fuzzy-Regeln eine selektive Filterung einzelner Pixel. Die zu optimierenden Parameter $\pi_1, \pi_2 \in \mathbb{R}$, mit $0 \leq \pi_1 < \pi_2$, definieren die Fuzzy-Menge μ_{π_1, π_2} [5], mit der die Stärke der Filterung nicht-linear beeinflusst wird.

Detektion Auf der zweiten Pipelinestufe werden auf den gefilterten Bilddaten die einem Virus zugehörigen Pixel mittels Zeitreihenanalyse identifiziert. Die Ausprägungen Virus, Artefakt und Hintergrund werden über die Charakteristik im zeitlichen Verlauf unterschieden, beschrieben über die Funktion $f_i(t)$. Abb. 1 zeigt hierzu exemplarische Ausprägungen der Pixel-Zeitreihen für verschiedene Klassen auf. Für diese werden mithilfe des GA gemäß Abschnitt 2.2, Template-Zeitreihen $f_{\text{Template}}(t)$ bestimmt. Die Schwellwert-getriggerte Klassifikation erfolgt, ausgehend von der allgemeinen Form der Minkowski-Distanz, über das Distanzmaß $d(f_i(t), f_{\text{Template}}(t))$ [10].

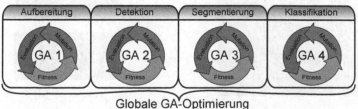

Globale GA-Optimierung

Abb. 2. Schematische Darstellung zur GPGPU-basierten Verarbeitungspipeline und zum inhärenten Konzept aus lokaler und globaler evolutionärer Optimierung

Segmentierung und Klassifikation In der dritten Pipelinestufe erfolgt die Aggregation der als Virus identifizierten Pixel, in zusammenhängende Segmente, über einen hoch parallelen Marching Squares Algorithmus. Abb. 3 zeigt einen Bildausschnitt mit als Virus identifizierten Pixeln (hell/gelb) und resultierenden Polygonen (dunkel/rot). Da sich die verschiedenen Strukturen neben ihrer zeitlichen Ausprägung auch durch ihre zweidimensionale polygonale Form unterscheiden (Abb. 4), wird in der abschließenden Pipelinestufe eine zusätzliche Klassifikation jedes Segments über Formfaktoren durchgeführt [9].

2.2 GA-basierte Parameteroptimierung

Im Hinblick auf den mehrdimensionalen Parameterraum, der durch die Stellgrößen der Algorithmen innerhalb der Pipelinestufen aufgespannt wird, ist eine manuelle Festlegung nicht tragfähig – dies auch in Anbetracht unterschiedlicher Szenarien (z.B. unterschiedliche Virusausprägungen). Daher wird die Parametrisierung über einen Genetischen Algorithmus (GA) [11] realisiert, welcher gemäß der Konfigurationen zum Fuzzy-Denoising und zur Zeitreihenanalyse aus einer Population mit zwei Chromosomen c_1 und c_2 besteht. Dabei repräsentieren die Gene von $c_1 = (\pi_1, \pi_2)$ die Stützstellen der unscharfen Entscheidungsfunktion und von $c_2 = (f_i(0), \ldots, f_i(T-1), r)$ die Funktionswerte der Pixelzeitreihen und den Schwellwert. Eine entsprechende Integration ist auch für die Parameter der weiteren Pipelinestufen gegeben. Dieser Aspekt geht aber über den Fokus der aktuellen Darstellung hinaus. Zur Bewertung der Optimierungsgüte kommt innerhalb eines automatischen Vergleichs eine Fitnessfunktion zum Tragen, die auf dem Klassifikationsmaß der Genauigkeit $acc = \frac{tp+tn}{tp+fn+fp+tn}$ beruht und auf einer Gegenüberstellung von falsch und richtig (true) Positiven gemäß des ROC-Ansatzes – manuell annotierte Daten wurden durch Experten zur Verfügung gestellt (Abschn. 3). Für die globale Optimierung wurden in einem ersten Schritt die Chromosomen von GA 1 bis GA 4 (Abb. 2) aggregiert und die Startpopulation mit den Ergebnissen aus den einzelnen Optimierungen konfiguriert. Für weitergehende globale Ansätze sei auch auf den Abschnitt 4 verwiesen.

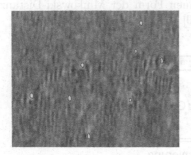

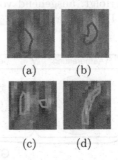

(a)   (b)

(c)   (d)

Abb. 3.   Darstellung   identifizierter „Virus-Pixel"und aggregierter Polygone

Abb. 4. Ausprägung von (a), (b) Virus- und (c), (d) Artefaktanhaftungen

3 Ergebnisse

Die Evaluierung erfolgte über einem Versuchsaufbau bestehend aus einer superlumineszenten Diode QSDM-680-9, einem 50nm Goldplättchen mit Prisma und einer Kappa DX40-1020FW Kamera respektive einem PC-Komplettsystem (Intel Q9550, 8GB RAM, GeForce GTX 480). Als Testdatenfundus standen drei exemplarische Typen von manuell segmentierten Datensätzen mit 4316 Bildern zur Verfügung. Zwei Typen von Datensätzen mit einer Auflösung von 1000×566 Pixeln respektive 1000×367 Pixeln beruhen auf synthetischen Partikeln der Größe 200nm bzw. 280nm. Für den dritten Typus mit einer Auflösung von 1000×295 Pixeln wurden 100nm große HIV-VLPs (Virus-like Particles) verwendet.

Ausgehend von dieser Testkonfiguration vermittelt Abb. 5 (a) die Klassifikationsrate, insbesondere die zunehmende Güte durch das evolutionäre Optimierungsverfahren. Hierbei wird mit acc_{man} die unoptimierte Genauigkeit referenziert, bei der alle Parameter manuell gesetzt wurden. Die Klassifikationsrate bei der optimierten Fuzzy-Rauschreduktion (GA 1) und angepassten Parametern für die Detektion (GA 2) wird durch acc_{fuzzy} und acc_{det} repräsentiert – die globale Optimierung referenziert acc_{glob}. In jedem Optimierungsschritt wurden jeweils in 800 Generationen 20.000 Individuen erzeugt. Obwohl die HIV-VLPs bei den vorliegenden Daten das schlechteste SNR-Verhältnis aufweisen, konnte eine Steigerung der Klassifikationsrate von 45 % auf 88 % erreicht werden. Bei den 200 nm Datensätzen zeigt sich die ausgeprägteste Verbesserung in den letzten Pipelinestufen. Eine Optimierung der beiden ersten Stufen steigerte die Güte von 21 % auf 36 %, während die Optimierung der letzten beiden Stufen die Genauigkeit auf 80 % erhöht hat. Bei den 280 nm Datensätzen waren die beiden letzten Pipelinestufen besser konfiguriert, sodass eine Steigerung von 74 % auf 86 % erreicht werden konnte. Schließlich zeigt die Laufzeit der Analyse der jeweils ca. 300 Bilder umfassenden Datensätze von unter einer Minute die Effizienz der vorgestellten Verfahren. Zudem vermittelt Abb. 5 (b) die Echtzeitfähigkeit und die gute Skalierung der Laufzeit in Abhängigkeit von der Bildgröße.

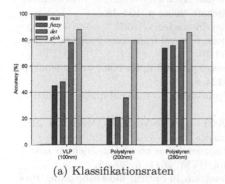

(a) Klassifikationsraten

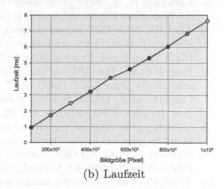

(b) Laufzeit

Abb. 5. (a) Prozentuale Klassifikationsraten bei unterschiedlichen Typen von Datensätzen und (b) Laufzeit in Millisekunden pro Frame im Verhältnis zur Bildgröße

4   Diskussion

Ausgehend von der Motivation, eine Echtzeit-konforme Detektion viraler Strukturen auch im außerklinischen Umfeld z.B. an Flughäfen zur Verfügung zu stellen, wurden in dieser Arbeit GPGPU-basierte Verarbeitungsalgorithmen und dessen evolutionäre Parameteroptimierung für Plasmonen-unterstützter Mikroskopiedaten vorgestellt. Es konnte dabei gezeigt werden, dass der neuartige 3D Fuzzy-Denoising-Algorithmus Verbesserungen der Klassifikation gewährleistet und insbesondere die automatische GA-gestützte Parametrisierung einen deutlichen Einfluss auf die Klassifikationsgüte hat. Die durchgängig OpenCL-gestützte Umsetzung erzielt zudem eine hochparallele und damit echtzeitkonforme Verarbeitung. In die globale Optimierung können zudem softwaretechnische als auch Hardware-assoziierte Ressourcenmodelle eingebracht werden, dies auch in Kombination mit Konzepten der Design Space Exploration – Trade-offs zwischen Hardwareeffizienz, Zeiteffizienz und Detektionsqualität sind dabei noch zu untersuchen. Weitere Betrachtungen tangieren die Fusion von zeitlicher und örtlicher Klassifikation und hybride Klassifikationsverfahren, die unüberwachte und überwachte Ansätze, z.B. Support Vector Machines, integriert betrachten.

Danksagung

Teile dieser Arbeit wurden von der Deutschen Forschungsgemeinschaft (DFG) im Sonderforschungsbereich SFB 876 „Verfügbarkeit von Information durch Analyse unter Ressourcenbeschränkung", Projekt B2, unterstützt.

Literaturverzeichnis

1. Erickson D, et al. Optofluidic, electrical and mechanical aproaches to biomolecular detection at the nanoscale. Microfluid Nanofluid. 2008;4:33–52.
2. Zybin A, et al. Real-time detection of single immobilized nanoparticles by surface plasmon resonance imaging. Plasmonics. 2010;5:31–5.
3. Karlovsky P. Moderne Diagnosemethoden und Nachweisverfahren. Schriftenreihe der Deutschen Phytomedizinischen Gesellschaft. 2006; p. 104–18.
4. Allen RL, Mills DW. Signal analysis. Wiley-Interscience; 2004.
5. Melange T, et al. Fuzzy random impulse noise removal from color image sequences. IEEE Trans Image Process. 2011;20(4):959–70.
6. Ruiz A, et al. The GPU on biomedical image processing for color and phenotype analysis. In: Proc IEEE ICBB; 2007. p. 1124–8.
7. Dasika G, et al. MEDICS: Ultra-portable processing for medical image reconstruction. In: Proc ICPA; 2010. p. 181–92.
8. Luke S. Essentials of metaheuristics; 2009. Online-Version (Dezember 2011) http://cs.gmu.edu/~sean/book/metaheuristics/.
9. Weichert F, et al. GPGPU-basierte Echtzeitdetektion von Nanoobjekten mittels Plasmonen-unterstützter Mikroskopie. Proc BVM. 2011; p. 39–43.
10. Timm C, et al. Improving nanoobject detection in optical biosensor data. Proc 5th BMIC Symp. 2011;2:236–40.
11. Man K, et al. Genetic algorithms: concepts and designs. Springer-Verlag; 2001.

Cell Tracking for Automatic Migration and Proliferation Analysis in High-Throughput Screens

Nathalie Harder[1], Richa Batra[1], Sina Gogolin[2], Nicolle Diessl[1], Roland Eils[1],
Frank Westermann[2], Rainer König[1], Karl Rohr[1]

[1]University of Heidelberg, BIOQUANT, IPMB and DKFZ Heidelberg
[3]Department of Tumor Genetics, DKFZ Heidelberg
n.harder@dkfz.de

Abstract. Systematic analysis of cell migration and proliferation in large-scale image-based screens is important for the final evaluation as well as for optimization of experimental conditions. We here present a tracking approach for high-throughput image data, and extract global movement and growth patterns on a large scale. In particular, we analyze between-spot movement on cell arrays to estimate the confidence of the phenotypic readout, we determine the cellular reproduction time, and we automatically detect multi-polar divisions to support the identification of target genes. A quantitative evaluation of our approach showed that high segmentation and tracking accuracies of 92% and 98% are reached.

1 Introduction

Image-based high-throughput experiments have become a widely-used technique since various types of cellular responses can be directly studied by observing the behavioral changes after experimental treatment. In particular, systematic gene knockdown, using RNA interference (RNAi), enables detailed studies of gene regulation. To obtain high quality image data the experimental and technical parameters need to be carefully selected which can be facilitated using image analysis techniques. In this work, we first present a robust tracking approach with mitosis detection suitable for large data sets, and second, we extract information on cell migration and proliferation to optimize automatic high-throughput experiments. In particular, we estimate the percentage of transfected cells staying within the siRNA treated regions of a cell array w.r.t. the number of leaving and entering cells (Fig. 2) to evaluate the true correlation of an observed phenotype with the respective siRNA: Only if a high percentage of cells transfected with the siRNA stay in the field of view we can be sure that the observation is correlated with the treatment at the spot. Also, non-transfected cells entering from the border of the cell array lead to a biased readout. Quantifying such migration effects is therefore essential to derive meaningful results. Moreover, we determine the cell division rate over time and estimate the doubling time to optimize the overall observation time. Finally, the trajectories are searched for rare events such as multi-polar mitoses (i.e., divisions into more than two daughter cells).

In previous work, different approaches for cell tracking have been used, depending on the diverse properties of live cell image data. Often, approaches for cell tracking are based on deformable models, such as active contours [1, 2]. Since usually the computed active contour of a frame is used in the subsequent frame to initialize the contour and establish the correspondence, the inter frame cell displacements need to be smaller than the cell diameter [1], which is not given for our images. Active contours have also been combined with other methods for correspondence finding, probabilistic methods [3]. Approaches using probabilistic methods without active contours are based, on Kalman filters [4] or particle filters [5]. However, such approaches are computationally expensive, and thus, less suited for large image sets. Other approaches use graph-based optimization [6, 7] which, however, has a high computational complexity for large cell numbers. An important requirement for successful cell tracking is the robust detection of cell divisions. Mitosis detection is either directly integrated into the tracking approach [7, 5] or performed as a separate step, based on morphological features [8, 2] or event classification [9].

In this contribution, we present an automatic tracking approach which is based on the distance in feature space, and which well copes with low temporal resolution of the data and high cell density. We have applied our approach to images of a large-scale study of cell migration and proliferation to optimize the experimental conditions for high-throughput screening (Fig. 1).

2   Materials and methods

We first perform segmentation of fluorescently labeled cell nuclei, followed by automatic tracking with mitosis detection, and trajectory analysis.

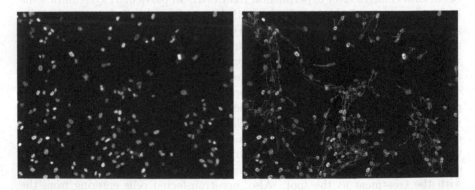

Fig. 1. Left: Example of an original image, right: overlay of computed trajectories

2.1   Cell nucleus segmentation and tracking

For cell nucleus segmentation we used a region adaptive, Otsu-based thresholding scheme which allows us to detect cells with varying contrasts and other types of phenotypic variations. To resolve clusters of cell nuclei we performed a Euclidean distance transform on the segmentation result, followed by watershed transform for cell splitting. Dense clusters of cells growing on top of each other could not be resolved with this approach and were treated as cluster objects in the subsequent analysis.

For robust tracking of cell nuclei we extended the approach in [8]. First, one-to-one correspondences are established, and second, mitosis events are detected and the respective trajectories are merged. In [8], a cost function evaluating the smoothness of trajectories was used for correspondence finding, which turned out to be not well suited for the here considered image data because of the low temporal resolution and densely growing cells. Instead, we determine correspondences based on a combination of feature similarity and spatial distance. For all candidates within a limited Euclidean distance $d_{\max}$ (maximum possible displacement) we compute the Euclidean distance in a three-dimensional, normalized feature space using the features mean intensity, standard deviation of intensities, and area. All feature values are scaled to the interval $[0, 1]$ resulting in a distance value in $[0, \sqrt{3}]$, which is transformed to the range $[0, d_{\max}]$ and combined with the spatial distance $D_{ij} = ||\mathbf{c}_i - \mathbf{c}_j|| + \alpha ||\mathbf{f}_i - \mathbf{f}_j|| d_{\max}/\sqrt{3}$, where $\mathbf{c}_i, \mathbf{c}_j$ are the centroid position vectors, $\mathbf{f}_i, \mathbf{f}_j$ are the feature vectors of two objects i, j in subsequent frames, and α is a positive weight (here we used $\alpha=1$). Afterwards, mitosis events are identified based on the size and mean intensity of mother and daughter cell nuclei [8]. To avoid false positive detections of multi-polar divisions we added a constraint considering only bright objects above a threshold, which is computed based on the mean object intensity of the respective frame.

2.2   Motion analysis

After tracking, we systematically analyze the resulting cell lineage trees (Fig. 1, right). To estimate the fraction of cells remaining in the spot area until the end of the observation period, we analyze trajectories w.r.t. their start and end points. First, we define a border region in the images of width $d_{\max}$ (maximum possible displacement, Fig. 2, middle). Trajectories starting within the border region in frames later than the first frame and ending within the inner image region are counted as entering cells n_e (type (a), Fig. 2, middle). Correspondingly, trajectories ending within the border region before the last frame are identified as cells leaving the spot region n_l (types (b),(c)). For leaving cells we check whether there exists an entering cell very close to the leaving position in the subsequent frame, which is identified as leaving and re-entering cell (type (d)). A third measure can be directly determined: the number of cells in the final frame n_{end}. However, the number of cells which leave the spot region and re-enter after some time $n_{l,e}$ (type (e)) cannot be directly measured but these cells are included in the leaving cells n_l together with cells definitely leaving the spot $n_{l,\text{final}}$. Correspondingly, the entering cells n_e include re-entering cells $n_{l,e}$. We assume $n_{l,e}=n_{e,l}$ and formulate three equations: (1) $n_{\text{end}} = n_{\text{orig}} - n_l + n_e$, (2) $n_l = n_{l,e} + n_{l,\text{final}}$, and (3) $n_{\text{orig}}/n_{l,\text{final}} = n_e/n_{l,e}$, where n_{orig} is the number of cells originating from the spot region. Using these equations we can compute the fraction of cells remaining in the spot region $R = (n_{\text{orig}} - n_{l,\text{final}})/n_{\text{end}}$.

2.3   Detection of multi-polar divisions

Since multi-polar divisions (splits into more than two daughter cells) are rare events which are very difficult to identify manually in a large data set, we automatically analyze cell lineage trees to find such events. In our tracking approach, mitosis detection is not limited to two daughter cells. Consequently, we are able to detect normal as well as multi-polar divisions based on the same mitosis detection criterion. For the identified multi-polar divisions we provide a visualization, which helps the biologists to quickly find and approve potential multi-polar divisions.

3   Results

Our approach was applied to 4400 image sequences (180–220 frames) of two neuroblastoma cell lines (SH-EP and SK-N-BE2c expressing GFP-labeled histones), acquired with a widefield fluorescence microscope (10x objective). 16 cell arrays with 275 spots each were imaged over five days (acquisition interval: 35–40 min, spatial resolution 1344×1024 pixels). A typical image contained 100–300 cells (Fig. 1). The average computation time for tracking for one image sequence was

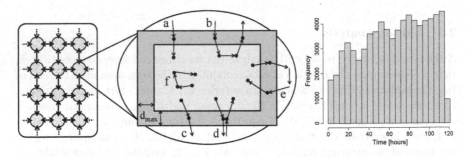

Fig. 2. Cell array and imaging region. Left: Cells grow on the whole cell array and take up siRNA when they are located on a spot. Images are acquired at each spot. During the experiment cells move from the border region into spot regions (dotted arrows) and between spot regions (solid arrows). Middle: Types of cell movement (dark gray: image border region). a) Entering, b) entering and leaving, c) leaving, d) immediately re-entering, e) leaving and re-entering later, f) staying within the spot region. Right: Histogram of mitosis events based on four cell arrays

ca. 2 min on an AMD Opteron 2220 processor. Using manually labeled ground truth (1145 cells, 10681 correspondences) we obtained a segmentation accuracy of 92% (1% oversegmentations, 3% undersegmentations, 4% false negatives), and a tracking accuracy of 98% (1% missing, 0.5% wrong correspondences).

3.1   Evaluation of cell motility and proliferation

To avoid systematic errors (bias) in the quantitative results caused by global cell migration behavior, we analyzed the global movement of the cells over the entire cell array. Such global migration patterns might be caused, by a gradient of the growth medium. Fig. 3 (left) shows the average displacement for each spot of a cell array (averaged over eight cell arrays). The motility turned out to be higher in the border regions of the cell array. This finding is used to correct bias effects by selecting adequate normalization schemes for the final statistical analysis. Furthermore, we determined the percentage of cells remaining in the spot where they took up siRNA. This allows us to judge the confidence of the experimental observations with respect to the treatment. Fig. 3 (right) shows the result for all spots, which allows us to quickly identify and discard spots with low confidence.

Based on the tracking results, we next analyzed the global proliferation behavior for the entire data set. Fig. 2 (right) shows the mitosis frequency over the observation period (based on four cell arrays), which reveals a periodic increase and decrease of mitosis frequencies, corresponding to the doubling time of the cells. Upon seeding in fresh medium, a subset of cells are synchronized w.r.t. their cell cycle, leading to partially synchronized cell divisions. The estimated doubling time of the observed cells allows us to verify general experimental settings (total observation time). Moreover, the trajectories were automatically searched for potential multi-polar divisions, resulting in a hit list which (after manual approval) can be used to identify genes related to this rare event.

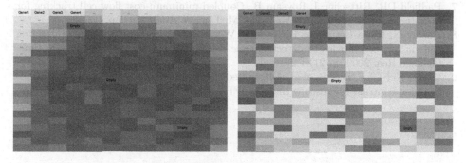

Fig. 3. Left: Average velocities of cells (range [red, yellow] corresponds to [4.0, 7.0] pixels), right: fraction of cells remaining at a spot (range [red, yellow] corresponds to [0.83, 0.95]). Both results are based on eight cell arrays

4   Discussion

We have presented a tracking approach with mitosis detection which, in comparison to previous work, is particularly suited for large image data sets with low temporal resolution and high object density, and handles normal as well as multi-polar cell divisions. Our approach has been applied to large scale data from a high-throughput screen on neuroblastoma cell lines and yields high accuracies of 92–98%. The resulting trajectories have been analyzed regarding global cell motility and proliferation behavior to optimize experimental parameters. In future work, the tracking results will be further analyzed to gain new biological insights, by automatic detection of more complex temporal phenotypes.

Acknowledgement. Support by the BMBF projects ENGINE (NGFN+) and FANCI (SysTec) is gratefully acknowledged.

References

1. Zimmer C, Zhang B, Dufour A, et al. On the digital trail of mobile cells. IEEE Signal Proc Mag. 2006; p. 54–62.
2. Dzyubachyk O, van Cappellen WA, Essers J, et al. Advanced level-set-based cell tracking in time-lapse fluorescence microscopy. IEEE T Med Imag. 2010; p. 852–67.
3. Li K, Miller ED, Chen M, et al. Cell population tracking and lineage construction with spatiotemporal context. Med Image Anal. 2008; p. 546–66.
4. Ong LLS, Ang MH, Asada HH. Tracking of cell population from time lapse and end point confocal microscopy images with multiple hypothesis Kalman smoothing filters. In: IEEE CVPR Workshops (CVPRW); 2010. p. 71–8.
5. Delgado-Gonzalo R, Chenouard N, Unser M. A new hybrid Bayesian-variational particle filter with application to mitotic cell tracking. In: Proc IEEE ISBI; 2011. p. 1917–20.
6. Mosig A, Jäger S, Wang C, et al. Tracking cells in live cell imaging videos using topological alignments. Algorithm Mol Biol. 2009; p. 10.
7. Padfield DR, Rittscher J, Roysam B. Coupled minimum-cost flow cell tracking for high-throughput quantitative analysis. Med Image Anal. 2011; p. 650–68.
8. Harder N, Mora-Bermúdez F, Godinez WJ, et al. Automatic analysis of dividing cells in live cell movies to detect mitotic delays and correlate phenotypes in time. Genome Res. 2009; p. 2113–24.
9. Huh S, Ker DFE, Bise R, et al. Automated mitosis detection of stem cell populations in phase-contrast microscopy images. IEEE Trans Med Imaging. 2011; p. 586–96.

Model Dependency of RBMCDA for Tracking Multiple Targets in Fluorescence Microscopy

Oliver Greß, Stefan Posch

Institute of Computer Science, Martin Luther University Halle-Wittenberg
gress@informatik.uni-halle.de

Abstract. The analysis of the dynamics of sub-cellular structures is of great interest to bio-medical research. We propose to use probabilistic tracking techniques to analyze the dynamics of stress granules (SGs) to avoid the problems of manual analysis. A crucial challenge in multi-target tracking is the association of observations to underlying targets. Rao-Blackwellized Monte Carlo Data Association (RBMCDA) based on sampling of association variables avoids the combinatorics of this association problem. We propose the use of a parametric data association prior for sampling of association variables and evaluate tracking results with regard to the impact of parameter deviations on synthetic data.

1 Introduction

An important part of systems biology is concerned with the dynamic behavior of cellular components under varying conditions. As an example we consider aggregation of stress granules (SGs) observed in the cytoplasm of eukaryotic cells in response to environmental stress [1]. Elucidation of their role in cellular processes requires analysis of features like quantity per cell, sizes as well as dynamic properties like accumulation, motion and interaction. Time lapse images of SGs in living cells are acquired by fluorescence microscopy. Analysis of SGs dynamics requires tracing of trajectories for numerous SGs over a number of frames. Manual analysis of these data is time-consuming and error-prone, because SGs may move fast or are densely arranged. In contrast automatic analysis allows high throughput of large data sets and also ensures reproducibility of results.

SGs are detected as spot-like structures of different and changing size (Fig. 1). Tracking SGs is difficult, as their visual appearance contains few clues to identify individual SGs and SGs suddenly start or stop moving and change their direction. Thus employing probabilistic tracking techniques which incorporate a dynamic

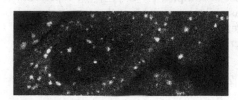

Fig. 1. Clip of a confocal laser scanning microscopy image with fluorescently labeled SGs in eukaryotic cell

model may be beneficial to track SGs. Here the state distribution of targets, SGs in our case, is predicted in each time step using a dynamic model and previous estimates. Subsequently this estimate is corrected using an observation of the target, a detected spot. The major issue in multi-target tracking is the combinatorial problem to associate observations per frame to underlying targets.

Various approaches exist to cope with the complexity of this task. The Joint Probabilistic Data Association filter [2] uses observations in the vicinity of a predicted target to update its state distribution and merges the resulting distributions to avoid exponential growth, but is intended to track a constant number of targets in presence of clutter. Multi-Hypothesis Tracking [3] provides an optimal solution in theory, but the resulting tree of hypotheses must be reduced by heuristics for practical application. Sequential Monte Carlo (MC) methods approximate distributions by a set of samples. In multi-target tracking a large number of samples is necessary to avoid overly sparse representation in high dimensions. A MC method for multi-target tracking is presented in [4]. An overview of tracking approaches is given in [5] with focus on microscopy image analysis.

The RBMCDA approach presented in [6] circumvents the combinatorial problem of data association by sampling in the space of association variables, while distributions of targets' states are kept in analytical form. We propose to use RBMCDA for tracking SGs as it allows integration of the Interacting Multiple Models (IMM) filter [2] required to account for the changing dynamics of SGs.

Contributions of this work comprise the investigation of RBMCDA tracking based on a parametric data association prior presented in [7]. Furthermore, dynamic models for SG tracking are specified. The tracking technique is evaluated on synthetic data with focus on the performance of tracking with regard to varying degree of agreement between parameters for tracking and data generation.

2   Materials and methods

2.1   Parametric data association prior for RBMCDA

Probabilistic tracking of multiple targets requires to estimate the joint distribution of the number of targets, their states and associations. The number of targets and observations may vary and a detector may produce clutter observations. $\mathbf{X}^t$ describes the set of target states, $\mathbf{Z}^t$ the vector of observations and $\mathbf{C}^t$ the vector of association variables at time t. The latter associate each observation in $\mathbf{Z}^t$ to an existing target, to a newborn target, or to clutter. The RBMCDA approach [6] avoids the combinatorial explosion of all possible associations by MC approximation. A finite set of samples $\{^{(s)}\mathbf{C}^t\}_{s=1,...,S}$ represents the joint distribution in the space of association variables whereas analytical form is maintained in the space of targets' states (Eq. (1)). A set of variables from time 1 to t is denoted by a superscript $1:t$, $\mathbf{Z}^{1:t} := \{\mathbf{Z}^1,\ldots,\mathbf{Z}^t\}$

$$p(\mathbf{X}^t, \mathbf{C}^t | \mathbf{Z}^{1:t}) \approx \frac{1}{S} \sum_{s=1}^{S} p(\mathbf{X}^t | \mathbf{Z}^{1:t}, {}^{(s)}\mathbf{C}^{1:t}) \cdot \delta(\mathbf{C}^t - {}^{(s)}\mathbf{C}^t) \tag{1}$$

where $^{(s)}\mathbf{C}^t$ is sampled from $p(\mathbf{C}^t|\mathbf{Z}^{1:t},{}^{(s)}\mathbf{C}^{1:t-1})$ A RBMCDA sample $^{(s)}$ comprises sampled associations $^{(s)}\mathbf{C}^{1:t}$ and corresponding state distribution $p(\mathbf{X}^t|\mathbf{Z}^{1:t},\ {}^{(s)}\mathbf{C}^{1:t})$. To sample $^{(s)}\mathbf{C}^t$ we decompose the previous equation

$$p(\mathbf{C}^t|\mathbf{Z}^{1:t},\mathbf{C}^{1:t-1}) \propto p(\mathbf{Z}^t|\mathbf{Z}^{1:t-1},\mathbf{C}^{1:t})p(\mathbf{C}^t|M^t,\mathfrak{N}^t_-) \tag{2}$$

The first term in Eq. (2) corresponds to the likelihood of observations for given associations. The second term in Eq. (2) is the joint data association prior, which can be shown to only require information about the number of observations M^t and the set of target IDs $\mathfrak{N}^t_-$ that exist prior to the association step, i.e. before targets are born or die in time step t. More details are given in [6, 7].

In the following the time parameter t is omitted. In [7] a joint data association prior is proposed that models the formation of M observations, composed of k observations from existing targets detected with probability P_D, b observations from newborn targets where the number of newborn targets is distributed with $\nu(b)$, and u observations from clutter distributed according to $\mu(u)$, such that $k+b+u = M$. The fraction in Eq. (3) gives the probability of the configuration $\mathbf{C}$ given k and b. The number of existing targets is denoted by $N = |\mathfrak{N}_-|$

$$p(\mathbf{C}|M,\mathfrak{N}_-) \propto p(\mathbf{C}|\mathfrak{N}_-) = \frac{1}{\binom{M}{k}\binom{N}{k}k!\binom{M-k}{b}}\binom{N}{k}P_D^k(1-P_D)^{N-k}\nu(b)\mu(u) \tag{3}$$

For experiments we choose $\nu(b)$ and $\mu(u)$ as Poisson distributed with λ_B and λ_c.

2.2 Modeling of dynamics and observations

Observations are defined by position and size of detected SGs, a target's state additionally contains its previous location. A linear model describes the relation of observations to underlying targets with additional Gaussian measurement noise with covariance matrix R, a diagonal matrix with different variances for position and size. The dynamic process is modeled by two linear models with additional Gaussian process noise with covariance matrix Q, again a diagonal matrix that determines the variances of current and previous position and the variance of size. The dynamic models represent random walk (rw) with no deterministic movement and directional motion (fle) by extrapolation of the next position from the current and last position [5]. We use IMM filters [2] to model state distributions with Gaussian mixtures employing both dynamic models. P_{rw} and P_{fle} denote the probabilities to stay with the rw model and fle model respectively.

3 Results

Suitable parameters for tracking SGs are typically unknown. In the following we evaluate how sensitive the proposed method is with regard to deviations between tracking parameters and characteristics of the data. We generate synthetic data with the (generative) model used for tracking and superscript parameters used for data generation with ^{G} and parameters for tracking by ^{T}, λ_B^G vs λ_B^T.

As targets of different RBMCDA samples do not relate to each other nor to ground-truth data the trajectories of RBMCDA samples cannot be compare directly. Therefore we base the evaluation on track graphs, which comprise all observations of a (synthetic) time-lapse sequence as nodes. To define edges, for each target all associated observations are considered. These observations are ordered with respect to time and neighboring observations in this sequence are connected by an edge. An example is given in Fig. 2, where ground-truth connects the observations horizontally, but observations 2|1 and 2|2 are switched by the tracker and observations 4|2 and 6|1 are wrongly associated to clutter. Edges common to both graphs are considered as true positives (TP), edges only in the ground truth graph as false negatives (FN) and edges only in the graph from the current sample as false positives (FP). We use precision $\mathcal{P} := \frac{\text{TP}}{\text{TP}+\text{FP}}$ and recall $\mathcal{R} := \frac{\text{TP}}{\text{TP}+\text{FN}}$ to characterize the quality of tracking. Evaluation assesses only neighboring associations which may underestimate the performance. In Fig. 2 observation 6|1 is associated to clutter by the tracker resulting in two FN and one FP, while the association of observations 4|1 to 7|1 is obviously correct. We still prefer this measure here, as it is well defined and the focus is on comparing different parameter setting.

For evaluation we investigate the influence of λ_B, λ_c, Q, R, and P_{rw} and P_{fle} in turn. Synthetic sequences are generated where one of these parameter was varied. Comparable numbers of dead and newborn targets are enforced except when varying λ_B^G. Each sequence is tracked with the same variations of parameters as used for generation. In all experiments 100 RBMCDA samples are used. Fig. 3(a) shows $\mathcal{R}$ and $\mathcal{P}$ for different tracker birth parameters λ_B^T for data generated with varying λ_B^G. Analogously results are presented in Fig. 3(b) for clutter parameter λ_c. Deviations of noise variances in generator and tracker model are evaluated by scaling fixed noise covariance matrices Q and R by factors s_Q and s_R respectively. The impact of scaling Q is presented in Fig. 3(c), and for R in Fig. 3(d). $\mathcal{R}$ and $\mathcal{P}$ for varying IMM parameters P_{rw} and P_{fle} are given in Fig. 4.

4   Discussion

We discuss $\mathcal{R}$ and $\mathcal{P}$ of the different experiments in the following to gain insight into the sensitivity of parameters with regard to tracking quality. Images are

Fig. 2. Evaluation of track graphs: Circles correspond to observations. Continuous edges represent the ground truth track graph, dashed edges represent track graph from a RBMCDA sample

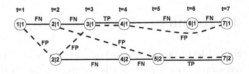

more densely populated by observations when λ_B^G is increased as more targets are born and wrong associations become more likely. Thus, for identical parameters $\lambda_B^G = \lambda_B^T$ both $\mathcal{R}$ and $\mathcal{P}$ decrease for increasing λ_B^G. If λ_B^T deviates from λ_B^G the performance is hardly influenced. Also increasing λ_c^G increases the number of observations in the image. Again, $\mathcal{R}$ and $\mathcal{P}$ decrease for increasing λ_c^G (Fig. 3(b)). In this case deviations between generation and tracker parameter have a considerable impact on performance. If λ_c^T is chosen too high, observations originating from targets easily get associated to clutter, which results in a decrease of $\mathcal{R}$. Otherwise, if λ_c^T is too low, clutter observations are often associated to targets which decreases $\mathcal{P}$. Interestingly, $\mathcal{R}$ for $\lambda_c^G = 1$ is high independently of the choice of λ_c^T. In this case, association is barely interfered by clutter observations and thus target observations get correctly associated.

The increase of noise variances with s_Q^G and s_R^G allows to generate observations which are increasingly distant from their expected mean. Thus the problem gets harder and performance decreases also given correct tracker parameters. If variances for tracking are chosen too low, the likelihood of an observation decreases very fast with distance from the expected mean and thus rather clutter or a new target are associated. This effect can be observed for values of $\mathcal{R}$ and $\mathcal{P}$ for $s_Q^G = 5$ and $s_R^G = 5$ in Fig. 3(c) and Fig. 3(d). If tracker variances are chosen too large, observations more distant to a target's location are more likely to be associated. This leads to wrong associations to targets resulting in a slight decrease of $\mathcal{R}$ and $\mathcal{P}$ when s_Q^T and s_R^T exceed s_Q^G and s_R^G.

P_{rw}^G and P_{fle}^G control the dynamic behavior of observations in the generated data. If targets are likely to stay in the fle model (large P_{fle}^G), they permanently

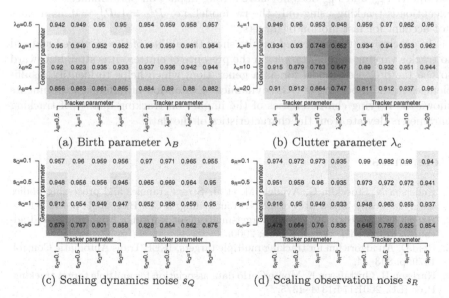

(a) Birth parameter λ_B (b) Clutter parameter λ_c

(c) Scaling dynamics noise s_Q (d) Scaling observation noise s_R

Fig. 3. $\mathcal{R}$ (left) and $\mathcal{P}$ (right) for deviating parameters in generator and tracking model

Fig. 4. $\mathcal{R}$ (left) and $\mathcal{P}$ (right) for varying model switching probabilities P_{rw}, P_{fle}

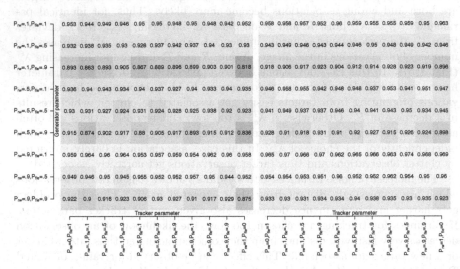

move across the image and often approach others, therefore provoking wrong associations. For this reason a decrease in $\mathcal{R}$ and $\mathcal{P}$ can be observed in Fig. 4 when P_{rw}^{G} is fixed and P_{fle}^{G} increases. In contrast if targets frequently move according to rw, they do not move far and thus are mostly associated correctly. Therefore $\mathcal{R}$ and $\mathcal{P}$ increase when P_{rw}^{G} increases. In all cases the choice of tracker parameter P_{rw}^{T} and P_{fle}^{T} does not have strong impact on performance. The only exception is tracking using only the rw model, i.e. $P_{\mathrm{rw}}^{T} = 1, P_{\mathrm{fle}}^{T} = 0$, as it does not account for fast motion of targets.

In conclusion, the presented results show the ability of the employed method to track a varying number targets in the presence of clutter. It is straightforward to use the proposed model for data generation, which helps to identify insufficiencies in the modeling of SGs' dynamics. Evaluation of different experiments shows the varying characteristics of the impact on tracking quality, if tracking parameters deviate from the characteristics of the data.

References

1. Kedersha N, Stoecklin G, Ayodele M, et al. Stress granules and processing bodies are dynamically linked sites of mRNP remodeling. J Cell Biol. 2005; p. 871–84.
2. Bar-Shalom Y, Blair WD. Multitarget-multisensor tracking: Applications and advances. Volume III. Artech House; 2000.
3. Reid D. An algorithm for tracking multiple targets. IEEE Trans Automatic Control. 1979; p. 843–54.
4. Karlsson R, Gustafsson F. Monte Carlo data association for multiple target tracking. Proc IEE. 2001;174:13/1–13/5.

5. Genovesio A, Olivo-Marin J. Particle tracking in 3D+t biological imaging. In: Microscopic Image Analysis for Life Science Applications. Artech House; 2008. p. 223–82.
6. Särkkä S, Vehtari A, Lampinen J. Rao-Blackwellized particle filter for multiple target tracking. J Inform Fusion. 2007; p. 2–15.
7. Greß O, Posch S. Parametric data association prior for multi-target tracking based on Rao-Blackwellized Monte Carlo Data Association. In: Proc ICCV; 2012. p. accepted.

Segmentierung von Blutgefäßen in retinalen Fundusbildern

Sebastian Gross, Monika Klein, Alexander Behrens, Til Aach

Lehrstuhl für Bildverarbeitung, RWTH Aachen University
sebastian.gross@lfb.rwth-aachen.de

Kurzfassung. Blutgefäßstrukturen im Auge sind bei der Diagnose einer Vielzahl von Krankheiten von herausragender Bedeutung. Arteriosklerose, Retinopathie, Mikroembolien und Makuladegeneration z.B. gehen mit einer Veränderung der Blutgefäßstruktur im Auge einher. Das vorgestellte Verfahren zur Segmentierung von Blutgefäßen nutzt unter anderem eine angepasste Variante der Phasensymmetrie nach Kovesi und einen Hystereseschritt. Der Algorithmus wurde auf Basis der öffentlichen Bilderdatenbanken DRIVE und STARE evaluiert und die Ergebnisse (DRIVE: $94,92\%$, Sensitivität $71,22\%$ und Spezifität $98,41\%$, STARE: $95,65\%$, Sensitivität $71,87\%$ und Spezifität $98,34\%$) wurden mit anderen Verfahren aus der Literatur verglichen.

1 Einleitung

Die Beurteilung von Retinafundusbildern ist in der heutigen Medizin eine wichtige Methode zur Diagnose vieler Krankheiten. Arteriosklerose, Retinopathie, Mikroembolien und Makuladegeneration z.B. gehen mit einer Veränderung der Blutgefäßstruktur im Auge einher. Im Folgenden wird ein Verfahren zur automatisierten Segmentierung von Blutgefäßen vorgestellt und mit Ansätzen aus der Literatur verglichen.

Der Text gliedert sich in mehrere Abschnitte: Abschnitt 2 gibt einen Überblick über den Stand der Technik. In Abschnitt 3 wird das Verfahren zur Segmentierung von Blutgefäßen beschrieben. Danach werden die genutzten Bilddaten eingeführt und die Auswertungskriterien erläutert. Abschnitt 4 geht auf die Ergebnisse der Evaluierung ein, und in Abschnitt 5 werden die abschließende Diskussion geführt und Schlussfolgerungen gezogen.

2 Stand der Forschung

Für die Segmentierung von Blutgefäßen in Fundusbildern werden insbesondere Richtungsinformationen häufig genutzt [1, 2, 3, 4, 5]. Hierbei wird die Hesse-Matrix bestimmt und der Vektor der maximalen Ausrichtung mit Hilfe einer Eigenwertanalyse gesucht. Auch Matched Filter werden oft zum Einsatz gebracht [3, 4, 5, 6, 7]. Um hier den Rechenaufwand zu reduzieren, schlagen viele

Veröffentlichungen vor, die Gefäßrichtung erst mit der Hesse-Matrix zu bestimmen und dann das Gefäß mit Matched Filtern zu lokalisieren [3, 4, 5]. Weiterhin wurden Merkmalsextraktion und Klassifikation [8] (u.a. auf Basis von Local Binary Patterns sowie morphologischen Operationen) und Linienoperatoren [9] eingesetzt.

3   Material und Methoden

Für die Segmentierung von Blutgefäßen wird der Grünkanal der Bilder ausgewählt, weil dieser den besten Kontrast zwischen Blutgefäßen und Hintergrund bietet [9, 10]. Um den Hintergrund zu unterdrücken, wird der Grünkanal nun mit einem 11 × 11 Min-Max-Filter gefiltert und das Ergebnis vom ursprünglichen Bild abgezogen. Damit Filteroperationen auch im Randbereich des Bildes ausgeführt werden können, wird die Retina nach außen dilatiert, indem die Pixel radialsymmetrisch fortgesetzt werden [10].

Bei Betrachtung des Grauwertverlaufs im Gefäßquerschnitt wird deutlich, dass es sich bei dem rechteck-förmigen Verlauf des Schnittbildes bezogen auf den Mittelpunkt um eine symmetrische Struktur handelt. Für die Detektion und Analyse von symmetrischen und asymmetrischen Strukturen hat Peter Kovesi einen Algorithmus vorgeschlagen [11], der nach charakteristischen Strukturen mit Hilfe einer Waveletzerlegung basierend auf komplexen, logarithmischen Gaborfunktionen sucht. Mit $e_n(\boldsymbol{x})$ und $o_n(\boldsymbol{x})$ beschreibt er die relle bzw. imaginäre Filterantwort einer Skalierung n, die als Teile einer komplexwertigen Frequenzkomponente interpretiert werden kann.

$$A_n = \sqrt{e_n(\boldsymbol{x})^2 + o_n(\boldsymbol{x})^2} \qquad (1)$$

ergibt dann die Amplitude. Kovesi schlägt vor, die Beträge von $e_n(\boldsymbol{x})$ und $o_n(\boldsymbol{x})$ skalenweise zu subtrahieren, die Ergebnisse aufzusummieren und auf die Amplitude A_n zu normieren. Desweiteren wird in der Formel

$$sym(\boldsymbol{x}) = \frac{\sum_n \lfloor |e_n(\boldsymbol{x})| - |o_n(\boldsymbol{x})| - T \rfloor}{\sum_n A_n(\boldsymbol{x}) + \epsilon} \qquad (2)$$

der Rauschanteil T subtrahiert, um die durch Rauschen erzeugte Symmetrie zu unterdrücken. Da $A_n \geq 0$, wird ausserdem $\epsilon > 0$ addiert, um eine Division durch 0 zu verhinden. Allerdings zeigen die Ergebnisse, dass die so gefundenen Blutgefäße deutlich zu dünn sind. Dies wird vor allem durch den imaginären Anteil ausgelöst, der im Randbereich der Gefäße betragsmäßig groß ist (Abb. 1). Um diesen störenden Einfluß zu unterbinden, wird der Beitrag von $o_n(\boldsymbol{x})$ ignoriert. Die modifizierte Formel

$$sym(\boldsymbol{x}) = \frac{\sum_n \lfloor |e_n(\boldsymbol{x})| - T \rfloor}{\sum_n A_n(\boldsymbol{x}) + \epsilon} \qquad (3)$$

verdeutlicht dies. Die Ergebnisse der Vorverarbeitung und der Symmetriefilterung sind in Abb. 1 zu sehen.

Für die binäre Klassifikationsentscheidung steht das Front-Propagation-Verfahren Fast Marching [12] zur Verfügung. Für dieses werden ausgedünnte Ergebnisse des Phasensymmetriefilters als Saatpunkte genutzt. Alternativ kann ein Verfahren mit Hystereseschritt zum Einsatz kommen. Hierzu werden ein Strukturbild und ein Detailbild, die jeweils mit unterschiedlichen Parametersätzen und Schwellwerten, T_1 und T_2, erzeugt werden, zu einem Gesamtergebnis kombiniert.

Zum Vergleich der Performance der Segmentierungsalgorithmen werden zwei speziell zu diesem Zweck veröffentlichte Datensätze herangezogen, für die neben den Bilddaten auch Handsegmentierungen als Ground Truth vorliegen. Die im Jahr 2004 unter dem Namen DRIVE [13] veröffentlichte Bilddatenbank besteht aus 20 Test- und 20 Trainingsbildern. Für jedes Bild gibt es eine Maske, die das zu analysierende Field of View (FOV) angibt. Die STARE-Datenbank wurde im

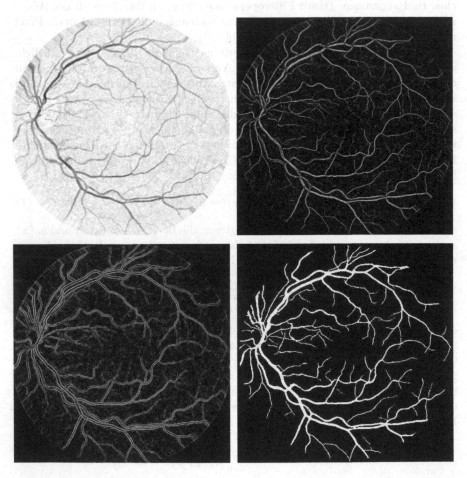

Abb. 1. links oben: vorverarbeitetes Bild, rechts oben: Betrag des Realteils $e_n(\boldsymbol{x})$, links unten: Betrag des Imaginärteils $o_n(\boldsymbol{x})$ und rechts unten: fertige Segmentierung

Jahr 2000 von Adam Hoover vorgestellt [7] und enthält 20 Bilder, von denen 10 pathologische Befunde dokumentieren. Ein FOV steht hier nicht zur Verfügung und wurde nachträglich handsegmentiert. Weiterhin existieren jeweils zwei Handsegmentierung, die von geschulten Beobachtern bestimmt wurden. Die jeweils erste wird - wie in der Literatur üblich - als Goldstandard verwendet, um die Performance des Segmentierungsverfahrens zu bestimmen. Es werden die gleichen Methoden zur Auswertung verwendet, die auch in den bereits vorgestellten Veröffentlichungen [1, 2, 3, 4, 5, 6, 7] genutzt wurden. Hierzu werden die Verfahren auf die Bilder der beiden Datenbanken angewendet. Die Segmentierungen werden anschließend mit den jeweils ersten Handsegmentierungen, die als Goldstandard dienen, verglichen.

4   Ergebnisse

Die Paramter T_1 und T_2 wurden hinsichtlich ihres Einflußes auf das Klassifikationsergebnis der DRIVE-Datenbank untersucht. Das Verfahren reagiert stabil, auch wenn die Parameter deutlich geändert werden (Abb. 2). Mit den Parametern $T_1 = 0,18$ und $T_2 = 0,62$ wird das beste Ergebnis bezüglich der Erkennungsrate erzielt. Der Algorithmus erreicht kombiniert mit Fast Marching eine Gesamtklassifikationsrate von 94,74% (Sens = 73,07%, Spez = 97,99%). Demgegenüber liefert die Kombination mit einem Hystereseansatz eine leicht bessere Gesamtklassifikationsrate von 94,92%. Dies wird aufgrund der hohen Anzahl an Hintergrundpixeln vor allem durch eine verbesserte Spezifität (Spez = 98,41%) erzielt, wogegen die Sensitivität (Sens = 71,22%) abnimmt. Die Gesamtergebnisse aus der Literatur sind zusammen mit den neuen Ergebnissen in Tab. 1 aufgeführt. Die Daten der STARE-Datenbank [7] wurden genutzt, um die Ergebnisse von gesunden und pathologischen Bildern mit den ermittelten Schwellwer-

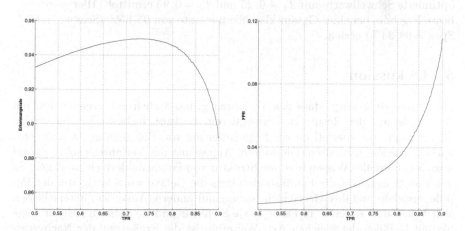

Abb. 2. Verhalten der Erkennungsrate und der False Posivit Rate bei Änderung der Parameter T_1 und T_2

Tabelle 1. Ergebnisse für DRIVE [13] und STARE [7] mit Gesamtklassifikationsrate (GKR), Sensitivität (Sens) und Spezifität (Spez) im Vergleich

Autor	DRIVE			STARE		
	GKR	Sens	Spez	GKR	Sens	Spez
PS+FM	0,9474	0,7307	0,9799	-	-	-
PS+Hysterese	0,9492	0,7122	0,9841	0,9565	0,7187	0,9834
Budai [2]	0,9490	0,7509	0,9680	0,9380	0,6510	0,9750
Wu [3]	-	0,9023	0,9518	-	-	-
Soares [10]	0,9466	-	-	0,9480	-	-
Staal [1]	0,9441	0,7194	0,9773	0,9516	-	-
Ricci [9]	0,9595	-	-	0,9646	-	-
Niemeijer [13]	0,9416	0,6898	0,9696	-	-	-
Rezatofighi [8]	0,9462	0,7358	0,9767	-	-	-
Alonso-Montes [14]	0,9180	-	-	-	-	-
Farzin [15]	0,9370	-	-	0,9480	-	-
Fraz [16]	0,9352	-	-	0,9384	-	-
Hoover [7]	-	-	-	0,9275	-	-
Lam [17]	-	-	-	0,9474	-	-
manuell [8, 13]	0,9473	0,7761	0,9725	0,9349	0,8951	0,9572
nur Hintergrund [13]	0,8727	0,0000	1,0000	0,8958	0,0000	1,0000

ten zu vergleichen. Für gesunde Bilder ergab sich eine Gesamtklassifikationsrate von $94,80\%$ (Sens $= 79,56\%$, Spez $= 96,38\%$). Die Erkennungsrate für Bilder mit Krankheitsbefund veränderte sich demgegenüber nur leicht auf $94,85\%$ (Sens $= 79,22\%$, Spez $= 96,47\%$). Auf der STARE-Datenbank wurde ebenfalls optimierte Schwellwerte mit $T_1 = 0,25$ und $T_2 = 0,95$ ermittelt. Hier wurde das beste Ergebnis bei einer Gesamtklassifikationsrate von $95,65\%$ (Sens $= 71,87\%$, Spez $= 98,34\%$) erzielt.

5 Diskussion

Die Auswertung zeigt, dass das Verfahren grundsätzlich gut geeignet ist, um Blutgefäße auf der Retina zu segmentieren. Es kann insbesondere mit vielen Algorithmen, die speziell für die Segmentierung von Blutgefäßen im Auge entwickelt wurden, mithalten. Die weitere Anpassung des Verfahrens sollte darauf abzielen, spezielles Wissen über die Struktur von Fundusbildern einzupflegen. So gilt zum Beispiel für die Fundusbilder, dass die Gefäße wurzelartig von der Papille ausgehen und ihre Größe nicht sprunghaft ändern. Außerdem unterscheiden sich Venen und Arterien in Farbe sowie Struktur und sie kreuzen sich im Auge nie mit Gefäßen der gleichen Art. Weiterhin ist die Ergänzung der Nachverarbeitung der Segmentierung um einen Schritt, der Artefakte lokalisiert und aus der Segmentierung entfernt, ein möglicher Ansatzpunkt.

Danksagung. Die Autoren danken dem Bundesministerium für Bildung und Forschung (Förderkennzeichen 01EZ1006B) sowie der Exzellenzinitiative des Bundes und der Länder für die Förderung.

Literaturverzeichnis

1. Staal J, Abramoff MD, Niemeijer M, et al. Ridge-based vessel segmentation in color images of the retina. IEEE Trans Med Imaging. 2004;23(4):501–9.
2. Budai A, Michelson G, Hornegger J. Multiscale blood vessel segmentation in retinal fundus images. In: Proc BVM; 2010. p. 261–5.
3. Wu CH, Agam G, Stanchev P. A hybrid filtering approach to retinal vessel segmentation. In: Proc ISBI; 2007. p. 604–7.
4. Sofka M, Stewart CV. Retinal vessel centerline extraction using multiscale matched filters, confidence and edge measures. IEEE Trans Med Imaging. 2006;25(12):1531–46.
5. Sofka M, Stewart CV. Erratum to "Retinal vessel centerline extraction using multiscale matched filters, confidence and edge measures". IEEE Trans Med Imaging. 2007;26(1):133.
6. Chaudhuri S, Chatterjee S, Katz N, et al. Detection of blood vessels in retinal images using two-dimensional matched filters. IEEE Trans Med Imaging. 1989;8(3):263–9.
7. Hoover AD, Kouznetsova V, Goldbaum M. Locating blood vessels in retinal images by piecewise threshold probing of a matched filter response. IEEE Trans Med Imaging. 2000;19(3):203–10.
8. Rezatofighi SH, Roodaki A, Pourmorteza A, et al. Polar run-length features in segmentation of retinal blood vessels. In: Proc. IDIPC; 2009. p. 72–5.
9. Ricci E, Perfetti R. Retinal blood vessel segmentation using line operators and support vector classification. IEEE Trans Med Imaging. 2007;26(10):1357–65.
10. Soares JVB, Leandro JJG, Cesar RM, et al. Retinal vessel segmentation using the 2-D Gabor wavelet and supervised classification. IEEE Trans Med Imaging. 2006;25(9):1214–22.
11. Kovesi P. Symmetry and asymmetry from local phase. In: Proc 10th Australian JCAI; 1997. p. 2–4.
12. Sethian JA. A fast marching level set method for monotonically advancing fronts. In: Proc Nat Acad Sci; 1995. p. 1591–5.
13. Niemeijer M, Staal JJ, van Ginneken B, et al. Comparative study of retinal vessel segmentation methods on a new publicly available database. Proc SPIE. 2004;5370:648–56.
14. Alonso-Montes C, Vilariño DL, Dudek P, et al. Fast retinal vessel tree extraction: a pixel parallel approach. Int J Circuit Theory Appl. 2008;36:641–51.
15. Farzin H, Moghaddam HA, Moin MS. A novel retinal identification system. EURASIP J Adv Sig Proc. 2008.
16. Fraz MM, Javed MY, Basit A. Evaluation of retinal vessel segmentation methodologies based on combination of vessel centerlines and morphological processing. In: Proc. Emerging Technologies ICET; 2008. p. 232–6.
17. Lam BSY, Yan H. A novel vessel segmentation algorithm for pathological retina images based on the divergence of vector fields. IEEE Trans Med Imaging. 2008;27(2):237–46.

3D Optic Nerve Head Segmentation in Idiopathic Intracranial Hypertension

Ella Maria Kadas[1], Falko Kaufhold[1], Christian Schulz[2], Friedemann Paul[1], Konrad Polthier[2], Alexander U. Brandt[1]

[1]NeuroCure Clinical Research Center, Charité-Universitätsmedizin Berlin
[2]Mathematical Geometry Processing Group, Freie Universität Berlin
ella-maria.kadas@charite.de

Abstract. Patients with idiopathic intracranial hypertension (IIH) often present papilledema at the optic nerve head (ONH), associated with visual field losses. In order to quantify the edema, the computation of its volume is needed. Optical coherence tomography (OCT) is a non-invasive method for spatial imaging of retinal layer composition. However, current algorithms fail to segment the ONH in IIH patients satisfactorily. We developed an automatic method for segmenting the retinal pigment epithelium layer (RPE) from spatial high-resolution OCT ONH scans with robust performance in IIH patients. Using a hypothetical extension of the RPE through the ONH we were able to compute ONH height and volume. Using this algorithm we could automatically detect differences in ONH volume and height between healthy controls and IIH patients. Quantifying ONH edema in IIH is potentially important for diagnosis and especially for monitoring progression and treatment effectiveness.

1 Introduction

Modern spectral domain optical coherence tomography (OCT) allows non-invasive, spatial imaging of retinal layers and is being established in several neurological disorders. However, automatic segmentation methods most often fail in identifying complex structures like the optic nerve head (ONH), where retinal nerve cells meet to form the optic nerve connecting eye and brain.

Segmentation is especially challenging in diseases that show profound ONH alterations like idiopathic intracranial hypertension (IIH). IIH is characterized by increased intracranial pressure leading – among others – to papilledema, a sometimes severe swelling of the ONH. The neurologist has to rely on clinical symptoms and direct measurement of intracranial pressure by lumbar puncture alone for monitoring treatment effects and disease progression. It had been shown [1] that OCT can provide useful information in patients with IIH using indirect measures like the peripapilly nerve fiber layer thickness (RNFLT) in a circular peripapillary scan. Direct ONH quantification has never been investigated.

The swelled ONH region in scans from IIH patients appears as a "hill" (Fig. 1(a)) or a "volcano" (Fig. 1(b)) with varying sizes. In this region the retinal layers or other structures, like the neural canal opening, are hardly recognizable. Other approaches [2] that asses the detection of the ONH structural change in 3D OCT scans use the neural canal opening as a basis for a longitudinally stable reference plane. In IIH patients this structure is not visible. Therefore our main assumption was that the papilledema is enclosed by the inner limiting membrane (ILM) and RPE. These layers are used by other 3D retinal layers segmentation algorithms [3, 4], that do, however, not work in IIH. While the ILM is provided by the OCT device's software, the RPE is detected with the presented algorithm. The objective of this work was then to develop a segmentation algorithm that is (a) working in IIH and (b) can be used as a robust basis for ONH quantification.

2   Materials and methods

19 IIH patients and 19 matched healthy controls were included. Optical Coherence Tomography scans were acquired using a spectral-domain OCT (Spectralis SD-OCT, Heidelberg Engineering, Germany). Spatial ONH scans were performed using a custom protocol for high-resolution optic nerve head imaging with 145 B-scans focusing the optic nerve head with a scanning angle of 15×15 degrees and a resolution of 384 A-scans per B-scan. Algorithm development was done using Matlab R2011A with Spline library (Mathworks, Germany). Comparisons of ONH in IIH patients and controls were performed with generalized estimating equation models (GEE) accounting for inter-eye/intra-patient dependencies using SPSS (IBM SPSS Version 19, IBM, NY, USA).

2.1   Algorithm development

: To compute the volume and the height of the edema, B-scan and corresponding ILM position have to be given. ILM information is provided by the device software. The key ingredient is the RPE layer. It separates the other layers from the choroid (Fig. 2). In the presented algorithm, we detect the RPE around the ONH and extend it through the ONH as a theoretical lower bound to volume and height measurements.

1. *Preprocessing*: Given a B-scan from the 3D OCT scans, the intrinsic speckle noise is reduced by denoising each B-scan using anisotropic diffusion as described in [5], with iteration step set to 10. Then a relative homogeneous

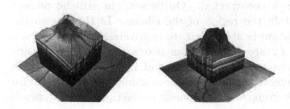

Fig. 1. 3D SDOCT volume of two different swelled regions. Left: hill form; right: "volcano" shape

region from the corresponding ILM to the inner nuclear layer (INL) is created by dilating the ILM with a disc structure of radius 4. After that, each B-scan is smoothed with a large Gaussian filter, size $[7, 7]$, with $\sigma = 5$. The resulting image contains three regions in the following order from top to bottom: light grey, black and grey.

2. *RPE region*: The regions we assumed to contain the RPE are the two lower ones. Two curves are detected to bound the search area for the RPE from these regions. The candidate pixels for the construction of the curves are found per column for the upper one from top to bottom, starting at the ILM

$$\{p(x_i, y_j) \,|\, I(p(x_i, y_j) < 60, 0 < i < m, ILM(i) < j < n\} \qquad (1)$$

and for the lower one from bottom to top

$$\{p(x_i, y_j) \,|\, I(p(x_i, y_j)) > 20, 0 < i < m, ILM(i) < j < n, \} \qquad (2)$$

where $m \times n$ is the total number of pixels in each B-scan, and $I(p)$ the intensity value at a point p. The two intensity threshold values were found by experiments with our data set such that RPE regions with low intensity values are also taken into account. Fitting a cubic polynomial to the set of top and lower resulting pixels two boundary curves C_1 (Fig. 2(a)) and C_2 are created. (Fig. 2(b)).

3. *RPE initial pixels*: Having the two curves C_1 and C_2 from the previous step, RPE pixels candidates within the bounded region are now chosen. Previous reports [3] defined RPE consisting of pixels having the highest intensity value among all other layers. In the present data this observation is not reliable due to strong artifacts from ONH swelling. To ensure a spatial choice that respects the anatomical position of this layer, we use information about pixel intensity and position in the grey value profile of each column in a B-scan. For each profile the set P of peaks is detected. From each of these sets, a point p with $d(p, C_1) > 20px$ is added to a list L which meets the conditions

$$\begin{cases} p = \min\limits_{h(p) \in M} M, M = \{x, |h(x) - h(s)| < 10, \forall s \in P\} \\ p = \max\limits_{h(p) \in M} M, M = \{x, |h(x) - h(s)| > 10, \forall s \in P\} \end{cases} \qquad (3)$$

where $d(p, C_1)$ represents the distance from the candidate point p to the corresponding point of the upper bounding curve C_1, $h(p)$ the grey value of a point in the intensity profile.

From the list L of each B-scan the final selection of points to create the curve, describing the RPE layer is constructed. Outliers might still be present in L in B-scans that contain the region of the edema. In this region the only reliable RPE information is at the left, respectively right side of each scan. Two lists $L1$ and $L2$ are created from pixels in L. For each side a point $p(x_i, y_i)$ in the first quarter from left and right of the scan with minimal y_i coordinate is detected. These give the starting reference height for creating two lists. Starting from these seed points to the right and left, pixels are added iteratively to the corresponding list if they meet the following conditions (Fig. 2(c))

$$\begin{cases} |x_i - x_{i-1}| < 5\text{px, for } |y_i - y_{i-1}| < 5\text{px} \\ |x_i - x_{i-1}| < 10\text{px, for } |y_i - y_{i-1}| < 15\text{px} \end{cases} \quad (4)$$

In case of missing image information, RPE segmentation data from the previous scan is taken into account.

4. *RPE curve*: Finally having the two lists, a least square spline approximation is applied to $L1 \bigcup L2$, with knots and order of the spline, quadratic or cubic, depending on the number of pixels of $L1$, respectively $L2$. The scan alignment step is performed by column shifting as described in [4].

5. *ONH volume and height*: For the volume measurement a threshold of 20 pixels was applied from the reference height computed at the right side and left side of each B-scan. The areas found on each B-scan, multiplied by the spatial spacing were summed up to obtain the final volume. The threshold of 20 pixels was found due experiments to provide a satisfying result in images from IIH patients as well from healthy controls (Fig. 3).

3   Results

Optic nerve head volume (ONHV) was significantly increased in IIH patients (2.3 ± 1.3 mm^3) compared to healthy controls (1.1 ± 0.5 mm^3, GEE, B = 1.2, SE = 0.3, p < 0.001). Maximal optic nerve head height (ONHH) was elevated in IIH (108.0 ± 17.5 μm) compared to healthy controls (102.5 ± 6.9 μm), however, this difference was statistically not significant (GEE $p = 0.101$).

GEE models with ICP as independent and either ONHV or ONHH as dependent variable were weakly significant for ONHV (B = 0.02, SE = 0.01, p = 0.045) and highly significant for ONHH with a negative association (B = -0.85, SE = 0.12, p < 0.001).

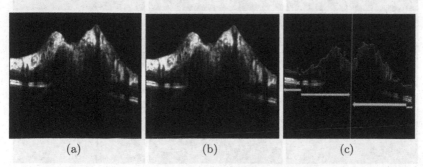

(a)   (b)   (c)

Fig. 2. (a) upper border (b) lower border. (c) The processed image containing the RPE region and the two starting points mark by crosses. Green points contain the upper boundary, and blue ones the initial RPE pixels. The arrow suggests the search direction for RPE pixels included into the list before the spline fitting step

3.1 Evaluation

To determine the accuracy of the RPE detection we conducted an automatic versus manual segmentation validation study. This study included five randomly selected healthy controls and five IIH patients. In total, 3D scans from 20 eyes, each with 145 B-scans, were manually segmented by two expert graders and compared to the results of the automatic segmentation. The results in Table 1 show that the automatic algorithm accurately detected the RPE in healthy control scans as well as in scans from IIH patients (Tab. 1). The quantitative results indicate a very good agreement and high correlation between the manual graders and our sets of measurements. Furthermore, the agreement was comparable to the agreement between two manual graders.

4 Discussion

We developed an automatic segmentation approach for computing ONH volume and maximal height from 3D spectral domain OCT scans that is robust and applicable in IIH patients. Our algorithm provided good results in IIH patients as well as healthy controls and was able to detect pronounced and significant differences between the groups. The discriminatory ability between untreated

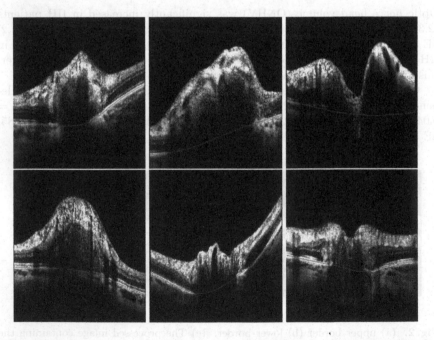

Fig. 3. These images belong to different patients at different position relative to the ONH, and are representative of the different changes that occur in this region. The blue line represents the ILM, while the red one stands for RPE

Table 1. Differences in RPE detection for 1450 B-scans of healthy controls and 1450 B-scans of IIH patients, between the first expert manual grader compared to the proposed algorithm (Column I), between the second expert manual grader compared to the proposed algorithm (Column II). Column III reports the differences between the two manual graders. Each pixel is 3.8717 μm.

RPE Differences	Manual Grader 1 vs. Algorithm	Manual Grader 2 vs. Algorithm	Manual Grader 1 vs. Manual Grader 2
Healthy controls:			
Mean Difference	1.1515	1.2265	1.1284
Standard deviation	0.1628	0.1813	0.1725
intraclass correlation coeff.	0.9996	0.9999	0.9998
IIH patients:			
Mean Difference	1.3478	1.4093	1.3859
Standard deviation	0.3724	0.392	0.3578
intraclass correlation coeff.	0.9979	0.9983	0.9998

patients and healthy controls was indeed very good, with only very few patients and controls overlapping. In contrast, control measurements using RNFLT did not show differences between the groups (data not shown).

These findings disclose several possibilities for using quantified ONH volume in practice. OCT could aid in diagnosis of IIH, providing an easy tool to quantify ONH swelling in patients with unclear symptoms. Automated 3D ONH assessment could also be useful for monitoring therapeutic effects of IIH treatment or for quantifying disease progression.

The development of our algorithm focuses now on studying follow-up data from IIH patients and further improving the algorithm's reliability in repeated measurements.

References

1. Heidary G, Rizzo JF. Use of optical coherence tomography to evaluate papilledema and pseudopapilledema. IEEE Trans Pattern Anal Mach Intell. 2010; p. 25(5–6):198–205.
2. Hu Z, Michael DA, Young HK, et al. Automated segmentation of neural canal opening and optic cup in 3D spectral optical coherence tomography volumes of the optic nerve head. Invest Ophthalmol Vis Sci. 2010;51.
3. Chiu JS, Li XT, Nicholas P, et al. Automatic segmentation of seven retinal layers in SDOCT images congruent with expert manual segmentation. Optic Express 19413. 2010;18.
4. Rossant F, Ghorbel I, Bloch I, et al. Automated segmentation of retinal layers in OCT imaging and derived ophthalmic measures. Biomedical Imaging. 2009; p. 1370–73.
5. Perona P, Malik J. Scale-space and edge detection using anisotropic diffusion. IEEE Trans Pattern Anal Mach Intell. 1990;12.

Skull Extraction from MR Images Generated by Ultra Short TE Sequence

Mohamad Habes[1][2], Elena Rota Kops[3], Hans-Gerd Lipinski[2], Hans Herzog[3]

[1]Institute for Community Medicine, University of Greifswald
[2]Biomedical Imaging Group, Dortmund University of Applied Sciences
[3]Institute of Neuroscience and Medicine, Jülich Research Centre
mohamad.habes@uni-greifswald.de

Abstract. We developed two methods for the virtual extraction of the skull from the ultra short echo time MR images: i) an interactive and a semi-automatic scatterplot based segmentation as well as ii) a support vector machine (SVM) based segmentation. Both interactive and semi-automated procedures allow for good segmentation results. On the other hand it was possible to full automate the skull segmentation process with the SVM which delivered slightly better results. Four datasets were evaluated with the corresponding registered CT images using the Dice coefficients (D). The interactive scatterplot based method reached a mean D of 0.802 ± 0.070, the semi automatic one yielded a mean D of 0.791 ± 0.042 and the SVM based segmentation delivered a mean D of 0.828 ± 0.053.

1 Introduction

Attenuation correction of positron emission tomography (PET) data acquired by hybrid MR-PET scanners is still one of the main problems for this new technique. This correction may be done by using the segmented T1-weighted images [1]. For the segmentation of these images the separation of the cortical bone and the air filled cavities represents the major problem. The ultra short echo time (UTE) sequence was developed to visualize in MRI tissues with very short T2 time as ,e.g., the cortical bone. In this way with this sequence one is able to still measure some signal coming from such tissues [2, 3].

Morphological operations were used in [4] for automatic skull segmentation from MR images, while Neural Networks were used in [1] to realize a knowledge based approach. Because the UTE image components have very low visualization quality, the application of such methods would not yield reliable results. Therefore new segmentation methods are needed. We took advantage of the bone visualization in the UTE images and developed skull segmentation methods by generating images primarily containing cortical bone tissue and background only.

2   Material and methods

2.1   Preliminary work

The ultra short echo time (UTE) sequence was developed to visualize tissues with short T2 time, for example for ligament [2]. Furthermore tissues like cortical bone have also shorter T2 time (table 1). In fact tissues in human body can be divided in different classes dependent on their T2 time. They vary between long (> 200 ms) and very short (0.05 ms). The UTE sequence used in this work provides two 3D image components by setting the parameters at TR=200 ms, flip angle 15°, TE_1=0.07 ms and TE_2=0.46 ms respectively (Fig. 1). The resulting resolution is $1.67 \times 1.67 \times 1.67$ mm^3.

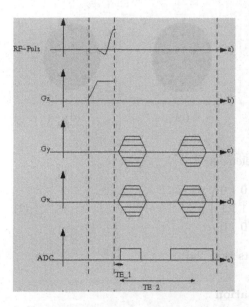

Fig. 1. Pulse sequence diagram for a basic double echo UTE sequence: (a= Radio Frequency pulse (RF), b,c,d= space encoding gradients,e= sampling window)

While the first image component (TE_1) visualizes the compact bone, the second image component (TE_2) with the longer echo time is no more able to. Due to the measurement parameters the TE_1 image appears usually more blurred than the TE_2 image showing wider head edges. To eliminate the influence of these edges on the final segmented images, a correction mask is used.

The main aim of this mask is to label all outside voxels as background. The mask was created as following (Fig. 2): The image component TE_1 was selected (Fig. 2, a) and thresholded (Fig. 2, b). The threshold value was automatically detected with the Iso-Data thresholding technique calculated for every slice independently. The remaining cavities were then filled using region growing algorithm (Fig. 2, c). Finally a 2D morphological operation "Erosion" was

Table 1. Approximate mean T2 time of short T2 tissues [2]. The values were taken from adult subjects and estimated using 1.5 T scanner

Tissue	Mean T2
Ligaments	4−10 ms
Cortical bone	0.42−0.50 ms
Dentine	0.15 ms
Protons in solids (e.g., calcium hydroxy appatite)	1 μs or less

Fig. 2. Creation of the correction mask. (a) TE_1 image component, axial view; (b) iso data thresholded; (c) region growing; (d) correction mask after applying the morphological erosion

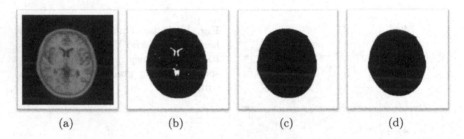

(a)   (b)   (c)   (d)

applied with the following structure element

$$\begin{pmatrix} 0\ 1\ 0 \\ 1\ 1\ 1 \\ 0\ 1\ 0 \end{pmatrix} \tag{1}$$

,which empirically leads to best results (Fig. 2,d).

2.2   Scatter plot based segmentation

From both UTE image components a scatter plot (voxel intensities of the image TE_1 vs. voxel intensity of the image TE_2) was generated. The scatter plot is a useful tool for descriptive intensity detection (Fig. 3).

To classify the cortical bone from the scatter plot two methods were applied: (i) a user interactive and (ii) a semi-automatic marker-based one. The first method requires that the user, which is expected to be an expert, selects the cortical bone class directly on the scatter plot. This selection is based on a priori information about the characteristics of the UTE sequence which leads to higher intensity values for cortical bone in the TE_1 image than the corresponding values in the TE_2 image. For the semi-automatic method (Fig. 3) seed points have to be selected on the scatter plot with just one point for the cortical bone class and several points for the background. From these seed points regions will spread with the region growing algorithm creating the two required classes.

Fig. 3. Steps of semi automatic selection of the bone class in the scatter plot; ordinates axis: voxel intensities of the image component TE_1; abscissa axis: voxel intensities of the image component TE_2. (a) scatter plot of image component TE_1 and TE_2 with seed points; (b) bone class with region growing detected; (c) labeling the results on original scatter plot)

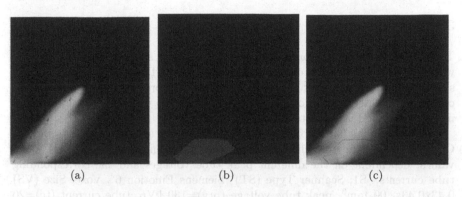

(a)   (b)   (c)

Next, for both methods (i and ii) the image components TE_1 and TE_2 will be traversed and only the voxels with the intensities belonging to the bone region will be classified as cortical bone.

2.3   SVM-based segmentation

For the fully automatic segmentation the support vector machine (SVM) [5] algorithm was used. SVM are supervised learning systems usually used for binary classification. The start point of the SVM is a training dataset

$$T = (\{x_i, y_i\} : i = 1..L, y_i \in \{-1, +1\}, x_i \in R^D\} \qquad (2)$$

where the vectors x_i are from the d dimensional room R^D and are labeled in two classes $y_i = -1$ or $y_i = +1$, i.e., background class or bone class. The SVM finds he best hyper plane, which optimally divides the two classes. By tuning the hyper plane just the support vectors (i.e., the nearest vectors to the hyper plane) will play a role in the segmentation procedure. Again, the priori information about the cortical bone characteristics in both UTE images has to be used by the expert for training the machine. As consequence the expert decides whether a voxel intensity belongs to cortical bone or not. The training pool for N participants can be formulated as following

$$T = (\{x_{(i,j)}, y_{(i,j)}) : i = 1..L, y_{(i,j)} \in \{-1, +1\}, j = 1..N\} \qquad (3)$$

The training vectors will be determined from the corresponding intensities in the image components T_1 and T_2, respectively. The training sets were built from 100 vectors for the cortical bone class and 100 vectors for the background class. The voxel classification starts as soon as the optimal hyper plane is found and the whole volumes will be traversed building the test vectors ,i.e., vectors to be classified in new images not included in the training pool).

All the methods introduced in this paper were implemented in the java based framework ImageJ [6].

3 Results

To evaluate the methods presented here data of four subjects were used which were acquired in the Siemens MAGNETOM Trio 3T MR scanner. Figure 4 shows the segmentation results of the SVM based approach ((a) transversal, (b) coronal, (c) sagittal view) of one of the subjects. To validate the methods CT images were used as gold standard.

For each of the four subjects (S) a CT image was acquired, but on different CT scanners, leading to different resolutions and eventually different HU bone values, dependent on the different peak tube voltages and the corresponding tube currents. S1; Scanner Type (ST) "Siemens Emotion 6", Voxel Size (VS) 0.43x0.43x2.00 mm^3, peak tube voltage (ptv)=130 kVp, tube current (tc)=20 mAs. S2; ST: "Siemens Emotion", VS: 0.66x0.66x2.00 mm^3, ptv=120 kVp, tc=20 mAs. S3 and S4; ST: "Philips Gemini TOF 16", VS: 1.17x1.17x1.00 mm^3, ptv=120 kVp, tc=20 mAs. All images (CT and MR) were firstly transformed to the Voxel Size of 1.00x1.00x1.00 mm^3 via trilinear interpolation. After that the CT images were linear registered with SPM5 [7] to the corresponding MR images and then segmented into cortical bone and background by setting a threshold at HU greater than 400.

For validation the Dice coefficients (D) were calculated between the final segmentation and the segmented corresponding gold standard. A Dice coefficient averaged over the whole segmented volume of each subject was calculated. The mean over these four D values for each segmentation method is presented.

The interactive scatter plot based segmentation with heuristically selected regions in the scatter plot reached D of 0.802±0.070 (mean ± SD). The marker

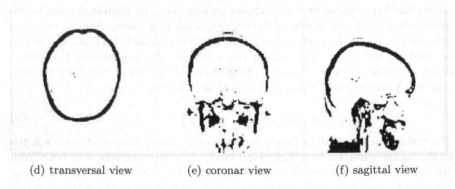

(d) transversal view   (e) coronar view   (f) sagittal view

Fig. 4. Segmentation results of the SVM based approach

based scatter plot segmentation yielded a D of 0,791±0,042 and finally the fully automatic segmentation method with well-trained SVM reached a D of 0,828±0,053. The values of the Dice coefficients were normal distributed (tested with Shapiro-Wilk tests). No significant differences between the values could be found (Tukey test).

4 Discussion

To solve the problem of attenuation correction in brain PET images acquired by hybrid MR-PET scanners, it is mandatory to account for the cortical bone. UTE sequence images can be interesting as anatomical reference. The virtual extraction of the skull was realized by developing two methods (an interactive and a semi-automatic) based on the generated scatter plot. With these methods it was possible to segment the cortical bone with good segmentation result. More important for the practice, however, is to obtain a fully automatic segmentation procedure. The SVM based segmentation yielded slightly better results than the semi-automatic one and may be used for this purpose. In conclusion, it was possible to show that the use of the SVM based segmentation can fully automate the cortical bone extraction process yielding an acceptable quality at the same time.

Acknowledgement. We would like to thank Siemens AG for their cooperation in this project.

References

1. Rota Kops E, Wagenknecht G, Scheins J, et al. Attenuation correction in MR-PET scanners with segmented T1-weighted MR images. IEEE Nucl Sci Symp Conf Rec. 2009; p. 2530 – 3.
2. Robson MD, Gatehouse PD, Bydder M, et al. Magnetic resonance: an introduction to ultrashort TE (UTE) imaging. J Comput Assist Tomogr. 2003;27(6):825–46.
3. Tyler DJ, Robson MD, Henkelman MR, et al. Magnetic resonance imaging with ultrashort TE (UTE) PULSE sequences: Technical considerations. J Magn Reson Imaging. 2007;25(2):279–89.
4. Dogdas B, Shattuck DW, Leahy RM. Segmentation of skull and scalp in 3-D human MRI using mathematical morphology. Hum Brain Mapp. 2005;26(4):273–85.
5. Begg R, Lai DTH, Palaniswami M. Computational Intelligence in Biomedical Engineering. CRC; 2007.
6. Abramoff MD, Magelhaes PJ, Ram SJ. Image Processing with ImageJ. Biophotonics International. 2004;11(7):36–42.
7. Ashburner J, Friston KJ. Rigid body registration. In: Frackowiak RSJ, et al, editors. Human Brain Function. 2nd ed. Academic Press; 2003.

Ein semiautomatischer Ansatz zur Flächenbestimmung von Wirbeln in MRT-Aufnahmen

Jan Egger[1,2,3], Thomas Dukatz[2], Bernd Freisleben[3], Christopher Nimsky[2]

[1]SPL, Dept. of Radiology, BWH, Harvard Medical School, Boston, MA, USA
[2]Klinik für Neurochirurgie, Philipps-Universität Marburg
[3]Fachbereich Mathematik und Informatik, Philipps-Universität Marburg
egger@bwh.harvard.edu

Kurzfassung. Graphbasierte Verfahren verteilen die Knoten des Graphen gleichmäßig und äquidistant auf einem Bild. Hinzugefügt wird ein sog. Smoothness Term, um dem Segmentierungsergebnis eine gewisse Steifigkeit zu verleihen und es so zu beeinflussen. Diese Vorgehensweise erlaubt dem Cut (Trennung von Objekt und Hintergrund) allerdings nicht, eine bestimmte (komplexere) Struktur zu bevorzugen, insbesondere, wenn Bereiche des Objekts nicht vom Hintergrund zu unterscheiden sind. Zur Evaluierung unseres Ansatzes verwendeten wir Magnetresonanztomographie (MRT)-Aufnahmen der Wirbelsäule, um die zeitaufwendige Schicht-für-Schicht-Konturierung der Ärzte zu unterstützen. Die quantitative Auswertung erfolgte mit dem Dice Similarity Coefficient (DSC) und ergab bei einem direkten Vergleich mit manuellen Expertensegmentierungen einen Wert von 90,97±2,2% für neun Wirbel (bei einer Rechenzeit von ca. einer Sekunde).

1 Einleitung

Degenerative Erkrankungen der Wirbelsäule, insbesondere durch Veränderungen der ligamentären und ossären Strukturen, sind weit verbreitet. Die konsekutive Zunahme der Spinalkanalstenose hat vermehrt Einschränkungen der Patienten im Alltag zur Folge. Die demographische Entwicklung führt zu einem höheren Anteil älterer Patienten, die eine operative Maßnahme erfahren [1, 2]. Die bildgebende Diagnostik der spinalen Strukturen spielt für die Entscheidungsfindung der adäquaten Therapie und das Ausmaß der operativen Behandlung eine maßgebliche Rolle. Die MRT-Bildgebung ist für die Evaluation spinaler Erkrankungen besonders geeignet, da spinale Strukturen wie Bandscheibengewebe, Nervenwurzeln und Bandstrukturen ohne Strahlenbelastung in hoher Auflösung dargestellt werden können. Dennoch können bestimmte ossäre Veränderungen der Wirbelsäule besser über eine Computertomographie (CT)-Aufnahme diagnostiziert werden, wie es z.B. bei Osteoporose oder Frakturen im Wirbelsäulenbereich der Fall ist [3]. Mit diesem Beitrag soll die Möglichkeit der MRT-Segmentierung im Hinblick auf die Rekonstruktion der Wirbelkörper demonstriert werden. Dies bedeutet eine reduzierte Anzahl von Untersuchungen vor operativen Eingriffen und Schonung der interdisziplinären Ressourcen bei Vermeidung einer potentiell gefährdenden Strahlenbelastung für den Patienten. In der Literatur finden sich mehrere 2D-Algorithmen für die (semi-)automatische Segmentierung von Wirbeln. Huang et al. [4] nutzten einen normierten Cut-Algorithmus mit Nyström-Approximation und erzielten einen DSC [5] von 93% bis 95% für sechs Patienten. Michopoulou et al. [6] registrierten Bandscheiben mit einem Atlas und erreichten einen DSC zwischen 84% und 92%. Das Verfahren von Shi et al. [7] ist ein top-down-Ansatz, der statistische Mustererkennung für die Rückenmarksextraktion verwendet. Ein manuell definiertes Fenster wird hierbei als Initialisierung für eine Bandscheibenerkennung eingesetzt, die Autoren berichten über eine 96%ige Detektionsrate. Huang et al. [4] und Michopoulou et al. [6] vermeiden aufwendige Rechenoperationen und brauchen für eine Segmentierung wenige Sekunden, der Ansatz von Shi et al. [7] dagegen benötigte ca. 40 Sekunden.

2 Material und Methoden

Das vorgestellte Verfahren lässt sich in zwei Schritte unterteilen: Zuerst wird von einem benutzerdefinierten Saatpunkt aus (der innerhalb des Wirbels liegt) ein gerichteter 2D-Graph aufgebaut. Dann wird der minimale s-t-Schnitt auf diesem Graphen berechnet und damit der Wirbel vom Hintergrund getrennt (Abb. 1). Die Knoten des Graphen werden durch Abtasten von Strahlen gewonnen, die durch die Kontur einer rechteckigen Vorlage verlaufen (Mittelpunkt der Vorlage ist der Saatpunkt). Die abgetasteten Punkte sind die Knoten $n \in V$ vom Graphen $G(V, E)$, und $e \in E$ ist ein Satz von Kanten. Es gibt zwei Arten von Kantentypen: Kanten, die den Graphen mit einer Quelle s und einer Senke t verbinden, und Kanten innerhalb des Graphen. Bei den Kanten innerhalb des Graphen gibt es wiederum mehrere Arten. Die Kanten $< v_i, v_j > \in E$ des Graphen G verbinden immer zwei Knoten v_i, v_j innerhalb des Graphen. Dabei gibt es unter anderem zwei ∞-gewichtete Kanten: z-Kanten A_z und r-Kanten A_r. Dabei ist Z die Anzahl der abgetasteten Punkte entlang eines Strahls $z = (0, \ldots, Z-1)$ und R ist die Anzahl der Strahlen, die durch die Kontur des Rechtecks gesendet

Rechteck   **Graph**   **Wirbel**   **Segmentierungs-ergebnis**

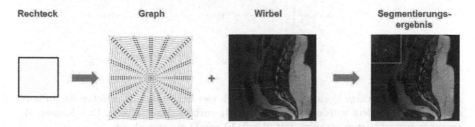

Abb. 1. Prinzipieller Ablauf des Verfahrens: Anhand einer rechteckigen Vorlage wird der Graph konstruiert und an der Position des benutzerdefinierten Saatpunktes im Bild positioniert. Anschließend liefert der s-t-Schnitt die Wirbelkontur bzw. Fläche zurück

werden $r = (0, \ldots, R - 1)$, wobei $V(x_\text{n}, y_\text{n})$ ein Nachbarpunkt von $V(x, y)$ ist (Abb. 2)

$$A_\text{z} = \{\langle V(x, y), V(x, y - 1)\rangle \mid y > 0\} \tag{1}$$

$$A_\text{r} = \{\langle V(x, y), V(x_\text{n}, \max(0, y - \Delta_\text{r}))\rangle\} \tag{2}$$

Die Kanten zwischen zwei Knoten entlang eines Strahls A_z stellen sicher, dass alle Knoten unterhalb einer Kontur im Graphen in einem closed set enthalten sind. Die Kanten A_r zwischen den Knoten der unterschiedlichen Strahlen schränken die Anzahl der möglichen Segmentierungen ein und erzwingen eine Glätte der resultierenden Kontur mit Hilfe eines Parameters Δ_r. Je größer Δ_r ist, desto mehr mögliche Segmentierungen gibt es. Nach der Graphkonstruktion wird das Closed Set des Graphen mit minimalen Kosten anhand eines s-t-Schnittes berechnet [8]. Dieser liefert eine optimale Segmentierung des Wirbels unter dem Einfluss des Parameters Δ_r, der die Steifigkeit der Kontur beeinflusst (Abb. 3). Ein Deltawert von 0 stellt sicher, dass das Segmentierungsergebnis ein Rechteck ist. Die Kosten $w(x, y)$ für die Kanten $v \in V$ zur Quelle und Senke werden folgendermaßen berechnet: Gewichte haben einen Wert von $c(x, y)$, wenn z Null oder maximal ist, ansonsten $c(x, y) - c(x, y - 1)$, wobei $c(x, y)$ der Betrag der Differenz zwischen einem durchschnittlichen Grauwert (GW) des Wirbels und dem GW des Voxels an Position (x, y) ist [9]. Der durchschnittliche GW zur Berechnung der Kosten ist essentiell für die Segmentierung. Basierend auf der Annahme, dass der benutzerdefinierte Saatpunkt innerhalb des Wirbels sitzt, kann der durchschnittliche GW allerdings automatisch bestimmt werden. Dazu wird über eine Region der Dimension d (ca. 1 cm) um den Saatpunkt (s_x, s_y) integriert [10]

$$\int_{-d/2}^{d/2} \int_{-d/2}^{d/2} T(s_\text{x} + x, s_\text{y} + y) \, \text{d}x \, \text{d}y \tag{3}$$

und anschließend durch die Voxelanzahl geteilt (Mittelwert).

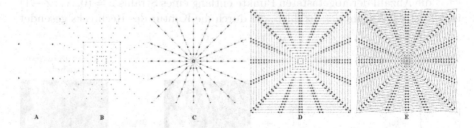

Abb. 2. A: rechteckige Vorlage, definiert durch vier Eckpunkte. B: Knoten die anhand der Vorlage generiert wurden. C: z-Kanten A_z entlang der Strahlen. D: r-Kanten A_r zwischen benachbarten Strahlen mit $\Delta_\text{r}=0$. E: wie D nur mit $\Delta_\text{r}=1$

3   Ergebnisse

Die Realisierung erfolgte mit C++ innerhalb von MeVisLab (www.mevislab.de). Die Graphkonstruktion und die Berechnung eines s-t-Schnitts benötigten in unserer Implementierung ca. eine Sekunde (Intel Intel Core i5-750 CPU, 4x2.66 GHz, 8 GB RAM, Win. XP Prof. x64, 2003, SP 2). Dagegen nahm eine Segmentierung, von Ärzten manuell vorgenommen, ca. eine Minute in Anspruch. Zum Testen des Ansatzes standen vierzehn Datensätze von zwölf Patienten zur Verfügung, wobei nicht für alle Wirbel manuelle Expertensegmentierungen vorhanden waren. Tab. 1 listet detailliert die Evaluationsergebnisse für Segmentierungen von neun Wirbeln auf. Neben dem Volumen in Kubikmillimetern und der Anzahl der Voxel ist der DSC [5] angegeben

$$DSC = \frac{2 \cdot V(A \cap B)}{V(A) + V(R)} \tag{4}$$

wobei A die Binärmaske der automatischen Segmentierung und R die Binärmaske der Referenzsegmentierung ist. V ist das Volumen (in mm^3) der Voxel in einer Binärmaske. Dazu wird die Anzahl der Voxel in einer Binärmaske gezählt und mit der Voxelgröße multipliziert (Abb. 4).

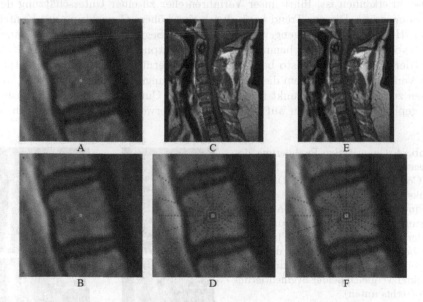

Abb. 3. Schritt-für-Schritt-Konstruktion eines Graphen und anschließende Segmentierung eines Wirbels. A: Saatpunkt (weiß) und die Ecken einer Vorlage (pink). B: Schnittpunkte der ausgesandten Strahlen mit der Vorlage (grün). C und D: abgetastete Knoten für den Graphen (blau). E und F: Segmentierungsergebnis (rot)

Tabelle 1. Evaluationsergebnisse: min., max., Mittelwert μ und Standardabw. σ

	Volumen in mm^3		Anzahl der Voxel		DSC (%)
	manuell	automatisch	manuell	automatisch	
min.	247,803	242,92	1015	995	87,37
max.	510,498	490,723	2091	2010	94,93
$\mu \pm \sigma$	420,41±72,22	404,30±72,98	1722	1656	90,97±2,2

4 Diskussion

In diesem Beitrag wurde ein graphbasierter Segmentierungsalgorithmus für Wirbel vorgestellt. Das Verfahren nutzt eine rechteckige Vorlage, um den Graphen aufzubauen. Bei dieser Vorgehensweise bevorzugt ein s-t-Schnitt eine rechteckige Struktur. Unseres Wissens nach ist dies das erste Mal, dass bei einem graphbasierten Verfahren die Knoten des Graphen nicht gleichmäßig und äquidistant auf einem Bild verteilt wurden, sondern anhand einer rechteckigen Vorlage. Der präsentierte Ansatz kann auch zur Segmentierung anderer rechteckiger Objekte genutzt werden und eignet sich besonders, wenn Bereiche des Objekts nicht vom Hintergrund zu unterscheiden sind (Abb. 5). Wie anhand der Evaluationsergebnisse zu erkennen ist, führt unser Verfahren eher zu einer Unterschätzung der Regionengröße. Diesem Trend kann durch eine höhere Gewichtung der Kanten zum "Hintergrund" entgegengewirkt werden. Das Segmentierungsergebnis hängt auch von der Position des benutzerdefinierten Saatpunktes ab. Allgemein gilt: je zentrierter im Objekt, desto besser die Segmentierung. Evtl. ist ein mehrstufiges Verfahren besser, indem das erste Segmentierungsergebnis genutzt wird, um einen zentrierteren Saatpunkt für einen weiteren Cut zu erhalten. Als nächstes ist geplant, das Verfahren auf einen Kubus zu erweitern, um Wirbel auch in

Abb. 4. Quantitative Evaluierung des Ansatzes anhand des Dice Similarity Coefficients (DSC): MRT-Datensatz (links oben), Fläche eines Wirbels (grün), die aus der manuellen Konturierung von einem Neurochirurgen generiert wurde (rechts oben), Fläche des Wirbels (rot), berechnet mit dem vorgestellten Verfahren (links unten), und direkter Vergleich beider Segmentierungen (rechts unten)

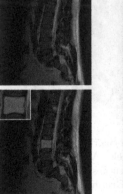
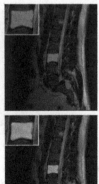

Abb. 5. Das vorgestellte Verfahren kann auch zur Segmentierung anderer rechteckiger Objekte genutzt werden, die subjektive Konturen aufweisen: zu segmentierendes Objekt (schwarz), wobei nicht nur eine gerade Kante, sondern auch eine Ecke fehlt (links), benutzerdefinierter Saatpunkt (blau) innerhalb des Objektes (Mitte) und Segmentierungsergebnis (rot), bei dem die fehlende Ecke rechts unten rekonstruiert wurde (rechts)

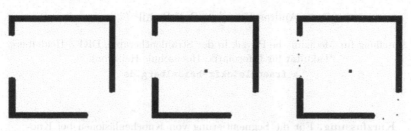

3D zu segmentieren. Dieser Ansatz soll anschließend aktuellen 3D-Verfahren zur Wirbelsegmentierung gegenübergestellt werden.

Literaturverzeichnis

1. Joaquim AF, et al. Degenerative lumbar stenosis: update. Arq Neuropsiquiatr. 2009;67(2):553–8.
2. Hicks GE, et al. Degenerative lumbar disc and facet disease in older adults: prevalence and clinical correlates. Spine (Phila Pa 1976). 2009;34(12):1301–6.
3. Richards PJ, et al. Spine computed tomography doses and cancer induction. Spine (Phila Pa 1976). 2010;35(4):430–3.
4. Huang SH, et al. Learning-based vertebra detection and iterative normalized-cut segmentation for spinal MRI. IEEE Trans Med Imaging. 2009;28(10):1595–605.
5. Zou KH, et al. Statistical validation of image segmentation quality based on a spatial overlap index. Sci Rep Acad Radiol. 2004;11(2):178–89.
6. Michopoulou SK, et al. Atlas-based segmentation of degenerated lumbar intervertebral discs from MR images of the spine. Trans Biomed Eng. 2009;56(9):2225–31.
7. Shi R, et al. An efficient method for segmentation of MRI spine images. IEEE ICME. 2007; p. 713–7.
8. Boykov Y, et al. An experimental comparison of min-cut/max-flow algorithms for energy minimization in vision. IEEE Trans Pattern Anal Mach Intell. 2004;26(9):1124–37.
9. Egger J, et al. Graph-based tracking method for aortic thrombus segmentation. Proc 4th Euro Congr MBEC, Engineering for Health. 2008; p. 584–7.
10. Egger J, et al. Nugget-Cut: a segmentation scheme for spherically- and elliptically-shaped 3D objects. Proc DAGM. 2010; p. 383–92.

Automatische Segmentierung und Klassifizierung von Knochenmarkhöhlen für die Positionierung von Formmodellen

Andrea Fränzle[1], Rolf Bendl[1,2]

[1]Abteilung für Medizinische Physik in der Strahlentherapie, DKFZ Heidelberg
[2]Fakultät für Informatik, Hochschule Heilbronn
a.fraenzle@dkfz-heidelberg.de

Kurzfassung. Für die Segmentierung von Knochenläsionen bei Knochenmetastasen und Multiplem Myelom sollen automatische Verfahren entwickelt werden. Als Teilschritt ist die Segmentierung der einzelnen Knochenstrukturen notwendig. Formmodelle erscheinen hier erfolgversprechend, da diese bereits Informationen über die Gestalt des Knochens beinhalten. Um diese Modelle automatisch im Bild zu positionieren, sollen die Knochenmarkhöhlen verwendet werden. Diese sind in Lage und Orientierung den Knochen selbst ähnlich und lassen sich leicht abtrennen. Durch Zuordnen der Markhöhlen zu den entsprechenden Knochen mit Hilfe von Mustererkennung kann das richtige Formmodell ausgewählt und positioniert werden. Anwenden lässt sich das Verfahren auf Röhrenknochen.

1 Einleitung

Die quantitative Analyse von Knochenläsionen, wie sie beispielsweise bei Knochenmetastasen oder beim Multiplen Myelom auftreten, ist eine sehr komplexe Aufgabe und ohne automatisierte Segmentierung der Läsionen kaum zu bewältigen. Im Falle des Multiplen Myeloms ist derzeit eine quantitative Angabe der gesamten Tumormasse aufgrund des in der Regel systemischen Befalls des gesamten Skelettes nicht möglich. Dafür wird eine exakte Segmentierung der Läsionen benötigt, die allerdings nicht manuell bewerkstelligt werden kann. Daher sollen Verfahren entwickelt werden, die diese Läsionen automatisch in 3-dimensionalen Schichtaufnahmen des Körpers detektieren und segmentieren. Dies soll durch einen Vergleich der veränderten Knochenstruktur mit einem gesunden Modell geschehen. Dafür ist zunächst eine Abgrenzung einzelner Knochen notwendig. In der Literatur finden sich vor allem interaktive Ansätze [1] oder atlasbasierte Verfahren, die auf bestimmte Körperregionen begrenzt entwickelt wurden,z.B. bei [2, 3, 4]. Aufgrund der großen Bilddatenmenge bei Ganzkörper-Aufnahmen beim Multiplen Myelom soll jedoch hier soweit wie möglich Benutzerinteraktion vermieden werden und ein Verfahren entwickelt werden, das auch auf Ganzkörper-Tomographien anwendbar ist. Für die Segmentierung der Knochen hier sollen statistische Formmodelle verwendet werden. Eine Übersicht über statistische Formmodelle findet man bei [5]. Damit diese ein zuverlässiges Segmentierungsergebnis liefern, müssen die Modelle initial in der Nähe der entsprechenden Knochenstruktur positioniert werden. Um eine vollständig automatisierte Lösung für die Detektion von Knochenläsionen zu erhalten, soll diese initiale Position automatisch gefunden werden. In diesem Beitrag wird ein Verfahren vorgestellt, das die Knochenmarkhöhlen in 3D-Low-Dose-Ganzkörper-CTs automatisch segmentiert und klassifiziert, so dass anschließend das richtige Formmodell für die Knochenstruktur ausgewählt und positioniert werden kann.

2 Material und Methoden

Während die Segmentierung des gesamten Skelettes in CT-Aufnahmen mit einem einfachen Schwellwertverfahren möglich ist, ist die Abgrenzung einzelner Knochenstrukturen komplexer. Hier ist der Kontrast zwischen benachbarten knöchernen Strukturen entweder zu gering oder die Struktur der Knochen ist zu komplex, um Bildregionen mit Hilfe von Region-Growing-Verfahren oder Kantendetektionsalgorithmen einem bestimmten Knochen zuordnen zu können. Erfolgversprechend scheint hier der Einsatz von Formmodellen zu sein, da diese bereits die Gestalt eines Knochens abbilden. Um ein zuverlässiges Segmentierungsergebnis zu erhalten, sind diese Modelle in der Nähe der entsprechenden Knochen zu positionieren. Als Anhaltspunkt für die Lage einer bestimmten Knochenstruktur sollen die Knochenmarkhöhlen verwendet werden, die sich im Gegensatz zu den Knochen eindeutig trennen lassen (Abb. 1) und ähnliche Eigenschaften hinsichtlich Position und Orientierung aufweisen.

2.1 Datenmaterial

Der vorgestellte Algorithmus zur Segmentierung der Markhöhlen und der Zuordnung der gefundenen Markhöhlen zu der zugehörigen Knochenstruktur wurde an 14 Low-Dose-Ganzkörper-CTs von Patienten mit Multiplem Myelom getestet. Die Übereinstimmung von Lage und Position von Knochen und ihrer Markhöhle beim Menschen wurde exemplarisch an einem Patienten gezeigt.

2.2 Segmentierung der Knochenmarkhöhlen

Die Segmentierung der Knochenmarkhöhlen wird durch folgende Bildverarbeitungsschritte erreicht:

1. Binarisierung des Bildes mit einem Schwellwert, um die knöchernen Strukturen vom Hintergrund zu trennen

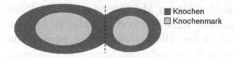

☐ Knochen
☐ Knochenmark

Abb. 1. Abgrenzung der Markhöhlen. Während die Knochen (dunkel) sich nicht eindeutig trennen lassen, sind die Markhöhlen (hell) eindeutig abgetrennt

2. Entfernen aller Objekte im Bild, deren Größe 1000 Voxel unterschreitet
3. 3d-Closing um kleinere Lücken zu schließen
4. Füllen der Höhlen innerhalb der Knochen mit Flood-Fill-Algorithmus
5. Differenzbild aus gefülltem und nicht gefülltem Knochenbild liefert Knochen-markhöhlen
6. Entfernen aller Objekte im Bild, deren Größe 500 Voxel unterschreitet
7. Markieren der einzelnen Knochenmarkhöhlen mit Connected Component Labeling

2.3 Klassifikation der segmentierten Markhöhlen

Um das richtige Formmodell für jeden Knochen auswählen zu können, ist es notwendig, die gefundenen Markhöhlen den entsprechenden Knochenstrukturen zuzuordnen. Hierzu wird Mustererkennung eingesetzt. Folgende Merkmale der Markhöhlenobjekte werden verwendet:

- Volumen
- Abstand des Schwerpunktes zur Medianebene des Körpers
- Abstand des Schwerpunktes zur mittleren Koronalebene des Körpers
- Relative Position des Schwerpunktes im Bilddatensatz in kranial-kaudaler Richtung

Die Markhöhlen werden anhand der genannten Merkmale mit einem Random-Forest-Klassifikator klassifiziert. Ein Random-Forest-Klassifikator ist eine Zusammenfassung von einzelnen Entscheidungsbäumen, die jeweils mit einer unterschiedlichen Stichprobe aus der ursprünglichen Trainingsmenge erstellt wurden. Ein neues Objekt wird zunächst von allen Entscheidungsbäumen klassifiziert. Die endgültige Klasse ist die am häufigsten von den Bäumen gelieferte Klasse. Details zur Klassifikation mit Random Forests beschreibt [6]. Um die Güte des Klassifikationsverfahrens zu beschreiben, wurde die Fehlerrate nach der Leave-one-out-Methode bestimmt. Dazu wurden in drei Durchgängen mit unterschiedlicher Anzahl von Bäumen (10, 25 und 100) je 14 Random-Forests auf Markhöhlen von jeweils 13 Ganzkörper-CTs trainiert und mit dem jeweils übrigem Patientendatensatz getestet. Die Fehlerrate wird dabei folgendermaßen bestimmt

$$\text{Fehlerrate} = \frac{\text{Anzahl falsch klassifizierter Elemente}}{\text{Stichprobenumfang}} \quad (1)$$

3 Ergebnisse

3.1 Lage und Position von Markhöhle und Knochen

Exemplarisch wurden an einem menschlichen Skelett der Abstand der Schwerpunkte von Knochen und automatisch segmentierter Markhöhle sowie der Winkel zwischen der erste Hauptkomponente von Knochen und Markhöhle bei den Röhrenknochen bestimmt. Im Mittel beträgt der Abstand der Schwerpunkte von Knochen und Markhöhle 21,68mm bei einer Standardabweichung von 15,37mm.

Tabelle 1. Fehlerraten der Markhöhlenklassifikation in Röhrenknochen

Klasse	10 Bäume	25 Bäume	100 Bäume
Femur links	0,21	0,14	0,07
Femur rechts	0,13	0,13	0,13
Tibia links	0,27	0,13	0,27
Tibia rechts	0,29	0,21	0,14
Fibula links	0,21	0,07	0,14
Fibula rechts	0,40	0,27	0,27
Humerus links	0,07	0,00	0,00
Humerus rechts	0,13	0,20	0,13
Radius links	0,50	0,50	0,33
Radius rechts	0,57	0,57	0,29
Ulna links	0,45	0,45	0,45
Ulna rechts	0,69	0,62	0,62
Sonstige	0,03	0,01	0,01

Die Position variiert hier entlang des Knochens. Der durchschnittliche Winkel zwischen der erste Hauptkomponente der Röhrenknochen und ihrer Markhöhle beträgt $1{,}54°$ bei einer Standardabweichung von $0{,}94°$. Die Orientierung des Knochens lässt sich also recht gut anhand der Markhöhle ermitteln. Somit lässt sich eine ungefähre Position und Lage des eigentlichen Knochens bestimmen und ein Formmodell initialisieren. Abb. 2 zeigt automatisch segmentierte Markhöhlen innerhalb von Arm- und Unterschenkelknochen. Hier ist zu erkennen, dass sich ausgehend von der Markhöhle gut auf die Lage des Knochens schließen lässt.

3.2 Klassifikation der Markhöhlen

Die Klassifikation der Markhöhlen wurde anhand der Klassen „Femur links" „Femur rechts" „Tibia links" „Tibia rechts" „Fibula links" „Fibula rechts" „Humerus links" „Humerus rechts" „Radius links" „Radius rechts" „Ulna links" „Ulna rechts" und „sonstige" durchgeführt. Unter „sonstige" werden Objekte zusammengefasst, die ebenfalls automatisch segmentiert wurden, sich aber keinem Röhrenknochen zuordnen lassen. Tab. 1 zeigt die Fehlerraten für die einzelnen Klassen für drei Durchgänge mit unterschiedlicher Baumanzahl. Generell am zuverlässigsten werden die großen Röhrenknochen Femur und Humerus erkannt, die Unterarmknochen Radius und Ulna werden nur unzureichend erkannt. Die Fehlerrate über alle Objekte beträgt für Random Forests mit 10 Bäumen 0,14, mit 25 Bäumen 0,11 und mit 100 Bäumen 0,09. Hier führt eine größere Baumanzahl zwar zu geringeren Fehlerraten insgesamt, das gilt jedoch nicht für alle Knochenklassen gleichermaßen, in den Klassen Radius und Ulna wird durch Erhöhung der Baumanzahl keine Verbesserung erreicht.

284   Fränzle & Bendl

4 Diskussion

Es wurde gezeigt, dass es prinzipiell möglich ist, zur Initialisierung von Formmodellen für die Knochensegmentierung eine Segmentierung der Knochenmark-

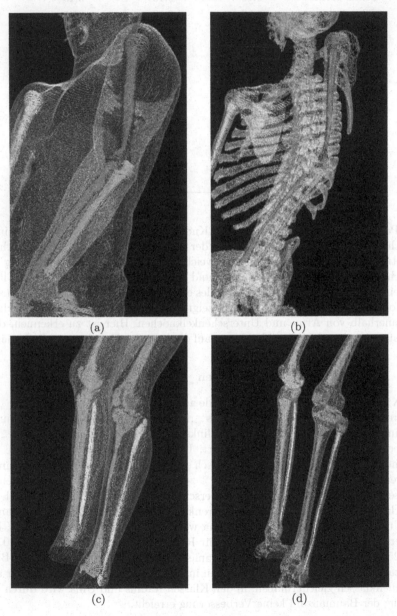

Abb. 2. Knochen und automatisch segmentierte Markhöhlen. (a) Armknochen innerhalb der Anatomie (b) Markhöhlen in den Armknochen (c) Unterschenkelknochen innerhalb der Anatomie (d) Markhöhlen in den Unterschenkelknochen

höhlen zu verwenden. Diese lassen sich bei den Röhrenknochen einfach segmentieren und weisen ähnliche Eigenschaften hinsichtlich Position und Orientierung wie die eigentliche Knochenstruktur auf. Ist eine Knochenmarkhöhle gefunden und identifiziert, kann anhand des Schwerpunktes und der 1. Hauptkomponente, die mit Principal Component Analysis ermittelt werden kann, ein Formmodell ausgewählt und automatisch positioniert werden.

Mit Mustererkennung können zumindest die großen Röhrenknochen Femur und Humerus, sowie die Unterschenkelknochen Tibia und Fibula erkannt werden, so dass hier ein entsprechendes Formmodell automatisch ausgewählt werden kann. Um die Unterarmknochen Radius und Ulna zu erkennen, ist es möglicherweise ausreichend, die Position des Humerus zu kennen und ausgehend davon auf die Position von Radius und Ulna zu schließen. Getestet wurde an 14 Low-Dose-Ganzkörper-CTs, die Random Forests wurden jeweils mit 13 Patientendaten trainiert. Es wurden drei Durchgänge mit unterschiedlicher Baumanzahl durchgeführt. In einigen Klassen wird durch die Verwendung einer größeren Anzahl von Bäumen eine Verbesserung erreicht, eine allgemeine Tendenz kann jedoch nicht klar erkannt werden. Um aussagekräftige Ergebnisse zu erzielen, ist der Stichprobenumfang von 14 Patienten vermutlich nicht ausreichend und ist für den Einsatz für ein vollautomatisches Segmentierungsverfahren zu erhöhen. Des weiteren ist zu testen, ob andere Klassifikatoren zuverlässigere Klassifikationsergebnisse, d.h. geringere Fehlerraten, liefern.

Bei Wirbelkörpern ist es schwierig, das Knocheninnere abzutrennen, da sich die Deckplatten der Wirbelkörper unter anderem auf Grund von Partialvolumeneffekten und des relativ geringen Kontrastes bei Low-Dose-CTs nicht stark genug vom restlichen Wirbelkörper und der Bandscheibe unterscheiden. Um das Modell auf die Wirbelkörper zu erweitern, sind Anpassungen nötig, um die Markhöhlen dort zuverlässig zu erkennen, wenn dort auf die gleiche Art und Weise Formmodelle initialisiert werden sollen.

Literaturverzeichnis

1. Liu L, Raber D, Nopachai D, et al. Interactive separation of segmented bones in CT volumes using graph cut. Med Image Comput Comput Assist Interv. 2008;11(1):296–304.
2. Ehrhardt J, Handels H, Malina T, et al. Atlas-based segmentation of bone structures to support the virtual planning of hip operations. Int J Med Inform. 2001;64(2-3):439–47.
3. Haas B, Coradi T, Scholz M, et al. Automatic segmentation of thoracic and pelvic CT images for radiotherapy planning using implicit anatomic knowledge and organ-specific segmentation strategies. Phys Med Biol. 2008;53(6):1751–71.
4. Wu C, Murtha PE, Jaramaz B. Construction of statistical shape atlases for bone structures based on a two-level framework. Int J Med Robot. 2010;6(1):1–17.
5. Heimann T, Meinzer HP. Statistical shape models for 3D medical image segmentation: a review. Med Image Anal. 2009;13(4):543–63.
6. Breiman L. Random Forests. Mach Learn. 2001;45(1):5–32.

Anisotropic Diffusion for Direct Haptic Volume Rendering in Lumbar Puncture Simulation

Andre Mastmeyer[1], Dirk Fortmeier[1,2], Heinz Handels[1]

[1]Institute of Medical Informatics, University of Lübeck
[2]Graduate School for Computing in Medicine and Life Sciences, University of Lübeck
mastmeyer@imi.uni-luebeck.de

Abstract. The segmentation of patient data often is mandatory for surgical simulations to enable realistic visual and haptic rendering. The necessary preparation time lies in the range from several hours to days. Here we augment a direct haptic volume rendering approach for lumbar punctures by edge-preserving smoothing preprocessing. Evaluation is carried out on user defined paths. Compared to our reference system force output can be improved over non-preprocessed image data.

1 Introduction

Surgical simulators help surgeons to develop and refine skills in a risk-free environment. They are applied in preoperative planning, anatomic education and training of surgical procedures. The goal is to achieve real-time performance for volume visualization, elastic tissue deformation and haptic feedback. The preparation phase mainly consists of the segmentation of patient data which is a major bottleneck and takes time within a range of several hours to days.

In [1] a comprehensive survey about "needle insertion" is given. The simulations carried out must mimic stiffness, cutting and friction force at the needle tip and shaft. Tissue deformation and needle bending in real-time are major challenges.

Previously [2, 3] has presented AcusVR as a system for the simulation of needle punctures which achieves highly realistic visual and haptic rendering using a Sensable Phantom 6DOF HF (Fig. 1) and the segmentation of all relevant structures. This system proves to be a valuable tool for the training of medical students.

However, expert segmentation of patient image data consumes up to 40 hours of work time per patient. Therefore in [4] we propose a direct haptic volume rendering with partially segmented data. Statistically determined gray value intervals with haptic transfer functions and the segmentation of some structures are combined to perform force calculation without the need of a complete segmentation.

Here we support the latter setup by preprocessing the patient image data by median and anisotropic diffusion filtering and evaluate the improvement on several manually defined puncture paths.

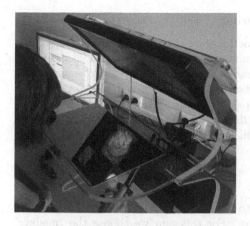

Fig. 1. Haptic device and workbench

The paper is organized as follows: First, the used data set is described. Force calculation is briefly repeated as presented in [4] and [5]. Then we describe the image preprocessing algorithms, the output of which replaces the original gray value data. Evaluation is done quantitatively by comparing force output from the reference system AcusVR and the new approach.

2 Methods

We use a standard abdominal CT patient data set with isotropic voxel size 1.0 mm and 240 slices (Fig. 3(a)). In the complete virtual patient bone, ligaments, spinal canal, inter-vertebral disks, fat, muscle, skin and liver are manually segmented by experts and used for haptic rendering [2, 3]. The AcusVR system described there is the reference we compare our new algorithms to. In contrast, the new system [4] only uses a subset of the segmentations.

Briefly summarizing [5, 4], in proxy based haptic rendering the device tip x_t is connected via a virtual spring with stiffness parameter k to a proxy x_p. According to Hooke's law the force output is determined depending on the proxy position and stiffness (Fig. 2).

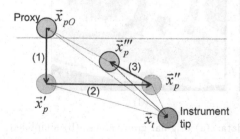

Fig. 2. Proxy-based haptic rendering. First the proxy position x_p' for the surface penetrability along the normal vector of a virtual surface is determined. Then the position x_p'' tangentially to the surface is calculated. Finally, a viscosity term retracts the proxy to the position x_p''' which is used to calculate the virtual spring force at the instrument tip x_t

2.1 Direct haptic volume rendering

In the new approach [4], transfer functions are used to obtain the haptic parameters used in the three calculation steps. A color-coded axial slice is given below to show the adequacy of the transfer function's intervals to separate tissues (axial slice in Fig. 3(b)). As can be seen the separation of skin (orange), fat (yellow), muscle (red) and bone (white) is plausible. However, the spinal canal and inter-vertebral disk as well as the flavum ligaments are often misclassified as muscle. These important parts are still present as segmentations in the reduced segmentation set.

2.2 Edge-preserving smoothing

In our application it is mandatory to preserve the edges of the image while smoothing more homogeneous regions. For this aim we choose the "median" with radius parameter r and "anisotropic diffusion" filter algorithms.

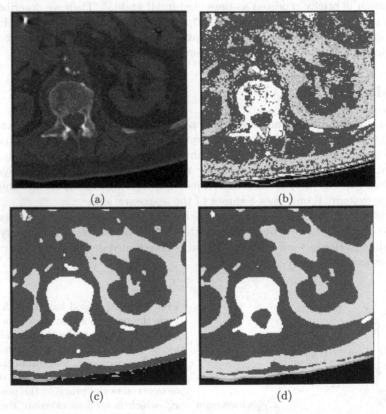

Fig. 3. An axial slice of the reference data: (a) original gray values, (b) simplified visual transfer function applied, (c) result using best anisotropic diffusion filter, (d) result using best median filter

Anisotropic diffusion has been described in the literature extensively. In the framework proposed by [6] a non-linear PDE is iteratively solved

$$\frac{\partial I}{\partial t} = \nabla \cdot c\left(\|\nabla I\|\right) \cdot \nabla I \tag{1}$$

This equation reduces to the isotropic heat diffusion if $c\left(\|\nabla I\|\right)$ is chosen constant. Now to preserve edges reliably while denoising the image data I, we use the sigmoidal and monotonically decreasing "conductance term" c

$$c\left(\|\nabla I\|\right) = e^{-\left(\frac{\|\nabla I\|}{K}\right)^2} \tag{2}$$

as a local-adaptive weight. It contains the conductance parameter K controlling the sensitivity of the diffusion process to edge contrast. Large gradient magnitude image parts $\|\nabla I\|$ (edges) result in lower smoothing, whereas homogeneous image regions with $\|\nabla I\| \simeq 0$ are smoothed comparably to isotropic diffusion.

Numerically, the time step parameter t together with number of iterations n are important and determine the length and stability of the diffusion process. They have a similar effect as σ in Gaussian smoothing.

In summary, the combined heuristic approach from [4] is further refined. Partially segmented patient data and haptic transfer functions are combined with preprocessed patient image data. This minimizes the effect of isolated falsely classified voxels that occur spuriously distributed over the image.

2.3   Evaluation

For the automatic quantitative evaluation we implement a path steering along twelve predefined vectors ("reference paths"). From a start point the virtual needle is penetrating the body along the line towards the end point assuming a constant velocity. The needle then is retracted to the start position again (Fig. 4(a)). This way we are able to obtain reproducible results for comparing different haptic force calculation algorithms.

Puncture simulations with 140 parameter settings for anisotropic diffusion are compared:

- Number of iterations: $n = 3,\ 5,\ 8,\ 25,\ 50,\ 75,\ 100$
- Time step: $t = 0.0550,\ 0.0575,\ 0.0600,\ 0.0625\ [s]$
- Conductance parameter: $K = 1,\ 2,\ 3,\ 4,\ 5$

On the other hand, the median filter at different kernel radii r from 1 to 10 mm is used.

We evaluate the direct haptic volume rendering with 12 paths (Fig. 4(a)) that reflect trainee experience with the system. The valid paths $v_{1,0}$ to $v_{2,4}$ reach the spinal canal target (10 paths) respectively collide with bony risk structures in case of b_0 and b_1 (2 paths).

Along a reference path at a needle position the force output is calculated twice: (1) by the algorithm used in AcusVR and (2) the new method respectively.

As measures to compare the paired force output values the sum of squared differences (SSD) and maximum absolute error (MAE) and p-value from paired t-tests are used.

3   Results

In Table 1 the errors for the force ouputs along the reference paths are shown for three types of input data.

In three cases the paths show significantly different force feedback from the reference system AcusVR (Fig. 4(b)), two of which can be attributed to our new method's higher force output for bone.

One-way ANOVA comparing the force feedback errors from the three algorithms shows no statistical differences ($p < 0.72$). Comparing the error sums, there is a tendency to choose the anisotropic diffusion. Superiorly, it preserves the important risk structure of the ribs which can be clearly seen comparing Fig. 3(c) and Fig. 3(d).

4   Discussion

In [4] we present a new approach that considerably reduces the segmentation preparation workload from days to hours. Additionally, in this paper edge-preserving smoothing is shown to be a valuable tool to further improve direct haptic rendering. Resistance of important structures such as bone and ligaments is clearly reproduced by the simulation. The errors for the valid paths are very small, consequently for the field of lumbar puncture simulation our enhanced transfer function approach yields very good results. For the bone paths higher

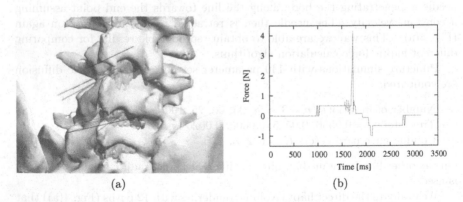

(a)   (b)

Fig. 4. Reference paths. (a) Valid paths (green) and invalid paths with bone contact (red). (b) Force curves for valid path $v_{2,1}$ using best anisotropic diffusion: AcusVR calculated force (green) vs. new algorithm (red): The force outputs for the valid paths are overall very similar, but clothing near the body surface which is not included in the full-segmentation based approach, leads to significant differences

Table 1. Comparison of force output values calculated by AcusVR to new algorithm using original and preprocessed data. Asterisks indicate significantly different force feedback

Path	Original Data (unpreprocessed)			Best Diffusion Data ($n = 25$, $t = 0.06$, $K = 4$)			Best Median Data ($r = 4$)		
	SSD [N²]	MAE [N]	p<	SSD	MAE	p<	SSD	MAE	p<
b_0	47.7555	2.5328	0.0668	24.2742	1.4063	0.8454	32.7637	2.6459	0.0014*
b_1	26.1108	2.7748	0.1139	17.5851	2.6036	0.0003*	25.8936	2.7320	0.1022
$v_{1,0}$	6.2548	1.8078	0.8012	5.2065	1.6295	0.7435	4.1973	1.1672	0.9421
$v_{1,1}$	3.8126	1.0552	0.8168	3.0034	0.5669	0.8574	2.1612	0.7746	0.4747
$v_{1,2}$	9.4194	1.4549	0.1951	3.5786	0.7587	0.5396	4.5091	0.7587	0.7891
$v_{1,3}$	2.4296	0.7030	0.6219	1.7169	0.7030	0.5493	1.7746	0.7006	0.8250
$v_{1,4}$	2.0289	0.5785	0.2394	1.0291	0.5785	0.2313	2.3452	0.7977	0.2850
$v_{2,0}$	2.8679	1.1038	0.3549	1.2756	0.5407	0.5718	4.7546	1.2975	0.2204
$v_{2,1}$	2.3950	0.5	0.1261	1.7104	0.5000	0.0326*	1.2371	0.5	0.4275
$v_{2,2}$	2.9520	0.6337	0.0806	2.9396	0.6817	0.7643	2.0454	0.6337	0.1040
$v_{2,3}$	3.2452	0.5494	0.7070	2.9201	0.5494	0.5200	3.2553	0.5494	0.6040
$v_{2,4}$	1.7968	0.66484	0.1920	2.3572	0.6805	0.8542	1.6131	0.6727	0.4694
Sum	111.0685	14.3588	N/A	67.5967	11.1988	N/A	86.5503	13.2301	N/A

errors occur which can be attributed to a different force rendering for bone structures([4]). An interesting outlook of the presented concepts would be to use more sophisticated transfer functions to cope with inner organs which are classified incorrectly in the current set up.

Acknowledgement. This work is supported by the German Research Foundation (DFG, HA 2355/10-1).

References

1. Abolhassani N, Patel R, Moallem M. Needle insertion into soft tissue: a survey. Med Eng Phys. 2007;29(4):413–31.
2. Färber M, Hoeborn E, Dalek D, et al. Training and evaluation of lumbar punctures in a VR-environment using a 6DOF haptic device. Stud Health Technol Inform. 2008;132:112–4.
3. Färber M, Hummel F, Gerloff C, et al. Virtual reality simulator for the training of lumbar punctures. Methods Inform Med. 2009;48(5):493–501.
4. Mastmeyer A, Fortmeier D, Handels H. Direct Haptic Volume Rendering in Lumbar Puncture Simulation. In: Medicine Meets Virtual Reality 19; 2012.
5. Lundin K, Ynnerman A, Gudmundsson B. Proxy-based haptic feedback from volumetric density data. Eurohaptics Conference. 2002; p. 104–9.
6. Perona P, Malik J. Scale-space and edge detection using anisotropic diffusion. IEEE Trans Pattern Anal Mach Intell. 1990;12:629–39.

Quality-Guided Denoising for Low-Cost Fundus Imaging

Thomas Köhler[1,2], Joachim Hornegger[1,2], Markus Mayer[1,2],
Georg Michelson[2,3]

[1]Pattern Recognition Lab, University Erlangen-Nuremberg, Germany
[2]Erlangen Graduate School in Advanced Optical Technologies, SAOT, Germany
[3]Department of Ophthalmology, University Erlangen-Nuremberg, Germany
Thomas.Koehler@informatik.uni-erlangen.de

Abstract. The restoration of noisy images is an essential pre-processing step in many medical applications to ensure sufficient quality for diagnoses. In this paper we present a new quality-guided approach for denoising of eye fundus images that suffer from high noise levels. The denoising is based on image sequences and an adaptive frame averaging approach. The novelty of the method is that it takes an objective image quality criteria to assess the different frames and tries to maximize the quality of the resulting image. It can be implemented in an incremental manner which allows real-time denoising. We evaluated our approach on real image sequences captured by a low-cost fundus camera and obtained competitive results to a state-of-the-art method in terms of signal-to-noise ratio whereas our method performs denoising about four times faster.

1 Introduction

Fundus imaging provides high-resolution photographs with good signal-to-noise ratio (SNR) of the human eye fundus. It is a common modality used by ophthalmologists to diagnose eye diseases. In contrast to high-end cameras, a low-cost fundus device is a mobile solution which suffers from high noise levels in the captured images. Denoising is an essential pre-processing step to analyze such images and to recognize structures like blood vessels. In this work we focus on temporal filtering based on image sequences to acquire a denoised image.

Most approaches for temporal filtering are based on frame averaging [1] where an average image of a sequence of frames showing the same scene is calculated. The average image is an estimation for the ideal image of this scene. A common goal is to make this average more robust and adaptive to the frames of the sequence [2, 3]. One potential error source is imperfect alignment of the frames which causes blur in the denoised image. An adaptive approach proposed by Dudek et al. [4] uses optical flow to compensate motion and errors in the motion field are detected to avoid blur in the result image. However, optical flow is sensitive to varying illumination which is a main limitation for fundus images. Multiframe wavelet denoising as described by Borsdorf et al. [5] and Mayer et al. [6] are robust denoising methods. Here noise is identified by analyzing wavelet coefficients and deriving different kind of weights e. g. by correlation analysis. A good SNR gain can be achieved, but this approach has a higher asymptotic run time of $O(n^2)$ for n images. We propose a frame averaging method due to its simplicity and low computational effort. This makes it suitable for a real-time application in a low-cost fundus camera system.

2   Materials and methods

2.1   Adaptive and incremental frame averaging

The proposed denoising method works in an incremental manner and consists of two stages (Fig. 1). First, a new frame is aligned with the denoised image estimated in the previous time step. Afterwards, an adaptive average between both frames is calculated. This average takes the relative quality of the two images into account and avoids motion blur caused by inaccurate registration.

Frame averaging Let $\mathbf{Y}^{(1)}\ldots\mathbf{Y}^{(n)} \in \mathbb{R}^{M \times N}$ be a sequence of n images of dimension $M \times N$ which show the same content. Frame averaging calculates a denoised image $\mathbf{X}^{(n)} \in \mathbb{R}^{M \times N}$ according to

$$x_{ij}^{(n)} = \sum_{k=0}^{n} v_{ij}^{(k)} y_{ij}^{(k)} \qquad (1)$$

with adaptive weights $v_{ij}^{(k)}$ for each pixel (i,j) in each frame $\mathbf{Y}^{(k)}$. For $v_{ij}^{(k)} = 1/n$ and additive white Gaussian noise this provides an unbiased estimate for the ideal image. Motion during image acquisition must be compensated using image registration to avoid motion blur. It is well known that the average is sensitive to outliers, e. g. due to varying and inhomogeneous illumination. One possible

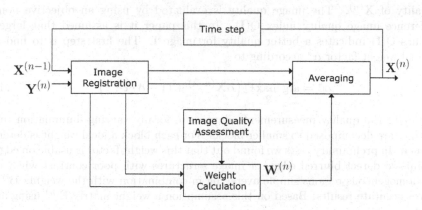

Fig. 1. The flowchart of the proposed denosing algorithm for $n > 1$

solution is the application of robust estimators like median or RANSAC [7]. Unfortunately, these approaches have higher computational effort. Instead we modify equation 1 and provide an incremental solution for image denoising.

Incremental frame averaging A recursive formulation of frame averaging with adaptive weights $w_{ij}^{(n)}$ for each pixel (i, j) is given by

$$x_{ij}^{(n)} = w_{ij}^{(n)} x_{ij}^{(n-1)} + \left(1 - w_{ij}^{(n)}\right) y_{ij}^{(n)} \tag{2}$$

A new frame $\mathbf{Y}^{(n)}$ at the current time step n refines the previous estimation $\mathbf{X}^{(n-1)}$ based on the frames 1 to $n-1$ to the new estimation $\mathbf{X}^{(n)}$. The weight factors $w_{ij}^{(n)}$ are adjusted such that $\mathbf{X}^{(n)}$ is a usable estimation in terms of an objective quality criteria and outliers are suppressed. This allows an incremental refinement of the denoised image over time as shown in Fig. 1.

Weight matrix calculation The weight matrix $\mathbf{W}^{(n)} \in \mathbb{R}^{M \times N}$ in equation 2 is composed as a multiplication $w_{ij}^{(n)} = b_{ij}^{(n)} e_{ij}^{(n)}$. First, we use temporal weights for corresponding pixels of $\mathbf{X}^{(n-1)}$ and $\mathbf{Y}^{(n)}$ to suppress outliers in homogeneous regions or blurring caused by inaccurate registration on edges. Using a Gaussian filter kernel G_σ the first weight matrix $\mathbf{B}^{(n)}$ is calculated as follows

$$b_{ij}^{(n)} = \frac{1}{1 + G_\sigma \left(x_{ij}^{(n-1)} - y_{ij}^{(n)} \right)} \tag{3}$$

For $n > 1$ the denoised image $\mathbf{X}^{(1)}$ is initialized with a slightly smoothed version of $\mathbf{Y}^{(1)}$ using a bilateral filter [8]. The standard deviation σ of G_σ has to be adjusted to the noise level, since a large σ filters noise effectively whereas a small σ suppresses motion blur.

The second weight matrix $\mathbf{E}^{(n)}$ is calculated in order to maximize the image quality of $\mathbf{X}^{(n)}$. The image quality is evaluated by using an objective non-reference image quality index $Q(\mathbf{I})$. In this paper it is assumed that larger values $Q(\mathbf{I})$ indicates a better quality for image $\mathbf{I}$. The first step is to find a global weight factor α^* according to

$$\alpha^* = \arg \max_\alpha Q \left(\alpha \mathbf{X}^{(n-1)} + (1 - \alpha) \mathbf{Y}^{(n)} \right) \tag{4}$$

To make the quality measurement adaptive to locally varying illumination the images are decomposed to smaller blocks. For each block a local weight is determined. In preliminary tests we found out that this weight factor is usable on edge points to detect blurred edges or image structures with poor contrast whereas in homogeneous regions simple averaging in combination with the weights $\mathbf{B}^{(n)}$ gives accurate results. Based on this assumption a weight matrix $\mathbf{E}^{(n)}$ using an edge strength measurement τ_{ij} for each pixel (i, j) is derived

$$e_{ij}^{(n)} = \begin{cases} \alpha^* & \text{if } \tau_{ij} > \tau_u \\ m\tau_{ij} + t & \text{if } \tau_l \leq \tau_{ij} \leq \tau_u \\ \frac{n-1}{n} & \text{if } \tau_{ij} < \tau_l \end{cases} \qquad (5)$$

The edge strength τ_{ij} is determined using edge detection and the thresholds τ_l and τ_u are used to classify into homogeneous points and strong edge points respectively. Between homogeneous and strong edge pixels linear interpolation is performed which is denoted by the linear term $m\tau_{ij} + t$.

Image quality index The function $Q(\mathbf{I})$ is used to give an objective assessment of the quality of an image $\mathbf{I}$. We choose the so called *edge magnitude distribution*. It was already applied to evaluate the quality of low-cost scanning laser ophthalmoscope images [9]. For an image $\mathbf{I}$ the index $Q(\mathbf{I})$ is calculated as follows: First, the gradient magnitude image $\mathbf{G}$ is calculated. The quality index $Q(\mathbf{I})$ is the skewness of the histogram of $\mathbf{G}$. A large positive skewness indicates a right-skewed distribution which means that there is a good separation between sharp and weak edges. In this case for fundus images background and structures like blood vessels or the optic disc can be discriminated, thus the image has a good quality.

2.2 Experiments

The denoising method is evaluated using real image sequences captured by a low-cost fundus camera. We compare our quality-guided approach with the state-of-the-art wavelet multi-frame denoising described in [6] and simple median estimation. For spatial alignment of the frames we use rigid registration based on mutual information [10]. This compensates the motion between the frames caused by the movement of the human eye during image acquisition. We adjusted the parameters of our algorithm as follows: For the Gaussian kernel to determine $\mathbf{B}^{(n)}$ we use the standard deviation $\sigma = 15$ to compensate slow varying illumination. The edge weights $\mathbf{E}^{(n)}$ are calculated in blocks of size 50×50 pixels whereas the ratio of eigenvalues of the structure tensor is used to determine edge strength. For classification of strong and weak edge points we use $\tau_l = 3\tilde{\tau}$ and $\tau_u = 5\tilde{\tau}$ as thresholds where $\tilde{\tau}$ is the median edge strength. For wavelet denoising we use Haar wavelets and three decomposition levels. We provide qualitative as well as quantitative results for the SNR to measure noise suppression. The different methods were implemented in MATLAB and run times were measured on an Intel Xeon 2.80 GHz Quad Core CPU with 4 GB RAM.

3   Results

The qualitative evaluation of the denoising methods is based on a sequence of eight frames. Denoising results and a comparison between the different methods is shown in Fig. 2. We evaluated the SNR in a homogeneous image region for the different denoising methods. The SNR is determined for varying number of frames taken as input for denoising and plotted in Fig. 3. The edge preservation can be observed by visual inspection of the denoised images shown in Fig. 2.

If we exclude the run time required for image registration, our proposed algorithm needs 23.5 seconds to denoise eight frames of size 296×200. This outperforms the multi-frame wavelet approach which takes 96.1 seconds. Compared to the median method that takes 2.5 seconds there is an overhead caused by the assessment of the image quality during each step.

4   Discussion

The SNR evaluation in Fig. 3 shows that our approach outperforms traditional frame averaging although robust median estimation is used. It gives competitive results to the wavelet multi-frame method with respect to SNR for longer sequences ($n \geq 5$). If the steady state for the SNR is reached ($n \geq 10$), our approach is slightly better than the multi-frame wavelet method whereas the latter one gives better results for short sequences in the present case. Edges are preserved by temporal filtering which can be observed by visual inspection of structures like the optic disc border in Fig. 2. Our proposed method is about four times faster than multi-frame wavelet denoising and performs incremental filtering with competitive results. This makes it more feasible to provide real-time denoising. However, there is still a high potential to speed up this method by parallelizing different steps like the weight calculation.

In our future work we plan to evaluate other image quality indices or combinations of them. This should make the image quality assessment more robust and a variety of criteria concerning contrast or blur can be taken into account.

Acknowledgement. The authors gratefully acknowledge funding of the Erlangen Graduate School in Advanced Optical Technologies (SAOT) by the German National Science Foundation (DFG) in the framework of the excellence initiative.

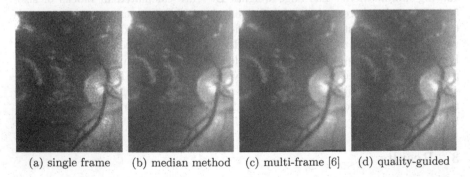

(a) single frame   (b) median method   (c) multi-frame [6]   (d) quality-guided

Fig. 2. Results of different denoising methods for a region of interest (ROI) in eight frames after contrast enhancement

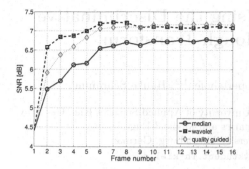

Fig. 3. Evaluation of SNR vs. frame number to be used for denoising

References

1. Buades T, Lou Y, Morel JM, et al. A note on multi-image denoising. In: Proc Int Workshop Local and Non-Local Approximation in Image Processing; 2009. p. 1–15.
2. Saeidi M, Motamedi SA, Behrad A, et al. Noise reduction of consecutive images using a new adaptive weighted averaging filter. In: Proc IEEE Workshop Signal Processing Systems Design and Implementation; 2005. p. 455–60.
3. Shen B, Perry S, Fraser D. Adaptive motion-compensated temporal filtering of sector scan sonar image sequences. In: proc IEEE OCEANS; 2010. p. 1–6.
4. Dudek R, Cuenca C, Quintana F. Image sequences noise reduction: an optical flow based approach. In: Proc EUROCAST. vol. 5717. Springer Berlin / Heidelberg; 2009. p. 366–73.
5. Borsdorf A, Raupach R, Hornegger J. Wavelet based noise reduction by identification of correlations. In: Pattern Recognition. vol. 4174. Springer Berlin / Heidelberg; 2006. p. 21–30.
6. Mayer M, Wagner M, Hornegger J, et al.. Wavelet denoising of multiple-frame OCT date enhanced by a correlation analysis; 2010.
7. Fischler MA, Bolles RC. Random sample consensus: a paradigm for model fitting with applications to image analysis and automated cartography. Commun ACM. 1981;24:381–95.
8. Tomasi C, Manduchi R. Bilateral filtering for gray and color images. In: Proc ICCV. IEEE Computer Society; 1998. p. 839–46.
9. Murillo S, Echegaray S, Zamora G, et al. Quantitative and qualitative image quality analysis of super resolution images from a low cost scanning laser ophthalmoscope. Proc SPIE. 2011;7962:4T.
10. Hahn DA, Daum V, Hornegger J. Automatic parameter selection for multimodal image registration. IEEE Trans Med Imaging. 2010;29(5):1140–55.

Femur Localization Using the Discriminative Generalized Hough Transform

Francesco Boero[1], Heike Ruppertshofen[1,2], Hauke Schramm[1]

[1]Institute of Applied Computer Science, University of Applied Sciences Kiel, Germany
[2]Chair for Healthcare Telematics and Medical Engineering,
Otto-von-Guericke-University Magdeburg, Germany
francesco.boero@student.fh-kiel.de

Abstract. The Discriminative Generalized Hough Transform, a method for object localization and training of suitable models, is employed here for the localization of the femur in long-leg radiographs. The method is extended to improve the robustness of the procedure by integrating anatomical knowledge. This is achieved by combining the femur localization with the more robust knee localization. To this end, a region of interest is extracted from the original image, based on the result of the knee localization, in which the femur is initially localized. In addition, the procedure focuses on the target by extracting smaller regions of interest around the previously found coordinates and repeating the localization with smaller models. By this means, the precision of the first coarse localization is refined. The presented method is tested here on a large set of long-leg radiographs, where it achieves a localization rate of 94 % on femurs not showing pathological conditions.

1 Introduction

Automatic object localization is a useful feature in many fields of computer-aided diagnosis. An example is the automatic segmentation of bone structures in digital radiographs [1], used as a prerequisite for quantitative orthopedic examinations, like the measurement of length and angles of bones, or for the acquisition of further information required for preoperative planning. The initialization of these procedures often still requires the manual positioning of the segmentation model in the image.

For an automatic initialization a robust localization of some anatomical landmarks is desiderable. Interesting results in automatic joint and bone localization were achieved using the Discriminative Generalized Hough Transform (DGHT) [2]. Here, a model, automatically trained with a rather small set of images of radiographs showing the legs and the pelvic region, proved to be able to locate the knee joint with an accuracy within 11 mm in about 97 % of the images showing knees without pathological conditions. Less optimal results were gained with a model targeting the upper extremity of the femur. Here, the successful localizations were only 74.8 %. A result that worsens to 67 % when the model is used on images showing anomalies or femur prostheses.

In order to improve these performances two main problems need to be dealt with. First of all the images tend to be darker in the region surrounding the pelvis. As a result the canny edge detector, which is a key component both during the training of the model and the localization, tends to miss a lot of useful details in the region of interest, focusing instead on the lower parts of the legs. Second, the anatomical target exhibits large variability concerning shape, size and appearance, which is also influenced by the patient posture. Furthermore, the rotational freedom of the femur poses another challenge.

In this paper we will address these challenges by two measures. On the one hand, we employ the results of the knee localization to restrict the search region of the femur and to increase the robustness of the search. On the other hand, we will refine the results of the localization by successively searching the upper part of the femur in a region of ever decreasing size.

In some aspects the method is similar to the multi-level approach [3] used to speed up the localization of anatomical structures. While the multi-level approach employs multiple models trained for different image resolutions, here multiple models are used to refine the localization of the structure of interest by targeting at each step a smaller region using a constant resolution.

2   Method

The GHT [4] is a widely used shape detection technique, able to localize an arbitrary object in an image using a point model. It works by generating a Hough space reflecting at each point the degree of matching between the edges extracted from that region and the points of the model. The Hough cell showing the highest value is assumed to indicate the object location. In the DGHT the employed models additionally contain an individual weight for each point, which is used during the voting procedure. The model and the weights are automatically generated and trained on a number of images with a discriminative training algorithm, making them robust towards individual variability, noise or partial occlusions.

For more detailed information on the employed iterative training technique and the standard DGHT procedure, we refer the reader to [2].

A DGHT model, trained for the knee, was able to locate its target in $\sim 97\%$ of the images [2], making the knee a potentially helpful reference point in finding the femur. For this reason the first step of the localization procedure consists of searching for the knee. Subsequently, the femur is searched for with a large model of the hip. The Hough spaces obtained with the knee and with the femur model are normalized, and overlapped using the average offset of the knee and the femoral neck observed in the training images.

In this combined Hough space a new maximum is searched for, which is expected to be a point close to the femur. Around the maximum, found in the combined Hough space, a smaller region is cut from the original input image with variable size. In case the right femur is searched for, the region includes the left and the upper image boundary and, starting from the coordinates of the former maximum, it extends in direction of the right and the bottom of the image three times the standard deviation of the distance between the femoral neck and the knee. The opposite applies if the left femur is searched for. This is done in order to ensure that the upper part of the femur is always present in the image, despite the fixed offset used for the Hough space combination and possible mislocalization of the knee. In this area a smaller model is employed as a first attempt to coarsely locate the femur. During two successive iterations the localization is refined by cutting smaller regions around the previously found coordinates from the image, and conducting the search in these reduced regions with ever smaller growing models of the femoral neck.

Before each localization step a histogram equalization is performed on the examined image region. The use of small models in small regions improves the precision since the equalization, if applied locally in a restricted area with a more uniform brightness, allows the Canny edge detector to return more details. Moreover, restricting the considered search region mostly avoids the competition of other joints or further structures.

3 Material and experimental setup

The experiments were conducted on a large set of radiographs containing 705 images showing the legs and the pelvic region. Some images show only one leg, while others contain prostheses of the femur or the knee. The original images were downsampled for faster processing. In the experiments each image has a size of approximately 380×1000 pixels and an isotropic resolution of 1.14 mm. As target landmark to represent the femur a point on the upper boundary of the femur medial of the greater trochanter was chosen, which can be consistently annotated by a human observer. A localization procedure is considered successful if the system is able to localize the target within 5 Hough cells (11.4 mm) from the manually annotated point.

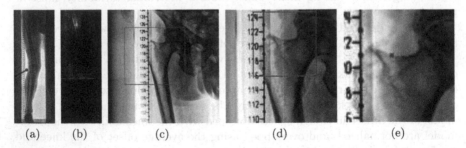

(a)   (b)   (c)   (d)   (e)

Fig. 1. An example of the localization procedure. In the original image (a), the knee is localized and the femur head is searched for using the *large* model. The maximum in their combined Hough space (b) is found, and around those coordinates a smaller region (c) is extracted. Here the *medium* model is localized, and an even smaller area is cut (d). A more accurate search for the landmark is performed with the *small* model, bringing to the final step, where the *tiny* model is localized in the small region (e)

All the models for the femur and for the knee were trained using a single training set composed of 54 radiographs showing healthy joints, which was also employed in [2]. The initial *large* femur model (220×160 px) is trained on the upper part of the training images (~378×360 px). The next three smaller femur models are trained over smaller regions of the training images, having the same size of the area in which they will be employed. A *medium* model (120×150 px) is trained over regions of the training images with variable size, extracted by cutting around the target point a region as explained in the previous section. The average size is 190×260 px. This is done in the attempt to replicate as close as possible the conditions in which the model will operate. A *small* model (60×60 px) is trained over smaller square images (140×140 px), centered at the target point. During the last step a very small *tiny* model (50×40 px) is employed, trained over a region of only 80×80 px. In these small images there are not many chances to miss the target, provided that the previous steps were succesful in approaching it.

At first the localization of the right femur was tested on 553 radiographs for which annotations were available. Then all the models were horizontally flipped and tested again, searching the left femur in a set composed of 659 images. Overall the test image set showed 1130 normal joints and 82 femurs containing artificial replacements or anomalies.

4   Results

The presented system manages to locate the femur with an error (distance between the localized point and the manually annotated landmark) of less than 11.4 mm (=5 Hough cells) in 94.1 % of the images showing normal joints.

The 3 localization steps are effective in reducing the localization error: after the first localization with the *medium* model, the percentage of femurs localized

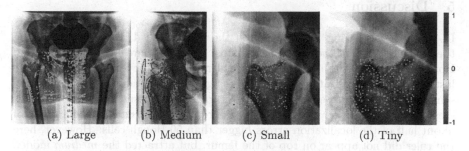

(a) Large   (b) Medium   (c) Small   (d) Tiny

Fig. 2. The femur models employed during the localization procedure with their target point. The *large* model is used for generating the Hough space that will be combined with the one generated by the knee. The other models are used in the successive steps. The colors show the weight of the model points. For the *medium* model the weighting of model points was not really successful. Nevertheless, this did not prevent the model to operate with an acceptable accuracy

Table 1. Localization errors for 1130 healthy joints expressed in Hough cells (1 Hough cell = 2.28 mm). For errors larger than 5 Hough cells the reason of error is given. The values in parenthesis state the errors which occurred due to wrong knee localizations

Error	Total	%	Regression	Ruler superimposed	Ruler mistaken for femur	Other
0→5	1064	94.1	0	0	0	0
5→10	13	1.1	2	9	0	1(1)
10→30	26	1.3	6	14	1	5
30→50	11	0.9	4	1	2(1)	4
>50	16	1.4	0	0	9(6)	7(1)

with an error of less than 5 Hough cells is 74.6 % . This percentage improves to 83.6 % after the second step performed with the *small* model, and reaches 94.1 % after the third and last step.

Since the models are trained on healthy joints, they cannot be expected to perform well on the 82 images showing replaced hip joints. Nevertheless, the percentage of correct localizations is 51.2 % for those cases.

It is interesting to note that 51.3 % of the normal joints and 21.9 % of the joints with implants or replacements are localized with an accuracy of one Hough cell (=2.28 mm) or less.

While, in general, this technique manages to reduce the localization error step by step, in few cases a regression can be observed in the localization precision. Meaning that a joint, which was close to a correct localization during the first localization step(s), suddenly is mislocalized in the next one(s). This result is probably due to the reason that smaller models are less robust against the various disturbances that can be present in the images.

5 Discussion

In the images showing normal femurs, the system failed in correctly locating the femur in 5.9 % of the images. The most common source of errors within 30 Hough cells or less is the presence of the ruler on top of the femur (Table 1). The last steps of the localization procedure, using very small models, tend to be very sensible to this disturbance and often return a worse result than the previous step(s) which use bigger models. Furthermore, the ruler seems to be the cause of about half of the localization errors bigger than 50 Hough cells. However, here the ruler did not appear on top of the femur, but attracted the *medium* model, causing a big localization error already in the second step.

Given that the first step of the femur localization makes use of the model of the knee, the result of the procedure can be negatively influenced by the failed localization of the latter. During the test the evidence of a wrongly localized knee appears in 2.3 % of the images, but results in a localization error for the femur only in one out of three cases. Such that the number of errors in presence of a mislocalized knee is below 1 %. This can be considered good news because the mislocalized knee is often associated with the biggest errors (more than 50 Hough cells).

In any case such large errors occur rarely, and the achieved localization rate constitutes a remarkable step forward if compared with the former 74.8 %.

Acknowledgement. The authors would like to thank the Dartmouth-Hitchcock Medical Center and Diagnostic X-Ray, Philips Healthcare for providing the radiographs used in this study.

References

1. Gooßen A, Hermann E, Weber GM, et al. Model-based segmentation of pediatric and adult joints for orthopedic measurements in digital radiographs of the lower limbs. Comp Sci Res Dev. 2011;26(1):107–116.
2. Ruppertshofen H, Lorenz C, Schmidt S, et al. Discriminative generalized Hough transform for localization of joints in the lower extremities. Comp Sci Res Dev. 2011;26(1):97–105.
3. Ruppertshofen H, Künne D, Lorenz C, et al. Multi-Level approach for the discriminative generalized Hough transform. Proc CURAC. 2011; p. 67–70.
4. Ballard DH. Generalizing the Hough transform to detect arbitrary shapes. Pattern Recognit. 1981;13(2):111–122.

Mikro-CT basierte Validierung digitaler Tomosynthese Rekonstruktion

Aileen Cordes[1], Yulia M. Levakhina[1,2], Thorsten M. Buzug[1]

[1]Institut für Medizintechnik, Universität zu Lübeck
[2]Graduate School for Computing in Medicine and Life Sciences, Lübeck
cordes@imt.uni-luebeck.de

Kurzfassung. Die digitale Tomosynthese ist ein röntgenbasiertes Verfahren zur Generierung von tomographischen Schnittbildern auf der Grundlage einer begrenzten Anzahl von zweidimensionalen Projektionen. Aufgrund der prinzipbedingten unvollständigen Abtastung des zu untersuchenden Objektes ergeben sich deutliche Vorteile hinsichtlich der Strahlenbelastung. Eine mathematisch exakte dreidimensionale Bildrekonstruktion ist jedoch nicht möglich. In diesem Beitrag wird überprüft, inwieweit die Tomosynthese- Rekonstruktion trotz einer unvollständigen Datenerfassung korrekte Informationen über die zu untersuchenden anatomischen Strukturen liefern. Hierzu wurde eine Tomosynthese-Aufnahme mit Hilfe eines Mikro-CT-Rohdatensatzes simuliert. Da die Tomosynthese- und Mikro-CT-Rekonstruktionen die gleichen Strukturen abbilden, können die beiden Datensätze qualitativ und quantitativ verglichen werden. Die Ergebnisse zeigen bei geeigneter Wahl der Akquisitionsparameter eine sehr gute Übereinstimmung mit den Mikro-CT-Rekonstruktionen. Qualitativ hochwertige realistische Bilder können trotz einer eingeschränkten Anzahl von Projektionen generiert werden.

1 Einleitung

Bei konventionellen Röntgenaufnahmen führt die für ein Projektionsverfahren typische Überlagerung von Gewebestrukturen zu einem Verlust an räumlicher Information und einer eingeschränkten Sensitivität und Spezifität. Die digitale Tomosynthese (DT) verspricht durch eine Verbesserung der Detailerkennbarkeit mehr Sicherheit in der medizinischen Diagnostik [1]. Bei dieser Technologie werden jeweils mit niedriger Dosis eine begrenzte Anzahl von Projektionen aus unterschiedlichen Betrachtungswinkeln akquiriert und zu Schichtbildern des Gewebes rekonstruiert [2, 3]. Der Scan-Winkel ist in den meisten Anwendungen auf maximal 50° beschränkt. Die Dosis einer Untersuchung liegt in der Größenordnung einer herkömmlichen Röntgenaufnahme und ist bedeutend geringer als bei der Computertomographie (CT). Die Kombination von dreidimensionaler Bildgebung und einer geringen Strahlenbelastung machen die Tomosynthese zu einer vielversprechenden Technologie. Bevorzugte Anwendung finden die Systeme insbesondere in der Mammadiagnostik. Nachteil dieser Modalität ist jedoch, dass die begrenzte Rotationsbewegung eine vollständige Datenerfassung verhindert.

Eine mathematisch exakte Bildrekonstruktion und eine artefaktfreie dreidimensionale Darstellung sind nicht möglich [4]. Im Rahmen dieser Arbeit wurde daher überprüft, inwieweit die Rekonstruktionen trotz einer unvollständigen Datenerfassung korrekte Informationen über die tatsächlich vorhandenen anatomischen Strukturen liefern. Eine Beantwortung dieser Frage erfordert die Kenntnis des idealen Bildes. Da derartige Referenzen in der klinischen Praxis jedoch im Allgemeinen nicht verfügbar sind, wurden Mikro-CT- Projektionsbilder zur Simulation einer Tomosynthesemessung verwendet. Die Tomosynthese- und Mikro-CT Rekonstruktionen repräsentieren auf diese Weise identische Strukturen. Dies erlaubt eine Verwendung der Mikro-CT-Bilder als Referenz und ermöglicht eine qualitative sowie eine quantitative Evaluation der Rekonstruktionsgenauigkeit.

2   Material und Methoden

2.1   Simulation von Tomosynthese-Projektionen

Für die Mikro-CT-Daten wurde das Kegelstrahlröntgensystem SkyScan 1172 verwendet. In Abb. 1 ist der Aufbau eines solchen Systems schematisch dargestellt. Die beiden entscheidenden Komponenten sind die Röntgenröhre und ein 1,3 MP Flat-Panel-Detektor. Das zu untersuchende Objekt wird im etwa 2 cm^3 großen Messfeld auf einem Drehteller platziert. Aufgrund der sehr feinen inneren Strukturen wurde im Rahmen dieser Arbeit als Testobjekt ein Fingerknochen[1] gewählt. Auch in der klinischen Praxis müssen im Allgemeinen sehr feine Abnormalitäten und Strukturveränderungen abgebildet und diagnostiziert werden. Bei einer Röhrenspannung von 59 kV und einem Anodenstrom von 167 μA wurden zweidimensionale Projektionsbilder dieses Fingerknochens in 0,7° und 0,9° Schritten über 360° akquiriert.

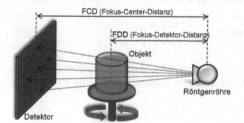

Abb. 1. Schematischer Aufbau eines Mikro-CTs

Die Mikro-CT-Rohdaten wurden anschließend zur Simulation von Tomosynthese-Projektionen verwendet. In diesem Beitrag wurde eine Tomosynthese-

---

[1] Die Leichname der Körperspender – beziehungsweise die verwendeten Körperteile (in diesem Fall die Fingerknochen) – wurden unter Genehmigung durch das „Gesetz über das Leichen-, Bestattungs- und Friedhofswesen (Bestattungsgesetz) des Landes Schleswig-Holstein vom 04.02.2005, Abschnitt II, $ 9 (Leichenöffnung, anatomisch)" untersucht. In diesem Fall ist es gestattet, die Körper von Körperspendern/innen zu wissenschaftlichen Zwecken und/oder Lehraufgaben zu sezieren.

Sequenz simuliert, bei der sich die Röntgenröhre während der Bildakquisition auf einer bogenförmigen Trajektorie über einem stationären Detektor bewegt. Eine Simulation dieser Modalität erfordert demzufolge eine Projektion der Mikro-CT Rohdaten auf einen virtuellen stationären Detektor (Abb. 2). Eine Spalte einer Mikro-CT-Projektion im Abstand c vom Detektorzentrum wird gemäß folgender Gleichung auf einen virtuellen Detektor, der sich im Abstand k vom Rotations-zentrum befindet, projiziert

$$s = \frac{k(c\cos(\gamma) + FDD\sin(\gamma)) + cFCD}{FDD\cos(\gamma) - c\sin(\gamma)} \tag{1}$$

wobei γ der Projektionswinkel in Bezug auf die z-Achse, FDD die Fokus--Detektor-Distanz, FCD die Fokus-Center-Distanz und s der Abstand vom Zentrum des virtuellen Detektors sind. Sich durch die Transformation ergebende Längenunterschiede der einzelnen Spalten in y-Richtung werden durch folgenden Skalierungsfaktor realisiert

$$\text{scale}(c) = 1 + \frac{c\sin(\gamma) + k - \cos(\gamma)(FDD - FCD)}{\cos(\gamma + \tan^{-1}(\frac{c}{FDD}))\sqrt{FDD^2 + c^2}} \tag{2}$$

2.2 Shift-and-Add-Rekonstruktion

Der verwendete Rekonstruktionsalgorithmus basiert auf dem traditionellen Shift-and-Add-Verfahren [1]. Durch geeignetes Verschieben und Summieren der Projektionsbilder werden die Strukturen einer bestimmten Ebene scharf abgebildet, während alle Fremdstrukturen außerhalb der zu rekonstruierenden Schicht durch Verschmierung unterdrückt werden. Die notwendige Verschiebung zur Rekonstruktion einer Ebene im Abstand a vom Rotationszentrum ist gegeben durch

$$\text{shift}(a, \gamma) = FCD\sin(\gamma)\frac{k + a}{FCD\cos(\gamma) - a} \tag{3}$$

Um Vergrößerungsunterschiede aufgrund variierender Abstände zwischen dem Röntgenfokus und dem Detektor auszugleichen, ist zusätzlich ist eine Skalierung

Abb. 2. Projektion der Mikro–CT-Rohdaten auf einen virtuellen stationären Detektor zur Simulation von Tomosynthese-Projektionen

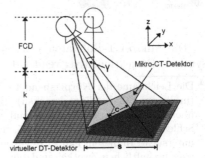

der einzelnen Projektionsbilder erforderlich. Der notwendige Skalierungsfaktor ist gegeben durch

$$\text{scale}(a, \gamma) = \frac{FCD + k}{FCD} \cdot \frac{FCD\cos(\gamma) - a}{FCD\cos(\gamma) + k} \tag{4}$$

Das resultierende Schnittbild ergibt sich schließlich als Mittelwert aller verschobenen und skalierten Projektionsbilder. Nachteil dieses Algorithmus ist, dass die Informationen von Objekten ober- und unterhalb der zu rekonstruierenden Schicht nicht eliminiert werden, sondern als verwischte Bilder die scharfe Abbildungsebene überlagern. Zur Reduktion dieser Fremdschichtartefakte wurde eine Filterung entlang der Zeilen der Projektionsbilder mit einem Rampenfilter durchgeführt.

2.3 Ähnlichkeitsmaß

Eine geeignete Metrik zur Bestimmung der Ähnlichkeit der Mikro-CT- und Tomosynthese-Rekonstruktionen ist die Mutual Information. Die Verwendung dieses informationstheoretischen Maßes als Gütekriterium wird dadurch motiviert, dass kein Vorwissen über die Abhängigkeiten zwischen den Intensitätswerten in beiden Datensätzen erforderlich ist. Die Berechnung der Mutual Information erfolgt auf Basis der Entropien der zu vergleichenden Bilddatensätze [5]. Die Entropie eines Bildes I mit den Intensitäten $a_1, \ldots, a_n$ ist definiert durch

$$H(I) = -\sum_{i=1}^{n} p(a_i) ln(p(a_i)), \quad \sum_{i=1}^{n} p(a_i) = 1 \tag{5}$$

wobei $p(a_i)$ die Wahrscheinlichkeit des Auftretens der Intensität a_i beschreibt. Analog kann die gemeinsame Entropie eines Bildes I und eines Referenzbildes I_{ref} mit den Intensitäten $b_1, \ldots, b_m$ aus den Wahrscheinlichkeiten des gemeinsamen Auftretens der Intensitäten a_i und b_j bestimmt werden

$$H(I, I_{ref}) = -\sum_{j=1}^{m} \sum_{i=1}^{n} p(a_i, b_j) ln(p(a_i, b_j)) \tag{6}$$

Die Mutual Information ist dann gegeben durch

$$MI(I, I_{ref}) = H(I) + H(I_{ref}) - H(I, I_{ref}) \tag{7}$$

Eine Zunahme der Ähnlichkeit zweier Bilddatensätze geht mit einer Reduktion der gemeinsamen Entropie und demzufolge mit einer Erhöhung der Mutual Information einher.

3 Ergebnisse

Abb. 3 zeigt beispielhaft rekonstruierte Schnittbilder des Fingerknochens. Die Berechnung dieser Schnittbilder erfolgte mit einem konstanten Rotationsschritt

Abb. 3. (a) Mikro-CT-Referenzbild eines Fingerknochens. (b)-(d) Entsprechende Tomosynthese-Rekonstruktionen bei variierendem tomografischen Winkel α

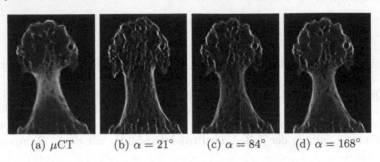

(a) μCT   (b) $\alpha = 21°$ (c) $\alpha = 84°$ (d) $\alpha = 168°$

von $\Delta\alpha = 0,7°$ und variierendem tomographischen Winkel α von 21°-168°. Während die Detailerkennbarkeit in Abb. 3(b) durch die Überlagerung von Fremdschichtartefakten deutlich reduziert ist, kann bei größeren Winkelbereichen eine sehr gute Übereinstimmung der abgebildeten Strukturen mit der Mikro-CT-Referenz festgestellt werden. Eine quantitative Analyse durch Berechnung der Mutual Information bestätigt die zunehmende Rekonstruktionsgenauigkeit bei Erhöhung des tomografischen Winkels (Abb. 4). Die in Abb. 4(a) und 4(b) analysierten Schichten unterscheiden sich durch eine unterschiedliche Orientierung innerhalb des Fingerknochens. Die Größe des Objektes senkrecht zur rekonstruierten Schicht beträgt in Abb. 4(a) 5,6 mm und in Abb. 4(b) 18,4 mm. In Abb. 4(b) zeigt sich ein deutlich stärkerer Qualitätsverlust bei einer Erhöhung des Rotationsschrittes der Röntgenröhre als in Abb. 4(a). Der Grund dafür liegt darin, dass das Vorhandensein von Strukturen in größerem Abstand zur rekonstruierten Schicht das Auftreten von Artefakten begünstigt. Bei einer zu geringen Abtastdichte ist die Verschiebung zwischen zwei aufeinander folgenden Projektionen zu groß um eine ausreichende Verwischung der weiter entfernt liegenden Strukturen zu ermöglichen. Das Ausmaß der verbleibenden Artefakte ist somit stark von Form und Orientierung des Objektes in Bezug auf die verwendete Systemgeo-

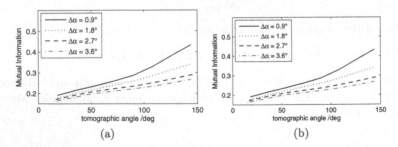

(a)   (b)

Abb. 4. Mutual Information in Abhängigkeit des tomografischen Winkels α und des Rotationsschrittes $\Delta\alpha$. Die Objektgröße senkrecht zur rekonstruierten Schicht beträgt in (a) 5,6 mm und in (b) 18,4 mm

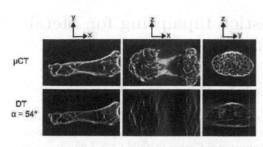

Abb. 5. Anisotrope räumliche Auflösung der digitalen Tomosynthese (DT)

metrie abhängig. Abb. 5 illustriert die durch die unvollständige Datenerfassung bedingte anisotrope räumliche Auflösung der Tomosynthese. Die dargestellten Schichten in der x/z- und y/z-Ebene wurden aus dem primär rekonstruierten Bilderstapel der x/y-Schichten berechnet.

4 Diskussion

Mit der Simulation von Tomosynthese-Projektionen aus einem Mikro-CT-Rohdatensatz wird eine Methode bereitgestellt, die hervorragend für eine Validierung bereits bestehender sowie zukünftiger Strategien zur Verbesserung der Bildqualität geeignet ist. Es wird sowohl eine qualitative Evaluation durch einen visuellen Vergleich mit den Mikro-CT-Rekonstruktionen als auch eine quantitative Bewertung mittels referenzbasierter Metriken ermöglicht. Die Ergebnisse bestätigen, dass die digitale Tomosynthese ein erhebliches Potenzial für eine Verbesserung der medizinischen Diagnostik besitzt. Auch wenn die Tomosynthese prinzipbedingt keine isotrope exakte dreidimensionale Bildgebung liefern kann (Abb. 5), zeigen die rekonstruierten Schichtbilder bei geeigneter Wahl der Akquisitionsparamter eine sehr gute Übereinstimmung mit den Mikro-CT-Rekonstruktionen. Trotz einer unvollständigen Datenerfassung können alle relevanten Strukturen differenziert dargestellt werden. Die Tomosynthese verspricht somit zuverlässige Diagnosen auf der Basis von dreidimensionalen Datensätzen und das bei einer deutlich geringeren Strahlendosis als bei der Computertomographie. Auch auf der Grundlage einer begrenzten Anzahl von Projektionen können qualitativ hochwertige realistische Bilder rekonstruiert werden.

Literaturverzeichnis

1. Niklason LT, Christian BT, Niklason LE, et al. Digital tomosynthesis in breast imaging. Radiology. 1997;205:399–406.
2. Dobbins JT. Tomosynthesis imaging: at a translational crossroads. Med Phys. 2009;36(6):1956–67.
3. Dobbins JT, Godfrey DJ. Digital x-ray tomosynthesis: current state of the art and clinical potential. Phys Med Biol. 2003;48:65–106.
4. Machida H, Yuhara T, Mori T, et al. Optimizing parameters for flat-panel detector digital tomosynthesis. RadioGraphics. 2010;30:549–62.
5. Handels H. Medizinische Bildverarbeitung. Wiesbaden: Vieweg+Teubner; 2009.

Modified Eulers Elastica Inpainting for Metal Artifact Reduction in CT

Julia Hamer[1,2,3], Bärbel Kratz[1], Jan Müller[1], Thorsten M. Buzug[1]

[1]Institut für Medizintechnik, Universität zu Lübeck
[2]Graduate School for Computing in Medicine and Life Sciences, Univ. zu Lübeck
[3]Molecular Imaging North Competence Center (MOIN CC), Lübeck
hamer@imt.uni-luebeck.de

Abstract. In computed tomography (CT) metal causes strong streak artifacts in the reconstructed images, which may hinder the correct diagnosis of patients. In this work, metal artifacts are reduced using the modified Eulers elastica and curvature based sinogram inpainting (EECSI). The inconsistent data is deleted from the sinogram and replaced by a two-dimensional interpolation strategy based on the surrounding data information using partial differential equations. The inpainting domain is defined by a binary mask that is calculated using a thresholding method in the preliminary reconstructed image with a following forward projection of the metal-only image. Here, the EECSI is modified by a statistic weighting function that regulates the time step size depending on the probability of a gray value. Additionally, the connectivity principle is strengthened by applying a different strategy in the numerical implementation compared to prior methods. The measurements are realized on a Philips Tomoscan M/EG scanner using a torso phantom with the physical properties of an average male torso, suitable for medical experiments. For evaluation, the results are compared to the ones achieved by using the original EECSI and the classically used one-dimensional linear interpolation method. It is demonstrated that the performed modifications result in a better metal artifact suppression.

1 Introduction

Metal objects lead to inconsistencies in the Radon space, which cause streak artifacts in the reconstructed images. Commonly, this is corrected by replacing the inconsistent data in the Radon space with artificially generated data or by using iterative reconstruction methods. The state-of-the art method of metal artifact reduction (MAR) in computed tomography (CT) in the Radon space, i.e. sinogram domain, is the one-dimensional linear interpolation (LI) method where metal data is deleted from the sinogram and filled from the linear interpolated boundary information under a fixed angle [1].

In this work, the correction step is performed in the sinogram domain by using a two-dimensional interpolation method adapted from image inpainting. It has been shown that image inpainting can be applied for MAR in CT [2, 3].

The application of Eulers elastica and curvature based image inpainting [4] for MAR in CT was first performed by Gu et. al in 2006 [5] as the so called Eulers elastica and curvature based sinogram inpainting (EECSI). The interpolation is based on the minimization of the elasticity energy using partial differential equations (PDE), modeling an elastic data progression of the surrounding image information for replacing inconsistent data. In this work, the concept of using the EECSI for MAR in CT is further elaborated with real data measurements of a torso phantom on a Philips Tomoscan M/EG scanner. Furthermore, the numerical implementation of the algorithm is modified for the application of MAR in CT and an adaptive time step size is introduced into the iteration scheme of the EECSI, taking into account histogram information of the sinogram.

The results are compared to the ones received by using the originally proposed EECSI and the classically used one-dimensional artifact suppression technique, i.e. the linear interpolation method.

2 Material and methods

2.1 Data

The measurements were carried out on a Philips Tomoscan M/EG scanner. The torso phantom (CIRS Inc, Norfolk, USA) is designed with the physical proper- ties of an average male torso, suitable for medical experiments. The phantom simulates the attenuation values of actual tissue within 2% of the diagnostic en- ergy range. The simulated rib cage and the vertebral column are embedded into muscle material and the exterior coating consists of 30% adipose and 70% muscle tissue. Three steel markers are attached onto the phantom in order to create the metal artifacts. For evaluation, a measurement was carried out without steel markers to serve as ground truth.

2.2 Methodology

Segmentation of the metal trace For defining the inpainting domain in the sinogram, a segmentation of the metal data is necessary. Therefore, a standard filtered backprojection (FBP) reconstruction is used to slightly over-segment the metals by a simple thresholding method in the image domain. Afterwards, the metal-only image is forward projected into the Radon domain in order to calculate the sinogram mask. The sinogram mask is chosen to be binary, i. e. all sinogram values that have a value unequal to zero are labeled as the inpainting domain.

Image inpainting Originally, image inpainting was used for the restoration of old paintings by museum restoration artists. In 2000 Bertalmio et al. first introduced digital inpainting into image processing and demonstrated its broad field of applications, effects in movies, film restoration, text removal and scratch removal [6]. In the application of MAR in CT, image inpainting is used for replacing inconsistent projection data in the Radon domain by the surrounding sinogram information in the way that isophotes, lines with the same pixel values, are continued into the inpainting domain in an intelligent way. In this work, the MEECSI is introduced, which is based on the minimization of the elasticity energy by using partial differential equations. The elasticity energy can be written as

$$E(\gamma) = \int_\gamma \left(a + b\kappa(s)^2\right) ds \tag{1}$$

with ds the arc length element, $\kappa(s)$ the scalar curvature, and a,b two positive constant weights. Derived from the Euler-Lagrange equation, the update term for the iteration process can be calculated to

$$\frac{du}{dt} = \nabla \cdot \boldsymbol{V} \tag{2}$$

with

$$\boldsymbol{V} = \left(a + b\kappa^2\right)\boldsymbol{n} - \frac{2b}{|\nabla u|}\frac{\partial \kappa\,|\nabla u|}{\partial t}\boldsymbol{t} \tag{3}$$

where u is the gray value, $\boldsymbol{n}$ the normal direction and $\boldsymbol{t}$ the tangential direction to the isophotes of the sinogram.

Adaptive time step size The update term is modified by a weighting function $W(u^n)$ that takes the frequency of the sinogram value into account in order to adjust the time step in a reasonable way. The iteration scheme can therefore be written as

$$\frac{du}{dt} = W(u^n)\nabla \cdot \boldsymbol{V} \tag{4}$$

For calculating the weighting function $W(u^n)$ five different steps are needed:

1. The no-metal sinogram is calculated by deleting the values in the metal trace, i.e. by setting the values in the inpainting domain to zero.
2. The histogram of the no-metal sinogram is calculated.
3. A threshold of $u_\epsilon = 0.4$ is chosen for cutting the small values off the histogram to exclude the inconsistent sinogram data in the metal trace and the background information from the statistical considerations.
4. The histogram data is fitted by a standard Fourier fit, which shows good results under the condition of reasonable computational expenses

$$\mathrm{fit}(u^0) = a + b \cdot \cos(c \cdot u^0) + d \cdot \sin(c \cdot u^0) \tag{5}$$

   where $a = 459.1$, $b = 271.0$, $c = 1.5$, $d = -222.6$.
5. Every iteration step, the probability of the image data is calculated

$$\mathrm{fit}(u^n) = (a + b \cdot \cos(c \cdot u^n) + d \cdot \sin(c \cdot u^n))/A(fit(u^0)) \tag{6}$$

   where $a = 459.1$, $b = 271.0$, $c = 1.5$, $d = -222.6$. $A(\mathrm{fit}(u^0))$ is the integral over the original fit of the histogram.

6. $W(u^n)$ is defined as an increasing function with values in the range of $W(u^n)=[0,...,m]$

$$W(u^n) = w(1 - fit(u^n)) = m \cdot (1 - fit(u^n)) \tag{7}$$

Here, m=2 is chosen.

D. Numerical implementation: An iterative process is used to calculate the updated sinogram value $u_{(i,j)}^{n+1}$ at the pixel position (i,j) at the iteration step $n = 0, 1, ...$

$$u_{(i,j)}^{n+1} = u_{(i,j)}^n + hW(u^n)(|\nabla u|\nabla \cdot V) \tag{8}$$

The time step size h will be chosen to be $h = 0.25$ with an adaptive regularization if the update term of the equation exceeds a certain value. The factor $|\nabla u|$ leads to a faster convergence and is calculated by the central differencing

$$|\nabla u_{(i,j)}| = \frac{1}{2}\sqrt{\left(u_{(i+1,j)} - u_{(i-1,j)}\right)^2 + \left(u_{(i,j+1)} - u_{(i,j-1)}\right)^2} \tag{9}$$

With $V = (V^1, V^2)$, the normal direction $n = (n^1, n^2) = (\frac{u_x}{|\nabla u|}, \frac{u_y}{|\nabla u|})$, and the tangential direction $t = (t^1, t^2) = (-\frac{u_y}{|\nabla u|}, \frac{u_x}{|\nabla u|})$ the x-component of V can exemplarily be calculated to

$$V^1 = (a + b\kappa^2)n^1 - \frac{2b}{|\nabla u|}(t^1 D_x(\kappa |\nabla u|) + t^2 D_y(\kappa |\nabla u|))t^1 \tag{10}$$

$$= (a + b\kappa^2)\frac{D_x u}{|\nabla u|} + \frac{2b}{|\nabla u|^3}\left(-D_y u D_x(\kappa |\nabla u|) + D_x u D_y(\kappa |\nabla u|)\right)D_y u \tag{11}$$

For the computation of

$$\nabla \cdot V = D_x V_{(i,j)}^1 + D_y V_{(i,j)}^2 = \left(V_{(i+\frac{1}{2},j)}^1 - V_{(i-\frac{1}{2},j)}^1\right) \tag{12}$$

the half-point values of the used quantities need to be specified. For this purpose, the application of the min-mod function was suggested for the calculation of κ, $D_y u$ and $D_y(\kappa |\nabla|)$ at pixel position $(i+\frac{1}{2}, j)$, which realizes an edge-preserving characteristic. However, in this work, the max-mod function is proposed instead of the min-mod function for strengthening the connectivity principle to overcome the difficulty of fine structures in the sinogram and a proportionally large inpainting domain caused by the metal. The mentioned quantities can then be computed

$$\kappa_{(i+\frac{1}{2})} = \text{maxmod}\left(\kappa_{(i+1,j)}, \kappa_{(i,j)}\right) \tag{13}$$

$$D_y u_{(i+\frac{1}{2},j)} = \text{maxmod}(\frac{1}{2}(u_{(i+1,j+1)} - u_{(i+1,j-1)}), \frac{1}{2}(u_{(i,j+1)} - u_{(i,j-1)})) \tag{14}$$

with

$$\text{maxmod}(a,b) = \frac{\text{sign}(a) + \text{sign}(b)}{2}\text{max}(|a|, |b|) \tag{15}$$

$D_y(\kappa |\nabla|)$ can be calculated accordingly.

3   Results

In Fig.1 and in Fig. 2, the sinograms and the reconstructed images are shown before and after the metal artifacts have been corrected.

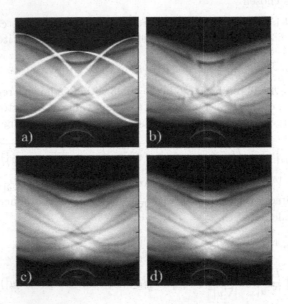

Fig. 1. Sinograms: a) without MAR, b) MAR with LI, c) MAR with EECSI, d) MAR with MEECSI

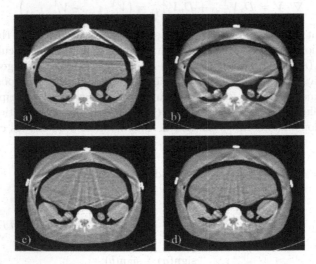

Fig. 2. Reconstructed images with FBP: a) without MAR, b) MAR with LI, c) MAR with EECSI, d)MAR with MEECSI

Table 1. Evaluation of the results. Sum of the absolute differences between the gray values and the reference values, normalized by the absolute sum of the gray values of the reference

	no MAR	MAR & LI	MAR & EECSI	MAR & MEECSI
Sinogram	0.539	0.042	0.028	0.023
Reconstructed image	0.281	0.149	0.151	0.144

4 Discussion

It can be seen in Fig. 1 that, compared to the LI, the EECSI fills the sinogram in a smoother and more accurate way. By modifying the numerical implementation with the max-mod function and the integration of an adaptive time step, a further improvement can be achieved for the MAR in CT. Fig. 2 shows that the MEECSI leads to superior results compared to the LI and the EECSI. For the evaluation process, the normalized absolute sum of differences between the considered sinograms as well as the reconstructed images and the ground truth are listed in Table 1. The values confirm the conclusions drawn from Fig. 1 and Fig. 2. It can be calculated that the MEECSI leads to an improvement of about sixteen percent in the sinogram and about five percent in the reconstructed image compared to the EECSI. As a limiting factor of the study the long iteration time can be mentioned. Additionally, the MEECSI algorithm needs to be further evaluated for different sizes of inpainting domains, i.e. metallic objects.

Acknowledgement. This work was supported by the European Union, the State of Schleswig-Holstein (MOIN CC: grant no. 122-09-053) and by the Graduate School for Computing in Medicine and Life Sciences funded by Germany's Excellence Initiative [DFG GSC 235/1].

References

1. Kalender WA, Hebel R, Ebersberger J. Reduction of CT artifacts caused by metallic implants. Radiology. 1987; p. 576-7.
2. Oehler M, Buzug TM. An image inpainting based surrogate data strategy for metal artifact reduction in CT images. In: Proc IFMBE; 2008. p. 651-4.
3. Oehler M, Buzug TM. Evaluation of surrogate data quality in sinogram-based CT metal artifact reduction. In: Proc SPIE; 2008. p. 1-10.
4. Chan T, Kang SH, Shen J. Euler's elastica and curvature based inpaintings. SIAM J Appl Math. 2002; p. 564-92.
5. Gu J, Zhang L, Yu G, et al. Metal artifact reduction in CT images through Euler's elastica and curvature based sinogram inpainting. In: Proc SPIE. vol. 6144; 2006. p. 65.
6. Bertalmio M, Sapira G, Caselles V, et al. Image inpainting. In: Proc SIGGRAPH; 2000. p. 417-24.

Sparse Principal Axes
Statistical Surface Deformation Models
for Respiration Analysis and Classification

Jakob Wasza[1], Sebastian Bauer[1], Sven Haase[1], Joachim Hornegger[1,2]

[1]Pattern Recognition Lab, Department of Computer Science
[2]Erlangen Graduate School in Advanced Optical Technologies (SAOT)
Friedrich-Alexander-Universität Erlangen-Nürnberg
jakob.wasza@cs.fau.de

Abstract. Detection, analysis and compensation of respiratory motion is a key issue for a variety of medical applications, such as tumor tracking in fractionated radiotherapy. One class of approaches aims for predicting the internal target movement by correlating intra-operatively captured body surface deformations to a pre-operatively learned deformable model. Here, range imaging (RI) devices assume a prominent role for dense and real-time surface acquisition due to their non-intrusive and markerless nature. In this work we present an RI based statistical model built upon sparse principal axes for body surface deformations induced by respiratory motion. In contrast to commonly employed global models based on principal component analysis, we exploit orthomax rotations in order to enable the differentiation between distinctive and local respiratory motion patterns such as thoracic and abdominal breathing. In a case study, we demonstrate our model's capability to capture dense respiration curves and the usage of our model for simulating realistic distinctive respiratory motion patterns.

1 Introduction

The internal movement of tissue, organs or anatomical structures due to respiratory motion is a crucial problem for a variety of medical applications, such as tomographic reconstruction or fractionated radiotherapy. For the latter, current systems employ gating techniques based on 1-D respiration signals acquired by dedicated sensors attached to the body surface [1] or non-intrusive range imaging (RI) devices [2]. Addressing the low duty cycle of these techniques, current research aims for real-time tumor tracking solutions that re-position the radiation beam dynamically with respect to the internal target motion. Here, the tumor movement is predicted by correlating intra-operatively captured 3-D body surface deformations with a pre-operatively trained 3-D volumetric model [3, 4, 5]. However, conventional approaches rely on global models obtained from standard principal component analysis that may fail to describe local deformations and that hinder an intuitive interpretation of the model's inherent variations. In this work, we propose an RI based statistical model for local and distinctive body surface deformations induced by respiratory motion. The basic idea of our approach is to relate local deformations to sparsity of the model's principal axes. Therefore, we build on the orthomax class of statistical methods to derive sparse principal modes of variation. Eventually, this enables the differentiation and intuitive interpretation of local respiratory motion patterns such as thoracic and abdominal breathing. In experiments on real data we demonstrate our model's ability to capture 1-D respiration curves of disjoint anatomical regions without the need to explicitly define the thorax and abdomen regions as proposed in [2]. We further show the usage of our model for simulating patient specific realistic respiratory motion patterns.

2   Materials and methods

The statistical model generation in this work relies on RI devices that deliver dense depth information of the captured body surface in real-time. We denote f as a range image with $f(\boldsymbol{x})$ holding the geometric depth at position $\boldsymbol{x} = (x, y)^T$ in the discrete 2-D sensor domain $\Omega : N \times M \mapsto \mathbb{R}$, where N and M denote the image width and height, respectively. Without loss of generality, any 2-D range image f can be linearized as a vector $\boldsymbol{g}$

$$f \equiv \boldsymbol{g} = \left(f(\boldsymbol{x}_1), \ldots, f(\boldsymbol{x}_{N \cdot M}) \right)^T, \quad \boldsymbol{g} \in \mathbb{R}^{N \cdot M} \tag{1}$$

We note that this naturally applies for all subregions $\widehat{\Omega} \subseteq \Omega$. A set of linearized RI training frames

$$\mathcal{G} = \{\boldsymbol{g}_i\}_{i=1}^K, \quad f_i \in \widehat{\Omega} \tag{2}$$

is then used to generate the proposed statistical model using the techniques described in Sec. 2.1 and 2.2. For visualization and analysis purposes, it is often desirable to transform a range image f into a triangulated 3-D point using the intrinsic RI device parameters. Fig. 1 illustrates a body surface acquired from a male subject using an off-the-shelf Microsoft Kinect RI device.

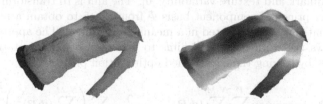

Fig. 1. Body surface of a male subject captured by the Microsoft Kinect RI device. RGB color overlay (left) and color coded depth information (right) where blue and red tones denote closeness and remoteness to the camera, respectively

2.1   Principal component analysis

Principal component analysis (PCA) is a commonly used technique for the extraction of variations along a given set of training samples and has proven to be a powerful tool in medical image analysis. As a first step, the training set $\mathcal{G}$ is arranged in the configuration matrix L

$$L = [g_1 - \overline{g}, \; g_2 - \overline{g}, \; \ldots, \; g_K - \overline{g}], \quad L \in \mathbb{R}^{N \cdot M \times K} \tag{3}$$

with the sample mean $\overline{g}$ defined as $\overline{g} = \frac{1}{K} \sum_{i=1}^{K} g_i$. Applying PCA to $\widetilde{L} = L^T L$ yields a set of eigenvectors $\{\widetilde{e}_i\}_{i=1}^{K}$ describing the principal modes of variation in the training data as $e_i = L\widetilde{e}_i$, $e_i \in \mathbb{R}^{N \cdot M}$. The mutually orthogonal modes of variation e_i are then sorted in descending order of their respective eigenvalues λ_i. By using the sample mean $\overline{g}$ and the modes that belong to the $P \ll K$ largest eigenvalues, a linear combination of the P principal modes of variation spans a subset of linearized RI frames composed of the given modes of variation

$$g^* = \overline{g} + \Phi b \tag{4}$$

Here, the principal component basis is stored in the matrix Φ defined as

$$\Phi = [e_1, \; e_2, \; \ldots, \; e_P], \quad \Phi \in \mathbb{R}^{N \cdot M \times P} \tag{5}$$

and $b \in \mathbb{R}^P$ defines the weighting factors for the modes of variation. We note that PCA yields an orthonormal system that maximizes the variance of the input data along the basis vectors. Hence, applying PCA to the training data usually results in global modes of variation as sparsity in the basis vectors is sacrificed for the sake of variance maximization. By design, this is a crucial drawback with respect to modeling of local and distinctive respiration patterns.

2.2   Orthomax rotations

The orthomax criterion is a technique that is commonly used in factor analysis. Among others, orthomax rotations where successfully employed in sparse modeling of landmark and texture variability [6]. The aim is to transform the global and abstract principal component basis Φ from Eq. 5 to obtain a more simple structure that can be interpreted in a meaningful manner. The approach in this paper follows the work of [6] and aims to find the orthomax rotation matrix $R_O \in \mathbb{R}^{P \times P}$ by solving the constrained optimization problem

$$R_O = \underset{R}{\operatorname{argmax}} \sum_{j=1}^{P} \sum_{i=1}^{N \cdot M} (\Phi R)_{ij}^4 - \frac{\gamma}{N \cdot M} \sum_{j=1}^{P} \left(\sum_{i=1}^{N \cdot M} (\Phi R)_{ij}^2 \right)^2 \tag{6}$$

subject to $R^T = R^{-1}$ and $\det(R) = 1$. Furthermore, R_{ij} denotes the element in the ith row and j^{th} column of R. The orthomax type is denoted by γ. This work investigates the varimax rotation only ($\gamma = 1$), thus allowing to solve

Eq. 6 by using an iterative scheme employing singular value decompositions [6]. To substantiate the use of varimax rotations in this work, we note that R_O transforms the principal component basis Φ from Eq. 5 as $\Phi_O = \Phi R_O$ in a way that maximizes the variances in the squared variation loadings across all modes. Inherently, this favors sparse modes of variation with several loadings close to zero and others large. This coincides with the aim of this paper to relate local and distinctive respiratory motion patterns to sparsity of the model's modes.

2.3 Experiments

For our experiments, we captured RI data from four male subjects using a Microsoft Kinect structured light sensor at 30 Hz. To account for sensor noise we perform edge-preserving denoising. The subjects where asked to perform thoracic, abdominal and regular breathing over several respiration cycles. In order to restrict the statistical model to the torso region $\widehat{\Omega}$ only, we applied a fast marching segmentation [7] on the acquired range images. The segmented RI stream of thoracic and abdominal breathing is then sampled with a temporal resolution of 300 ms to form the training set $\mathcal{G}$ from Eq. 2. We then performed standard PCA as explained in Sec. 2.1 yielding Φ with the number of modes P chosen such that the model accounts for $\geq 99\%$ of the total variance in the training data. Finally, as proposed in Sec. 2.2, the sparse varimax model Φ_O is built upon the standard PCA approach. As application scenarios, we demonstrate our model's capability to simulate selective respiratory motion patterns and to generate 1-D respiration curves of disjoint anatomical regions. For the latter, we project instantaneous RI frames g onto the model's principal axes e_i yielding a scalar value $\alpha_i = g^T e_i$ that can be interpreted as a 1-D respiration surrogate.

3 Results

For each of the four subjects of this study, two principal modes of variation accounting for $\geq 99\%$ of the total variance were identified. Fig. 2 depicts the two principal modes of variation as obtained from standard PCA and the varimax model. The PCA based modes exhibit global and meaningless variations, whereas the principal axes obtained from the orthomax model feature local deformations that are highly correlated to thoracic and abdominal breathing, respectively. Simulated respiratory motion patterns as obtained from our models are depicted in Fig. 3. The varimax model enables the selective simulation of thoracic and abdominal breathing whereas deformations obtained from standard PCA are of no relevance with respect to the human respiration system. Respiration curves generated with our models are illustrated in Fig. 4. For abdominal breathing, the first mode obtained from the orthomax model exhibits a smaller total variation and amplitude compared to the standard PCA approach. A similar behavior is observable for thoracic breathing and the second mode. This indicates that a varimax model is better suited for analysis of local and disjunct motion patterns. With regard to regular breathing, the PCA modes are not interpretable in an intuitive manner. In contrast, the varimax modes indicate that the subject mainly performed abdominal respiration with some thoracic movement superimposed.

4 Discussion

We have shown that the orthomax class of statistical methods can be used to generate a model for local surface deformations induced by respiratory motion. Our experimental study revealed that, in contrast to a standard PCA approach, distinctive and local respiratory motion patterns can be analyzed and classified. However, we note that orthomax methods only represent a small class of sta-

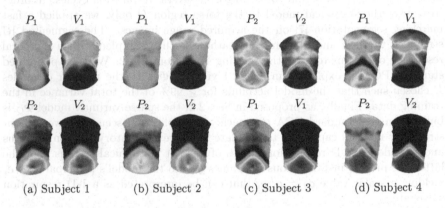

(a) Subject 1   (b) Subject 2   (c) Subject 3   (d) Subject 4

Fig. 2. Modes of variation obtained from standard PCA (P) and varimax rotation (V). The subscripts 1 and 2 denote the first and second principal variation, respectively. The magnitude of variation is color coded from blue (low loadings) to red (high loadings)

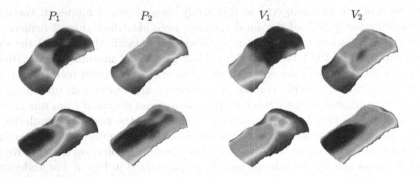

Fig. 3. Effect of varying the modes of variation for Subject 4. The weights are increased from top ($-\sqrt{\lambda_i}$) to bottom ($+\sqrt{\lambda_i}$) for the individual modes. Depth information is color coded where blue and red tones denote closeness and remoteness, respectively

Fig. 4. Using the statistical model to generate 1-D respiration curves. For the varimax model, the first principal mode accounts for thoracic and the second mode for abdominal breathing

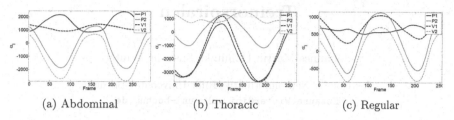

(a) Abdominal   (b) Thoracic   (c) Regular

tistical methods for respiration analysis. Therefore, ongoing work investigates alternative statistical methods and non-linear techniques for model generation.

Acknowledgement. J. Wasza and S. Bauer gratefully acknowledge the support by the European Regional Development Fund (ERDF) and the Bayerisches Staatsministerium für Wirtschaft, Infrastruktur, Verkehr und Technologie (StM-WIVT), in the context of the R&D program IuK Bayern under Grant No. IUK338. S. Haase is supported by the Deutsche Forschungsgemeinschaft (DFG) under Grant No. HO 1791/7-1.

References

1. Keall PJ, Mageras GS, Balter JM, et al. The management of respiratory motion in radiation oncology, report of AAPM Task Group 76. Med Phys. 2006;33(10):3874–900.
2. Müller K, Schaller C, Penne J, et al. Surface-based respiratory motion classification and verification. Proc BVM. 2009; p. 257–61.
3. Fayad H, Pan T, Roux C, et al. A patient specific respiratory model based on 4D CT data and a time of flight camera (TOF). In: Proc IEEE NSS/MIC; 2009. p. 2594–8.
4. Hoogeman M, Prévost JB, Nuyttens J, et al. Clinical accuracy of the respiratory tumor tracking system of the cyberknife: assessment by analysis of log files. Int J Radiat Oncol Biol Phys. 2009;74(1):297–303.
5. Ehrhardt J, Werner R, Schmidt-Richberg A, et al. Statistical modeling of 4D respiratory lung motion using diffeomorphic image registration. IEEE Trans Med Imaging. 2011;30(2):251–65.
6. Stegmann MB, Sjöstrand K, Larsen R. Sparse modeling of landmark and texture variability using the orthomax criterion. In: Proc SPIE. vol. 6144; 2006. p. 61441G1–61441G.12.
7. Sethian JA. Level Set Methods and Fast Marching Methods. 2nd ed. Cambridge University Press; 1999.

Merkmale aus zweidimensionalen Orientierungshistogrammen zur Beurteilung von Tremorspiralen

Johannes-Martin Dolnitzki, Susanne Winter

Institut für Neuroinformatik, Ruhr-Universität Bochum
Susanne.Winter@ini.ruhr-uni-bochum.de

Kurzfassung. Das Ausmaß von krankhaftem Tremor kann anhand einfacher Zeichentests, bei denen der Patient eine Spirale auf einem Blatt Papier zeichnet, beurteilt werden. In dieser Arbeit wurden zweidimensionale Orientierungshistogramme für solche Tremorzeichnungen erstellt. Die Untersuchung von Merkmalen, welche aus diesen Histogrammen berechnet wurden ergab, dass einige der Merkmale mit dem Schweregrad des Tremors korellieren und somit eine Beurteilung des Tremors anhand dieser Merkmale möglich ist. Um das Verhalten der Merkmale systematisch untersuchen zu können, wurden zusätzlich künstliche Spiralbilder erzeugt, die Zeichnungen mit Tremor unterschiedlicher Amplitude und Frequenz simulieren.

1 Einleitung

Als Tremor wird das rythmische Zittern von Muskelgruppen bezeichnet. Neben dem physiologischen Tremor gibt es auch krankhaftes Zittern, welches zum Beispiel bei der Parkinsonerkrankung auftritt. Die Diagnostik und Einteilung von Tremortypen und Schweregraden erfolgt klinisch anhand unterschiedlicher Methoden [1, 2]. Dabei erfordern z. B. die Nutzung eines Digitizing Tablets [3] oder die Elektromyographie [4] das entsprechende Instrumentarium.

Eine wesentlich einfachere und kostengünstigere Methode ist ein Zeichentest, bei dem der Patient eine Spirale auf ein Blatt Papier zeichnet. Nach der Methode von Bain und Findley [1] wird die Stärke des Tremors anhand der Zeichnungen visuell beurteilt und in eine von 10 Stufen eingeteilt. Um eine automatische Auswertung zu ermöglichen wurden Methoden entwickelt, die auf digitalisierten Spiralzeichnungen eine automatische Analyse der Tremoramplitude vornehmen [5]. Dieses Verfahren erfordert allerdings eine automatische Verfolgung des Zeichengangs entlang der Spiralwindungen. Probleme ergaben sich bei dieser Methode, wenn der Tremor so stark ist, dass sich Überkreuzungen in den Linien ergeben, oder aber Lücken in der Zeichnung entstehen. In dieser Arbeit wurde daher einen Ansatz verfolgt, der unabhängig von diesen Störungen in der Lage ist, eine Beurteilung der Tremorstärke vorzunehmen. Dabei wird das Bild als Gesamtes verarbeitet ohne die Spiralwindungen berücksichtigen zu müssen.

2   Material und Methoden

2.1   Daten

Als Bilddaten lagen eine Reihe eingescannter Spiralzeichnungen von Patienten mit unterschiedlich ausgeprägtem Tremor vor. Die Verteilung der Daten bezüglich des Schweregrades des Tremors war sehr inhomogen, so dass eine Abbildung auf die von Bain und Findley [1] eingeführte Skala von 1 bis 10 nicht vorgenommen werden konnte. Die Zeichnungen wurden daher vier Gruppen verschiedener Schweregrade, mit einer Gruppengröße von jeweils 10, zugeordnet. Dabei entsprach die Gruppe 1 in etwa den Schweregraden 0 bis 2 der Skala von Bain und Findley, die Gruppe 2 den Schweregraden 3 bis 4, die Gruppe 3 den Schweregraden 5 bis 6 und die Gruppe 4 den Schweregraden 7 bis 9 (Abb. 1, oben). Die Zeichnungen wurden nach einem Einscanvorgang in Form von Bitmap-Dateien in Schwarz/Weiß mit einer Auflösung von 1664 × 2338 Pixeln gespeichert.

Zusätzlich wurden künstliche Spiralzeichnungen erstellt, indem eine archimedische Spirale mit einer Sinusschwingung überlagert wurde. Dies geschah unter der Annahme, dass die Winkelgeschwindigkeit der Spirale beim Zeichnen konstant ist und das resultierende Spiralbild von derselben Größe ist, wie eine Originalzeichnung.

2.2   Zweidimensionales Orientierungshistogramm und Merkmale

Auf den Bildern wurde mit einer Sobelfilterung der Gradient und nachfolgend die Orientierung des Gradienten bestimmt. Es erfolgte eine Einteilung in 8 verschiedene Sektoren, in denen jeweils ein Histogramm über die verschiedenen

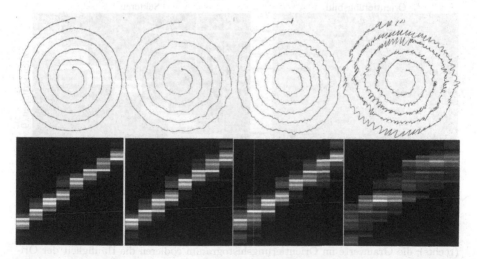

Abb. 1. Spiralzeichnungen und die dazugehörigen zweidimensionalen Orientierungshistogramme; Beispiele von links nach rechts für die Gruppen 1 bis 4

Orientierung berechnet wurde (Abb. 2). In jedem Sektor wurde die Orientierung auf einen Bereich der Größe 180° abgebildet. Das Zentrum dieses Bereichs entsprach der mittleren Orientierung einer Spirale ohne Tremor, in dem jeweiligen Sektor. Die 8 Histogramme wurden zu einem 2D-Orientierungshistogramm zusammengefasst, auf dem nachfolgend Merkmale berechnet wurden.

Da unterschiedliche Ausprägungen der Abweichung der Werte von der Diagonalen im 2D-Orientierungshistogramm, abhängig vom Grad des Tremors, zu erwarten sind, wurden Merkmale erzeugt, die diese Verteilungen beschreiben. In Anlehnung an die Texturmerkmale Entropie, Energie, Kontrast und Homogenität, wie sie auf Cooccurrence Matrizen berechnet werden [6], wurden die im Folgenden dargestellten Merkmale gewählt. Dabei beschreibt $H_{i,j}$ den normierten Histogrammeintrag

$$M_{\mathrm{ERG}} = \sum_i \sum_j H_{i,j}^2$$

Die Energie M_{ERG} ist ein Maß, welches die Stärke der Konzentration auf wenige Werte beschreibt

$$M_{\mathrm{ENT}} = -\sum_i \sum_j H_{i,j} \cdot \log(H_{i,j})$$

Die Entropie M_{ENT} beschreibt den Informationsgehalt in einem Bild

$$M_{\mathrm{KON}} = \sum_i \sum_j |i - j| \cdot H_{i,j}^2$$

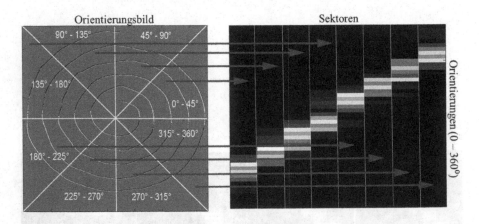

Abb. 2. Orientierungsbild einer Spiralzeichnung mit Aufteilung in 8 Sektoren (links) und der jeweiligen Zuordnung (Pfeile) zu den Spalten im 2D-Orientierungshistogramm (rechts); die Grauwerte im Orientierungshistogramm codieren die Häufigkeit der Orientierungen

Der Kontrast M_{KON} beschreibt, wie stark die Werte von der Hauptdiagonalen abweichen

$$M_{\text{HOM}} = \sum_i \sum_j \frac{H_{i,j}}{1 + |i - j|}$$

Die Homogenität M_{HOM} ist am größten bei geringen Abweichungen der Werte von der Diagonalen.

3 Ergebnisse

Die Untersuchungen wurden einerseits auf den künstlichen Spiralen und andererseits auf den realen Zeichnungen von Patienten durchgeführt. In Abb. 1 sind vier Beispiele der verschiedenen Gruppen mit unterschiedlicher Tremorstärke und jeweils das dazugehörige zweidimensionale Orientierungshistogramm abgebildet. Abb. 3 zeigt im Vergleich zwei künstliche und zwei reale Spiralen mit unterschiedlicher Tremorstärke. Es ist zu erkennen, dass sich bei vorhandenem Tremor die Einträge im Histogramm stärker um die Hauptdiagonale streuen, je stärker der Tremor in den Zeichnungen ausgeprägt ist.

Anhand der Bilder mit den künstlichen Spiralen wurde untersucht, wie sich die einzelnen Merkmale bei Veränderung der Parameter Frequenz und Amplitude des Tremors darstellen. Bei gleichbleibender Amplitude von 4 mm wurde die Frequenz des Tremors von 0 Hz bis 80 Hz in Schritten von 20 Hz variiert. Die Amplitude wurde, bei einer Frequenz von 30 Hz, mit Schrittweiten von je 2 mm von 0 mm bis 8 mm verändert. Es zeigte sich, dass M_{KON} und M_{ENT} sowohl bei Erhöhung der Amplitude, als auch bei Erhöhung der Frequenz anstiegen. Im Gegenzug dazu nahmen M_{ERG} und M_{HOM} ab (Tab. 1).

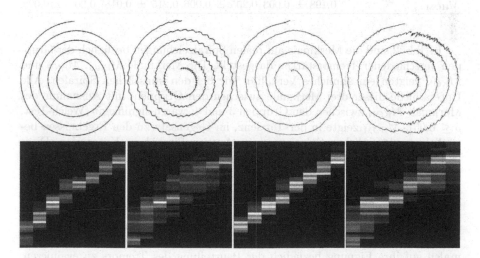

Abb. 3. Spiralzeichnungen und die dazugehörigen zweidimensionalen Orientierungshistogramme; links zwei künstlich erstellte Spiralen; rechts zwei reale Spiralen

Tabelle 1. Merkmale berechnet auf künstlichen Spiralen. Es wurde einmal die Frequenz des Tremors in 20 Hz Schritten erhöht (oben) mit einer festen Amplitude von 4 mm und einmal wurde die Amplitude des Tremors in 2 mm Schritten erhöht (unten) bei einer festen Frequenz von 30 Hz

Merkmal \ Frequenz	0 Hz	20 Hz	40 Hz	60 Hz	80 Hz
M_{ERG}	0,026	0,022	0,019	0,018	0,017
M_{ENT}	1,69	1,80	1,88	1,92	1,94
M_{KON}	33,18	35,96	39,48	42,72	45,10
M_{HOM}	0,179	0,179	0,175	0,170	0,166

Merkmal \ Amplitude	0 mm	2 mm	4 mm	6 mm	8 mm
M_{ERG}	0,026	0,024	0,021	0,020	0,019
M_{ENT}	1,69	1,75	1,84	1,88	1,90
M_{KON}	33,18	34,50	37,58	39,95	42,51
M_{HOM}	0,179	0,180	0,177	0,173	0,170

Tabelle 2. Mittelwerte und Standardabweichungen der Merkmale, berechnet auf verschiedenen Gruppen von Tremorspiralen mit unterschiedlicher Tremorstärke; Gruppe 1: kein bis wenig Tremor; Gruppe 4: starker Tremor

Merkmal \ Gruppe	1	2	3	4
M_{ERG}	0,025 ± 0,005	0,020 ± 0,001	0,015 ± 0,002	0,014 ± 0,003
M_{ENT}	1,69 ± 0,01	1,81 ± 0,03	1,94 ± 0,04	1,99 ± 0,06
M_{KON}	32,71 ± 0,41	35,28 ± 0,99	43,29 ± 3,95	52,31 ± 9,17
M_{HOM}	0,198 ± 0,003	0,205 ± 0,006	0,215 ± 0,018	0,206 ± 0,022

In Tab. 2 sind die Merkmale auf realen Spiralzeichnungen bezüglich der Gruppen verschiedener Tremorstärken dargestellt. Die Merkmale M_{ERG}, M_{ENT} und M_{KON} zeigten ein ähnliches Verhalten wie bei den künstlichen Spiralen. Alle Unterschiede dieser drei Merkmale zwischen den Gruppen, mit Ausnahme des Merkmals M_{KON} zwischen den Gruppen 3 und 4, waren signifikant (Welch-Test, $p \leq 0,05$). M_{HOM} zeigte in der Tendenz, im Gegensatz zu den Ergebnissen bezüglich der künstlichen Spiralen, einen Anstieg für höhere Kategorien. Diese Unterschiede waren allerdings nicht signifikant.

4   Diskussion und Ausblick

Die erstellten künstlichen Spiralen eigneten sich sehr gut dazu, echte Spiralen mit Tremor unterschiedlicher Stärke nachzubilden, um darauf die Güte von Merkmalen auf ihre Eignung bezüglich der Beurteilung des Tremors zu evaluieren. Die auf den künstlichen und den realen Bildern berechneten zweidimensionalen Histogramme zeigen große Ähnlichkeiten.

Bei den Merkmalen, die auf den 2D-Orientierungshistogrammen von künstlichen Spiralen gerechnet wurden, fiel M_{ERG} mit wachsendem Tremor (wachsender Frequenz oder Amplitude) wie erwartet ab, da sich die Werte weniger stark auf die Diagonale konzentrierten. Die Entropie M_{ERG} stieg bei stärkerem Tremor an, da durch die stärker werdende Unordnung im Bild der Informationsgehalt geringer wurde. Ebenfalls stieg M_{KON} an, da sich der Kontrast bezüglich der Orientierungen der Kanten in den Bildern erhöhte. Aus demselben Grund nahm die Homogenität M_{HOM} ab.

Die Ergebnisse auf den realen Spiralbildern zeigten einen ähnlichen Verlauf wie die der künstlichen Spiralen. Das Merkmal der Homogenität M_{HOM} lieferte hier keine zur Unterscheidung des Tremorgrades geeigneten Ergebnisse, aber die drei anderen Merkmale zeigten zwischen allen Gruppen signifikante Unterschiede. Auch wenn diese Merkmale alleine noch keine lineare Klassifikation zulassen, so erscheinen sie doch geeignet die Ausprägung eines Tremors abzubilden.

Die Berechnung der hier vorgestellten Merkmale war störungsfrei auf allen Spiralbildern möglich. Die Ergebnisse erscheinen bezüglich der Beurteilung der Tremorstärke nutzbringend, unabhängig davon, ob die Bilder Störungen, wie Unterbrechungen in den Zeichnungen oder Überschneidungen benachbarter Spiralgänge, aufwiesen.

Abschließend lässt sich sagen, dass mit der Methode der Merkmalsberechnung auf 2D-Orientierungshistogrammen eine Möglichkeit gefunden wurde, automatisch das Ausmaß eines Tremors in Spiralzeichnungen zu beurteilen, ohne zuvor ein störungsanfälliges Abwickeln der Spirale durchführen zu müssen. Gegenstand weiterer Forschung wird es sein, eine automatische Klassifikation anhand von Merkmalskombinationen zu untersuchen.

Danksagung. Wir bedanken uns bei PH Kraus, Abteilung Neurologie des St. Josef-Hospitals in Bochum, für die freundliche Überlassung der Bilder.

Literaturverzeichnis

1. Bain PG, Findley LJ. Assessing Tremor Severity: A Clinical Handbook. Smith-Gordon, London; 1993.
2. Bain PG, Findley LJ, Atchison P, et al. Assessing tremor severity. J Neurol Neurosurg Psych. 1993;56:868–73.
3. Pullman SL. Spiral analysis: a new technique for measuring tremor with a digitizing tablet. Mov Disord. 1998;13(Supplement 3):85–9.
4. Milanov I. Electromyographic differentiation of tremors. Clin Neurophysiol. 2001;112(9):1626–32.
5. Kraus PH, Hoffmann A. Spiralometry: computerized assessment of tremor amplitude on the basis of spiral drawing. Mov Disord. 2010;25(13):2164–70.
6. Haralick RM, Shapiro LG. Computer and Robot Vision. Addison Wesley Verlag; 1993.

Regularisierung lokaler Deformation im probabilistischen Active Shape Model

Matthias Kirschner, Stefan Wesarg

Graphisch-Interaktive Systeme, TU Darmstadt
matthias.kirschner@gris.tu-darmstadt.de

Kurzfassung. Zur robusten und präzisen Segmentierung von Organen in medizinischen Bilddaten werden oft Varianten des Active Shape Models (ASM) verwendet, die über eine Energieminimierung einen Kompromiss zwischen Bildinformation und Vorwissen über die zu erwartende Organform bestimmen. Im probabilistischen ASM (PASM) wird die Plausibilität einer Form mit Hilfe einer Wahrscheinlichkeitsverteilung bewertet. Da diese lediglich globale, nicht aber lokale Formvariation ausreichend modelliert, kann der PASM ungleichmäßige und damit unplausible Segmentierungskonturen erzeugen. In dieser Arbeit wird der PASM um ein lokales Deformationsmodell erweitert, welches zu glatten Segmentierungskonturen führt. Das lokale Deformationsmodell wird an einem linearen PASM zur Lebersegmentierung und einem nichtlinearen PASM zur Wirbelsegmentierung evaluiert. Die Ergebnisse zeigen, dass die Erweiterung quantitativ wie qualitativ bessere Segmentierungen liefert.

1 Einleitung

In der medizinischen Bildverarbeitung wird häufig Vorwissen über die Form eines Organs verwendet, um dieses trotz geringen Kontrastes zu benachbarten Strukturen und geringer Bildqualität robust zu segmentieren. Das Vorwissen kann durch ein landmarkenbasiertes statistisches Formmodell (SFM) beschrieben werden, das die typische Variation eines Organs aus einer Menge von Trainingsdaten gelernt hat. Als SFM-basierter Segmentierungsalgorithmus hat sich das Active Shape Model (ASM) [1] etabliert, das zur Segmentierung einer Vielzahl von anatomischen Strukturen erfolgreich eingesetzt wurde.

Zur robusten Segmentierung ist ein spezifisches SFM notwendig, welches unplausible Organformen während des Segmentierungsprozesses verbietet. Anderseits muss das SFM flexibel eingesetzt werden, so dass auch Organe präzise segmentiert werden können, die leichte Abweichungen von den Trainingsdaten aufweisen. Da das klassische ASM-Verfahren zu restriktiv ist, wird die Genauigkeit oft durch eine nachgeschaltete Freiformdeformation verbessert [2]. Alternativ dazu wurden flexible Varianten des ASM entwickelt, die einen Energieminimierungsansatz verfolgen [3, 4], welcher Bildinformation und Vorwissen über die Organform mittels einer Energiefunktion gegeneinander abwägt.

Wir haben kürzlich [5, 6] einen probabilistischen ASM (PASM) vorgestellt, welcher auf dem Energieminimierungsansatz beruht. Im Gegensatz zu anderen

Verfahren [3, 4] ist die dort verwendete Formenergie aus einer Wahrscheinlichkeitsfunktion abgeleitet, die die Plausibilität einer Organform beurteilt. Dadurch lassen sich in den PASM nichtlineare SFMs integrieren – beispielsweise auf Basis von Kernel Principal Component Analysis (KPCA) [6] – so dass sich Organe mit komplexer Formvariation spezifischer modellieren lassen. Der PASM erlaubt jedoch unplausible lokale Deformationen, die sich in einer ungleichmäßigen Segmentierungskontur widerspiegeln (Abb. 1).

In dieser Arbeit wird der PASM um ein lokales Deformationsmodell erweitert, welches die Energieminimierung derart regularisiert, dass er glatte Segmentierungskonturen erzeugt. Die Erweiterung wird an einem linearen PASM zur Lebersegmentierung und an einem nichtlinearen PASM zur Wirbelsegmentierung quantitativ und qualitativ evaluiert.

2 Material und Methoden

Wir betrachten die Segmentierung dreidimensionaler medizinischer Bilddaten mit Hilfe des ASMs. Zunächst wird initial das Durchschnittsmesh des SFMs grob auf die zu segmentierende Struktur im Bild platziert. Das Mesh sei repräsentiert durch N Landmarken $x^{(i)} \in \mathbb{R}^3$, die über eine Triangulierung miteinander verbunden sind. Die Konkatenation der Landmarken zu einem Vektor bezeichnen wir mit $x = (x^{(1)}, \ldots, x^{(N)}) \in \mathbb{R}^{3N}$. Der ASM passt das Mesh iterativ an das Bild an: In jeder Iteration wird zunächst in der Nachbarschaft jeder Landmarke i mit Hilfe eines Erscheinungsmodells nach einem optimalen Merkmal im Bild gesucht, und die Landmarke wird auf die Position $\hat{x}^{(i)}$ dieses Merkmals verschoben. Die Güte des optimalen Merkmals wird vom Erscheinungsmodell durch ein Gewicht $w_i > 0$ abgeschätzt. Da das deformierte Mesh nicht notwendigerweise eine plausible Organform hat, wird es anschließend durch das SFM beschränkt.

2.1 Berechnung plausibler Formen durch Energieminimierung

Im PASM erfolgt die Beschränkung der Segmentierung auf plausible Formen durch Minimierung der Funktion

$$\tilde{E}(x; \hat{x}, w) = \alpha \cdot \tilde{E}_{\text{Bild}}(x; \hat{x}, w) + E_{\text{Form}}(x) \tag{1}$$

Dabei ist $\tilde{E}_{\text{Bild}}(x; \hat{x}, w)$ die Bildenergie, $E_{\text{Form}}(x)$ die Formenergie und α ein freier Parameter. Die Energieminimierung findet im Koordinatensystem des SFMs

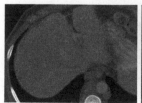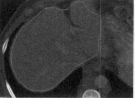

Abb. 1. Der PASM kann ungleichmäßige Segmentierungskonturen generieren (links), die durch Integration des lokalen Deformationsmodells verhindert werden (rechts)

statt. Die rigide Transformation zwischen diesem Koordinatensystem und dem Koordinatensystem des Bildes wird wie im klassischen ASM berechnet [1].

Im linearen SFM kann die Formvariabilität durch eine multivariate Gaussverteilung beschrieben werden. Als Formenergie wird die negative Log-Wahrscheinlichkeit (unter Vernachlässigung konstanter Terme) verwendet, also

$$E_{\text{Form}}(\boldsymbol{x}) = \sum_{i=1}^{t} \frac{b_i}{\lambda_i} + \frac{S-t-1}{\sum_{i=t+1}^{S-1} \lambda_i} \|\boldsymbol{r}\|^2 \qquad (2)$$

wobei die Form $\boldsymbol{x}$ zerlegt wird in $\boldsymbol{x} = \bar{\boldsymbol{x}} + \boldsymbol{P}\boldsymbol{b} + \boldsymbol{r}$. Hierbei ist $\bar{\boldsymbol{x}} = \frac{1}{N}\sum_{i=1}^{S}\boldsymbol{x}_i$ die aus der Trainingsmenge $\mathcal{S} = \{\boldsymbol{x}_1,\ldots,\boldsymbol{x}_S\}$ berechnete Durchschnittsform, $\boldsymbol{P} \in \mathbb{R}^{3n \times t}$ die Matrix der ersten t Eigenvektoren der Kovarianzmatrix $\boldsymbol{C} = \frac{1}{S-1}\sum_{i=1}^{S}(\boldsymbol{x}_i - \bar{\boldsymbol{x}})(\boldsymbol{x}_i - \bar{\boldsymbol{x}})^T$, $\boldsymbol{b} = \boldsymbol{P}^T(\boldsymbol{x} - \bar{\boldsymbol{x}})$ der Vektor der Principal Components (PCs), und $\lambda_1 \geq \ldots \geq \lambda_{S-1}$ die von 0 verschiedenen Eigenwerte von $\boldsymbol{C}$. Die Formenergie für ein nichtlineares, KPCA-basiertes SFM hat die gleiche Struktur, wobei die PCs b_i durch die Kernel-PCs β_i und $\|\boldsymbol{r}\|^2$ durch die Norm des Residualvektors im KPCA-Merkmalsraum ersetzt werden [6].

Über die Bestrafung der Norm von $\boldsymbol{r}$ erlaubt der PASM, den von den ersten t Eigenvektoren aufgespannten Vektorraum kontrolliert zu verlassen, so dass eine bessere Anpassung an Bildmerkmale möglich wird. Der Vektor $\boldsymbol{r}$ kann eine konsistente Bewegung benachbarter Landmarken zur tatsächlichen Organkontur, oder aber das Ausreißen einzelner Landmarken beschreiben. Solange beide Deformationen die gleiche Norm besitzen, ist ihre Formenergie identisch. Da die letztgenannte Deformation nicht ausgeschlossen ist, können bei Verwendung des PASM daher ungleichmäßige und somit unplausible Segmentierungskonturen auftreten. Um dies zu verhindern, muss das Modell um die zusätzliche Annahme, dass Organkonturen überwiegend glatt sind, erweitert werden. Eine Glättung mit dem Laplace-Verfahren nach der Energieminimierung [6] ist methodisch nicht sauber, da die Glattheitsannahme nicht mit den anderen Annahmen simultan betrachtet wird, und kann zudem mit einem ungewollten Volumenverlust einhergehen.

Wir schlagen stattdessen vor, die Energiefunktion um einen lokalen Modellterm $E_{\text{Lokal}}(\boldsymbol{x})$ zu ergänzen. Die neue Energiefunktion ist dann durch

$$E(\boldsymbol{x}; \hat{\boldsymbol{x}}, \boldsymbol{w}) = \alpha \cdot (E_{\text{Bild}}(\boldsymbol{x}; \hat{\boldsymbol{x}}, \boldsymbol{w}) + E_{\text{Lokal}}(\boldsymbol{x}; \boldsymbol{w})) + E_{\text{Form}}(\boldsymbol{x}) \qquad (3)$$

gegeben, wobei $E_{\text{Bild}}(\boldsymbol{x}; \hat{\boldsymbol{x}}, \boldsymbol{w})$ eine modifizierte Bildenergie ist.

2.2 Lokale Modellenergie

Zur Regularisierung der Deformation führen wir als zusätzliche Modellbedingung ein, dass sich eine Landmarke nicht weit von seinen Nachbarn entfernen darf. Dies wird durch den lokalen Modellterm

$$E_{\text{Lokal}}(\boldsymbol{x}; \boldsymbol{w}) = \sum_{i=1}^{N} \sum_{j \in \mathcal{N}(i)} \hat{w}_i^2 \|\boldsymbol{x}^{(i)} - \boldsymbol{x}^{(j)} - \boldsymbol{\mu}^{(i)}\|^2 \qquad (4)$$

erreicht. Hier bezeichne $\mathcal{N}(i)$ die Menge der Indizes der Landmarken, die mit Landmarke i durch eine Meshkante verbunden sind. Für jede Landmarke i wird der Offset $\boldsymbol{\mu}_i$ aus den Trainingsdaten gelernt, indem die durchschnittliche Position von i relativ zum Mittelpunkt der Nachbarn gebildet wird, das heißt

$$\boldsymbol{\mu}^{(i)} = \bar{\boldsymbol{x}}^{(i)} - \frac{1}{|\mathcal{N}(i)|} \sum_{j \in \mathcal{N}(i)} \bar{\boldsymbol{x}}^{(i)} \qquad (5)$$

Durch die Offsets $\boldsymbol{\mu}^{(i)}$ wird erreicht, dass die Segmentierungsergebnisse an der Landmarke i tendenziell eine ähnliche Krümmung haben wie in den Trainingsdaten beobachtet. Die Gewichte $\hat{w}_i$ sind gegeben durch $\hat{w}_i = C \cdot (w_{\max} - w_i + w_{\min})$ mit $w_{\max} = \max_{k=1...N} w_k$ und $w_{\min} = \min_{k=1...N} w_k$. Der Glättungseffekt schwächt sich also bei hohem Texturgewicht w_i ab. Durch den Normalisierungsfaktor $C = \sum_{k=1}^{N} \frac{w_k}{w_{\max} - w_k + w_{\min}}$ gilt $\sum_{k=1}^{N} w_k = \sum_{k=1}^{N} \hat{w}_k$, so dass Bildenergie und lokale Modellenergie automatisch balanciert sind.

2.3 Modifikation der Bildenergie

Die lokale Modellenergie bevorzugt tendenziell kleiner skalierte Formen. Dies führt zu einem Schrumpfen des Meshes, wenn die lokale Modellenergie mit der Bildenergie $\tilde{E}_{\text{Bild}}(\boldsymbol{x}; \hat{\boldsymbol{x}}, \boldsymbol{w}) = \sum_{i=1}^{N} w_i \|\boldsymbol{x}^{(i)} - \hat{\boldsymbol{x}}^{(i)}\|^2$ kombiniert wird, die wir in vorherigen Arbeiten [5, 6] verwendeten. Dadurch wird bei der Rücktransformation vom Modell- ins Bildkoordinatensystem ein zu kleiner Skalierungsfaktor verwendet, so dass das Organ untersegmentiert wird. Wir schlagen daher

$$E_{\text{Bild}}(\boldsymbol{x}; \hat{\boldsymbol{x}}, \boldsymbol{w}) = \sum_{i=1}^{N} \|w_i(\boldsymbol{x}^{(i)} - \hat{\boldsymbol{x}}^{(i)}) + \sum_{j \in \mathcal{N}(i)} w_j(\boldsymbol{x}^{(j)} - \hat{\boldsymbol{x}}^{(j)})\|^2 \qquad (6)$$

als neue Bildenergie vor, die die gewichtete Summe der Abstände benachbarter Landmarken von ihren jeweils optimalen Bildmerkmalen bestraft. Die Idee hierbei ist, das immer, wenn eine Landmarke während der Optimierung in eine bestimmte Richtung wandert, Kräfte auf die benachbarten Landmarken wirken, die diese genau in die entgegengesetzte Richtung drücken. Wandert eine Landmarke also in Richtung des Ursprungs, gleichen die Nachbarn den hierbei entstehenden Volumenverlust durch eine entgegengesetzte Bewegung wieder aus.

2.4 Evaluation

In der Evaluation setzen wir den PASM mit und ohne lokalem Deformationsmodell jeweils zur Segmentierung von Lebern und Wirbeln ein, um beide Varianten miteinander zu vergleichen. Bei der Lebersegmentierung verwenden wir ein lineares SFM. Wir haben insgesamt 34 Trainings- und Testdaten, die wir im Leave-One-Out-Verfahren segmentieren. Bei der Wirbelsegmentierung verwenden wir ein KPCA-basiertes SFM mit Kern $k(\boldsymbol{x}, \boldsymbol{y}) = \exp(\frac{\|\boldsymbol{x}-\boldsymbol{y}\|^2}{2\sigma^2})$, das aus 23 Thorax- und Lendenwirbeln (Th10-Th12; L1-L3) von insgesamt fünf Patienten

332 Kirschner & Wesarg

Tabelle 1. Segmentierungsergebnisse des PASM mit und ohne lokalem Deformations-modell. Die Tabelle zeigt Durchschnittswerte und Standardabweichung (SA)

		VÜF [%]		DOA [mm]		HD [mm]	
	Initialisierung	21.81	SA: 8.38	4.42	SA: 2.15	35.36	SA: 14.65
Leber	PASM	9.74	SA: 2.93	1.73	SA: 0.75	27.20	SA: 11.57
	PASM-lokal	9.00	SA: 2.85	1.71	SA: 0.81	30.27	SA: 12.60
	Initialisierung	60.66	SA: 7.01	3.83	SA: 0.82	16.40	SA: 2.97
Wirbel	PASM	17.91	SA: 5.41	0.61	SA: 0.28	7.64	SA: 3.73
	PASM-lokal	16.97	SA: 5.14	0.58	SA: 0.26	7.40	SA: 3.07

gelernt wurde. Als Testdaten stehen elf zusätzliche Wirbel von zwei weiteren Patienten zur Verfügung. In allen Testszenarien wurde das SFM initial manuell im Bild platziert. Da die Qualität der Segmentierung vom Balancierungsparameter α abhängt, wurden pro Energiefunktion mehrere Testreihen durchgeführt, um jeweils einen möglichst guten Balancierungsparameter zu bestimmen. Die Güte der Segmentierung wird durch einen Vergleich mit Expertensegmentierungen über die Maße volumetrischer Überdeckungsfehler (VÜF), symmetrischer durchschnittlicher Oberflächenabstand (DOA) und Hausdorff-Abstand (HD) bewertet.

3 Ergebnisse

Die quantitativen Ergebnisse unserer Experimente sind in Tab. 1 aufgeführt, wobei PASM-lokal der in dieser Arbeit vorgeschlagenen erweiterten Methode entspricht. Aufgeführt sind dabei die Werte, die mit dem für das Organ und die verwendete Energiefunktion jeweils besten Balancierungsparameter α erzielt wurden. Die Ergebnisse zeigen, dass durch Integration des lokalen Deformations-

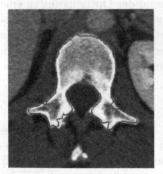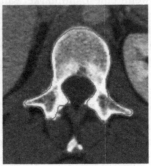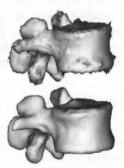

Abb. 2. Segmentierungsergebnis eines L1-Wirbels mit PASM (links) und PASM-lokal (mitte). Rechts: Darstellung der finalen vom PASM (oben) und PASM-lokal (unten) berechneten Meshes desselben Wirbels

modell der VÜF und der DOA leicht verringert werden (Abb. 1, 2). Der PASM erzeugt eine ungleichmäßige, der PASM-lokal eine glatte Segmentierungskontur.

4   Diskussion

In dieser Arbeit haben wir ein neues lokales Deformationsmodell vorgestellt, durch das der PASM glatte Segmentierungskonturen erzeugt. Wie das globale SFM greift auch das lokale Deformationsmodell auf aus den Trainingsdaten gelernte Information zurück, und benötigt keine zusätzlichen Modellparameter. Da die lokale Modellenergie automatisch mit der Bildenergie balanciert wird, ist zudem kein zusätzlicher Balancierungsparameter erforderlich. In unserer Evaluation haben wir gezeigt, dass sich durch die Integration des lokalen Deformationsmodells die Segmentierungsqualität gegenüber dem PASM leicht verbessert. Wir erklären dies damit, das durch unsere Erweiterung Ausreißer des Erscheinungsmodells besser erkannt werden können. Vor allem erzielt der Algorithmus aber qualitativ bessere Ergebnisse, da glatte Segmentierungskonturen deutlich plausibler sind. Die Evaluation an zwei sehr unterschiedlichen Organen – Leber und Wirbel – zeigt die breite Anwendbarkeit unserer Erweiterung in verschiedenen Applikationen. Darüber hinaus kann das lokale Deformationsmodell sowohl für lineare als auch für nichtlineare SFMs eingesetzt werden. Dies ist bei den Deformationsmodellen von Weese et al. [3] oder Heimann et al. [4] nicht möglich, die im Wesentlichen den Residualvektor r regularisieren. Dieser ist im Fall der KPCA im Allgemeinen aber weder bekannt – sondern nur seine Norm – noch lässt er sich als Vektorfeld auf den Landmarken interpretieren. In zukünftigen Arbeiten werden wir untersuchen, ob die Segmentierungsqualität weiter verbessert werden kann, wenn zusätzliche statistische Information aus den Trainingsdaten im lokalen Deformationsmodell ausgenutzt wird.

Literaturverzeichnis

1. Cootes TF, Taylor CJ, Cooper DH, et al. Active shape models: their training and application. Comp Vis Image Underst. 1995;61(1):38–59.
2. Kainmueller D, Lange T, Lamecker H. Shape constrained automatic segmentation of the liver based on a heuristic intensity model. Proc MICCAI Workshop on 3D Segmentation in the Clinic: A Grand Challenge. 2007; p. 109–16.
3. Weese J, Kaus M, et al CL. Shape constrained deformable models for 3D medical image segmentation. Proc IPMI. 2001; p. 380–7.
4. Heimann T, Münzing S, Meinzer HP, et al. A shape-guided deformable model with evolutionary algorithm initialization for 3D soft tissue segmentation. Proc IPMI. 2007; p. 1–12.
5. Kirschner M, Wesarg S. Active shape models unleashed. Proc SPIE. 2011;7962:11-1–11-9.
6. Kirschner M, Becker M, Wesarg S. 3D active shape model segmentation with nonlinear shape priors. Proc MICCAI. 2011; p. 492–9.

Identification of Prostate Cancer Cell Nuclei for DNA-Grading of Malignancy

David Friedrich[1], Chen Jin[2], Yu Zhang[1], Chen Demin[2], Li Yuan[2],
Leonid Berynskyy[3], Stefan Biesterfeld[3], Til Aach[1], Alfred Böcking[3]

[1]Institute of Imaging and Computer Vision, RWTH Aachen University, Germany
[2]Motic China Group Co. Ltd., Xiamen, Peoples Republic of China
[3]Dep. of Pathology, Division Cytopathology, University Düsseldorf, Germany
David.Friedrich@lfb.rwth-aachen.de

Abstract. DNA Image Cytometry is a method for early cancer diagnosis and grading of cancer, using a photomicroscopic system to measure the DNA content of nuclei. Specifically for the prostate, this method can be used to distinguish between clinically insignificant, non-aggressive tumors, and those which need to be removed or irradiated. This decision is based on the analysis of the DNA distribution among examined nuclei. However, even trained personnel usually requires more than 40 minutes for collecting the requested number of nuclei. Considering a shortage of skilled personnel, reducing the interaction time with the system is desired. Towards this end, a training set consisting of 47982 Feulgen stained nuclei and features mainly based on the nucleus morphology are used to train a Random Forest classifier. A motorized microscope was used to automatically scan ten slides from a test set and classify their nuclei. Using the leaving one out strategy, the classifier achieved a classification rate of 90.93% on the training set. For the test set, the resulting DNA distribution of each measurement was evaluated by a pathological expert. The DNA grades of malignancy of the automated measurement were identical to the grades of the corresponding manual reference measurements in all cases. Interaction time required for grading was reduced to approximately five minutes per case for manually validating the classified nuclei in diagnostically relevant DNA ranges.

1 Introduction

Thanks to developments in the early detection of cancer and cancer treatment, the chance of survival has increased in the past years [1]. However, recent studies show that especially for the prostate, the established PSA test leads to overdiagnosis and overtreatment of prostate cancer [2]. Unnecessary prostate resections with the risk of leaving the patient impotent or incontinent result. An approach to reduce overtreatment is the Active Surveillance approach: Only if progression of a cancer has been identified by regular clinical follow-up, curative therapy is recommended.

DNA Image Cytometry (DNA-ICM) may be a suitable technique for grading prostate cancer malignancy in Active Surveillance [3], it is based on estimating the DNA content of hundreds of cancer cell nuclei. To prepare the specimens, cancer cell nuclei are extracted via enzymatic cell separation from core biopsies, sedimented, fixated on glass slides and stained according to Feulgen. For this specific stain, the uptake of dye in the nucleus is proportional to its DNA content. By measuring the attenuation of light when passing through Feulgen stained nuclei with a microscope system and a digital camera, an estimate of the integrated optical density of the nuclei can be computed [4]. If the system is calibrated with nuclei of normal DNA content, for instance with fibroblasts or cells of the immune system, the DNA content of cells under analysis can be estimated. The grading of prostate cancer is then based on the DNA distribution of the cells on the slide. A DNA distribution of a non-aggressive tumor shows only a peak at the normal DNA content. Cancers which grow faster reveal a second significant peak at two times the normal DNA distribution, as the cells have to replicate the DNA content before cleavage. Even more aggressive cases contain cells with DNA content higher than 2.2 times the normal DNA content, or a significant scatter of DNA contents.

A prognostic DNA-ICM measurement consists of examining all fields of view (FOV) on the glass slide which contain nuclei, focusing on each of these FOVs and deciding whether an object can be used for calibration, should be analyzed or needs to be rejected (Fig. 1). If a nucleus is to be included in the conventional, manual measurement, the examiner clicks on the corresponding nuclei in a live view of the camera image, and then automated segmentation and DNA content estimation of this nucleus are performed in software. For a valid DNA-ICM measurement, the consensus report of the European Society for Analytical Cellular Pathology prescribes that at least 300 cancer cell nuclei and 30 reference nuclei for calibration need to be collected [4]. However, even trained personnel requires usually more than 40 minutes for this task. With most of the schools for cytotechnicians in Germany being already closed, a shortage of skilled personnel can be foreseen. Consequently, a reduction of the interaction time of cytopathological experts with the system is desired.

We therefore developed a classifier for Feulgen stained nuclei of the prostate in order to identify nuclei from cancerous cells among reference nuclei and artifacts. Our classifier was first trained on a training set which has been classified by a pathological expert (A.B.). Subsequently, the classifier was applied to classify test set data which has been collected with a motorized microscope with an autofocus system. Diagnostically relevant nuclei were presented in an image gallery and manually reviewed, before the DNA distribution was used for grading the malignant potential of the respective cancer. Finally, grading results of automated and manual measurements on the test set were compared.

2   Methods and material

Prostate cells of microdissected cancer foci in core needle biopsies from 19 patients were deposited on glass slides by centrifugation and stained according to Feulgen. From this dataset, nine slides were declared as training set and scanned

manually. All objects in each field of view on the slides were collected using a
Motic BA410 microscope with 40x objective (NA=0.65), a Motic 285A camera
(1360x1024) and the MotiCyte-I software for segmentation and estimation of
the DNA of the nuclei. The collected nuclei were classified by a cytopathologist
into the classes: Cancer cell, Granulocyte, Lymphocyte, Fibroblast and Artifact. This gold standard, comprising a total of 47982 objects, and features from
Rodenacker et al. [5] were used to train a Random Forest classifier [6]. For this
classifier, several subsets of the gold standard are selected and a Decision Tree
is induced for each of these subsets, forming a Random Forest. For an object
to be classified, the classification results for all Decision Trees in the Random
Forest are computed and counted as a vote. The dominating class is then assigned as the classification result of the Random Forest classifier. The leaving
one out strategy on a slide basis was used for training, that is eight slides were
used for training a classifier, and the remaining slide was classified. This process
was repeated so that each slide was classified once, and the classification results

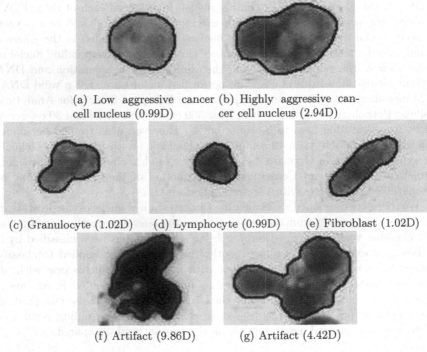

(a) Low aggressive cancer (b) Highly aggressive can-
cell nucleus (0.99D)   cer cell nucleus (2.94D)

(c) Granulocyte (1.02D)   (d) Lymphocyte (0.99D)   (e) Fibroblast (1.02D)

(f) Artifact (9.86D)   (g) Artifact (4.42D)

Fig. 1. Relevant types for classification. The first row shows two cancer cell nuclei,
whose DNA content is used for grading. The second row shows cells from the immune
system and a fibroblast, which can be used for the calibration of the system. The last
row shows artifacts which must be excluded from the measurements. The contours
extracted from the segmentation mask are shown in blue, the DNA content of the
nuclei after calibration is given in brackets and with suffix D

Table 1. Random Forest classifier on the training set

Classification	Ground truth				
	Cancer cell	Artifact	Figroglast	Granulocyte	Lymphocyte
Cancer cell	22389	657	192	15	1189
Artifact	818	15033	257	35	174
Figroglast	63	125	1083	1	14
Granulocyte	0	0	0	0	0
Lymphocyte	677	94	8	33	5125
Total	23974	15909	1540	84	6502
Error (%)	6.50	5.51	29.68	100.00	21.18

were compared to the gold standard to estimate the classification performance. The features used describe the morphology of nuclei, such as area, perimeter, jaggedness and bending of the contour, the intensity (mean and variance) and the texture (entropy, dark spots). For justifying the choice of the Random Forest classifier, this classifier is compared to an AdaBoost classifier [6], a k Nearest Neighbor classifier where the variables have been normalized for variance and a conventional Decision Tree [6].

A Motic BA600 motorized microscope with an auto focus system realized in software was used for the automated collection of the ten remaining slides from the clinical test set. During the scanning process, a classifier trained with the whole training set was used to classify the collected nuclei. After the automated classification of the nuclei, a cytopathological expert reviewed all nuclei in the diagnostically relevant range: Firstly, this included checking all cells which are classified as cancer cell nuclei and have a DNA content 2.2 times higher than the normal DNA content. This is because artifacts which have a high DNA value and are misclassified as cancer cell might lead to an overtreatment. Secondly, this includes checking all artifacts with 2.2 times larger the normal DNA content if they contain cancer cells, as missing cancer cells might lead to not treating a progressing cancer (chapter 1).

Furthermore, a conventional manual DNA-ICM measurement was performed for all slides from the test set. The DNA distributions from automated and manual measurements were graded according to the algorithms presented in [7], which allocates seven grades.

3   Results

The classification rate on the gold standard, using the leaving one out strategy as described in the previous section (Tab. 1). The Random Forest classifier achieves an overall correct classification rate of 90.93%. Misclassifications which are especially relevant for grading are the fraction of cancer cells, which were not classified as such (cancer cells lost, 6.51%) and the fraction of artifacts among all cells classified as cancer cells (2.69%). The correct classification rate and the

Table 2. Total correct classification rate and diagnostically relevant misclassification rates for the classifiers used in this study, given in percent

Classifier	Classification rate	Cancer Cells lost	Artifacts classified Cancer Cell
Random Forest	90.93	6.51	2.69
AdaBoost	89.83	7.81	3.63
Decision Tree	84.90	13.16	5.52
kNN	89.65	5.89	4.97

misclassification rates relevant for diagnosis are given in Table 2 for all classifiers used in this study.

After collection of the nuclei in the automated measurements, diagnostically relevant nuclei were reviewed by an expert. For each case, 75 objects classified as cancerous and 367 objects classified artifacts needed to be checked on average. To ascertain if the classification performance achieved is sufficient to confirm the grading, the DNA-distributions from automated and manual measurements were compared. The DNA-grades of the manual measurement could be confirmed in all 10 cases.

4 Discussion

We used the leaving one out strategy on all available data classified by an expert to train classifiers and estimate the classification performance, following Fukunaga's recommendation to use this strategy instead of the separation of training- and test set [8, page 312]. The Random Forest classifier outperformed the other classifiers tested. Decision Trees, which are the foundation for this classifier, have a built-in feature ranking: When inducing the Decision Tree, the most important features are used in vertices close to the root vertex. This explains the better performance compared to the other complex classifiers as the kNN and AdaBoost classifier on the same features. But unlike a conventional Decision Tree, the Random Forest classifier trains a collection of Decision Trees on subsets of the gold standard data, which prevents over fitting.

Among the five classes, abnormal and cancer cell nuclei are classified with a better performance as Fibroblasts, Granulocytes and Lymphocytes. This is due to the fact that a priori probabilities for these classes are much lower: cancer cell nuclei and artifacts together constitute 50.0% and 33.1% of the gold standard, while Fibroblasts, Granulocytes and Lymphocytes are just 3.2, 0.2 and 13.5%.

The most critical errors for the classification problem at hand are missed cancer cell nuclei, which might lead to not treating a progressing cancer, and the classification of artifacts as cancer cells, which might lead to over treatment. For the Random Forest classifier, these relevant misclassifications were lower than the misclassification rate on the whole dataset. A grading procedure was set up which included a verification of diagnostically relevant nuclei. By automatically collecting and classifying all nuclei on the slide, the interaction of the cytotechnician was reduced from the whole manual measurement of a slide (40 minutes/case) to the visual inspection of relevant nuclei. These are presented compactly in an image gallery, which reduces the interaction time to approximately five minutes per case. Applied on the test set, this grading procedure confirmed the DNA-grading of the manual reference in all ten cases.

As a future work, we intend to develop classifiers for other modalities such as for cells from the uterine cervix or the oral cavity. These cells can be extracted non-invasively using brush biopsies, which causes new challenges for classification: The samples extracted from brush biopsies are usually more contaminated with debris. Cells might, on the one hand, lie in different focus planes or, on the other hand, lie much closer to each other and touch or overlap. Thus strategies for the detection of defocused nuclei and these specific forms of artifacts need to be developed.

References

1. Schön D, Haberland J, Görsch B. Weitere Entwicklung der Krebssterblichkeit in Deutschland bis zum Jahr 2010. Der Onkologe. 2003;9:409–10.
2. Roemeling S, Roobol MJ, Postma R, et al. Management and survival of screen-detected prostate cancer patients who might have been suitable for active surveillance. Eur Urol. 2006;50:475–82.
3. Helpap B, Hartmann A, Wernert N. Anleitung zur pathologisch-anatomischen Diagnostik von Prostatatumoren. Bundesverband Deutscher Pathologen und Deutsche Gesellschaft für Pathologie; 2011.
4. Böcking A, Giroud F, Reith A. Consensus report of the ESACP-task force on standardization of diagnostic DNA-image cytometry. Anal Cell Pathol. 1995;8:67–74.
5. Rodenacker K, Bengston E. A feature set for cytometry on digitized microscopic images. Anal Cell Pathol. 2003;25:1–36.
6. Bradski G. The OpenCV library. Dr Dobb's Journal of Software Tools. 2000.
7. Engelhardt M. PSA-Kinetiken als Indikationsstelllung zur Prostata-Biopsie, to be published. Heinrich Heine University Düsseldorf; 2011.
8. Rheinboldt W, editor. Introduction to Statistical Pattern Recognition. Academic Press Limited; 1990.

Markerlose Navigation für perkutane Nadelinsertionen

A. Seitel[1], M. Servatius[2], A. M. Franz[1], T. Kilgus[1], N. Bellemann[2],
B. R. Radeleff[2], S. Fuchs[3], H.-P. Meinzer[1], L. Maier-Hein[1]

[1]Abt. Medizinische und Biologische Informatik, Deutsches Krebsforschungszentrum
[2]Abt. Diagnostische und Interventionelle Radiologie, Universität Heidelberg
[3]Institut für Robotik und Mechatronik, Deutsches Zentrum für Luft- und Raumfahrt
a.seitel@dkfz-heidelberg.de

Kurzfassung. Navigationssysteme für minimal-invasive Nadelinsertionen basieren häufig auf externen oder internen Markern zur Registrierung und Bewegungserfassung. Somit wird der bisherige klinische Workflow durch Verwendung zusätzlicher Hardware und speziell angefertigter Instrumente sowie teilweise durch erhöhte Invasivität drastisch verändert. Wir stellen das erste Navigationssystem für perkutane Nadelinsertionen vor, das, basierend auf der Time-of-Flight (ToF)-Kameratechnik, (1) ohne zusätzliche Marker auskommt und (2) sowohl Registrierung als auch Navigation mit einer einzigen Kamera ohne zusätzliche Hardware (z.B. Trackingsystem) ermöglicht. In einer ersten Phantomevaluation konnte eine Zielgenauigkeit im Bereich von 4 mm ermittelt werden.

1 Einleitung

Minimal-invasive Verfahren gewinnen mehr und mehr an Bedeutung bei der Diagnose und Behandlung von Krebserkrankungen. Viele dieser Verfahren wie z.B. Radiofrequenzablationen oder Biopsien erfordern das Einbringen eines nadelförmigen Instrumentes in die Zielstruktur wie z.B. die Leber. Ein grundlegendes Problem dieser Eingriffe ist die Übertragung des präoperativ bestimmten Zugangsweges auf die aktuelle Situation am Patienten (Registrierung). Während bei der konventionellen Vorgehensweise der Radiologe unter manueller Assistenz diese Übertragung herbeiführen muss, existieren computer-basierte Navigationsansätze, die ihn dabei, sowie bei der Nadelinsertion unterstützen [1]. Die Lokalisation des Instrumentes sowie die Registrierung und die Erfassung etwaiger Bewegungen der Zielregion wird meistens markerbasiert mit Hilfe eines Trackingsystems realisiert, wobei hier häufig externe (z.B. [2]) oder interne (z.B. [3]) Marker zum Einsatz kommen. Diese Marker können sowohl in den präoperativen Bilddaten als auch in den intraoperativen Trackingdaten lokalisiert werden. Solche markerbasierten Ansätze erfordern die Verwendung zusätzlicher Trackingsysteme sowie speziell angefertigter trackbarer Instrumente und erhöhen teilweise die Invasivität des Eingriffes durch zusätzliches Einbringen interner Marker. Wir stellen daher in dieser Arbeit einen Navigationsansatz basierend auf der neuartigen Time-of-Flight (ToF) Kameratechnik [4] vor, der eine navigierte Nadelinsertion ermöglicht, ohne dabei auf zusätzliche Marker oder ein Trackingsystem angewiesen zu sein.

2 Material und Methoden

Abb. 1 zeigt die Schritte des markerlosen Navigationsverfahrens.

- *Präoperative Datenaufnahme und Zugangsplanung:* Präoperativ wird ein CT Bild akquiriert, welches zur Bestimmung eines sicheren Zugangsweges sowie zur Erstellung einer Oberflächenrepräsentation der Hautoberfläche verwendet wird. Für die Zugangsplanung kommt ein in [5] vorgestelltes automatisches Planungssystem zum Einsatz, welches unter Berücksichtigung von kritischen Strukturen sowie Parametern wie Trajektorienlänge und Einstichswinkel geeignete Zugangswege berechnet.
- *Intraoperative Datenaufnahme:* Intraoperativ erfasst eine, oberhalb des Patienten angebrachte, ToF Kamera ebenfalls die Oberfläche des Patienten. Die Korrektur systematischer Fehler dieser ToF Aufnahmen sowie die Bestimmung der zur Erstellung der ToF-Oberfläche notwendigen intrinsischen Kameraparameter werden durch Anwendung der Kalibrierung von Fuchs et al. [6] vorgenommen. Die Unterdrückung systembedingten Rauschens geschieht durch Anwendung eines kantenerhaltenden Glättungsfilters.
- *Registrierung:* Die Übertragung des präoperativ geplanten Zugangsweges auf die intraoperative Situation am Patienten geschieht durch eine oberflächenbasierte Registrierung der CT und ToF Oberfläche. Hier wird zunächst eine

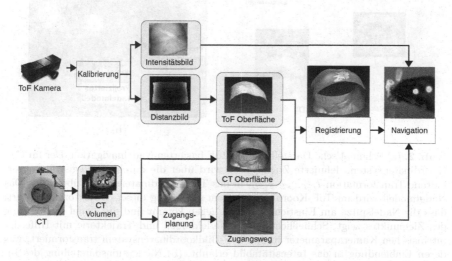

Abb. 1. Übersicht des Verfahrens zur markerlosen Nadelnavigation

initiale Transformation ermittelt, welche beide Oberflächen grob in Übereinstimmung bringt. Mit Hilfe eines Iterative Closest Point (ICP)-basierten Verfahrens wird die finale, möglichst exakte Transformation bestimmt.

– *Navigation:* Zur Navigation wird das Intensitätsbild der Kamera verwendet, welches in real-time mit Informationen zur Zielführung angereichert wird und dem Arzt auf einem Navigationsbildschirm dargestellt wird. Das Verfahren wird im folgenden Abschnitt 2.1 genauer erläutert.

2.1 ToF-basierte Nadelinsertion

Für die Zielführung des Instruments entlang des geplanten Zugangsweges werden lediglich die Bilder der ToF-Kamera genutzt. Abb. 2 zeigt das zugrundeliegende Verfahren.

Ein Oberflächenmodell der verwendeten Insertionsnadel wird, im Koordinatensystem der ToF-Kamera, virtuell auf den geplanten Einstichspunkt platziert und entlang der Trajektorie ausgerichtet. Unter Verwendung der intrinsischen Kameraparameter wird diese Oberfläche, sowie der geplante Zugangsweg in das Intensitätsbild der ToF Kamera zurückprojiziert und dient dort der Zielführung. Zur Nadelausrichtung wird das im Intensitätsbild sichtbare Instrument mit der überlagerten Projektion in Übereinstimmung gebracht. Für die Nadelinsertion wird das Nadelmodell sowie dessen Projektion entlang des Zugangsweges an den

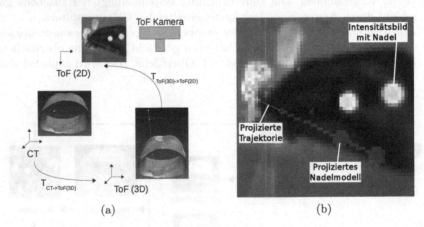

(a)   (b)

Abb. 2. (a) Schematische Darstellung der ToF basierten Nadelnavigation: Der im CT-Koordinatensystem definierte Zugangsweg wird über die durch die Registrierung erhaltene Transformation $T_{CT->ToF(3D)}$ in das ToF-Koordinatensystem überführt. Das Nadelmodell wird im ToF-Koordinatensystem so entlang dieser Trajektorie platziert, dass die Nadelspitze am Einstichspunkt zu liegen kommt und die Nadel in Richtung des Zielpunktes zeigt. Schließlich werden Nadelmodell und Trajektorie mit Hilfe der intrinsischen Kameraparameter in das ToF-Bildkoordinatensystem transformiert, was deren Einblendung in das Intensitätsbild erlaubt. (b) Navigationsdarstellung des Intensitätsbildes mit eingeblendeter Trajektorie und eingeblendetem Nadelmodell

Zielpunkt verschoben. Eine Führungsvorrichtung kann verwendet werden, um den eingeschlagenen Einstichswinkel beizubehalten.

2.2 Evaluation

Zur Bestimmung von Präzision und Genauigkeit der entwickelten Methode wurde anstelle eines CTs ein optisches Trackingsystem (Polaris Spectra®, Northern Digital Inc. (NDI); Waterloo, Ontario, Canada) zur Trajektorienbestimmung und Registrierung verwendet. Dies ermöglichte zudem die kontinuierliche Erfassung von Position und Orientierung der für diese Versuche verwendete, optisch trackbare Nadel [3]. Die eingesetzte ToF Kamera (CamCube 3, PMD Technologies, Siegen, Deutschland; Auflösung: 200×200) wurde bereits zwei Stunden vor Versuchsbeginn in Betrieb genommen um somit den temperaturabhängigen Distanzfehler in den Daten zu verringern. Die Registrierung von ToF- und Trackingkoordinatensystem wurde punktbasiert anhand neun korrespondierender Landmarken durchgeführt um von den durch die Oberflächenregistrierung entstehenden Fehlern zu abstrahieren.

Sowohl Präzisions- als auch Genauigkeitsexperimente wurden vom Entwickler des Systems (E) sowie von je zwei Informatikern (I1, I2) und zwei Medizinern (M1, M2) durchgeführt. Vor jedem Versuch und für jeden Studienteilnehmer wurde eine neue Registrierung durchgeführt. Das getrackte Instrument diente zur Trajektoriendefinition, wobei dieses hierfür senkrecht zur Phantomoberfläche ausgerichtet wurde. Der Einstichspunkt wurde definiert durch die initiale Position der Nadelspitze, davon ausgehende Trajektorien wurden unter verschiedenen Winkeln ($0°, 10°, 20°, 30°, 40°$) zur inital senkrecht zur Phantomoberfläche ausgerichteten getrackten Nadel bestimmt.

Für die Bestimmung der Präzision kam ein planares Phantom zum Einsatz, was eine möglichst stabile Rotation der Nadelspitze um einen definierten Punkt erlaubte. Jeder Benutzer führte die Ausrichtung der Nadel für jeden definierten Winkel in zufälliger Reihenfolge zehn Mal durch.

Zur die Bestimmung der Genauigkeit diente ein Phantom aus ballistischer Gelatine (GELITA AG, Eberbach, Deutschland). Nach der Registrierung wurde eine Führungsvorrichtung (SeeStar® Guiding Device, AprioMed, Uppsala, Schweden) auf der Phantomoberfläche fixiert. Jeder Benutzer führte für die Winkel $0°$, $20°$ und $40°$ zunächst die Nadelausrichtung durch und führte die Nadel schließlich sukzessive auf die Tiefen 50 mm, 60 mm und 70 mm ein. Dieser Vorgang wurde zufällig für jeden Winkel drei mal wiederholt.

3   Ergebnisse

Im Mittel konnte eine Präzision (Standardabweichung des Winkelfehlers) von $0.6°$ über alle angefahrenen Winkel ($n = 25$) bestimmt werden (Abb. 3). Abb. 4 zeigt die Ergebnisse der Genauigkeitsevaluation gemittelt über die drei Wiederholungen. Der mittlere Fehler der Nadelinsertion - gemessen als Euklidische Distanz zwischen geplanter Zielposition und getrackter Position der Nadelspitze lag bei 4.1±1.7 mm gemittelt über alle Studienteilnehmer, jeden Winkel, jede Tiefe und alle Wiederholungen ($n = 135$). Für die einzelnen Tiefen ($n = 45$) konnten Werte von 3.8±1.7 mm (Tiefe: 50 mm), 3.8±1.4 mm (Tiefe: 60 mm) und 4.7±1.8 mm (Tiefe: 70 mm) ermittelt werden. Die benötigte Zeit für die Nadelausrichtung betrug im Mittel 26±13 s, für die Nadelinsertion 12±10 s ($n = 45$).

4 Diskussion

Das in dieser Arbeit vorgestellte Nadelnavigationssystem ist unseres Wissens nach das erste CT basierte, markerlose Navigationssystem, das mit nur einer ein-

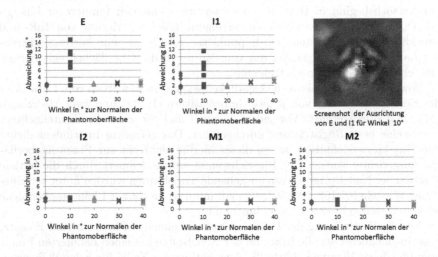

Abb. 3. Ergebnisse der Präzisionsanalyse für jeden Studienteilnehmer (E: Entwickler, I1: Informatiker 1, I2: Informatiker 2, M1: Mediziner 1, M2: Mediziner 2). Der Screenshot zeigt die problematische Ausrichtung für Winkel 10° bei E und I1

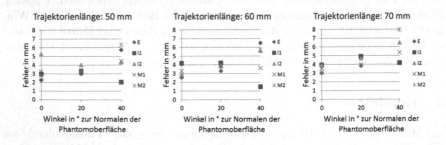

Abb. 4. Ergebnisse der Genauigkeitsanalyse für unterschiedliche Einstichswinkel, Trajektorienlängen sowie jeden Studienteilnehmer (E: Entwickler, I1: Informatiker 1, I2: Informatiker 2, M1: Mediziner 1, M2: Mediziner 2)

zigen Kamera sowohl zur Registrierung als auch zur Navigation auskommt. Wir konnten mit unserem Ansatz eine Genauigkeit im Bereich von 4 mm erreichen. Für kleine Einstichswinkel (0°, 20°) konnten alle Studienteilnehmer mit einer ähnlichen Genauigkeit die Nadelinsertion durchführen, was dafür spricht, dass die initiale Ausrichtung der Nadel mit Hilfe der Führungsvorrichtung während der Nadelinsertion gehalten werden konnte. Für den großen Einstichswinkel (40°) kam es zu einer größeren Streuung, was unseres Erachtens mit der nicht vollständig am Einstichspunkt fixierten Nadelspitze zusammenhängt. Die Ausrichtung des Instruments zeigt sich abhängig von dessen Geometrie, die zur Projektion verwendet wird. Besonders deutlich ist die Auswirkung für die Ausrichtung unter dem Winkel 10° für die Studienteilnehmer E und I1 zu erkennen (Abb. 3). Wir gehen davon aus, dass derartige Schwankungen in der Ausrichtungspräzision durch ein geeignetes Tooldesign vermieden werden können. Außerdem hat die Geometrie des Tools auch Auswirkungen auf die Genauigkeit des zur Evaluation verwendeten Trackingverfahrens was sich als zusätzliche Ungenauigkeit in den Ergebnissen wiederspiegelt. In zukünftigen Arbeiten soll daher der Einfluss des Tooldesigns auf die Genauigkeit des Navigationssystems untersucht werden. Zudem gilt es, das entwickelte Verfahren in einem klinisch realistischen Setup unter Verwendung oberflächenbasierter Registrierung weiter zu evaluieren.

Nichtsdestotrotz zeigen die Ergebnisse das enorme Potential der ToF-Technik navigierte Nadelinsertionen (1) markerlos und (2) unter Verwendung nur einer Kamera für Registrierung und Navigation zu ermöglichen. Das einfache Setup sowie die vergleichsweise geringen Hardware-Kosten unterstreichen zudem das klinische Potential des vorgestellten Verfahrens.

Danksagung. Die vorliegende Studie wurde im Rahmen des DFG-geförderten Graduiertenkolleg 1126 „Intelligente Chirurgie" durchgeführt. Die Software für dieses Projekt wurde innerhalb des Medical Imaging Interaction Toolkits (MITK) entwickelt.

Literaturverzeichnis

1. Wood BJ, Kruecker J, Abi-Jaoudeh N, et al. Navigation systems for ablation. J Vasc Interv Radiol. 2010;21(8 Suppl):S257–63.
2. Nicolau SA, Pennec X, Soler L, et al. An augmented reality system for liver thermal ablation: design and evaluation on clinical cases. Med Image Anal. 2009;13(3):494–506.
3. Maier-Hein L, Tekbas A, Seitel A, et al. In vivo accuracy assessment of a needle-based navigation system for CT-guided radiofrequency ablation of the liver. Med Phys. 2008;35(12):5386–96.
4. Kolb A, Barth E, Koch R, et al. Time-of-flight sensors in computer graphics. In: Proc Eurographics; 2009. p. 119–34.
5. Seitel A, Engel M, Sommer CM, et al. Computer-assisted trajectory planning for percutaneous needle insertions. Med Phys. 2011;38(6):3246–59.
6. Fuchs S, Hirzinger G. Extrinsic and depth calibration of ToF-cameras. Proc IEEE CVPR. 2008.

Kalibrierung elektromagnetischer Trackingsysteme
Vorstellung und Evaluation eines neuartigen vollautomatischen Systems

Johannes Gaa[1], Ingmar Gergel[1], Hans-Peter Meinzer[1], Ingmar Wegner[1]

Abteilung für Medizinische und Biologische Informatik, DKFZ Heidelberg

jogaa@gmx.de

Kurzfassung. Trackingsysteme, basierend auf elektromagnetischer Technologie (EMT), spielen eine immer wichtigere Rolle im Bereich der Image Guided Therapy. Ein Hauptproblem bezüglich EMTs ist jedoch die Anfälligkeit auf metallische Einflüsse. Es wurden bereits verschiedene Methoden vorgestellt, um EMT Systeme diesbezüglich evaluieren zu können. Allerdings sehen diese Systeme immer das manuelle Erstellen des Datensatzes vor. Dies ist im Allgemeinen eine sehr zeitaufwändige Aufgabe und kann nur durch die Verringerung des betrachteten Arbeitsraums beschleunigt werden. In dieser Arbeit wird ein vollautomatisches Kalibrierungssystem für diesen Zweck vorgestellt. Dieses System setzt eine programmierbare Positionierrobotik ein, der ein parallel-kinematisches Konzept zu Grunde liegt. Auf diese Weise wird es ermöglicht sehr viele Daten über den kompletten Arbeitsraum eines EMTs und anderer Trackingsysteme zu sammeln.

1 Einleitung

Elektromagnetische Tracking Systeme kommen in der Medizintechnik bereits vielseitig zum Einsatz. Gerade bei der Anwendung in flexiblen Instrumenten, wie beispielsweise Endoskope und Katheter, weisen sie große Vorteile auf. Im Gegensatz zu Trackingsystemen mit optischer Funktionsweise, muss das Problem der Line-of-Sight hier nicht beachtet werden. Dies ermöglicht auch den Einsatz innerhalb des Körpers. Allerdings sind EMTs anfällig auf äußere Einflüsse. Bei solchen Einflüssen handelt es sich vor allem um metallische Gegenstände (z.B. Operationstisch) durch die das erzeugt Magnetfeld gestört wird [1, 2].

Hummel et al. entwarfen ein Protokoll zur Evaluierung von EMT Systemen. Dafür wurde ein Platte aus PMMA bzw. Plexiglas®verwendet, die durch ein Stecksystem den Sensor des Trackingsystems in vordefinierte Stellen positioniert [3]. Das System erlaubt die Akquisition von Trackingdaten in einer ebenen Fläche von 500×500 mm. Der Abstand der Messpunkte beträgt dabei immer 50 mm. Da das Stecksystem für jeden Messpunkt manuell positioniert werden muss, ist die Aufnahme der Messdaten ein zeitaufwendiges Verfahren. Der Aufwand erhöht sich mit der Anzahl der Ebenen die innerhalb des Trackingvolumens untersucht werden sollen. Nafis et al. beschreiben in ihrer Arbeit eine schnellere Methode, das sogenannte Scribbling, zur Evaluierung von EMT vor [4]. Ähnlich wie in der Arbeit von Hummel et al. wurden dabei die Messdaten manuell gesammelt. Jedoch waren diese nicht fest vordefiniert, da in diesem System die Datenakquisition durch das willkürliche Verschieben des Sensors über eine Glasfläche, mit den Abmaßen 650×450 mm, geschieht. Die gesammelten Messpunkte wurden anschließend mit dem mathematischen Modell einer Ebene verglichen und entsprechend evaluiert. Auch in diesem Fall ist ein hoher zeitlicher Aufwand notwendig um das gesamte Trackingvolumen abzudecken, da wiederum mehrere Schichten manuell abgetastet werden müssen. Jiang et al. präsentierten in [5] einen Ansatz, der die Datenakquisition nicht auf eine Ebene beschränkte. Dazu verwendeten sie ein Tool, dass zum einen im entsprechenden Magnetfeld des EMT getrackt wird, aber zur selben Zeit auch von einem Referenz-Tracking-System. In der Arbeit der Autoren wurde ein optisches Trackingsystem (OT) zur Erzeugung der Referenz der Punkte bzw. der Ground Truth verwendet. Dieses Verfahren weist einen wesentlich geringeren zeitlichen Aufwand auf. Jedoch muss auf eine sehr präzise Synchronisierung der beiden verwendeten Trackingsysteme geachtet werden und weiter hängt diese Methode sehr stark von der Anzahl der gesammelten Messpunkte ab. Der Aussage der Autoren nach werden über 10^5 Messpunkte benötigt, um eine aussagekräftige Evaluierung durchführen zu können.

2   Materialien und Methoden

Es wurde ein Parallelmanipulator konstruiert, um in einem vollautomatischen Prozess, ein EMT System im Einsatz in einer idealen Umgebung zu evaluieren.

2.1   Beschreibung des Kalibrierungsroboter

Dem erzeugten Roboterarm liegt das parallel-kinematische Prinzip des sgn. Tripod zu Grunde. Dadurch wird eine hohe Positioniergenauigkeit, eine erhöhte Steifigkeit und ein sehr gutes Schwingungsverhalten erreicht. Um den Eigeneinfluss des Roboters auf das EMT System auf ein vernachlässigbares Maß zu verringern, wurden Materialien verwendet die keinen Störeinfluss auf Magnetfelder haben, wie z.B. Karbon und Polymere. Die drei parallelen Antriebe in jeder Strebe wurden als Spindelantriebe realisiert. Um die zu erreichende Genauigkeit zu erfüllen, wurden hier metallische Spindeln verwendet. Dabei handelt es sich jedoch um nicht magnetisierendes Metall. Außerdem lässt die Konstruktion es zu, dass die Antriebsspindeln nur teilweise in das Trackingfeld reichen. Der gesamte Arbeitsraum des Tripods entspricht dem Trackingvolumen gängiger EMT Systeme (> 500×500×500 mm) und geht auch darüber hinaus. Der Kopf lässt das einfache Montieren des EMT Sensors im sgn. Tool Center Point (TCP), also in der kinematisch relevanten Position der Tripodspitze, zu. Zusätzlich kann dieser mit einem OT System getrackt werden.

2.2 Kalibrierungssoftware

Alle Softwarekomponenten des Kalibrierungssystems wurden innerhalb des Medical Imaging Interaction Toolkit (MITK) entwickelt. Dabei handelt es sich um ein Open Source, Plattform unabhängige Softwarebibliothek zur Entwicklung von Anwendungen im Bereich medizinischer Bildverarbeitung [6]. Die implementierte Software teilt sich auf in einen Treiberbereich zur Steuerung und Kommunikation mit der Tripod-Hardware und in eine Benutzeroberfläche zur Programmierung und Befehlseingabe. Diese werden zusammen mit der Kommunikation mit dem EMT System, so wie einem eventuellen Referenz-Trackingsystem, innerhalb der Anwendung in verschiedenen Threads verarbeitet. Die Verknüpfung der Systeme geschieht hierbei durch das MITK Image Guided Therapy Filterkonzept. Auf diese Weise wird die Synchronisierung der Messdaten und Ground Truth Daten garantiert und keine weiteren Nachbearbeitungsschritte benötigt. Die Benutzeroberfläche lässt das Konfigurieren (Antriebsgeschwindigkeit, Rampenlänge) und direkte Senden von Befehlen an den Tripod zu. Aber es ist auch die Möglichkeit gegeben Abtastgitter mit unterschiedlichen räumlichen Strukturen, wie z.B. Quader oder Zylinder, mit frei definierbaren Parametern zu erzeugen.

2.3 Experiment

In einem einführenden Experiment sollte der Tripod zur grundlegenden Evaluierung eines Versuchsaufbaus dienen. Deswegen wurde in einem Experiment ein EMT in ungestörter Umgebung evaluiert. Als EMT System kam hierbei das Aurora Tabletop 50–70 von NDI zum Einsatz. Der Versuchsaufbau wurde auf Positionsgenauigkeit, Rauschen und Wiederholgenauigkeit untersucht. Dabei wurde ein quaderförmiges Volumen mit der Seitenlänge von 400 mm und einer Höhe von 225 mm betrachtet. Die Messpunkte wurde mit einem 5 Degrees of Freedom (5DoF) Sensor, ebenfalls von NDI, aufgenommen. Zur Akquisition der Messdaten wurde ein Abtastgitter in einem Tripod-eignem Koordinatensystem

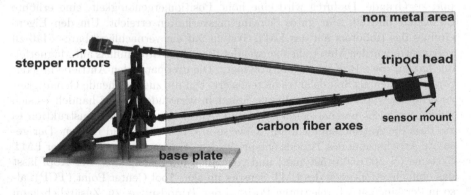

Abb. 1. Der Aufbau des parallelen Manipulators

angegeben. Das Abtastgitter selbst wies eine Dichte von insgesamt 2025 Punkten auf. Dabei wurden in Richtungen x, y jeweils 15 Messpunkte bestimmt. Zur Referenz und Positionsbestimmung wurde zusätzlich der TCP mit einem OT System verfolgt und protokolliert.

2.4 Datenanalyse

Wie Frantz et al. in ihrer Arbeit [7] beschreiben, werden bei der Abschätzung der Systemparameter mehrdimensionale Versuchs- und Messdaten auf ein quantitatives Maß reduziert. Als Beispiel kann der im Arbeitsraum allgemein gültige RMS (root-mean-square) Distanzfehler genannt werden. Obwohl Hersteller und Zertifizierer weitaus umfassenderer Messdaten aufnehmen und dadurch auch in der Lage sind Aussagen über Orts spezifische Positionsabweichungen zu machen, wird in vielen Fällen oftmals nur die maximale oder die gemittelte Positionsabweichung erfragt. Um jedoch die optimale Lage des Feldgenerators in einer spezifischen Anwendung zu bestimmen ist dies nicht ausreichend. Frantz et al. schlagen unter anderem ein volumetrisches Kalibrierungsprotokoll vor. Darin wird durch wiederholte (insgesamt 60 mal) Bestimmung von Position r_m und der Orientierung n_m in einer repräsentativen Anzahl m Messpunkten, zunächst die Positionsabweichung bestimmt. Ausgehend davon wird der jeweilig RMS-Fehler berechnet. Schließlich beschreibt das Protokoll, das schließen auf Trueness (Richtigkeit) τ und Precision (Präzision) ρ über das Ausgleichen von $\epsilon = \sqrt{\tau^2 + \rho^2}$ anhand des Datensatzes. Im Rahmen dieses Experiments wurden schließlich noch Untersuchungen des Jitters der Sensoren durchgeführt.

3 Ergebnisse

3.1 Genauigkeitsuntersuchungen Tripod

Um den Positionierroboter als Referenzsystem zur Evaluierung von EMT Systemen zu verwenden wurde eine Genauigkeitsanylyse des Tripod durchgeführt. In laufenden Versuchen konnte eine Positionier-Wiederholgenauigkeit von 0,228 mm, ausgehend von 1465 Messpunkten, gemessen werden. Diese Größenordnung ist ausreichend groß zur Evaluierung, üblicher EMT Systeme. Da derzeit die kinematische Analyse nicht vollständig abgeschlossen ist, wurde jedoch ein OT System zusätzlich als Ground Truth System hinzugezogen.

3.2 Evaluation EMT Feldgenerator

Anhand des Positionierroboters wurden insgesamt 2025 Messpunkte im EMT Volumen von 400×400×225 mm untersucht. Abb. 2 zeigt einen Teil der Ergebnisse. Es ist zu erkennen, dass das EMT System insbesondere zum Rand hin eine höhere Ungenauigkeit aufweist. Sehr starke Abweichungen rühren allerdings daher, dass sich der Sensor bereits außerhalb des Trackingsvolumens befand. Der durchschnittliche Fehler der Richtigkeit betrug 1,64 mm. Der maximale Präzisionsfehler über alle Punkte betrug 0,89 mm. Zur Bestimmung dieser Werte

wurden stark abweichende Werte, die an der Grenze des Trackingvolumens aufgenommen wurden, außer Acht gelassen, da hier kein Tracking erfolgte.

4   Diskussion

In dieser Arbeit wurde ein vollautomatisches System zur Kalibrierung von elektromagnetischen Trackingsystemen und zur Evaluierung ihrer Präzision in klinischer Anwendung vorgestellt. Der neu konstruierte Roboter kann auf einfache
Weise eine große Anzahl von Messpunkten sammeln und deckt dabei den kompletten Arbeitsraum verschiedener elektromagnetischer Trackingsysteme ab. Der

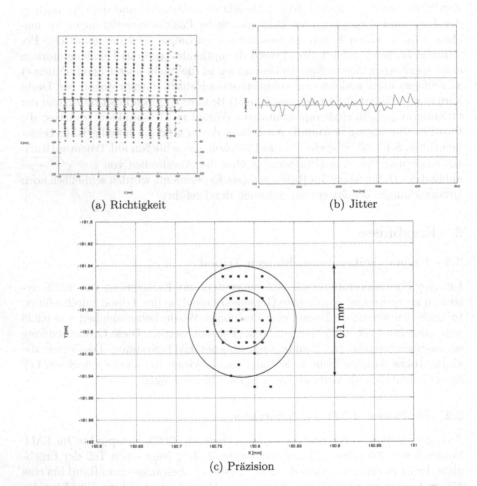

(a) Richtigkeit   (b) Jitter

(c) Präzision

Abb. 2. Darstellung der Richtigkeit über das Trackingvolumen (a), Verlauf des Jitters
eines Sensors in x-Richtung (b) und Präzision am Beispiel eines Messpunktes in der
(x, y)-Ebene (c)

größte Vorteil des Systems ist allerdings das eigenständige Arbeiten, das die zeitaufwendige manuelle Positionierung des jeweiligen Sensors unnötig macht und gleichzeitig das Erzeugen von großen Messdatensätzen ermöglicht. In dem beschriebenen Experiment konnte sich das Kalibrierungssytem bewähren. Obwohl momentan noch zusätzlich ein OT System zur Bestimmung der Ground Truth Positionen verwendet wird, deuten laufende Untersuchungen daraufhin, dass der Positionierroboter an sich alleine zur Ground Truth Bestimmung ausreicht. Eine detaillierte Ausarbeitung zur Analyse des Störeinflusses von metallischen Gegenständen auf EMT System anhand des Positionierroboters wird in zukünftigen Arbeiten präsentiert werden.

Da die Gesamtqualität von Genauigkeitsuntersuchungen für EMT-Systemen maßgeblichen von der Anzahl an aufgezeichneten Messpositionen abhängt, würden alle bekannten Evaluationsprotokolle von dem vorgestellten System profitieren. Nach abschließenden Untersuchungen, kann nach Absprache der Positionierroboter sowie die Ansteuersoftware, für andere Forschungsgruppen zugänglich gemacht werden.

Literaturverzeichnis

1. Birkfellner W, Watzinger F, Wanschitz F, et al. Systematic distortions in magnetic position digitizers. Med Phys. 1998;25.
2. Kirsch SR, Schilling C, Brunner G. Assessment of metallic distortions of an electromagnetic tracking system. Proc SPIE. 2006;6141:143–51.
3. Hummel Jb, Bax MR, Figl ML, et al. Design and application of an assessment protocol for electromagnetic tracking systems. Med Phys. 2005;32:2371–9.
4. Nafis Christopher JV, von Jako R. Method for evaluating compatibility of commercial electro-magnetic (em) microsensor tracking systems with surgical and imaging tables. Proc SPIE. 2008;6918:20.
5. Jiang Z, Mori K, Nimura Y, et al. An improved method for compensating ultratiny electro-magnetic tracker utilizing postion and orientation information and its application to a flexible neuroendoscopic surgery navigation system. Proc SPIE. 2009;7261:2T.
6. Wolf I, Vetter M, Wegner I, et al. The medical imaging interaction toolkit. Med Image Anal. 2005;9:594–604.
7. Frantz D, Wiles AD, Leis SE, et al. Accuracy assessment protocols for electromagnetic tracking systems. Phys Med Biol. 2003;48:2241–51.

SPECT Reconstruction with a Transformed Attenuation Prototype at Multiple Levels

Sven Barendt, Jan Modersitzki

Institute of Mathematics and Image Computing, University of Lübeck
sven.barendt@mic.uni-luebeck.de

Abstract. In this work, a novel multilevel approach to Single Photon Emission Computed Tomography (SPECT) reconstruction based on a so-called transformed attenuation prototype is presented. As our results indicate, the benefits of a multilevel strategy as known from literature can be observed as well. That is, we show results where a local minima of a single level reconstruction is avoided and a more preferable SPECT reconstruction is obtained.

1 Introduction

This work deals with an approach for Single Photon Emission Computed Tomography (SPECT) reconstruction based on a transformed attenuation prototype ([1, 2]). Such an approach uses an additional measurement, usually a Computed Tomography (CT) measurement, to obtain some information about the unknown attenuation properties of the tissue. See [2, 3] for benefits of such an approach and a discussion of alternative considerations with respect to the attenuation (see also recent work in [4]). The attenuation information gained from the additional measurement is then used as a prototype attenuation and is included in the SPECT reconstruction process. Due to repositioning of the patient between a SPECT and a CT scan or due to the different scanning times of the SPECT and the CT modality the attenuation prototype is in general inconsistent to the attenuation, underlying the SPECT scan. Thus, a multimodal correspondance problem exists. That is the motivation for allowing degrees of freedom on the attenuation prototype in the form of a transformation. This results in a SPECT reconstruction problem where the objective is to simultaneously reconstruct the density of radiation and a reasonable transformation of the attenuation prototype. However, often the reconstruction leads to unwanted transformations due to the existance of local minima. To reduce the existance of local minima in the objective, a family of continuous models for the attenuation prototype derived ([5] page 40 ff. and 145 ff.). A reconstruction of the density of radiation and the transformation of an attenuation prototype on the coarsest level is then used as an initial guess for the reconstruction on the next finest level and so forth. The next section describes the methodology of the proposed multilevel approach for SPECT reconstruction with a transformed attenuation prototype. Afterwards we show results that show the benefits of the multilevel approach with respect to the reduction of local minima compared to a single level reconstruction. Finally, the results are discussed and an outlook to future work is given.

2   Materials and methods

In this section, the proposed approach to SPECT reconstruction with a transformed attenuation prototype at multiple levels is explained. The reconstruction problem considered in this work is to find a minimizer f^* and ϕ^* of the objective

$$\|\mathcal{P}[f, \mu] - g\|_{L^2} + \alpha \mathcal{R}[\mu] \qquad \text{s.t. } \mu = \mu_{\text{CT}} \circ \phi \wedge f \geq 0 \qquad (1)$$

with $\mathcal{P}[f, \mu]$ as the attenuated ray transform, f as the density of radiation, μ as an attenuation map, μ_{CT} as a prototype for the attenuation, usually obtained by a CT scan, and ϕ as a transformation. To compensate for affine linear transformations as well as for nonlinear transformations of the attenuation prototype, configurations for ϕ are an affine linear transformation and a spline transformation. For readability, both transformations are parameterized by the unknown parameter vector c, where in the affine linear case the length of the parameter vector c is in general much smaller. By following a reduction approach and considering $\mathcal{R}$ as a Tikhonov regularization, the reconstruction problem is to find a minimizer f^* and c^* of

$$\mathcal{J}[f, c] := \|\mathcal{P}[f, \mu_{\text{CT}} \circ \phi_c] - g\|_{L^2} + \alpha \|c\|_2 \qquad \text{s.t. } f \geq 0 \qquad (2)$$

Note that the reconstruction model in (1) allows for an arbitrary, not necessarily parametric transformation as described in [2].

The problem of minimizing $\mathcal{J}$ in (2) is addressed with a "discretize then optimize" strategy. That is, after discretization of the objective in (2), a discrete nonlinear optimization problem of finding a minimizer of

$$J^\ell(f, c) := \|A_c^\ell f - g\|_2 + \alpha \|c\|_2 \qquad \text{s.t. } f \geq 0 \qquad (3)$$

with $A_c^\ell \in \mathbb{R}^{m,n}$ as a discretized version of $\mathcal{P}[f, \mu_{\text{CT}}^\ell \circ \phi_c]$ is derived. The identifier μ_{CT}^ℓ denotes a multilevel representation of the attenuation prototype at level ℓ (Fig. 1 for an illustration of μ_{CT}^ℓ). Note that there is a nonlinear dependence of the parameter c in A_c^ℓ. The discrete problem of finding a minimizer (f^{ℓ^*}, c^{ℓ^*}) of $J^\ell(f, c)$ at level ℓ is addressed with a coordinate search method ([6], page 229 ff.). The first coordinate to optimize is considered as the f coordinate. As f is linear in $A_c^\ell f$, a modified steepest descent method [7, 8], that takes the constraint $f \geq 0$ into account is choosen for finding a minimizer of (3) in the f direction. The second coordinate is considered as the c coordinate. As c is nonlinear in $A_c^\ell f$, a Gauss Newton method and an Armijo linesearch rule ([6], page 254 ff. and page 33) is choosen to find a minimizer of (3) in c direction.

The proposed multilevel reconstruction method is to find iteratively a minimizer (f^{ℓ^*}, c^{ℓ^*}) for $\ell = 1, 2, \ldots$ with the coordinate search method as described above based on the result $(f^{\ell-1^*}, c^{\ell-1^*})$ of the coarser $\ell - 1$-th level, starting with an initial (f^{0*}, c^{0*}). This methodology is used for obtaining a minimizer (f^*, μ^*). As it is common to reduce affine linear parts of the transformation before applying a nonlinear spline based motion compensation, two consecutive reconstructions are perforemed. The minimizer of the first reconstruction with the affine linear transformation model serves as an initial for the reconstruction with the spline transformation model.

The proposed method is tested on XCAT phantom data [9], that gives a density of radiation and an attenuation corresponding to a predefined photon energy of a synthetic human. This data is modified to simulate a higher concentration of a radiopharmaceutical in the surface area of a total hip endoprothesis due to an infection. In particular, the attenuation is enriched by a high attenuating region (the endoprothesis), whereas the density of radiation is enriched by a higher density in the surface area of the endoprothesis. The modified attenuation serves as an attenuation prototype μ_{CT} (Fig. 2).

A ground truth density of radiation f^{GT} and attenuation μ^{GT} is created by applying a transformation (with affine linear and nonlinear parts) on the aforementioned enriched density and attenuation images. The first two images of Fig. 2 show the ground truth density and attenuation. The linear transformation simulates in this example a repositioning of the patient, whereas the nonlinear transformation simulates a movement of one leg.

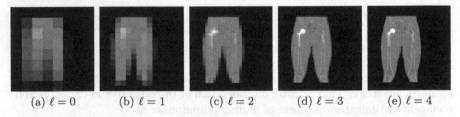

(a) $\ell = 0$ (b) $\ell = 1$ (c) $\ell = 2$ (d) $\ell = 3$ (e) $\ell = 4$

Fig. 1. The attenuation prototype μ_{CT}^{ℓ} at multiple levels ℓ

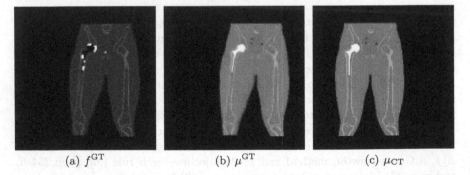

(a) f^{GT} (b) μ^{GT} (c) μ_{CT}

Fig. 2. Ground truth density of radiation and attenuation as well as the attenuation prototype

Table 1. Relative errors $\epsilon(f)$ and $\epsilon(\mu)$ between the ground truth (Fig. 2) and four different reconstructions are shown. The four reconstructions are differentiated by the considered transformation model and optimization strategy (single level (SL) versus multilevel (ML))

	$\epsilon(f) = \|f - f^{GT}\|_2 \,/\, \|f^{GT}\|_2$	$\epsilon(\mu) = \|\mu - \mu^{GT}\|_2 \,/\, \|\mu^{GT}\|_2$
Linear SL	45.04%	82.64%
Spline SL	34.48%	48.43%
Linear ML	13.23%	18.77%
Spline ML	8.22%	6.53%

A single level ($\ell = 4$) reconstruction and a multilevel reconstruction ($\ell = 0, 1, 2, 3, 4$) is then performed based on a simulated measurement g given by $\mathcal{P}[f^{GT}, \mu^{GT}]$ and an attenuation prototype μ^ℓ_{CT} (Fig. 1).

In the next section results of the proposed multilevel approach to SPECT reconstruction with a nonlinear attenuation prototype are shown in comparison with results of a single level reconstruction.

3   Results

Based on the testscenario explained in the previous section, single and multilevel reconstruction results are computed. The first two columns of of Fig. 3 show the single level reconstruction. The latter two columns the multilevel reconstruction. The relative error of the single and multilevel reconstructions to the ground truth is given in Table 1.

4   Discussion

The reconstruction results in Fig. 3 clearly indicate the benefits of the proposed multilevel reconstruction approach. That is, the ground truth attenuation μ^{GT} could not sufficiently be resembled with the computed transformed attenuation prototype of the single level reconstruction (see lower image in the second column of Fig. 3). However, the computed transformed attenuation prototype of the multilevel reconstruction shows a strong resemblence to the ground truth attenuation (see lower image in fourth column of Fig. 3). The same is true for the reconstruction of the density of radiation, as the difference images in the upper row of column two versus column four of Fig. 3 indicates (lower reconstruction error in the multilevel case). In Table 1 a relative error of the single level reconstructions and the multilevel reconstructions are shown. Again, the relative error indicates, that the proposed multilevel reconstruction is superior compared to a single level reconstruction.

These promising results of the proposed SPECT reconstruction with a transformed attenuation prototype at multiple levels of a synthetic human phantom

Fig. 3. The absolute error between the ground truth and four reconstructions are shown. The first row is related to the density, the second row to the attenuation. The columns show from left to right reconstruction errors of a single level reconstruction with an affine linear transformation model, a single level reconstruction with a spline transformation model, a multilevel reconstruction with an affine linear transformation model and a multilevel reconstruction with a spline transformation model. The reconstructions with a spline transformation model are computed based on the initials given by corresponding reconstructions with the affine linear transformation model

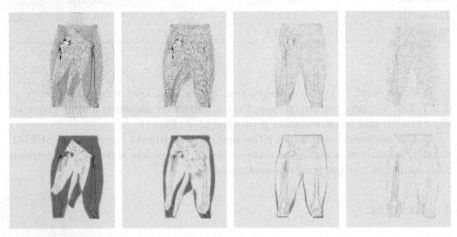

give rise to a 3D implementation. With such, the next step is to test the multilevel reconstruction on clinical data. Note that the 3D case is already provided by the theory.

Acknowledgement. We acknowledge the support of the European Union and the State of Schleswig-Holstein (MOIN CC: grant no. 122-09-053).

References

1. Natterer F. Determination of tissue attenuation in emission tomography of optically dense media. Inverse Probl. 1993;9:731–6.
2. Barendt S, Modersitzki J. SPECT reconstruction with a nonlinear transformed attenuation prototype. Proc BVM. 2011; p. 414–8.
3. Mennessier C, Noo F, Clackdoyle R, et al. Attenuation correction in SPECT using consistency conditions for the exponential ray transform. Phys Med Biol. 1999;44(10):2483–510.
4. Salomon A, Goedicke A, Schweizer B, et al. Simultaneous reconstruction of activity and attenuation for PET/MR. IEEE Trans Med Imaging. 2011;30(3):804–13.
5. Modersitzki J. Flexible Algorithms for Image Registration. Philadelphia: SIAM; 2009.
6. Nocedal J, Wright SJ. Numerical Optimization. Springer; 1999.

7. Bardsley J, Nagy J. Preconditioning strategies for a nonnegatively constrained steepest descent algorithm. Mathematics and Computer Science, Emory University; 2004. TR-2004-010.
8. Kaufman L. Maximum likelihood, least squares, and penalized least squares for PET. IEEE Trans Med Imaging. 1993;12:200–14.
9. Segars WP, Sturgeon GM, Mendonca S, et al. 4D XCAT phantom for multimodality imaging research. Med Phys. 2010;37:4902–15.

Experimentelle Realisierungen einer vollständigen Trajektorie für die magnetische Partikel-Bildgebung mit einer feldfreien Linie

Marlitt Erbe[1], Mandy Grüttner[1], Timo F. Sattel[1], Thorsten M. Buzug[1]

[1]Institut für Mediztechnik, Universität zu Lübeck
erbe@imt.uni-luebeck.de

Kurzfassung. In dieser Arbeit wird die Realisierung einer vollständigen Trajektorie für die magnetische Partikel-Bildgebung (MPI) mit einer feldfreien Linie vorgestellt. Dazu wird gleichzeitig sowohl das Selektionsfeld als auch das Anregungsfeld erzeugt, vermessen und im Bezug auf die Feldqualität ausgewertet. Damit konnte erstmals eine vollständige Trajektorie realisiert werden. Mittels dieser Trajektorie wird es möglich sein, sich effiziente Rekonstruktionsalgorithmen für MPI zu nutze zu machen.

1 Einleitung

Um eine schnelle, dynamische und nicht-invasive Bildgebung bereitzustellen wurde 2005 Magnetic-Particle-Imaging (MPI) vorgestellt [1, 2]. Bei diesem Verfahren werden magnetische Nanopartikel als Tracer injiziert und können mittels einer Kombination aus statischen und dynamischen Magnetfeldern lokalisiert werden. Vorteil dieser neuen Bildgebungsmodalität ist die Echtzeitfähigkeit, die Möglichkeit die Partikelverteilung in drei Dimensionen abzubilden, sowie die Tatsache, dass keinerlei Schädigung für den Patienten auftritt, da die Nanopartikel im Körper auf natürliche Weise abgebaut werden. Konventionell wird bei MPI ein sensitiver Punkt für die Bildgebung verwendet. Diese Methode hat jedoch zur Folge, dass die Auflösung und die Sensitivität des Verfahrens sich negativ beeinflussen. Der Grund dafür ist, dass die Auflösung mit dem Gradienten des applizierten Magnetfeldes steigt, da sich die Region verringert, in der Nanopartikel detektiert werden. Eine geringere Anzahl an signalgebenden Partikeln wirkt sich jedoch negativ auf die Sensitivität dieser Methode aus. Eine mögliche Lösung dieses Problems wird durch die Bildgebung mittels einer magnetischen feldfreien Linie (FFL) erreicht. Bei diesem Verfahren werden Partikel entlang einer Linie aufgenommen und aus dem empfangenen Signal ihre Verteilung rekonstruiert. Da in diesem Fall eine größere Anzahl an Nanopartikeln zum Signal beitragen, der Gradient jedoch erhalten werden kann, steigt das Signal-zu-Rausch-Verhältnis um bis zu einer Größenordnung und damit auch die Sensitivität [3]. Ein weiterer Vorteil der Bildgebung mittels einer FFL ist die Möglichkeit, sich effizienter Rekonstruktionsalgorithmen zu bedienen. Es konnte kürzlich in einer Simulationsstudie gezeigt werden, dass mittels Radon-basierter Rekonstruktion in der FFL-Bildgebung die Rekonstruktionszeit beträchtlich reduziert werden kann [4], was vor allem im Hinblick auf die Echtzeitbildgebung von fundamentaler Bedeutung ist. Bedingung hierfür ist jedoch die Tatsache, dass die Daten im Radonraum aufgenommen werden. Dazu ist sowohl die Rotation der FFL, die mittels eines Demonstrators bereits gezeigt werden konnte [5], als auch die Translation der FFL orthogonal zu ihrer Ausrichtung nötig. Eine vollständige Trajektorie für die FFL-Bildgebung wird in dieser Arbeit experimentell realisiert und evaluiert. Der verwendete Aufbau aus elektromagnetischen Spulen ist in Abb. 1 zu sehen.

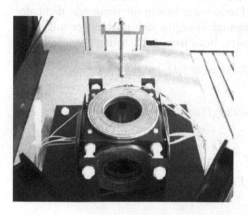

Abb. 1. Der FFL-Felddemonstrator sowie die Hallsonde, die zur Vermessung der Felder eingesetzt wurde

2 Material und Methoden

In dieser Arbeit wird die Realisierung aller zur Bildgebung mittels einer magnetischen FFL notwendigen Felder vorgestellt. Man unterscheidet bei MPI im Allgemeinen zwei magnetische Felder, das Selektionsfeld und das Anregungsfeld. Für das konventionelle MPI-Konzept eines feldfreien Punktes (FFP), ist das Selektionsfeld ein rein statischen Magnetfeld. Das Anregungsfeld dient dazu, den FFP entlang einer dedizierten Trajektorie zu bewegen und regt gleichzeitig die Partikel an, was zu einer Signalgenerierung führt. Für den Fall einer FFL ist die Situation anders. Das Selektionsfeld ist nicht mehr rein statischer Natur, sondern liefert eine FFL, die mit einer Frequenz f_S rotiert. Das bedeutet, dass das Selktionsfeld sowohl einen statischen, als auch einen dynamischen Anteil aufweist. Die Frequenz der Rotation f_S ist jedoch wesentlich geringer als diejenige, mit der das Anregungsfeld oszilliert. f_S liegt in etwa im Bereich von 100 Hz. Mittels eines Felddemonstrators konnte die Generierung des Selektionsfeldes gezeigt werden. Die zur Selektionsfeldgenerierung benötigten Komponenten sind rechts in Abb. 2 dargestellt. Alle verwendeten elektromagnetischen Spulen werden hierzu in Maxwell-Anordnung betrieben. Das bedeutet, dass gegenüberliegende Spulen von entgegengesetzt gleichem Strom durchflossen werden. So entsteht ein dynamisches Gradientenfeld. Für das Anregungsfeld hingegen, welches mit einer Frequenz von $f_A = 25000$ kHz oszilliert, muss ein räumlich homogenes und zeitlich dynamisches Magnetfeld erzeugt werden. Dies geschieht mittels zweier orthogonaler Helmholtz-Spulenpaare. Die Ströme sind in diesem Fall gleichgerichtet und identisch wie links in Abb. 2 dargestellt. Damit können die äußeren Selektionfeldspulen des Felddemonstrators gleichzeitig für die Generierung des Anregungsfeldes genutzt werden. Eine Überlagerung der beiden Stromanteile ergibt dann die angestrebte Trajektorie. Diese besteht in der FFL-Bildgebung somit aus einer langsamen Rotation und einer wesentlich schnelleren Verschiebung der FFL, die immer orthogonal zum Verlauf der FFL geschieht, und ist in Abb. 3 zu sehen. Das Verhältnis der Frequenzen bestimmt dann wie dicht der Bildbereich abgetastet wird. Das Anregungfeld ergibt sich mittels der folgenden Ströme in den orthogonalen Spulenpaaren in x- bzw. y-Richtung

$$I_{A,x}(t) = I_0 \sin(f_0 t) \cos(2\pi f_1 t) \quad \text{und} \tag{1}$$

$$I_{A,y}(t) = I_0 \sin(2\pi f_A t) \sin(2\pi f_S t) \tag{2}$$

mit

$$N_p = \frac{f_A}{f_S} \tag{3}$$

Die Abtastdichte wird also durch das Frequenzverhältnis N_p bestimmt.

3 Ergebnisse

Mittels des FFL-Felddemonstrators wurde zusätzlich zu der bereits gezeigten Rotation das Anregungsfeld für die FFL-Bildgebung erzeugt, vermessen und evaluiert. Um die Ergebnisse darstellen zu können, wurden exemplarisch drei Punkte der FFL-Trajektorie gewählt und vermessen. Dazu wurde eine horizontale, eine diagonale sowie eine vertikale FFL-Auslenkung generiert. Der Gradient senkrecht zur FFL liegt bei $0.25 \ \mathrm{Tm^{-1}}\mu_0^{-1}$. Der Messbereich umfasst eine Fläche von 28 x 28 mm^2 und setzt sich aus 15 x 15 Voxeln zusammen. Die Ergebnisse sind in Abb. 4 dargestellt. Die obere Reihe zeigt die mittels des Selektionsfeldes erzeugte, unausgelenkte FFL. In der unteren Bildreihe ist die zusätzliche Translation der FFL orthogonal zu ihrer Auslenkung zu sehen. Zur Feldvermessung wurde eine 3D-Hallsonde der Firma Lakeshore verwendet. Um die Ergebnisse auszuwerten, wurde die Abweichung der Messdaten von der Simulation anhand

Abb. 2. Das Anregungsfeld kann mittels zweier orthogonaler Helmholtz-Spulenpaaren realisiert werden (linke Seite). Damit können die äußeren Selektionsfeldspulen (rechte Seite, dunkelgrau) des Felddemonstrators gleichzeitig zur Erzeugung des Anregungsfeldes genutzt werden

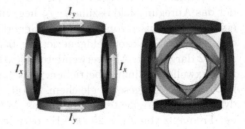

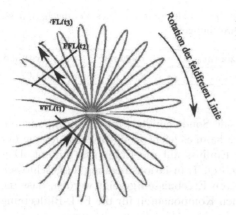

Abb. 3. Radiale Trajektorie für die FFL-Bildgebung

des *normalized root mean square deviation* (NRMSD) berechnet. Die Simulation der Felder erfolgt über eine numerischen Auswertung des Biot-Savart-Integrals. Die Ergebnisse sind in Tab. 1 zu finden. Der NRMSD liegt sogar noch unterhalb der Ergebnisse, die für die reine Rotation erzielt werden konnten. Grund dafür ist eine Optimierung des Messprozesses. So wurde für die Messung des Anregungsfeldes eine 3D-Hallsonde verwendet. Für die Messung der reinen Rotation,

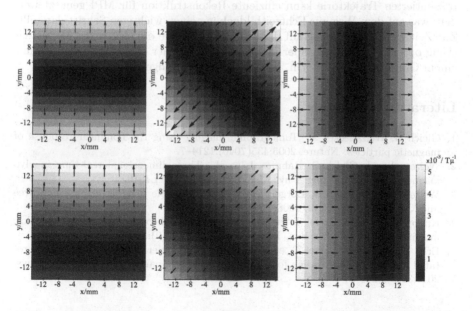

Abb. 4. Messergebnisse für das Selektions und das Anregungsfeld des FFL-Scanneraufbaus. In der oberen Reihe sind die Ergebnisse ohne Anregungsfeld zu sehen. Die untere Reihe zeigt nun zusätzlich implementierte Transkationder FFL, die orthogonal zu ihrer Ausrichtung geschieht

Tabelle 1. Eine Validierung der vermessenen Felder anhand eines Vergleichs mit simulierten Daten ergibt die folgenden Abweichungen

Richtung der Translation	horizontal	diagonal	vertikal
NRMSD in %	1,76	1,60	1,62

wurden eine axiale und eine transversale Sonde genutzt, um die Komponenten des Feldes einzeln zu vermessen. Dabei kann es leicht zu einer Verschiebung der Messpunkte kommen, was negativen Einfluss auf die Ergebnisse nimmt. Diese Fehlerquelle konnte bei der vorgestellten Translationsmessung ausgeschlossen werden. Es konnte mit den präsentierten Ergebnissen gezeigt werden, dass die Implementierung aller feldgenerierenden Komponenten für die FFL-Bildgebung möglich ist.

4 Diskussion

Es wurde ein Aufbau vorgestellt, der eine vollständige Trajektorie für die Bildgebung mit einer feldfreien Linie in MPI erzeugt. Drei beispielhafte Feldverläufe wurden vermessen und evaluiert. Die Abweichungen der Felder sind gering und werden zu einem großen Teil durch Messungenauigkeiten begründet. Mittels der präsentierten Trajektorie kann effiziente Rekonstruktion für MPI genutzt werden, was auf dem Weg zur Echtzeitbildgebung einen wichtigen Schritt darstellt. Zur Zeit wird ein in Bezug auf die Feldqualität sowie die elektrische Verlustleistung optimierter FFL-Scanner implementiert, welcher es ermöglichen wird mit einem Gradienten von $1.5 \ \mathrm{Tm}^{-1}\mu_0^{-1}$ dynamische Bildgebung zu betreiben.

Literaturverzeichnis

1. Gleich B, Weizenecker J. Tomographic imaging using the nonlinear response of magnetic particles. Nature. 2005;435(7046):1214–7.
2. Weizenecker J, Gleich B, Rahmer J, et al. Three-dimensional real-time in vivo magnetic particle imaging. Phys Med Biol. 2009;54(5):L1–10.
3. Weizenecker J, Gleich B, Borgert J. Magnetic particle imaging using a field free line. J Phys D Appl Phys. 2008;41(10):3pp.
4. Knopp T, Erbe M, Sattel T, et al. A Fourier slice theorem for magnetic particle imaging using a field-free line. Inverse Probl. 2011;27(9):095004.
5. Erbe M, Knopp T, Sattel T, et al. Experimental generation of an arbitrarily rotated magnetic field-free line for the use in magnetic particle imaging. Med Phys. 2011;38(9):5200–7.

Fast 3D Vector Field Multi-Frequency Magnetic Resonance Elastography of the Human Brain
Preliminary Results

Andreas Fehlner[1], Sebastian Hirsch[2], Jürgen Braun[1], Ingolf Sack[2]

[1]Institute of Medical Informatics, Charité – University Medicine Berlin, Germany
[2]Department of Radiology, Charité – University Medicine Berlin, Germany
andreas.fehlner@charite.de

Abstract. Magnetic resonance elastography (MRE) is capable of "palpating" the brain by measuring externally induced intracranial shear waves with high spatial and temporal resolution. Conventional MRE is limited as it either relies on two-dimensional multifrequency wave acquisition or three-dimensional vector field MRE at single frequencies. However, full assessment of spatially resolved viscoelastic constants requires both, the acquisition of full shear wave fields and broad dynamic range MRE at multiple frequencies. We therefore propose fast single-shot MRE at 3 Tesla magnetic field strength combined with continuous wave stimulation and interleaved image slice acquisition. By this protocol, a full three dimensional MRE data set is acquired within 60, which may readily be repeated for multifrequency data acquisition. The feasibility of the method is demonstrated in the brain of one healthy volunteer at 50 Hz mechanical excitation frequency. The measured complex modulus values are in agreement with results reported in the literature.

1 Introduction

Medical imaging modalities are important tools in clinical diagnosis. Most modalities such as magnetic resonance imaging (MRI) provide highly resolved morphological images but are limited in assessing the integrity and constitution of tissues. In contrast, manual palpation is a simple, yet highly efficient way of assessing soft tissue's mechanical constitution. Magnetic resonance elastography (MRE) combines MRI and palpation to a new and quantitative imaging modality [1]. To date, MRE is the only method capable of measuring intracranial viscoelastic parameters without intervention [2]. Clinical motivation of MRE of the brain is the diagnosis of diffuse neurodegenerative processes associated with various neurological disorders as Multiple sclerosis [3] or Alzheimer's disease [4]. In principle, MRE experiments combine three technical key-points: i) external stimulation of time-harmonic shear waves; ii) acquisition of wave fields by motion sensitive phase contrast MRI and iii) recovery of elasticity parameters using wave inversion algorithms. Currently, MRE is limited by long scan times and is therefore applied either by two-dimensional (2D) MRE at four drive frequencies [2] or by three-dimensional (3D) MRE at single frequency [5]. Multifrequency 2D MRE can assess the dynamics of the complex shear modulus but cannot provide field information. In contrast, 3D MRE provides the full vector field of the shear waves but is limited in dynamic information. We therefore seek to accelerate MRE of the human brain to ultimately combine 3D vector field acquisition with multifrequency MRE. The aim of this pilot study is to test the feasibility of rapid single-shot multislice wave field acquisition by continuous wave stimulation in a 3 Tesla MRI scanner and to compare the results to literature data. Vibration generation at 50 Hz is achieved by a novel non-magnetic driver based on piezo-electrical ceramics. If successful, the proposed cerebral MRE combines clinical requirements with a maximum of elastodynamic information deducible from intracranial shear wave fields.

2   Material and methods

All examinations were performed on a clinical 3 T scanner (Siemens Trio, Erlangen, Germany) (Fig. 1) using a single-shot spin-echo echo-planar imaging (EPI) sequence. The motion encoding gradient (MEG) of 59 Hz, one cycle, first moment nulling, was consecutively applied along the directions of all three Cartesian components of the scanner coordinate system. 15 transversal image slices were acquired for each field component within a total repetition time (TR) of 2500 ms while continuously stimulating the head by a harmonic vibration of 50 Hz frequency. A trigger pulse was sent to the wave generator at the beginning of each

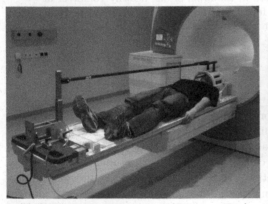
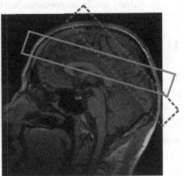
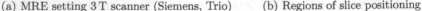

(a) MRE setting 3 T scanner (Siemens, Trio)   (b) Regions of slice positioning

Fig. 1. Experimental setup. (a) In the foreground the actor with the piezoelectric system is shown. The head is placed pivotable in a head cradle. The integrated waveform generator and amplifier, which is connected to the actor and the trigger of the scanner is located in the control room; (b) On day #1, a region containing the upper part of the the brain through the ventricular system (solid line) was used, whereas on day #2, more tiled slice positions (dashed lines) through the visual cortex, were selected

image acquisition. The dynamics of wave propagation was measured at 8 instances over a full vibration period (Fig. 2). Consequently, one full 3D MRE data

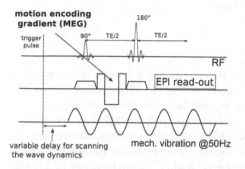

Fig. 2. Schematic of the MRE sequence. Different phases of the propagating wave are observed by varying the delay between the start of the vibration and the MEG

set including 8 time points, 3 components ("slice selection", "phase encoding", "read out" directions) consists of 24 volumes of 15 slices each. Further imaging parameters: Echo time (TE) = 48 ms, spatial resolution = $2.5 \times 2.5 \times 2.5 \,\text{mm}^3$, total measurement time = 60 sec, MEG amplitude = 30 mT/m, MEG slew rate = 100 mT/m/ms. The experiments were repeated 6 times at 2 different days on the same volunteer (age: 25) to estimate the reproducibility of the results.

The work flow for post-processing was as follows: The acquired phase images were spatially unwrapped by calculating the spatial derivatives of the spin phase from the raw wrapped phase data $\phi_k \in [0, 2\pi]$; $k \neq j \in \{1, 2, 3\}$

$$\frac{\partial \phi_k}{\partial x_j} = -i \exp(-i\phi_k) \frac{\partial \exp(i\phi_k)}{\partial x_j} \tag{1}$$

These oscillations $\partial \phi_k / \partial x_j$, were scaled to a strain quantity $\partial U_k / \partial x_j$ using a factor derived from fractional MRE [6]

$$\frac{\partial U_k}{\partial x_j} = \frac{\partial \phi_k}{\partial x_j} \cdot \frac{\pi(q^2 - 1)}{\gamma g_k \tau_g q \sin(\pi q)}; \quad q = \frac{\tau_g}{\tau_\nu} \tag{2}$$

The variable τ_ν denotes the vibration period $(2\pi/\omega)$; τ_g and g_k are the duration and amplitude of the MEG; γ stands for the gyromagnetic ratio. The index k refers to the different directions of the MEG. The resulting derivatives were Fourier transformed in time in order to calculate wave images at drive frequency. A spatial low pass filter was applied to reduce noise. To a minor portion, the vibration caused unwanted compression waves. Therefore, the curl-operator was applied to the total displacement vector field yielding pure deviatoric strain. Complex modulus images were obtained by a least squares wave inversion method [5] using all three vector field components. The complex shear modulus G^* was spatially averaged using the median of the entire parenchyma in three central image slices. Mean values and standard deviations of shear storage modulus $G' = \text{Re}(G^*)$ and shear loss modulus $G'' = \text{Im}(G^*)$

were tabulated for all experiments (Table 1). The real part G' of the complex modulus G^* relates to the restoration of mechanical energy due to the elastic properties of the material whereas the imaginary part G'' characterizes the loss of energy as a result of mechanical friction.

3 Results

The real and the imaginary parts of the curl components for one slice measured in the first experiment at day #2 are shown in Fig. 3. These maps display the oscillations without compression waves as used later for wave inversion.

Fig. 4 shows a typical complex modulus map. It is visible that the storage modulus is higher than the loss modulus. Fig. 5 and Table 1 demonstrate that the good reproducibility of the storage and loss modulus by low standard deviations of G' and G''. The mean relative error for G' and G'' is in the order of 5% and 7%. For day #1 an averaged storage modulus of 1.91(09) kPa and an averaged loss modulus of 0.96(05) kPa and for day #2 an averaged storage modulus of 1.85(09) kPa and an averaged loss modulus of 0.88(07) kPa were determined. The complex shear modulus values is in agreement to literature values reported for young healthy volunteers [2].

4 Discussion

By the proposed method, the scan time of 3D cerebral MRE could be reduced to 60 seconds corresponding to an acceleration factor of approximately 14 compared to conventional gradient echo based 3D MRE comprising seven slices [7]. This advancement was achieved by a short TE, single-shot EPI and 3 T MRI. 6 min

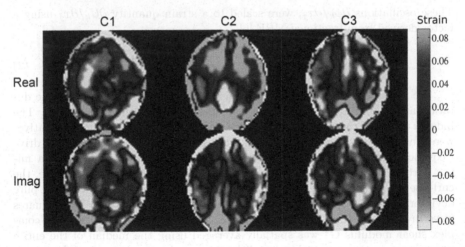

Fig. 3. Illustration of the curl components. $C1 = \partial U_3/\partial x_2 - \partial U_2/\partial x_3$, $C2 = \partial U_1/\partial x_3 - \partial U_3/\partial x_1$, $C3 = \partial U_2/\partial x_1 - \partial U_1/\partial x_2$

Table 1. Results for the real part G' and the imaginary part G'' of the complex storage moduli in kPa at 50 Hz for the repeated experiments (RX)

	R1	R2	R3	R4	R5	R6	Mean	std
G'(day #1)	1.81	1.94	1.80	1.98	2.04	1.92	1.91	0.09
G"(day #1)	0.91	1.04	0.95	0.96	1.00	0.89	0.96	0.05
G'(day #2)	1.80	1.97	1.72	1.83	1.91	1.90	1.86	0.09
G"(day #2)	0.82	0.89	0.83	0.91	1.02	0.83	0.88	0.07

are considered as the desired maximum MRE duration applied in addition to clinical MRI. Within this time one would be able to repeat 3D MRE at six different drive frequencies. Using conventional methods of the same duration, only two slices can be acquired by 2D MRE [2, 3] whereas 3D MRE is not feasible. The new 3D MRE method was proven very reproducible even though different 3D regions were considered. This method provides new perspectives for detailed investigations of mechanical alternations of the brain due to neurodegenerative processes in Multiple Sclerosis [3] or Alzheimer diseases [4].

References

1. Muthupillai R, Lomas D, Rossman P, et al. Magnetic resonance elastography by direct visualization of propagating acoustic strain waves. Science. 1995;269(5232):1854–7.

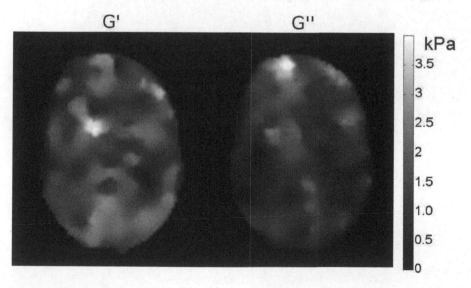

Fig. 4. Complex modulus images. G' and G'' denote real and imaginary part of G^*

Fig. 5. Variation of the storage and loss modulus of the complex modulus over 6 consecutive experiments. At the different days different positions of 3D regions were selected (Fig. 1b)

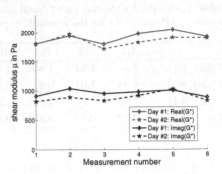

2. Sack I, Beierbach B, Wuerfel J, et al. The impact of aging and gender on brain viscoelasticity. Neuroimage. 2009;46(3):652–7.

3. Wuerfel J, Paul F, Beierbach B, et al. MR-elastography reveals degradation of tissue integrity in multiple sclerosis. Neuroimage. 2010;49(3):2520–5.

4. Murphy MC, Huston J, Jack CR, et al. Decreased brain stiffness in Alzheimer's disease determined by magnetic resonance elastography. J Magn Reson Imaging. 2011;34(3):494–8.

5. Oliphant TE, Manduca A, Ehman RL, et al. Complex-valued stiffness reconstruction for magnetic resonance elastography by algebraic inversion of the differential equation. Magn Reson Med. 2001;45(2):299–310.

6. Rump J, Klatt D, Braun J, et al. Fractional encoding of harmonic motions in MR elastography. Magn Reson Med. 2007;57(2):388–95.

7. Green MA, Bilston LE, Sinkus R. In vivo brain viscoelastic properties measured by magnetic resonance elastography. NMR Biomed. 2008;21(7):755–64.

Bildgestützte Formanalyse biomedizinisch relevanter Gold Nanorods

Dominic Swarat[1], Nico Sudyatma[1], Thorsten Wagner[1], Martin Wiemann[2],
Hans-Gerd Lipinski[1]

[1]Biomedical Imaging Group, Fachbereich Informatik, Fachhochschule Dortmund
[2]Institute for Lung Health (IBE R&D gGmbH), Münster
dominic.swarat@fh-dortmund.de

Kurzfassung. Gold Nanorods werden in der Medizin sowohl für experimentelle als auch für klinische Zwecke erfolgreich eingesetzt. Diese nanoskaligen Partikel sind mit Hilfe von Transmissionselektronenmikroskopen abbildbar und zeichnen sich in den Bildern durch eine einfache, ovale Grundstruktur aus. Mit Hilfe einer auf diese Geometrie abgezielten Formanalyse-Methode, können die Originalabbildungen der Nanorods durch ein einfaches, graphisches Modell beschrieben werden, dessen Geometrieparameter sich automatisch aus den Elektronenmikroskopiebildern extrahieren lassen. Nicht nur lässt sich mit dieser Methode eine Partikelcharge mit den Hersteller typischen Längen- und Durchmesserangaben kennzeichnen, sondern auch eine Formhomogenität charakterisieren. Eine solche zusätzliche Information über die Geometrie des Objektes erscheint sinnvoll, weil die geometrische Form das dynamische Verhalten dieser Partikel im biologischen System durchaus beeinflussen kann.

1 Einleitung

Zu den am häufigsten verwendeten nanoskaligen Materialien für die Biomedizin zählen so genannte Gold Nanorods [1, 2]. Es sind massive zylinderförmige Goldpartikel, die eine relativ einfache Geometrie besitzen und deren Länge üblicherweise zwischen 10 und 300 nm liegt. Damit sind diese Partikel mit optischen Methoden direkt nicht nachweisbar. Jedoch lassen sie sich mit Hilfe der Transmissionselektronenmikroskopie visualisieren.

Gold Nanorods werden in vielen Bereich der Biomedizin, z.B. in der Grundlagenforschung, zur Diagnoseunterstützung und auch für die Therapie, erfolgreich eingesetzt. So lassen sich diese Partikel für die Genforschung [3], für das Tumor-Targeting [4], die Krebstherapie [5] sowie in verschiedenen Bereichen der molekularen Biomedizin [1, 2, 6, 7] verwenden.

Beweglichkeit, chemische Reaktionsfähigkeit und weitere funktionelle Eigenschaften dieser Nanorods hängen u.a. auch von ihrer geometrischen Form ab [4]. Zwar erscheinen die industriell erzeugten, zumeist monodispersen Partikel in relativ gleichförmigen Kollektiven produzierbar zu sein, bei genauerem Hinsehen fallen jedoch durchaus individuelle Unterschiede hinsichtlich ihrer Form und Größe auf. Mit Hilfe einer einfachen, geometrischen Modellierung soll daher das Formverhalten von biomedizinisch-relevanten Gold Nanorods untersucht werden.

2   Material und Methoden

Mit Hilfe der Transmissionselektronenmikroskopie (TEM) lassen sich Gold Nano-rods (GNR) als zweidimensionale Bilder darstellen (verwendet wurden Materiali-en und deren elektronenmikroskopische Aufnahmen von der Fa. NanoRods LLC, Germantown/MD,USA). Die Abb. 1a zeigt, dass diese Art von Nanopartikeln eine relativ einfache geometrische Struktur besitzt, wobei bei der hier verwende-ten Bildgenerierung lt. Hersteller darauf geachtet wurde, dass alle abgebildeten GNR in einer Bildebene lagen. Industriell gefertigte GNR sollten weitgehend gleichgroß sein und ein festes Seitenverhältnis besitzen. Bei näherem Betrachten fällt jedoch auf, dass sie sich (u.a. produktionsbedingt) hinsichtlich Größe und Form durchaus unterscheiden (Abb. 1a).

In erster Näherung lässt sich ein GNR geometrisch als ein Oval interpretieren, das durch den Durchmesser D und die Länge L_0 festgelegt ist (Abb. 1b). Da sich die geometrische Form des Ovals durch die Kombination zweier Halbkreise mit dem Radius R und eines (zentral gelegenen) Rechtecks mit den Seitenlängen $D = 2R$ und $L = L_0 - 2R$ darstellen lässt, sind Fläche A und Umfang U eines solchen GNR-Modells einfach zu berechnen

$$A = 2 \cdot (\frac{\pi}{2} + \beta) \cdot R^2; \qquad U = 2 \cdot (\pi + \beta) \cdot R \qquad (1)$$

wobei $\beta = \frac{2 \cdot L}{D} = \frac{L}{R}$ ist. Dieser Faktor legt das Seitenverhältnis des zentralen Rechtecks eines GNR fest (Abb. 1b). Damit lässt sich die auf den Kreis normierte

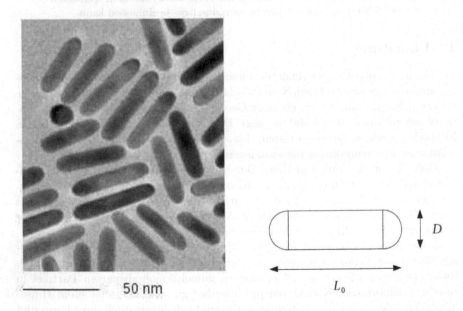

Abb. 1. Gold Nanorods. Original TEM-Registrierung (links); vereinfachtes geometri-sches Modell (Oval) mit Breite D und Länge L_0 (rechts)

Zirkularität c_M eines GNR-Modells durch den Ausdruck

$$c_M = \frac{1}{4\pi} \cdot \frac{U^2}{A} = 1 + \frac{\beta^2}{\pi \cdot (\pi + 2 \cdot \beta)} \qquad (2)$$

berechnen ($1 \leq c_M < \infty$).

Um die TEM-Registrierungen der GNR mit dem geometrischen Modell vergleichen zu können, werden von jedem GNR die Zirkularitätsfaktoren c_{GNR} und c_M bestimmt. Zu diesem Zweck müssen die Fläche und der Umfang eines GNR aus den Bilddaten extrahiert werden.

Ausgehend von der Originalregistrierung (Abb. 2a) wird in einem ersten Schritt, mit einem 5x5-Gaußfilter, eine Bildglättung im Ortsbereich durchgeführt. Aus dem so geglätteten Bild wird in einem zweiten Schritt, nach Anwendung einer einfachen schwellwertbasierten Segmentierung, daraus eine Binärszene erzeugt (Abb. 2b). Jedes Objekt dieser Szene entspricht einem GNR, der durch seine Lage eindeutig identifizierbar ist und dessen Fläche A_{GNR} bestimmt werden kann. In einem dritten Schritt wird auf die Binärszene ein Cannyfilter angewendet, mit dessen Hilfe die GNR-Konturen in 1-Pixelbreite erzeugt werden (Abb. 2c). Anhand der Konturen lässt sich nunmehr der Umfang U_{GNR} jedes einzelnen im Bild vorhandenen GNR ermitteln. Zusammen mit A_{GNR} lässt sich damit die empirische Zirkularität c_{GNR} analog zu (3) für jeden einzelnen GNR berechnen.

In einem letzten Schritt werden die Geometriedaten D und L_0 für jeden GNR automatisch detektiert. Dazu wird von jedem registrierten und identifizierten GNR der Mittelpunkt und seine Lage in der Ebene (Orientierung) bestimmt, von dem aus dann die Werte für die Parameter D und L_0-Wert ermittelt werden. Dazu wird, ausgehend vom Objektmittelpunkt, auf jeden GNR ein Rechteck derart gelegt, dass es die gleiche Ausrichtung wie der GNR in der Ebene hat.

Länge und Breite dieses Rechtecks werden dabei inkrementell so variiert, dass man das kleinste umschreibende Rechteck erhält. Dann stimmen Breite D_R und Länge L_R dieses Rechtecks (weitgehend) mit den Parametern D bzw. L_0 überein. Diese Parameter werden anschließend verwendet, um die Szene der GNR-Modelle zu generieren. Dabei werden die binären GNR in die korrespondierenden Modell-GNR überführt (Abb. 2d) und deren Zirkularität c_M abschließend nach (3) berechnet.

3 Ergebnisse

Mit Hilfe der oben beschriebenen Methoden konnten elektronenmikroskopische GNR-Bilddaten automatisch ausgewertet werden. Untersucht wurden 374 GNR in acht verschiedenen TEM-Aufnahmenserien, wobei zunächst nur solche GNR-Bilder herangezogen wurden, in denen die GNR eine offensichtlich ovale Struktur aufwiesen. Verglichen wurden dabei zunächst Umfang U und Fläche A der GNR, die den Binärszenen entnommen wurden, mit den Werten der korrespondierenden Modell-GNR, die mit Hilfe des kleinsten umschreibenden Rechtecks ermittelt wurden. Dabei zeigte sich, dass die Unterschiede der Parameter U und A von

Modell und korrespondierendem GNR normalverteilt (Test auf Normalverteilung mit D'Agostino-Test) sind. Die Anwendung des Differenz-t-Tests zeigte, dass keine signifikanten Unterschiede zwischen den GNR- und den Modell-Parametern bestehen ($p < 0.01$).

Anschließend wurde untersucht, ob eine signifikante Abweichung zwischen der empirischen Zirkularität und der Modell-Zirkularität besteht. Auch hier zeigten sich die Differenzwerte $c_{GRN} - c_M$ normalverteilt. Ein Differenz-t-Test ergab ebenfalls keinen Unterschied zwischen den beiden Formparameter-Werten c_{GRN} und c_M (p<0.01). Eine lineare Korrelationsanalyse zwischen den beiden Zirkularitätsparametern c_M und c_{GNR} ergab zudem einen Pearsonschen Korrelations-

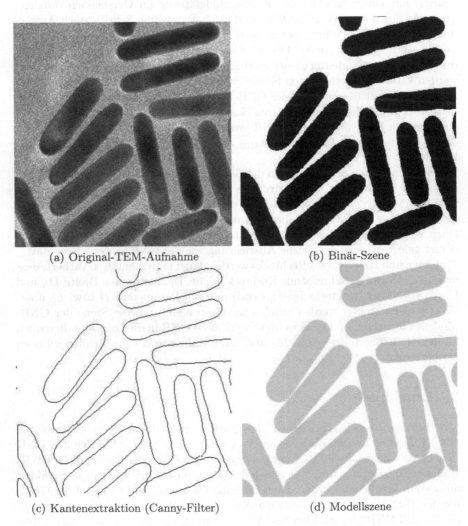

(a) Original-TEM-Aufnahme   (b) Binär-Szene

(c) Kantenextraktion (Canny-Filter)   (d) Modellszene

Abb. 2. Formanalyse einer Ansammlung von Nanorods

koeffizienten von 0.989. Schließlich wurden die von der jeweiligen GNR-Charge ermittelten Durchmesserwerte mit den Herstellerangaben verglichen, wobei zwischen den Herstellerangaben und den mit Hilfe des beschriebenen Algorithmus ermittelten Daten (Länge, Durchmesser, Aspect ratio) kein signifikanter Unterschied bestand ($p < 0.001$).

In einer weiteren Analyse wurde gezielt nach solchen Objekten in den TEM-Bildern gesucht, die sich auffällig von einer ovalen Form unterschieden. Diese ließen sich mit dem beschriebenen Algorithmus, aufgrund der ermittelten Geometrieparameter, leicht detektieren. Mit Hilfe ihres Anteils N an der Gesamtzahl N_g aller im Bild enthaltenen Partikel, wurde das Homogenitätskriterium H der Charge definiert: $H = 1 - \frac{N}{N_g}$. Für die acht ausgewählten Probenbilder betrug dieser Wert $H = 0.93 \pm 0.04$(mean $\pm$ SEM).

4 Diskussion

Es konnte gezeigt werden, dass es mit Hilfe eines einfachen Oval-Modells gelingt, die geometrische Form von Gold Nanorods in TEM-Bildern automatisch zu detektieren und zu analysieren. Dabei zeigte die direkte Gegenüberstellung der vom Original-GNR und dem korrespondierenden Oval-Modell ermittelten Parametern „Fläche" und „Umfang" keinen signifikanten Unterschied. Daher erscheint es sinnvoll, für weitere Bildanalysen von GNR-Szenen anstelle der Originalabbildungen mit den entsprechenden Geometriemodellen zu arbeiten.

Auch eine statistische Auswertung der Größenverteilungen der Partikel in einer Probenaufnahme lässt sich mit dieser automatischen, Form analysierenden Methode einfach durchführen. Zudem kann das Geometriemodell als Maske für die Analyse der TEM-Elektronendichte individueller GNR verwendet werden. Dadurch lassen sich die Dichteinhomogenitäten von GNR aufdecken, deren Kenntnis für das physikalische Verhalten der GNR (Diffusion, Verhalten während der Bestrahlung mit Laserlicht, Größenbestimmung mit Lasermikroskopiemethoden) wichtig ist [8, 9].

In den vorliegenden TEM-Bildern konnten zudem Objekte mit durchaus markanten Abweichungen von der idealen Ovalform beobachtet werden. Diese ließen sich mit Hilfe der genannten Geometrieparameter einfach detektieren. Somit konnten die jeweiligen GNR-Chargen nicht nur mit Hilfe der Hersteller typischen Angaben zum Längen- und Durchmesserverhalten der GNR charakterisiert werden, sondern auch hinsichtlich ihrer Formhomogenität.

Danksagung. Diese Arbeit wurde mit Mitteln des Bundesministeriums für Bildung und Forschung (BMBF / FKZ 17PNT026) gefördert.

Literaturverzeichnis

1. Pissuwan D, Valenzuela S, Cortie M. Prospects for gold nanorod partricles in diagnostic and therapeutic applications. Biotech Gen Eng. 2008;25(1):93–112.

2. Stone J, Jackson S, Wright D. Biological application of gold nanorods. Rev Nanomed Nanobiotechnol. 2011;3(1):100–9.
3. Cen CC, Lin Y, Wang C, et al. DNA-Gold nanorod conjugates for remote control of localized gene expression by near infrared irradiation. J Am Chem Soc. 2006;128(11):3709–15.
4. Maltzahn G, Park J, Lin K, et al. Nanoparticles that communicate in vitro to amplify tumor targeting. Nature Mat. 2011;10(1):545–52.
5. Huff T, Tong L, Zhao Y, et al. Hyperthermic effects of gold nanorods on tumor cells. Nanomed. 2007;2(1):125–32.
6. Hwang S, Tao A. Biofunctionalization of gold nanorods. Pure Appl Chem. 2011;83(1):233–41.
7. Ren X, Yang L, Ren J, et al. Direct interaction between gold nanorods and glucose. Nanosc Res Let. 2010;5(10):1658–63.
8. Jebb M, Pramod P, Thomas KG, et al. Ru(II) trisbipyridine functionalized gold nanorods: morphological changes and excited-state interaction. J Phys Chem B. 2007;111(24):6839–44.
9. Hernandez-Contreras M, Medina-Novola M. Brownian motion of interacting nonspherical tracer particles: general theory. Phys Rev E. 1996;54(6):6573–85.

Auffaltung von Gefäßbäumen mit Hilfe von deformierbaren Oberflächen

Anja Schnaars[1,2], Christian Tietjen[2], Grzegorz Soza[2], Bernhard Preim[1]

[1]Institut für Simulation und Graphik, Universität Magdeburg
[2]Siemens Healthcare Computed Tomography
peter.faltin@lfb.rwth-aachen.de

Kurzfassung. Follow-up assessment of pleural thickenings requires the comparison of information from different points in time. The investigated image regions must be precisely registered to acquire this information. Since the thickenings' growth is the target value, this growth should not be compensated by the registration process. We therefore present a non-rigid registration method, which preserves the shape of the thickenings. The deformation of the volume image is carried out using B-splines. With focus on the image regions located around the lung surface, an efficient way of calculating corresponding points combined with the reuse of information from different scale levels leads to the non-rigid registration, which can be performed within a short computation time.

1 Einleitung

Insbesondere in der Leber erlauben Kenntnisse über deren Gefäßbaumtopologien eine detaillierte Analyse, Planung sowie Durchführung von chirurgischen Eingriffen. Um die Versorgung von verbleibendem Gewebe nach einer Teilresektion der Leber weiterhin zu gewährleisten, sollte ebenfalls der Verlauf wichtiger Gefäße bekannt sein. Folglich ist eine Darstellung essentiell, die sowohl die Ausdehnung der Gefäße im Bereich der Resektion als auch übersichtlich die Verbindungs- sowie Verzweigungsstruktur wiedergibt. Die Verfolgung eines Pfades entlang des Lebergefäßsystems ist hingegen insbesondere im Bereich der Tumorbehandlung von großem Interesse. Bei einer Embolisation eines partiellen Gefäßbaumes muss das Embolisat über einen Katheter zielgerichtet verabreicht werden, um nur die Zielregion zu erreichen. Um eine möglichst einfache Navigation der Sonde zu ermöglichen, sollte der entsprechende Pfad in der Darstellung nicht durch andere Strukturen verdeckt werden.

Dabei stellt eine geeignete Visualisierung der Gefäßbäume eine essentielle Grundlage für eine qualitative Beurteilung dar. Sowohl existierende zweidimensionale als auch dreidimensionale Darstellungsverfahren geben jedoch nur einen bestimmten Ausschnitt des Gesamten Informationsgehalt der Daten zurück. Entweder entstehen Einbußen in der Übersichtlichkeit oder es können nur Teilausschnitte des Gefäßbaumes dem Betrachter präsentiert werden [1, 2]. Die Auffaltung eines Gefäßbaumes ermöglicht die Repräsentation seiner Topologie ohne

Überlagerungen von Strukturen in einer einzigen Darstellung und ist vielseitig einsetzbar. Zusätzlich kann diese Darstellung ideal zur Validierung und Editierung eines segmentierten Gefäßbaumes verwendet werden.

Voraussetzung für das in diesem Beitrag beschriebenen Verfahren ist, dass die Gefäße als segmentierte Baumstrukturen vorliegen, aus denen die Topologie als Centerline-Datenstruktur ermittelt werden kann.

2   Material und Methoden

Im Wesentlichen existieren zwei Verfahren, die versuchen einen Gefäßbaum aufgefaltet darzustellen [2, 3]. Bei der Multi-Path CPR werden Schnitte entlang der einzelnen Gefäß-Centerline erstellt, die in eine Ebene projiziert werden [2]. Anschließend erfolgt die Anordnung benachbarter Gefäßdarstellungen mit Hilfe von rekursiv umschreibenden Unterbäumen. In dem Ansatz von Kiraly et al. wird entlang jeder Gefäß-Centerline auf Grundlage der Gefäßoberfläche eine Intensity Projection erzeugt, die danach in einem Baumdiagramm angeordnet wird [3]. Beide Verfahren erzeugen eine sehr schematische Darstellung des Gefäßbaumes. Des Weiteren ist Multi-Path CPR eher für weniger komplexe Gefäßbäume geeignet. Anwendungsbeispiele hierfür wären Herzkranzgefäße oder periphere Gefäße. Ein weiteres relevantes Verfahren erzeugt mit Hilfe von Coons-Flächen einen Schnitt durch ein Gefäß [4]. Diese Fläche wird anschließend in einem Punkt bzw. in einer Curve-Of-Interest geebnet. Jedoch ist dieses Verfahren nur für ein Gefäß und nicht für einen Gefäßbaum konzipiert.

Die in diesem Beitrag verwendeten Ausgangsdaten beinhalten sowohl den originalen Volumendatensatz als auch einen segmentierten Gefäßbaum, der manuell bzw. automatisch gewonnen werden kann. Dieser Gefäßbaum liegt in einer Graphenstruktur vor, in der sowohl Informationen zum Gefäßverlauf als auch deren approximierten Gefäßkonturen der einzelnen Gefäßbaumäste vorliegen. Der Verlauf wird mittels der Gefäß-Centerlines, welche im Grunde eine in gleichmäßigen Abständen abgetastete, geordnete Punktefolge darstellen, beschrieben. Durch eine Kreisradiusvariable wird jedem Centerline-Punkt die Informationen zur lokalen Gefäßkontur zugeordnet.

3   Ergebnisse

Für die Auffaltung des Gefäßbaumes erzeugt das Verfahren eine Schnittfläche basierend auf der Topologie des Gefäßbaumes. Diese Schnittfläche wird anschließend so aufgefaltet, dass sie sich in einer planaren Ebene befindet. Eine Besonderheit des Verfahrens ist, dass es nicht nur auf ein Gefäß anwendbar ist, sondern auf Gefäßbäume mit beliebiger Verzweigungsanzahl. Somit ermöglicht das Verfahren einen Überblick über die komplette Topologie eines Gefäßbaumes. Aufgrund der Verwendung einer Schnittfläche werden nur geschnittene Strukturen dargestellt, so dass folglich keine Überlagerungen der Gefäßbaumstrukturen auftreten können.

Würde die resultierende Schnittfläche ohne weitere Verarbeitung aufgefaltet werden, so könnten insbesondere im Bereich der Centerline (je nach Differenz der Neigungswinkel zweier aufeinander treffenden Flächen) starke Verzerrungen auftreten. Im Wesentlichen zeichnen sich Verzerrungen bei der Auffaltung einer Fläche an starken Flächenkrümmungen ab. Um die Verzerrungen innerhalb des geschnittenen Gefäßes so gering wie möglich zu halten, sollte idealerweise die Krümmung an der Gefäß-Centerline gleich Null sein. Zu diesem Zweck erfolgt die Generierung eines Gefäßbandes auf Basis der bereits erzeugten Schnittfläche, welches als Skelett für die finalen Schnittfläche dient (Abb. 2(a)). Zwischen dem Gefäßband-Skelett werden abschließend Coons-Flächen aufgespannt.

In den nun folgenden Abschnitten werden die einzelnen Schritte zur Auffaltung eines Gefäßbaumes erläutert.

3.1 Spannen und Erzeugen einer Schnittfläche

Damit die gesamte Topologie von der Schnittfläche erfasst werden kann, wird diese aus mehreren Einzelflächen zusammengesetzt. Dafür werden Coons-Flächen verwendet, die sich auf Grundlage von vordefinierten Randkurven erzeugen lassen. Unter Einbindung der Centerline-Information in die Randkurve kann somit die Form der Fläche an den Verlauf des Gefäßes angepasst werden.

Mittels Pre-Order Traversierung werden auf dem Gefäßbaum Buchten erzeugt, in denen sich einzelnen die Coons-Flächen anordnen lassen (Abb. 1(a)). Die Fläche einer Bucht wird wiederum aus mehreren Einzelflächen zusammengesetzt. Dafür wird ein Schwerpunkt aus allen der Bucht umgebenden Centerline-Punkten berechnet, um den die einzelnen Flächen sternförmig angeordnet werden. Jede Fläche ist somit durch eine Centerline als Randkurve sowie den Schwerpunkt definiert (Abb. 1(b)). Je spitzer der Neigungswinkel der aufeinander treffenden Flächen an der Centerline ist, desto stärker ist bei der nachfolgenden Auffaltung die Verzerrung in dieser Umgebung. Dementsprechend wird auf Grund-

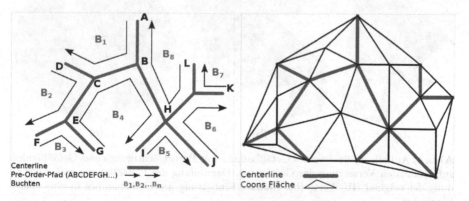

Abb. 1. Baumstruktur mit Eckpunkten $A - L$ und angeschlossenen Buchten $B_1 - B_8$ (links) und sternförmige Anordnung von Coons-Flächen (rechts)

lage der bereits erzeugten Schnittfläche ein Gefäßband generiert, welches das
Gefäß mit einer Geraden im Querschnitt schneidet.

3.2   Erzeugung eines Gefäßband-Skeletts

An jedem Punkt der Centerline wird eine Ebene erzeugt, die senkrecht zur lokalen Centerline-Richtung (lokaler Tangentenvektor) steht. Durch das Schneiden der Ebenen mit der bereits erzeugten Schnittfläche lassen sich die aktuellen
Austrittspunkte aus dem Konturbereich im Querschnitt entlang der jeweiligen
Centerline ermitteln. Anschließend werden diese Austrittspunkte jeweils mit gleichen Winkeln in den entsprechenden Ebenen um den Centerline-Punkt gedreht,
so dass sie mit dem Centerline-Punkt einen 180° Winkel einschließen (Abb. 2(a)).

Damit ein kontinuierlicher Übergang im Verzweigungsbereich entsteht, sollten die neu berechneten Punkte im Endbereich der jeweils aufeinander treffenden
Centerlines mittels eines Tiefpassfilters interpoliert werden. Basierend auf dem
Gefäßband-Skelett lässt sich die für die Auffaltung notwendige Schnittfläche erzeugen.

Anschließend müssen die Centerlines des Gefäßbaumes verbunden werden.
Statt der Gefäß-Centerline wird jedoch das Gefäßband-Skelett verwendet. Die
Flächen entlang der Centerline werden mit Coons-Flächen, bestehend aus vier
Randkurven, erzeugt. Dabei entspricht das Gefäßband-Skelett den jeweils gegen-
überliegenden Randkurven. Im Verzweigungsbereich werden die Flächen ähnlich
der in den Buchten erzeugt. Die Eckpunkte des Gefäßband-Skelettes dienen dabei
zur Generierung der Randkurven. Anschließend wird das generierte Flächenmo-
dell mit einem Laplacian-Filter geglättet und die Anzahl der Dreiecke für eine
effiziente Auffaltung reduziert.

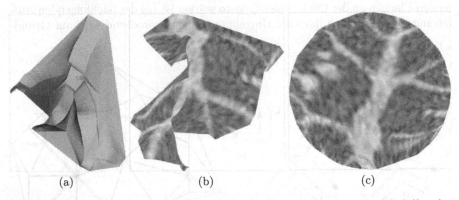

(a)   (b)   (c)

Abb. 2. Auffaltungsfläche eines Gefäßbaumes mit Berücksichtigung eines Gefäßbandes
zur minimalen Verzerrung der Gefäße (a). Darstellung des Gefäßbaumes mit Anwendung der original HU-Werte (b). Planare Einbettung des Gefäßbaumes in eine ebene
Fläche (c)

3.3 Planare Einbettung der Fläche

Die planare Einbettung der Fläche erfolgt mit Hilfe eines Optimierungsverfahrens aus dem Bereich der Mesh Parametrisierung. Aus Effizienzgründen wurde dabei ein Verfahren gewählt, welches den Rand der gesamten Fläche in eine bereits konvexe Region überträgt (zum Beispiel in eine Kreisregion). Bei der verwendeten Randbedingung wird dabei das Größenverhältnis einer einzelnen Kante zu allen Kanten in der Abbildung gewahrt (Abb. 2(c)). Für die Gewichte wurde der Mittelwert von [5] angewandt, aber es wäre das Einsetzen anderer Gewicht ebenenfalls denkbar. Das daraus resultierende lineare Gleichungssystem wurde mittels Gaußsches Eliminationsverfahren und LU-Zerlegung gelöst.

4 Diskussion

Für die Betrachtung der Gefäßbäume erstellt das Verfahren auf Grundlage der jeweiligen Centerline eine durchgehende Fläche, die alle Gefäße schneidet. Anschließend wird diese Fläche geebnet. Eine Besonderheit des Verfahrens ist, dass Gefäße eines Gefäßbaumes ohne Überschneidungen in einer Darstellung repräsentiert werden. Des Weiteren wird die angrenzende Umgebung des Gefäßbaumes mit dargestellt, wodurch benachbarte geschnittene Gefäßbäume ebenfalls in der Darstellung zu sehen sind.

Durch die Verwendung des Gefäßbandes wird sichergestellt, dass die Querschnitte der Gefäße korrekt wiedergegeben werden. Zur Darstellung pathologischer Gefäße sollte dieses Verfahren jedoch nicht verwendet werden, da hier nicht beliebig um die Centerline-Achse rotiert werden. Dafür müsste der Gefäßbaum an den Verzweigungen aufgebrochen werden. Sehr gut geeignet ist die Darstellung jedoch, wenn eine schnelle Orientierung in der Topologie des Gefäßbaumes erforderlich ist.

Literaturverzeichnis

1. Hahn HK, Preim B, Selle D, et al. Visualization and interaction techniques for the exploration of vascular structures. IEEE Visualization. 2001; p. 395–402.
2. Kanitsar A, Wegenkittl R, Fleischmann D, et al. Advanced curved planar reformation: flattening of vascular structures. IEEE Visualization. 2003; p. 43–50.
3. Kiraly AP, Naidich DP, Novak CL. 2D display of a 3D tree for pulmonary embolism detection. Proc CARS. 2005;1281:1132–36.
4. Saroul L, Figueiredo O, Hersch RD. Distance preserving flattening of surface sections. IEEE TVCG. 2006;12:26–35.
5. Floater MS. Parametrization and smooth approximation of surface triangulations. Comput Aided Geom Des. 1997;14(3):231–50.

Estimating Blood Flow Based on 2D Angiographic Image Sequences

Sepideh Alassi[1,2,3], Markus Kowarschik[2], Thomas Pohl[2], Harald Köstler[1], Ulrich Rude[1]

[1]Chair of System Simulation, University Erlangen-Nuremberg
[2]Siemens AG, Healthcare Sector, Forchheim, Germany
[3]NADA, The Royal Institute Of Technology, Stockholm, Sweden
alassi@kth.se

Abstract. The assessment of hemodynamics based on medical image data represents an attractive means in order to enhance diagnostic imaging capabilities, to evaluate clinical outcomes of therapies focusing on the patient's vascular system, as well as to guide minimally invasive interventional procedures in the catheter lab. We present a first evaluation along with comparisons of algorithmic approaches towards the quantitative determination of blood flow based on 2D angiography image data.

1 Introduction

For about 30 years, 2D imaging based on digital subtraction angiography (DSA) has been the method of choice for both the diagnosis of vascular disorders as well as the assessment of the therapeutic outcome of catheter-based interventional procedures [1]. The applications of 2D DSA imaging in the angiographic suite are manifold. In particular, they cover the minimally invasive treatment of neurovascular disorders (such as brain tumors and cerebral aneurysms), cardiovascular diseases (such as aortic aneurysms), and the peripheral occlusive disease, amongst others.

Recent trends in angiographic imaging concentrate on the interventionalists' needs of retrieving quantitative information regarding blood flow from 2D DSA data instead of inspecting the image series only visually. Besides the extraction of temporal blood flow information such as the pixel-specific time to peak opacification [2], for instance, the estimation of blood flow velocities represents a clinically relevant task. Example applications cover balloon dilation and stenting procedures in order to recanalize occluded blood vessels. In such scenarios, the quantification of the change in blood flow velocities or even volumetric blood flow rates before and after the procedure may play an essential role. In fact, velocity estimation based on videodensitometry has been a long-standing scientific challenge [3, 4], and there is no universal approach so far that is applicable to any clinical scenario. Alternative measurement approaches based on Doppler ultrasound or flow catheters, for example, are often not applicable due to the small calibers of the blood vessels under consideration.

Due to the lack of 3D information, it is only possible to estimate projected blood flow data. Note however, that there are alternative approaches towards the quantification of blood flow from X-ray based image data in 3D [5], which are not considered here. Hence, it often makes sense to consider pre/post ratios of projected blood flow velocities only, for example, to get rid of geometrical artifacts (due to vessel foreshortening [6]). A comprehensive overview of algorithms together with a broad list of references are given in [3]. So far, we have evaluated some of the most promising bolus tracking methods as well as their applicability to clinical applications. The validation of the estimated flow quantities particularly represents a challenging task. We therefore have concentrated on both synthetic image data as well as the retrospective analysis of clinical image data where also flow meter measurements are available as ground truth.

Our paper is structured as follows. In Section 2, we will give an overview of the velocity estimation methods we have implemented so far. Section 3 will cover first clinical results for a patient with a dialysis fistula. We will eventually discuss the current status of our research in Section 4.

2   Materials and methods

X-ray videodensitometric blood flow velocimetry in 2D is based on detection of movements of radio-opaque contrast material through the field of view of the X-ray scanner. In general, all approaches towards blood flow measurements using angiographic image sequences can be divided into two major classes; bolus tracking methods and computational methods based on suitable mathematical models of fluid mechanics [3].

Bolus tracking methods are based on tracking the contrast material as it travels along the blood vessel. Bolus transport time algorithms represent the main type of tracking algorithms. They are based on determining the transit time it takes for the bolus to travel the distance between two fixed regions of interest (ROIs). Typically, in bolus transit time algorithms, the bolus arrival times are determined by analyzing time-density curves. These curves show contrast density, which is a function of time, over the entire ROI: $P_{\mathrm{ROI}}(t) = \int_{\mathrm{ROI}} P(x,t)dx$.

The average blood flow velocity is then obtained as $v = \Delta x/\Delta t$, where Δx is determined from the axial coordinates of two ROIs chosen in the images, and Δt is determined by applying a proper algorithm to estimate bolus transport times (Sect. 2.1 and 2.2).

2.1   Bolus arrival time from time-density curve algorithms

For computing the bolus transport times, a criterion is needed to determine the bolus arrival times at the first and the second ROI using their corresponding time-density curves [3]. There are four criteria which have been implemented and evaluated so far:

- *Time of peak opacification*: The bolus is supposed to have arrived at the ROI once the time-density curve reaches its peak value.

- *Time of leading half peak opacification:* The bolus is considered to have arrived once the time-density curve reaches half of its peak density for the first time.
- *Time of trailing half peak opacification:* The bolus has arrived at the ROI if the time-density curve achieves its half peak value for the last time.
- *Time of peak gradient arrival:* The bolus is assumed to have arrived as soon as the gradient of the time-density curve reaches its maximum value.

2.2   Cross-correlation of time-density curves

This method is based on shifting the time-density curve obtained at the first ROI until it optimally matches the curve obtained at the second ROI [7]. The value $\Delta t \in [0, t_{\mathrm{end}}]$, which maximizes the cross-correlation function

$$\phi(\Delta t) = \int_0^{t_{end}} P_{ROI_1}(t - \Delta t) \cdot P_{ROI_2}(t) \, dt \tag{1}$$

is considered to be the time of bolus transport between the two ROIs [3].

2.3   Fitting time-density curves

The time-density curves which are used in the previously described methods, exhibit two significant drawbacks. First, their temporal resolution is determined by the chosen frame rate of the X-ray scanner. This limits the temporal accuracy of the curve features such as the peak value. Second, the inherent noise level in the time-density curves further degrades the accuracy of these curve features. One way to overcome both issues is to fit model curves to the given time-density curves. One commonly used type for curve fitting are gamma-variate curves [8]. Another self-evident choice would be polynomial curve fitting [9]. A further which tries to mimic the apparent features of a typical time-density curve as closely as possible is given by

$$I_{\mathrm{approx}}(t, I_{\max}, T_{\max}, s_{\mathrm{inc}}, s_{\mathrm{dec}}) = \begin{cases} I_{\max} \cdot \exp[-(\frac{t - T_{\max}}{s_{\mathrm{inc}}})^2 \cdot \ln 2] & \text{for} \quad t \leq T_{\max} \\ \\ I_{\max} \cdot \exp[-(\frac{t - T_{\max}}{s_{\mathrm{dec}}})^2 \cdot \ln 2] & \text{for} \quad t > T_{\max} \end{cases}$$
$$\tag{2}$$

For prolonged contrast injections, an additional parameter to model the sustained maximum contrast level was also evaluated in this work.

2.4   Synthetic data generation

In order to test the precision and the robustness of the previously described methods, synthetic image data sets were generated. In these data sets, vessels have simple geometric shapes (horizontal straight vessels), and blood flow in each vessel is given by a constant velocity v. For bringing the synthetic data closer to reality, Gaussian noise with constant mean μ_n and variance σ_n was added to the data and, in addition, diffusive transport of the contrast agent was introduced. One approach to model diffusion is given by

$$I(x, t, v, I_0) = I_0 \ F(x - v \ t, \mu, \sigma^2) \tag{3}$$

where the variance is $\sigma = \sigma(t) = \sigma_0 + \sigma_1 \ t$, and $F(x, \mu, \sigma^2)$ is the cumulative distribution function

$$F(x, \mu, \sigma^2) = \frac{1}{2} \left[1 + \mathrm{erf} \left(\frac{x - \mu}{\sigma \sqrt{2}} \right) \right] \tag{4}$$

3   Results

3.1   Patient data

The methods described in Section 2 were used to calculate an estimate for Δt corresponding to two different ROIs for two 2D DSA sequences as shown in Fig. 1. We evaluated data sets corresponding to a patient with a dialysis fistula in the arm, which represents a relatively simple vascular topology. In particular, we considered image data and flow measurement data prior to (pre) and after (post) the recanalization of the arterio-venous dialysis shunt. The volumetric flow measurements were obtained by using a thermodilution-based catheter device. To improve the temporal resolution of the image based flow estimates, gamma-variate curve fitting was applied as shown in Fig. 2.

Table 1 summarizes the time differences for each time-density curve feature. The most significant result is the ratio between these time differences for pre and post data sets which lies between 4.16 and 5. Based on the measured volumetric flow rates, the true ratio is expected to be 4.5.

3.2   Synthetic data

A synthetic data set covering two vessels was generated for testing the previously described methods. Based on the specified velocities, the exact ratio of bolus

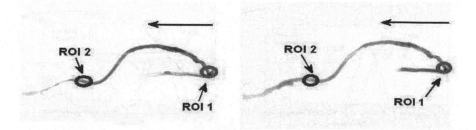

Fig. 1.   DSA images with ROIs; pre recanalization (left) and post recanalization (right). The arrows indicate the blood flow direction in the shunt

Table 1. Bolus transport time (Δt) for both pre and post recanalizations

	Peak	Leading half peak	Trailing half peak	Peak gradient	Cross-correlation
Pre	2.00s	2.44s	2.01s	2.47s	3.23s
Post	0.48s	0.53s	0.40s	0.54s	0.70s
Ratio	4.16	4.60	5.00	4.57	4.61

Table 2. Estimated ratios of the bolus arrival time differences for synthetic data

	Peak	Leading half peak	Trailing half peak	Peak gradient	Cross-correlation
Ratio	2.67	2.18	2.01	2.28	2.03

arrival time differences is 2. Analogous to Fig. 1, two ROIs were placed in each vessel. Gaussian noise (with $\mu_n = 0.1$ and $\sigma_n = 0.3$) and diffusion (with $\sigma_0 = \sigma_1 = 0.5$ and $\mu = 0$) were added to the images. Furthermore, the polynomial curve fitting method described in Section 2.3 was used for virtually enhancing the temporal accuracy of the curve features. Table 2 contains the estimated ratios of the bolus arrival time differences for each time-density curve feature.

The evaluation results show that the ratio between the bolus arrival time differences lies between 2.01 and 2.67. The severe deviations of the results for the time of peak opacification and the time of peak gradient arrival methods are attributed to noise.

4   Discussion

We have presented initial experiments regarding the quantification of blood flow from 2D angiographic image data. For the case of sufficiently simple vessel geometries, it appears possible to at least estimate ratios of pre/post volumetric blood flow rates. For the sake of simplicity, our current evaluations have focused on relatively straight vessel topologies such as arterio-venous dialysis shunts and vessels in the periphery, for example. Of course, such approaches towards the quantification of blood flow need to be investigated in much more detail before

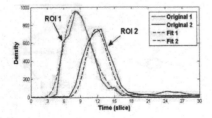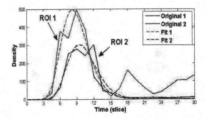

Fig. 2. Time-density curves of ROIs and their corresponding gamma-variate fits, pre recanalization (left), post recanalization (right)

they can be employed in clinical routine. However, their validation remains a challenging task since ground truth measurements based on Doppler ultrasound or flow catheters are not often available.

Acknowledgement. We would like to give special thanks to the staff of the Department of Interventional Radiology at the University of Virginia at Charlottesville, USA, for providing valuable clinical data and support.

References

1. Oppelt A. Imaging Systems for Medical Diagnostics. Fundamentals, Technical Solutions and Applications for Systems applying Ionizing Radiation, Nuclear Magnetic Resonance and Ultrasound. Erlangen: Publicis Kommunikations Agentur GmbH, GWA; 2005.
2. Strother C, Bender F, Deuerling-Zheng Y, et al. Parametric color coding of digital subtraction angiography. Am J Neuroradiol. 2010; p. 919–24.
3. Shpilfoygel D, Close A, Valentino J, et al. X-ray videodensitometric methods for blood flow and velocity measurement: a critical review of literature. Med Phys. 2000;27(9):2008–23.
4. Hilal S. Cerebral Hemodynamics Assessed by Angiography. St Louis: CV Mosby Co: Radiology of the Skull and Brain: Angiography; 1974.
5. Wächter I, Bredno J, Hermans R, et al. Model-based blood flow quantification from rational angiography. Med Image Anal. 2008;12(5):586–602.
6. Ahmed A, Deuerling-Zheng Y, Strother C, et al. Impact of intra-arterial injection parameters on arterial, capillary, and venous time concentration curves in a canine model. Am J Neuroradiol. 2009; p. 1337–41.
7. Rosen L, Silverman N. Videodensitometric measurement of blood flow using cross-correlation technique. Radiology. 1973; p. 305–10.
8. Thompson K, Starmer F, et al RW. Indicator transit time considered as a gamma variate. Circ Res. 1964; p. 502–15.
9. Kelley C. Iterative Methods for Optimization. Philadelphia: SIAM Press; 2004.

Cryo-Balloon Catheter Tracking in Atrial Fibrillation Ablation Procedures

Tanja Kurzendorfer[1], Alexander Brost[1], Felix Bourier[2], Martin Koch[1], Klaus Kurzidim[2], Joachim Hornegger[1], Norbert Strobel[3]

[1]Pattern Recognition Lab, University Erlangen-Nuremberg
[2]Klinik für Herzrhythmusstörungen, Krankenhaus Barmherzige Brüder, Regensburg
[3]Siemens AG, Healthcare Sector, Forchheim, Germany
Alexander.Brost@cs.fau.de

Abstract. Radio-frequency (RF) catheter ablation has become the standard treatment of atrial fibrillation if pharmacotherapy fails. As an alternative to traditional RF standard ablation catheters, single-shot devices have received more and more interest. One group of these devices are cryo-balloon catheters. Such catheters are designed to electrically isolate a pulmonary vein (PV) with only a few applications, ideally only one. Whereas standard radio-frequency ablation catheters operate point by point, cryo-balloon devices need to be positioned antrally to the pulmonary vein ostium before freezing. If a good seal can be achieved far enough outside of the pulmonary veins, the cryo-balloon is an effective and safe ablation device. The catheters are inserted through a transseptal sheath and are inflated using liquid nitrogen. Single-shot devices, when used successfully, promise a reduction of procedure time and X-ray exposure. Single-shot devices based on ablation energies other than RF, may not carry electrodes or electromagnetic sensors. This makes it difficult to visualize them using standard EP mapping systems. As a result, fluoroscopic imaging is needed. Unfortunately, the inflated balloon may be difficult to see under X-ray. To improve this situation, we propose a new method that tracks and enhances the visualization of a cryo-balloon catheter under fluoroscopic imaging. The method involves a 2-D template of the cryo-balloon that is manually initialized and then tracks the balloon device during live X-ray imaging. To improve visualization, a 2-D ellipse is overlaid onto the fluoroscopic imaging to highlight the position of the balloon catheter. The tracking error was calculated as the distance between the tracked catheter template and the manually segmented catheter. Our method achieved 2-D tracking error of 0.60 mm ± 0.32 mm.

1 Introduction

Radio-frequency (RF) catheter ablation to treat atrial fibrillation (AFib) has now become an accepted treatment option, in particular, when drug therapy fails [1]. Catheter ablation procedures are performed in electrophysiology (EP) labs usually equipped with modern C-arm X-ray systems. Augmented fluoroscopy, overlaying 2-D images rendered from either CT, MR, or C-arm CT 3-D data sets onto live fluoroscopic images, can facilitate more precise real-time catheter navigation and also reduce radiation [2, 3]. As an alternative to regular ablation catheters which operate on a point-wise ablation strategy, single-shot devices have attracted a significant amount of interest. Under ideal conditions, these devices can electrically isolate a pulmonary vein with a single application. One of these devices are cryo-balloon catheters. These catheters are inserted through a trans-septal sheath and can be inflated using liquid nitrogen [4]. Two different catheter types are currently available. They differ only in diameter, which is either 23 mm or 28 mm. The type of catheter is chosen depending on underlying patient anatomy. Since no mapping system is available yet for localizing cryo-balloon catheters without fluoroscopy, these devices are placed under X-ray. Unfortunately, the inflated balloon catheter may be difficult to see using traditional fluoroscopy imaging. Moreover, the diameter of the catheter can only be determined once the balloon is inflated. We propose a method to track and visualize a cryo-balloon device to simplify catheter placement.

2   Materials and methods

The proposed method uses a 2-D template that is manually initialized and then tracked during live X-ray imaging using template matching [5, 6]. Once the cryo-balloon catheter position has been found inside an X-ray image, a 2-D ellipse determined from manual initialization is superimposed onto the live fluoroscopic view to better visualize the position and the dimension of the catheter.

2.1   Tracking by template matching

On the first frame of the fluoroscopy sequence manual initialization is required to determine a 2-D tracking template. This template is denoted as $T \in \mathbb{R}^{n \times n}$ with $n \in \mathbb{N}$. Denoting the fluoroscopic images as $I_t \in \mathbb{R}^{N \times N}$ with $N \in \mathbb{N}$ and $t \in [0, F]$ the number of the frame in the sequence, a pixel of the image can be accessed by using $I_t(u, v)$. The same holds for the template. For simplicity, we assume quadratic images to be considered here, but our method was originally designed for coping with non-quadratic images. From manual initialization, the first position of the catheter in the first frame of the sequence $t = 0$ is known as $(u_0, v_0) \in \mathbb{N}$, with the image axis denoted as u and v. This information is used to constrain the search region to be of size $2M \times 2M$ with $M \in \mathbb{N}$. To find the catheter in the next frame $t = t + 1$, we use a multi-scale grid search and using the sum of squared distances (SSD) as cost function. The best translation in u-direction and v-direction such that the template matches best to the current observed fluoroscopic image is found by solving the following minimization problem

$$u_t, v_t = \underset{\substack{u \in [u_{t-1} - M, u_{t-1} + M] \\ v \in [v_{t-1} - M, v_{t-1} + M]}}{\arg\min} \sum_{\substack{i,j \\ \in [-\Delta, \Delta]}} (\boldsymbol{I}_t(u + i, v + j) - \boldsymbol{T}(i - \Delta, j - \Delta))^2$$

(1)

with the half size of the template denoted as $\Delta = \lfloor \frac{n-1}{2} \rfloor$ and the floor function $\lfloor \cdot \rfloor$ that maps to the largest integer smaller compared to the argument. Our approach is summarized in Fig. 1. The first frame of such a sequence is shown in Fig. 1 (a), the corresponding 2-D template is shown in Fig. 1 (b). The corresponding position in the successive frames is found by finding the best match for the template. The result for one frame is shown in Fig. 1 (c). Finally, the superimposed cryo-balloon position is shown in Fig. 1 (d).

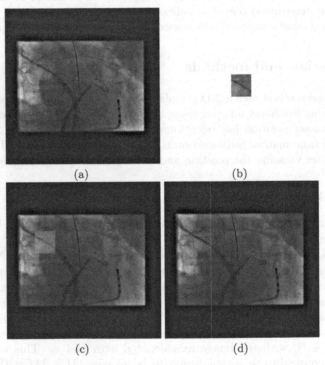

(a)   (b)

(c)   (d)

Fig. 1. (a) first image of one fluoroscopic sequence $t = 0$. (b) manually initialized 2-D template for tracking (c) matched template highlighted in red in the next frame of the sequence $t = 1$. (d) A superimposed ellipse was added to the fluoroscopic image to visualize position and dimensions of the cryo-balloon catheter

3 Evaluation and results

For the evaluation of the proposed method, 12 clinical sequences were available. The sequences were obtained at one clinical site from 10 patients and were acquired during regular EP procedures on an AXIOM Artis dBC C-arm system (Siemens AG, Forchheim, Germany). Although the data was acquired on a bi-plane system, our catheter tracking approach is not restricted to such a system and will work on a mono-plane device as well. As the sequences were acquired during standard EP procedures, our method is evaluated for a typical setup. It involves one circumferential mapping catheter, one catheter in the coronary sinus and a cryo-balloon catheter. In addition to that, some images show one ECG leads that were attached to the skin of the patient. The tracking error was calculated as the Euclidean distance between the translation vector from the tracking and translation vectors from the manually segmented catheter by a clinical expert. The expert was asked to pick the center of the tip of the cryo-balloon catheter. This is actually not a real tip, but the upper end of the catheter to which the balloon is attached. This upper end is also an opening through which contrast agent can be injected into the pulmonary vein. In contrast to the cryo-balloon itself, the opening can easily be seen as a dark spot in fluoroscopic images. Denoting the gold-standard segmentation by $u_t^\star$ and $v_t^\star$, the 2-D error ε_t in mm is calculated by

$$\varepsilon_t = \rho \cdot \sqrt{\left((u_t - u_{t-1}) - \left(u_t^\star - u_{t-1}^\star\right)\right)^2 + \left((v_t - v_{t-1}) - \left(v_t^\star - v_{t-1}^\star\right)\right)^2} \quad (2)$$

with $t > 0$ and the pixel spacing $\rho = 0.183$ mm/pixels. The magnification factor was not taken into account. Our proposed method achieved a 2-D tracking error of 0.60 mm $\pm$ 0.32 mm averaged of all frames of all sequences. The results for each sequence are given in Fig. 2. A total minimum error of 0.01 mm and a total maximum error of 1.64 mm was found.

4 Discussion and conclusions

Our proposed method successfully tracked a cryo-thermal balloon catheter in 12 clinical sequences. It is able to superimpose the position and diameter of the device onto live fluoroscopic images to enhance the visibility of the cryo-balloon catheter. Manual interaction is only required for the initialization of the template and the determination of the size of the cryo-balloon. After that, the catheter is tracked throughout the remainder of the sequence. The visualized outline of the cryo-balloon helps the physician to see the dimensions of the balloon catheter, otherwise hardly visible under X-ray. Our cryo-balloon catheter tracking method could also be combined with a motion-adjusted 3-D overlay rendered from preoperative data [7, 8]. Such an example is given in Fig. 3. By doing so, previous balloon catheter positions can be stored and recalled if a second freeze becomes necessary. In addition, a pre-planned cryo-balloon position, using AFiT [9], could be shown to guide the catheter placement. An example is presented in

Fig. 2. two-dimensional catheter tracking error, the proposed method achieves a 2-D accuracy of 0.60 mm ± 0.32 mm, a total minimum error of 0.01 mm and a total maximum error of 1.64 mm was found

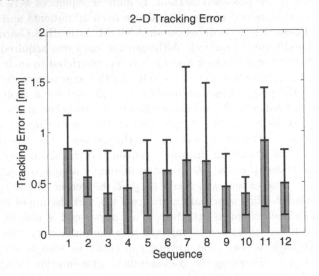

Fig. 3 (c). Future work will focus on tracking the catheter by other means than template matching. Learning based approaches such as in [8] and [10] provide a more robust framework for tracking. In addition, they might also be applicable without manual initialization.

Acknowledgement. This work has been supported by the German Federal Ministry of Education and Research (BMBF), project grant No. 01EX1012E, in the context of the initiative Spitzencluster Medical Valley – Europäische

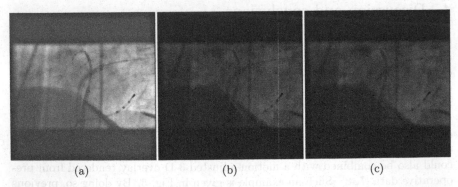

(a)   (b)   (c)

Fig. 3. Example: (a) fluoroscopic image of one sequence (b) the same fluoroscopic image with motion-adjusted overlay and tracked cryo-balloon (c) the same fluoroscopic image as in (b) with a pre-planned target position of the cryo-balloon (green)

Metropolregion Nürnberg. Additional funding was provided by Siemens AG, Healthcare Sector.

References

1. Calkins H, Brugada J, Packer D, et al. Expert consensus statement on catheter and surgical ablation of atrial fibrillation: recommendations for personnel, policy, procedures and follow-up. Europace. 2007; p. 335–79.
2. Sra J, Narayan G, Krum D, et al. Computed tomography-fluoroscopy image integration-guided catheter ablation of atrial fibrillation. J Cardiovasc Electrophysiol. 2007; p. 409–14.
3. De Buck S, Maes F, Ector J, et al. An augmented reality system for patient-specific guidance of cardiac catheter ablation procedures. IEEE Trans Med Imaging. 2005; p. 1512–24.
4. Koller M, Schumacher B. cryoballoon ablation of paroxysmal atrial fibrillation: bigger is better and simpler is better. Eur Heart J. 2009;30(6):636–7.
5. Schenderlein M, Rasche V, Dietmayer K. Three-dimensional catheter tip tracking from asynchronous biplane x-ray image sequences using non-linear state filtering. Proc BVM. 2011; p. 234–8.
6. Schenderlein M, Dietmayer K. Image-based catheter tip tracking during cardiac ablation therapy. Methods Inform Med. 2010; p. 1–5.
7. Brost A, Liao R, Strobel N, et al. Respiratory motion compensation by model-based catheter tracking during EP procedures. Med Image Anal. 2010; p. 695–706.
8. Brost A, Wimmer A, Liao R, et al. Constrained 2-D/3-D registration for motion compensation in AFib ablation procedures. In: Information Processing in Computer-Assisted Interventions. Springer Berlin / Heidelberg; 2011. p. 133–44.
9. Brost A, Bourier F, Kleinoeder A, et al. AFiT - Atrial fibrillation ablation planning tool. In: Proc VMV; 2011. p. 223–30.
10. Wu W, Chen T, Barbu A, et al. Learning-based hypothesis fusion for robust catheter tracking in 2D X-ray fluoroscopy. In: Proc IEEE CVPR; 2011. p. 1097–104.

Elektromagnetisches Tracking für die interventionelle Radiologie

Genauigkeitsuntersuchung und in-vitro Applikation eines neuen Feldgenerators

Alfred M. Franz[1], Mark Servatius[2], Alexander Seitel[1], Johann Hummel[3], Wolfgang Birkfellner[3], Laura Bartha[1], Heinz-Peter Schlemmer[4], Christof M. Sommer[2], Boris A. Radeleff[2], Hans-Ulrich Kauczor[2], Hans-Peter Meinzer[1], Lena Maier-Hein[1]

[1]Abteilung Medizinische und Biologische Informatik, DKFZ Heidelberg
[2]Abteilung Diagnostische und Interventionelle Radiologie, Uniklinikum Heidelberg
[3]Medizinische Universität Wien; [4]Abteilung Radiologie, DKFZ Heidelberg
a.franz@dkfz-heidelberg.de

Kurzfassung. Elektromagnetisches (EM) Tracking gewinnt zunehmend an Bedeutung in der interventionellen Radiologie, da es die Lokalisation von Instrumenten innerhalb des Körpers ermöglicht. Problematisch ist bei dieser Technik jedoch die Anfälligkeit gegenüber metallischen Gegenständen, die das Magnetfeld stören. Von der Firma NDI (Northern Digital Inc., Waterloo, Canada, www.ndigital.com) wurde kürzlich ein neuer Feldgenerator (FG) (s.g. Tabletop FG) für EM Trackingsysteme vorgestellt. Dieser schirmt das Magnetfeld nach unten hin ab und verhindert so Störungen durch den Patiententisch. Ziel dieser Studie war (1) die Untersuchung der Genauigkeit dieses Generators im CT nach einem standardisierten Evaluationsprotokoll sowie (2) die Einbindung dieses Generators in ein bestehendes markerbasiertes Navigationssystem für Nadelinsertionen. Die Ergebnisse zeigen eine wesentlich höhere Robustheit, Genauigkeit und Präzision im Vergleich zum herkömmlichen FG des Aurora-Systems (s.g. Planar FG). Der Tabletop FG wurde erfolgreich in das bestehende Navigationssystem eingebunden. Ein in-vitro Versuch ergab eine Insertionsgenauigkeit von 5,3±1,8 mm (n=5) verglichen mit 3,5±1,1 mm (n=20) bei optischer Navigation in einem Referenzversuch. Die Ergebnisse sollten aber durch weitere Versuche mit einer höheren Fallzahl bestätigt werden.

1 Einleitung

Eine zentrale Komponente bei Navigationssystemen in der Medizin ist das Trackingsystem. Es erfasst die Position und Orientierung medizinischer Instrumente im Raum, wobei verschiedene Trackingtechnologien zur Verfügung stehen. Optische Systeme lokalisieren unter Verwendung von Triangulationsalgorithmen spezielle Marker mit Hilfe von eingebauten Kameras. Sie bieten eine sehr hohe Genauigkeit und sind wenig störanfällig, benötigen allerdings eine freie Sichtlinie zum getrackten Instrument. Bei elektromagnetischen Systemen werden hingegen Sensoren innerhalb eines elektromagnetischen Felds lokalisiert. Dabei wird keine freie Sichtlinie benötigt, und es können Instrumente, wie zum Beispiel Katheter, Endoskope oder Nadelspitzen, innerhalb des Körpers getrackt werden. Ein Nachteil dieser Systeme ist eine hohe Störanfälligkeit durch Metalle und elektromagnetische Felder, was beispielsweise bei Eingriffen auf der Patientenliege eines Computertomographen (CT) zu hohen Ungenauigkeiten führt [1]. Um diesem Problem Rechnung zu tragen, wurde von der Firma NDI (Northern Digital Inc., Waterloo, Canada) kürzlich ein neuer elektromagnetischer Feldgenerator, bezeichnet als Tabletop FG und dargestellt in Abb. 1(a), vorgestellt.

Ziel dieser Studie war die Untersuchung der Genauigkeit des Tabletop FG nach einem standardisierten Protokoll unter Einsatzbedingungen im CT. Zum Vergleich sollten auch Werte eines herkömmlichen, als Planar FG bezeichneten, Feldgenerators der Firma NDI aufgezeichnet werden. Ein weiteres Ziel war der praktische Test des neuen Feldgenerators. Dazu sollte er in ein Navigationssystem zur navigierten Weichgewebepunktion eingebunden und im Rahmen eines in-vitro Versuchs unter klinischen Bedingungen getestet werden.

2 Materialien und Methoden

Der im Rahmen dieser Studie untersuchte Tabletop FG (Abb. 1(a)) schirmt das elektromagnetische Feld des Trackingsystems, wie in Abb. 2 dargestellt, nach unten hin ab. Dadurch wird ein praktischer Einsatz auf der CT-Liege, wie bei CT-geführten Punktionen in Weichgewebe benötigt, möglich. Der Bereich im elektromagnetischen Feld, in dem Instrumente lokalisiert werden können, wird als Trackingvolumen bezeichnet. Dieses Volumen ist für den Tabletop FG in Abb. 1(b) dargestellt und deckt die Arbeitsfläche eines üblichen Eingriffs ab. Der Feldgenerator ist 2,5 cm dick und lässt sich somit unter dem Patienten auf der Liege platzieren.

2.1 Vergleichende Genauigkeitsuntersuchung des Tabletop FG

Die Genauigkeitsuntersuchung wurde nach einem standardisierten, von Hummel et al. [2] vorgestellten, Protokoll durchgeführt. Das Protokoll umfasst Messungen

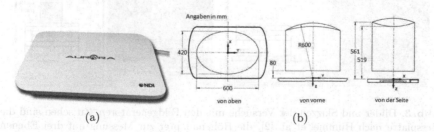

(a)   (b)

Abb. 1. Bild und Trackingvolumen des kürzlich vorgestellten Tabletop Feldgenerators der Firma NDI

Abb. 2. Skizze des Tabletop Feldgenerators im Einsatz. Der Feldgenerator wird zwischen Patient und CT-Liege platziert und schirmt das elektromagnetische Feld nach unten hin ab. Somit werden Störungen durch metallische Anteile der Liege vermieden und ein genaues Tracking ermöglicht

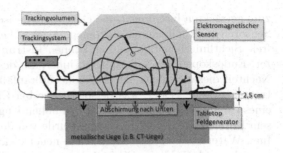

zur Genauigkeit und Präzision der Positionsbestimmung auf $9 \times 10 = 90$ Positionen einer 50 cm $\times$ 50 cm großen Messplatte. Des Weiteren werden mit einer Vorrichtung zur Rotationsmessung in der Mitte der Platte 32 verschiedene Orientierungen eines 5D-Sensors gemessen. Für einen elektromagnetischen 5D-Sensor lassen sich durch unterschiedliches Einspannen des Sensors in die Halterung Messungen bezüglich beider Freiheitsgrade der Orientierung (als ROT_1 und ROT_2 bezeichnet) durchführen. Da das Trackingvolumen des Tabletop FG nicht die ganze Messplatte abdeckt, wurden die äußeren Spalten und Reihen der Positionsmessung weggelassen. Somit ergeben sich für den Tabletop FG $7 \times 8 = 56$ Positionen auf der Messplatte.

Das Protokoll wurde für diese Studie auf drei Ebenen im Trackingvolumen erweitert. Über aus Holz gefertigte Höhenadapter, dargestellt in Abb. 3, können Messungen auf den Ebenen 15 cm, 25 cm und 35 cm über dem CT-Tisch durchgeführt werden. Die Ebene 25 cm über der CT-Liege, also 22,5 cm über dem Tabletop FG, wurde als Ausgangshöhe 0 cm (Mitte) definiert. Somit kann die Ebene darunter als Ausgangshöhe - 10 cm (Unten) und die darüber als Ausgangshöhe + 10 cm (Oben) bezeichnet werden. Bei den durchgeführten Vergleichsmessungen mit dem Planar FG wurde der Feldgenerator seitlich angebracht und die Ausgangshöhe in die Mitte des Trackingvolumens gelegt.

Auf diesen drei Ebenen wurden unter Einsatzbedingungen auf der CT-Liege für den Tabletop FG (I) 56 Messungen zur Sensorposition und (II) 64 Mes-

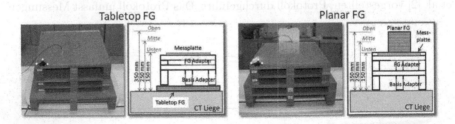

Abb. 3. Bilder und Skizzen der Versuche mit den Feldgeneratoren. Zu sehen sind die Messplatte nach Hummel et al. [2], die Höhenadapter zur Messung auf drei Ebenen und der an der Messplatte angebrachte optische Referenzsensor links vorne im Bild

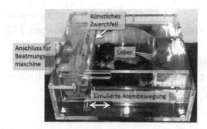

Abb. 4. Bild des Bewegungssimulators [4] mit eingebrachter Leber, der als Phantom für die in-vitro Versuche verwendet wurde. Die Leber wurde dazu an dem künstlichen Zwerchfell angenäht. An die Anschlüsse links im Bild kann eine Beatmungsmaschine angeschlossen und somit Atmung simuliert werden. Für die Versuche wurde auf dem Bewegungssimulator eine künstliche Haut aus Schaumstoff angebracht

sungen zur Sensororientierung (32 x ROT_1 und 32 x ROT_2) durchgeführt. Zum Vergleich wurden nach dem gleichen Protokoll (III) 90 Messungen zur Sensorposition (IV) 64 Messungen zur Sensororientierung mit dem herkömmlichen Planar FG durchgeführt. Um während der Messungen sicherzustellen, dass sich die Messplatte nicht bewegt, wurde zur Kontrolle ein optisch getrackter Referenzmarker an der Platte angebracht. Bei Bewegung des Referenzmarkers sollte eine Messreihe für ungültig erklärt und wiederholt werden.

2.2 In-vitro Versuch mit dem Tabletop FG

Um den Tabletop FG im praktischen Einsatz zu testen, wurde er in ein Navigationssystem für Weichgewebepunktionen, das in einer Vorarbeit vorgestellt wurde [3], eingebunden und ein in-vitro Versuch mit dem System durchgeführt. Dieser Versuch erfolgte unter Einsatz des ebenfalls in einer Vorarbeit entwickelten Bewegungssimulators [4]. Der Versuch wurde mit einer explantierten Schweineleber, die mit fünf künstlichen Zielen versehen war, durchgeführt (Abb. 4). Die Ziele bestanden aus in die Leber eingespritztem Agar, das mit Kontrastmittel angereichert war [5]. Sie wurden unter Einsatz des Tabletop FG punktiert, wobei der Eingriff auf der CT-Liege stattfand. Während des Versuchs wurde nach der Aufnahme des Planungs-CTs Atmung simuliert (25 Atemzüge mit einer Frequenz von $\frac{12}{min}$). Die eigentlichen Punktionen erfolgten unter Atemstillstand (Gating).

3   Ergebnisse

Die Genauigkeitsmessung nach dem Protokoll von Hummel et al. [2] ergab im Mittel eine Präzision (Rauschen) des Instruments von 0,19±0,19 mm ($\mu \pm \sigma$, gemittelt über alle gemessenen Positionen auf drei Ebenen) im Fall des Planar FG und 0,05±0,03 mm im Fall des Tabletop FG. Die Präzision unterschied sich dabei zwischen den Ebenen nicht wesentlich. Der Fehler der gemessenen 5cm-, 15cm- und 30cm-Distanzen (Hummel et al. [2]) ist als Boxplot in Abb. 3 dargestellt. Die akkumulierten Distanzen über die gesamte Messplatte (Hummel et al. [2]) sind in Abb. 3 als Diagramme aufgetragen. In beiden Fällen ist der hohe Fehler des Planar FG auf der CT-Liege, der nach unten hin zunimmt, deutlich zu sehen. Der Fehler des Tabletop FG nimmt nach oben hin, also mit größerem Abstand zum FG, leicht zu. Die Auswertung bezüglich der Genauigkeit der Sensororientierung ergab einen mittleren Winkelfehler von 1,5±1,5° für den Planaren FG und 1,3±1,9° für den Tabletop FG.

Das Ergebnis der in-vitro Punktionsversuche war für die fünf Punktionen mit dem Tabletop FG ein mittlerer Gesamtfehler von 5,3±1,8 mm. Darin enthalten ist ein Benutzerfehler von 4,1±2,2 mm.

4 Diskussion

Die Ergebnisse der Genauigkeitsuntersuchung zeigen deutlich bessere Werte sowohl bezüglich Präzision, als auch bezüglich Genauigkeit für den Tabletop FG im Vergleich zum Planar FG. Dabei ist eine deutliche Störungsanfälligkeit des

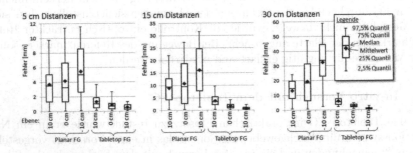

Abb. 5. Fehler der Distanzmessungen für 5 cm, 10 cm und 15 cm - Distanzen, jeweils auf drei Ebenen (Unten, Mitte, Oben) für den Planar FG und den Tabletop FG, dargestellt als Boxplot

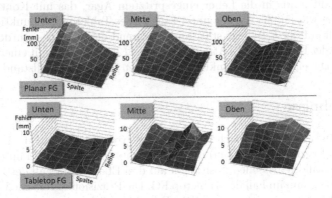

Abb. 6. Diagramme der Fehler der akkumulierten Distanzen für beide Feldgeneratoren auf drei Ebenen. x- und y-Achse bezeichnen die Spalte und Reihe auf der Messplatte, während die z-Achse den gemessenen Fehler in mm angibt. (Im Gegensatz zu Hummel et al. [2] wurde bei dieser Darstellung als Fehler der Betrag der Distanz zwischen gemessenem Wert und Referenz gewählt)

Planar FG bei der Positionsmessung beim Einsatz auf einer CT-Liege zu sehen. Diese Störanfälligkeit, die bereits von Yaniv et al. festgestellt wurde [1], ist beim Tabletop FG nicht zu beobachten. Hinsichtlich der Messung der Orientierung zeigen sich die Werte des neuen Feldgenerators in einer ähnlichen Größenordnung wie die des Planar FG.

Die in-vitro Versuche zeigen, dass ein Einsatz des Feldgenerators in klinischem Umfeld möglich ist. Die Ergebnisse sind mit einem mittleren Gesamtfehler von 5,3±1,8 mm (n=5) etwas schlechter als 3,5±1,1 mm (n=20) bei einem Referenzversuchs mit optischem Tracking [5]. Die ermittelte Genauigkeit bewegt sich dennoch im einstelligen Millimeterbereich und zeigt sich daher vielversprechend. Allerdings sind die Ergebnisse aufgrund der niedrigen Fallzahl nicht statistisch aussagekräftig. Es müssen weitere Versuche folgen, um den tatsächlichen Nutzen des Feldgenerators für den klinischen Einsatz zu zeigen.

Nach unserem Kenntnistand sind wir die ersten, die die Genauigkeit dieses Tabletop Feldgenerators standardisiert untersucht und ihn im Einsatz getestet haben. Die Studie zeigt das große Potential des Feldgenerators beim Einsatz im CT, da er bekannte Probleme des EM Tracking mit Störeinflüssen deutlich vermindert. Die Relevanz dieser Arbeit für den Bereich der computerassistierten Eingriffe in der interventionelle Radiologie ist daher hoch.

Danksagung. Dieses Projekt wurde im Rahmen des Graduiertenkollegs 1126: Intelligente Chirurgie durchgeführt. Der Prototyp des neuen Feldgenerators wurde freundlicherweise von der Firma NDI (Northern Digital Inc., Waterloo, Canada) für umfangreiche Tests zur Verfügung gestellt. Des Weiteren sei an dieser Stelle Martina Joachim erwähnt, die während der Versuche das CT bediente und Dank unermüdlichem Einsatz einen erfolgreichen Abschluss des Projekts ermöglichte.

Literaturverzeichnis

1. Yaniv Z, Wilson E, Lindisch D, et al. Electromagnetic tracking in the clinical environment. Med Phys. 2009;36(3):876–92.
2. Hummel JB, Bax MR, Figl ML, et al. Design and application of an assessment protocol for electromagnetic tracking systems. Med Phys. 2005;32(7):2371–79.
3. Maier-Hein L, Tekbas A, Seitel A, et al. In vivo accuracy assessment of a needle-based navigation system for CT-guided radiofrequency ablation of the liver. Med Phys. 2008;35(12):5386–96.
4. Maier-Hein L, Pianka F, Müller SA, et al. Respiratory liver motion simulator for validating image-guided systems ex-vivo. Int J CARS. 2008;2(5):287–92.
5. Maier-Hein L, Pianka F, Seitel A, et al. Precision targeting of liver lesions with a needle-based soft tissue navigation system. Lect Notes Computer Sci. 2007;4792:42–9.

Effect of Active Air Conditioning in Medical Intervention Rooms on the Temperature Dependency of Time-of-Flight Distance Measurements

Sven Mersmann[1], David Guerrero[2], Heinz-Peter Schlemmer[3],
Hans-Peter Meinzer[1], Lena Maier-Hein[1]

[1]Division of Medical and Biological Informatics, DKFZ Heidelberg
[2]McGill University, Montreal, Canada
[3]Division of Radiology, DKFZ Heidelberg
s.mersmann@dkfz-heidelberg.de

Abstract. Recently, Time-of-Flight (ToF) cameras have emerged as a new mean for intra-operative image acquisition. The ToF camera features co-registered depth and intensity image data from the observed scene in video frame rate. Due to systematic distance errors, depth calibration is crucially needed. One of the sources of error that so far received little attention in literature related to ToF camera calibration is the temperature of the camera's video chip. In this work we address the effect of active air conditioning in medically used rooms on the temperature related distance variability. The conducted experiments in which data were acquired over a long time indicate a reduction of the run-time related distance drift by up to factor five and a reduction of the measurement offset by factor three for certain examined ToF cameras in actively compared to passively climate controlled rooms. This has important implications on the ToF camera depth calibration process, for the calibration of the temperature related distance deviation in rooms with active air conditioning can be reduced to an easy to determine offset.

1 Introduction

In surgical navigation pre-operatively generated planning data are used to visualize anatomical structures and resection and risk margins to the surgeon. In order to use and update planning data in the operation room, an imaging modality is necessary that provides geometric data for intra-operative registration. Several modalities have been proposed so far for intra-operative image acquisition (in the context of navigated liver surgery [1, 2]).

Recently, continuous-wave Time-of-Flight (ToF) cameras have emerged as a new mean for intra-operative image acquisition [3]. This ToF camera uses a new type of video chip - the so called photo mixer device (PMD) chip [4]. Compared to established medical imaging modalities, ToF cameras are at the same time inexpensive, straightforward to use, do not result in patient or physician exposure to radiation and provide real-time images of the patient anatomy. The major benefit of the ToF technique in comparison to surface reconstruction methods based on triangulation (stereo, structured light, shape-from-motion) is the simultaneous generation of dense and co-registered distance and intensity image data by state-of-the-art cameras. The major drawback of the ToF technique compared to other techniques is the systematic depth errors which depend on different factors including temperature, intensity, and the distance to the object under observation. A comprehensive survey of sources of systematic errors in ToF cameras and an overview of proposed compensation methods can be found in Foix et al. [5].

In a previous study towards the use of ToF cameras in the context of navigated liver surgery we showed with human livers that - even in the rigid case - the target registration error (TRE), determined at introduced target marker, is about 10 mm [6]. This misalignment is caused to a high extend by systematic errors in the ToF distance measurement. Hence, ToF camera calibration is a crucial step towards clinical use of the new modality. While several studies exist on the assessment and compensation of errors related to intensity or distance to the object, the temperature related error has so far been given little attention.

Temperature dependency is a basic characteristic of semiconductor material as described by Gisolf [7]. The error in the distances measured by the ToF camera device is due to increasing temperature on the PMD chip caused by heat produced by the illumination unit and the resistance in the circuitry of the PMD chip. This temperature dependency has been investigated by Albrecht [8]. The effect of temperature on measured distances was investigated by Kahlmann et al. [9] and Rapp [10]. A viable solution to calibrate the temperature dependent distance error has been proposed so far only by Kahlmann et al. [9]. Their solution uses a glass fiber as a reference path mounted between the illumination unit and the PMD chip. Knowing the exact length and the refraction index of the glass fiber allows for determination of a correction parameter. However, incorporating this solution in state-of-the-art ToF cameras requires interference with the hardware of the camera.

In this work, we assume that the air conditioning in medically used rooms, like CT intervention rooms, is sufficient to compensate the temperature dependent distance drift. Therefore, we investigate the effect of active air conditioning on the distance measurement of a set of different ToF cameras and examine the runtime dependent measurement offset in the distance data.

2 Material and methods

In order to investigate the made assumption, we conducted a set of experiments in which we acquired data from three different ToF cameras, a Swiss Ranger 4000 (SR4000) (MESA Imaging AG, Zürich), a CamCube 2.0 (CC2), and a CamCube 3 (CC3) (both PMD Technologies GmbH, Siegen). The data acquisition took place in three different rooms:

1. a passive climate controlled lab room (pasLab);

2. an active climate controlled lab room (actLab);
3. and a CT intervention room (CTIR).

The pasLab room is the reference in which the temperature increase in the PMD chip is not compensated for. In the actLab room a continuously working climate control system is installed and in the CTIR a climate control system with feedback control is in use. These air conditioning systems transport the produced heat away from the cameras and provide a more constant environment towards temperature and humidity than in a passively climate controlled room.

2.1   Data acquisition

For each camera and room type, $n = 4$ experiments were performed. In navigated surgery the maximum runtime of an intra-operative imaging modality is assumed to be less than ten hours. Therefore, the runtime was set to ten hours with a sample interval of two minutes resulting in 300 sample points. Each acquired sample point was derived from an image stack of 500 distance images from the ToF camera with the size 30×30 pixels. The used image section was located in the middle of the distance images. The setup of the camera was perpendicular to a wall of the room at a distance of 1250 mm. This reflects a realistic distance between camera and a patient in a surgical navigation setup. The wall was covered with a uniformly reflecting white target. The settings of the ToF camera parameters were adapted for the different ToF cameras to avoid over- and under exposure of the pixels and reduce the measurement noise. The integration time was set to 500 μs for CC3, 700 μs for SR4000, and 2000 μs for CC2. The modulation frequency was set to 20 MHz for CC2 and CC3 and to 30 MHz for the SR4000. For demodulation of the ToF measurement signal, routines provided by the manufacturers were used.

2.2   Image processing and data evaluation

To evaluate the image data, initially the temporal median was calculated from the image stack, followed by the median of the image slice. From a highly accurate measurement gauge, the real distance from the camera to the target plane was known. The measurement offset of the sample points was determined as the difference between the measured distance and the real distance. For the distance data are generated without comprehensive calibration and the measurement gauge was used against a reference surface of the camera the determined offset value does not reflect an absolute error but it demonstrates the variability over the conducted experiments.

3   Results

The recorded data sets for the used ToF cameras and the three rooms are displayed in Fig. 1 ($n = 4$, colored curves). The black curves in the diagrams were determined as the least square fits to the mean of the sample points for the four measurements from a room for a linear model. These fits include all values recorded after a warm-up period of 30 minutes. The pitch of the linear function indicates the drift of the temperature dependent offset in the respective measurement. This pitch was in the pasLab up to five times higher than in the actLab or CTIR (Fig. 1 a, b, c and d, e, f). The variability of the offset over the recorded data sets for the evaluated ToF cameras is shown in Fig. 2. Again

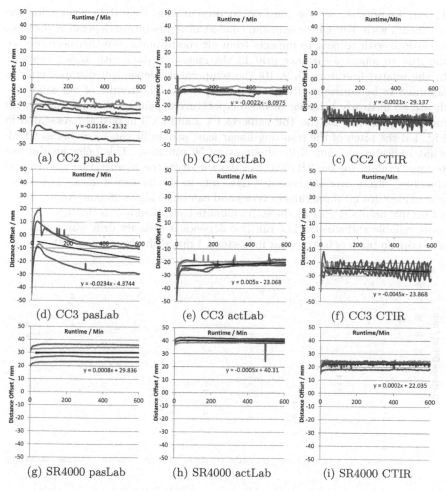

Fig. 1. The graphs show the distance offset of the measurements over time in the passively (pasLab) and actively (actLab) climate controlled lab room and the CT intervention room (CTIR) for the three used camera types. In the graphs the $n = 4$ data sets for each camera and room are represented by the colored curves. The black curves are the least square fits to the mean of the data sets after a warm-up period of 30 minutes. The linear functions in the diagrams are the results of the least square fit

402   Mersmann et al.

only the data after a warm-up period of 30 minutes are considered. The plot
indicates a higher variability of the measurement offset in the pasLab compared
to the actLab and the CTIR. The range from 25%-quantile to 75%-quantile for
the cameras in actLab and CTIR is between 2.1 mm and 4.6 mm, for the pasLab
this range is between 9.1 mm and 10.5 mm respectively.

4 Discussion

To our knowledge, we are the first to present long time data acquisition experiments with ToF cameras in the context of temperature dependent distance
deviations with respect to impacts from air conditioning. Furthermore, we are
the first to report a distance drift in the measured data with longer runtime.
In the related literature [5, 9, 10] the temperature dependent distance error is
assumed to be constant after a warm-up period. The results of our study indicate an unsteady behavior of the temperature dependent distance offset with
increasing runtime for the ToF cameras CC2 and CC3 in pasLab. As stated in
Fig. 1 d the pitch of the resulting linear least square fit can be as big as 0.023,
what indicates a 1 mm drift about every 50 minutes. This behavior did not
become evident for the SR4000. Besides the drift, the temperature also caused
changing offsets over the recorded data sets in the measured data. This effect
was evident for all three camera types and can be as big as 26 mm averaged over
all sample points (Fig. 1 a). In active climate controlled rooms the behavior was
more reliable and steady. The runtime dependent distance drift was reduced to
a maximum pitch of 0.005, what indicates a 1 mm drift about every 200 minutes.

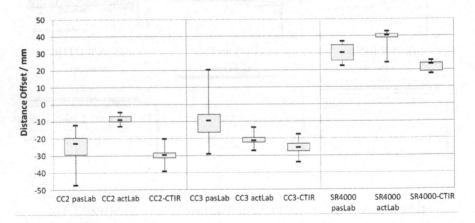

Fig. 2. Box-Whisker-Plot indicating the measurement offset over the recorded data
sets for the used cameras in the passively (pasLab) and actively (actLab) climate
controlled lab room and the CT intervention room (CTIR). The whiskers in the plot
represent the minimum and maximum offset determined by the experiments.The range
from 25%-quantile to 75%-quantile is about two to three times higher in the pasLab
than in the active climate controlled rooms

The variability of the offset over the recorded data sets was also reduced by a factor of two to three, according to Fig. 2. Comparing the measurement results from the actLab with that from the CTIR, a high jitter in the data sets from the CTIR is recognizable. This jitter can be as big as 8 mm from one sample point to the next (Fig. 1 c, f, i). As mentioned in Sec. 2, in the CTIR a feedback controlled air conditioning system is installed. The temperature feedback loop activates or deactivates the air conditioning, what causes a steady temperature rise and fall in that room. Due to the inhomogeneous temperature the distance offsets of the ToF cameras are also unsteady from one sample point to the next, causing the jitter in the data. Therefore, to profit from the influence of active climate control the settings of the air conditioning should be considered to work without temperature feedback loop to guarantee a steady heat transportation. Concluding, the use of active climate control has important implications on the depth calibration process of ToF cameras. Once ToF cameras are used in environments with active climate control, the temperature related distance error can be reduced after a warm-up period to an offset. In passively climate controlled environments, a drift in the measured distance data has to be compensated for additionally. This leads to a reduction of the number of calibration parameters needed, what eases the depth calibration process of ToF cameras.

Acknowledgement. The present study was conducted within the setting of Research Training Group 1126 funded by the German Research Foundation (DFG).

References

1. Lange T, et al. 3D ultrasound-CT registration of the liver using combined landmark-intensity information. Int J CARS. 2009;4(1):79–88.
2. Cash DM, et al. Concepts and preliminary data toward the realization of image-guided liver surgery. J Gastrointest Surg. 2007;11:844–59.
3. Mersmann S, et al. Time-of-Flight-Kameratechnik für die computerunterstützte Medizin. In: e-Health: Informationstechnologien und Telematik im Gesundheitswesen. Medical Future Verlag; 2011. p. 189–95.
4. Lange R. 3D Time-of-flight distance measurement with custom solid-state image sensors in CMOS/CCD-technology. University of Siegen; 2000.
5. Foix S, Alenya G, Torras C. Lock-in time-of-flight (ToF) cameras: a survey. IEEE Sens J. 2011;11(9):1917–26.
6. Mersmann S, et al. Time-of-flight camera technology for augmented reality in computer-assisted interventions. Proc SPIE. 2011;7964:2C.
7. Gisolf JH. Die Temperaturabhängigkeit des Widerstandes von Halbleitern. Ann Phys. 1947;436:3–26.
8. Albrecht M. Photogate-PMD-Sensoren. Universität Siegen; 2007.
9. Kahlmann T, Ingensand H. Calibration and development for increased accuracy of 3D range imaging cameras. J Appl Geodesy. 2008;2(1):1–11.
10. Rapp H. Experimental and theoretical investigation of correlating TOF-camera systems. University of Heidelberg; 2007.

A novel Real-Time Web3D Surgical Teaching Tool based on WebGL

Steven Birr, Jeanette Mönch, Dirk Sommerfeld, Bernhard Preim

Institut für Simulation und Graphik, Otto-von-Guericke-Universität Magdeburg
steven.birr@ovgu.de

Abstract. The purpose of this paper is the demonstration of a real-time Web3D surgical learning application. In contrast to existing medical e-learning portals, we provide interactive web-based 3D models derived from patient-specific image data. The 3D visualizations are accessible in real-time with our newly developed 3D viewer based on X3D and WebGL. Thus, no platform-specific browser plugin is required. Additional information, such as annotated 2D DICOM data, high-quality surgical movies and a quiz can be used by the learner to train his/her knowledge about human anatomy and surgical procedures. Our conclusion is that our presented Web3D e-learning application may support traditional educational methods like lectures and schoolbooks.

1 Introduction

E-learning systems increasingly support conventional medical education and training. They are applied to convey anatomical basics or to train therapy decision making and treatment. They allow an autonomous, time- and location-independent as well as active acquisition of knowledge. Graphics, movies, animations and 3D models illustrate complex anatomical relations much better than textbooks. The drawback of local software systems is their limited dissemination and content actuality. In contrast, web-based e-learning platforms can be accessed and updated easily.

There exist several offline and online e-learning systems for teaching anatomical basics by employing 3D models for interactive visualizations (PrimalPictures 3D Human Anatomy (http://www.primalpictures.com), VoxelMan Inner Organs [1], or VIRTUAL Liver [2]). The majority of web-based systems require special plugins, VRML [3], Flash [4] or QuicktimeVR [5] that have to be installed afore. Most of these systems are not based on individual patient data and offer no verification of the achieved knowledge gain for the learner.

Pape-Köhler et al. [6] have analyzed the five most important online and offline surgical e-learning portals in their study. It turned out that none of the reviewed systems fulfilled all criteria in terms of curricular integrity, currency of scientific content and validity. Therefore, our goal is the development of a surgical learning and communication platform which provides multimedia content and interactive web-based 3D visualizations.

In this paper we present an interactive Web3D tool for liver anatomy teaching based on WebGL (http://www.khronos.org/webgl). In contrast to previously existing medical e-learning tools, we abandon the usage of 3D modeling software to get high-detailed 3D graphics. Instead, our tool employs real patient-specific 2D and 3D data to show the variety of liver anatomy and to train its interpretation. An integrated quiz shall convey interaction with the 3D model and provide feedback concerning the learning success.

2 Materials and methods

We employed 13 abdominal DICOM CT datasets as basis for our interactive web application. Anatomical and pathological structures were segmented by several medical experts. In order to represent a typical clinical case, further information about radiological findings, preliminary investigation, diagnosis and surgical reports are provided. The generation of web-based medical 2D images and 3D models as well as the combination with a didactical concept is explained in the following sections.

2.1 Web-based 2D viewer

Typically, DICOM volume data are too large for fast online access. Furthermore, clinical DICOM data are often not anonymized adequately for online publishing. Thus, we chose the JPG image format to achieve a fast online access on anonymized patient data. The usage of compressed JPG images instead of high-detailed DICOM data is reasonable, since no exact diagnostics have to be accomplished on the web platform. Nevertheless, we loose the opportunity of interactive level-windowing when using JPG images. To overcome this issue, several image datasets with predefined window levels are provided and can be switched interactively by the user.

MeVisLab [7] is used to export the DICOM CT slices to JPG images. For educational purposes, the 2D slices are overlayed with colored segmented masks, e.g. vessels, tumors or organs serving as context information (Fig. 1). Images and overlays are scrollable by the user similar to a common radiological workstation. The segmented structures are exported as SVG (Scalable Vector Graphics) objects and mapped on the JPG images with the Raphaël JavaScript framework (http://raphaeljs.com). This procedure allows flexible scaling, coloring and usage of the overlays in our educational web application. Mouseover events on the SVG objects are used to dynamically display textual annotation labels. In addition, SVG enables the flexible integration of symbols, e.g. circles or arrows indicating important medical structures.

2.2 Web-based 3D viewer

We use X3D (http://www.web3d.org/x3d), an ISO Web3D standard, since it allows to export and represent 3D objects in a hierarchical scene graph via XML-based textual encoding. Furthermore, X3D content can be easily integrated and

Fig. 1. An interactive purely HTML-based 2D viewer for slicing through a medical image stack. Colored overlays and textual annotations indicate segmented anatomical and pathological structures

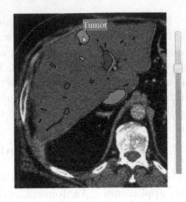

rendered in real-time with our interactive web application using the X3DOM [8] framework. The advantage of X3D is the simple integration into the HTML DOM since no additional transformation of 3D nodes is necessary to display 3D content on a website. WebGL is a JavaScript API and provides a platform-independent, plugin-free, scalable and GPU-supported access on dynamic 3D models. WebGL closely matches OpenGL ES 2.0 and uses GLSL as language for shader programs. By now, WebGL is supported by the most used web browsers in the latest releases (e.g. Mozilla Firefox or Google Chrome).

The segmented 2D structures are automatically transformed into 3D models (Fig. 2(a)) and exported as X3D files using MeVisLab. In addition, mesh simplification algorithms are used to decimate the number of polygons and thus reduce rendering time in the web-based 3D viewer. The X3D content is not embedded directly in HTML to assure fast access to the web application. Instead, the 3D elements are dynamically downloaded from the server and integrated on the client side into the website using AJAX (Asynchronous JavaScript and XML).

The medical 3D scenes rendered with WebGL can be rotated, tanslated and zoomed freely without the need of installing any additional browser plugin. However, free exploration of 3D scenes like rotating the scene, zooming in/out and enabling/disabling different structures can be a complex and tedious task for unfamiliar users. Therefore, we provide easy-to-learn interaction modes to ease the exploration of the 3D models and to reduce the learning effort. The rotation can be restricted to fixed axes to avoid unwanted viewpoints. Furthermore, we enable different levels of zooming by providing an interactive zoom slider.

Surgeons often want to manipulate only a few parameters of a 3D visualization. Therefore, we provide several visualization presets that can be used to adjust the visualization result depending on user's requirements. For example, a complex 3D liver model displaying the tumor, several vessels and territories can be simplified by one click to show just the tumor in its correlation to the portal vein. Thus, the 3D scene is less complex and gives the learner the possibility to concentrate on certain details. In particular, this is a beneficial feature if the learner wants to gain knowledge about surgical procedures. Therefore, we provide several 3D resection proposals made by medical experts, depending on the individual patient case. A 3D resection proposal consists of a resection and remnant volume visually separated by a resection plane. The tumor(s), vessel territories and the surrounding liver are also integrated into the 3D scene (Fig. 2(b)). The learner can interactively explore the 3D resection proposal and has to decide whether this surgical procedure (e.g. a left hemihepatectomy) is indicated or not. To support the learner's decision, the resulting resection and remnant volume measurements can be enabled. After choosing one of the proposed resection methods, the user receives an immediate feedback on his/her answer.

2.3   Anatomy quiz and additional multimedia content

X3D allows an easy combination of 3D content with simple HTML, CSS and JavaScript elements. In our case, we combine our educational application by providing a quiz beside the 3D viewer. Multiple choice questions can be used by the learner to reflect and test his/her anatomy knowledge. On the one hand, questions can be answered by simply choosing an option in the quiz (e.g. "What is the correct medical term for the blue vessel displayed in the 3D scene?"). On the other hand, interactive selections of certain 3D elements are also supported (e.g. "Please identify and click on the portal vein!"). This can be achieved by simple JavaScript *onClick* event handlers. If all questions were answered successfully, a new patient case with higher difficulty is selected and can be investigated by the learner.

Additional hyperlinks to relevant websites are provided to support the learning process of the user. Furthermore, each patient case is enhanced by a high-detailed surgical movie composed and annotated by a surgeon. Thus, the learner is able to gain insight typical workflows of surgical interventions, e.g. surgery preparation, resection techniques and potential complications.

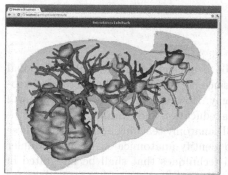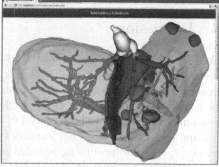

Fig. 2. High-quality X3D liver model with several colored tumors and vessels derived from individual patient anatomy (left) and 3D resection proposal of a hemihepatectomy (green: remnant, red: resection volume, orange: resection plane) displayed in our WebGL-based 3D viewer in Google Chrome 16 (right)

3   Results

We have presented a real-time Web3D surgical learning application which has many advantages for medical students. Web-based learning contents are accessible anywhere and anytime on demand. Compared to existing e-learning portals, we provide interactive medical 3D models that can be explored in common web browsers, without the need to install any plugin. The high-quality Web3D graphics derived from patient-specific anatomy allow for more realistic and detailed representations of anatomical and pathological structures. Since we use WebGL, every major web browser which implemented the forthcoming HTML 5 standard (e.g. Mozilla Firefox 8 or Google Chrome 16) can be employed. X3D as free file format enables easy exchange, reuse and integration of Web3D content in existing and future e-learning applications. A typical X3D scene is approximately 5 MB in size and is therefore accessible in a few seconds with high bandwidth. Our interactive web-based learning tool can be easily deployed in the classroom due to its simplicity. In order to improve the teaching and training process, the e-learning tool is supplemented by a web-based 2D DICOM image viewer and high-quality surgical movies.

Until now, we have carried out an informal evaluation with one radiologist. It turned out that the medical expert had no major problems to explore the web-based 2D data and 3D models. The physician favored the free exploration of high-detailed 3D graphics derived from individual patient data. However, the radiologist suggested that annotation labels might be essential for medical students to indicate anatomical structures. Furthermore, the radiologist claimed that interactive annotations of important structures is not possible, yet. A promising feature would be to highlight certain pathologies in order to collaborate with other learners about annotated findings and appropriate therapy strategies. Further evaluations with prospective users, which will investigate usability, knowledge gain and user acceptance of our application, are currently prepared.

4   Discussion

Our Web3D learning application can be beneficial to traditional educational methods like lectures and schoolbooks since it provides highly interactive web-based 3D visualizations of patient anatomy. However, further developments will be considered in order to enhance surgical education and training. Amongst others, annotations seem to be essential in 3D anatomy teaching applications. These textual annotations can help learners to identify anatomical structures. Mühler et al. [9] describe promising annotation techniques that shall be integrated in our e-learning application. Furthermore, WebGL is a promising technology for providing highly interactive surgical training tools online. It would be desirable to train surgical procedures [10] online without installing special browser plugins or applications. We will also concentrate on the development of an online authoring system for web-based 3D data. This authoring tool might give tutors the chance to update existing 3D models online, upload new cases and build questionnaires based on the uploaded content.

Further developments will also concentrate on medical visualization using mobile devices that are highly welcome by medical doctors. WebGL is basically a JavaScript binding of OpenGL ES 2.0 (http://www.khronos.org/opengles) and enables 3D renderings on portable devices like smartphones or tablets. Therefore, several hardware limitations and optimized shaders have to be considered carefully to assure high-quality performance on such devices.

Acknowledgement. We thank Fraunhofer MEVIS for advanced MeVisLab features. This work was supported by the BMBF in the framework of the SurgeryNet project (Promotional reference: 01PF08003E).

References

1. Höhne K, Pflesser B, Pommert A, et al. Voxel-Man 3D-Navigator: Inner Organs. New York: Springer Electronic Media; 2003.
2. Crossingham JL, Jenkinson J, Woolridge N, et al. Interpreting three-dimensional structures from two-dimensional images: a web-based interactive 3D teaching model of surgical liver anatomy. HPB. 2009;11(6):523-8.
3. Lu J, Pan Z, Lin H, et al. Virtual learning environment for medical education based on VRML and VTK. Comput Graph. 2005;29(2):283-8.
4. Jerath A, Vegas A, Meineri M, et al. An interactive online 3D model of the heart assists in learning standard transesophageal echocardiography views. Can J Anesth. 2011;58(1):14-21.
5. Friedl R, Preisack MB, Klas W, et al. Virtual reality and 3D visualizations in heart surgery education. Heart Surg Forum. 2002;5(3):17-21.
6. Pape-Köhler C, Chmelik C, Heiss MM, et al. E-learning in surgical procedure manuals and blogs. Chirurg. 2010;81(1):14-8.
7. Ritter F, Boskamp T, Homeyer A, et al. Medical image analysis. IEEE Pulse. 2011;2(6):60-70.
8. Behr J, Jung Y, Keil J, et al. A scalable architecture for the HTML5/X3D integration model X3DOM. Proc Web3D. 2010; p. 185-94.
9. Mühler K, Preim B. Automatische Annotation von 2D- und 3D-Visualisierungen. Proc BVM. 2009; p. 11-5.
10. Cordes J, Mühler K, Oldhafer KJ, et al. Evaluation of a training system of the computer-based planning of liver surgery. Proc CURAC. 2007; p. 151-4.

Rigid US-MRI Registration Through Segmentation of Equivalent Anatomic Structures

A Feasibility Study using 3D Transcranial Ultrasound of the Midbrain

Seyed-Ahmad Ahmadi[1], Tassilo Klein[1], Annika Plate[2], Kai Boetzel[2],
Nassir Navab[1]

[1]Computer Aided Medical Procedures, Technische Universitaet Muenchen, Germany
[2]Dept. of Neurology, Ludwig-Maximilians-University of Munich
ahmadi@cs.tum.edu

Abstract. Multi-modal registration between 3D ultrasound (US) and magnetic resonance imaging (MRI) is motivated by aims such as image fusion for improved diagnostics or intra-operative evaluation of brain shift. In this work, we present a rigid region-based registration approach between MRI and 3D-US based on the segmentation of equivalent anatomic structures in both modalities. Our feasibility study is performed using segmentations of the midbrain in both MRI and 3D transcranial ultrasound. Segmentation of MRI is based on deformable atlas registration while for 3D US segmentation, we recently proposed an accurate and robust method based on statistical shape modeling and a discrete and localized active surface segmentation framework. The multi-modal registration is performed through intensity-based rigid registration of signed distance transforms of both segmentations. Qualitative results and a demonstration of the basic feasibility of the region-based registration are demonstrated on a pair of MRI and challenging 3D transcranial US data volumes from the same subject.

1 Introduction

Multi-modal registration is a difficult and much-studied problem in computer-aided medical imaging. Among multi-modal registration problems, the registration of ultrasound (US) and magnetic resonance imaging (MRI) remains a particularly difficult challenge. Despite its difficulty, the problem is being studied intensively, due to a large number of possible applications, such as image fusion for diagnosis, US-based real-time imaging for intra-operative monitoring and deformation of a pre-operative plan for tissue shift correction. Several approaches have been proposed in literature, e.g. for non-linear registration in cardiac [1] and orthopedic surgery [2] as well as pre-operative planning [3]. In this paper, we are pursuing US-MRI registration for multi-modal fusion of brain volume images. Registration of 3DUS with MRI for the brain has been previously studied mainly in the area of brain shift detection. Brain shift occurs after craniotomy and cutting of the dura mater. The resulting change in intra-cranial pressure leads to a non-linear deformation of the brain tissue, often rendering the pre-operative plan inapplicable to the intra-operative situation. One exemplary approach for US-MRI registration is based on registration of segmented vessel structures from MR angiography and Doppler ultrasound [4]. Intra-operative 3D US and a biomechanical deformable model for detection of brain shift are used in [5]. Speckle-reduced US images are rigidly registered to MRI in [6] using mutual information (MI). In this work, we are demonstrating the feasibility of region-based rigid US-MRI registration using a pair of corresponding transcranial US and MRI image volumes, which can be used as an initialization for more complex, e.g. deformable registration. Transcranial US (TCUS) is a completely non-invasive method, which is regularly used in neuroradiology, e.g. for assessment of cranial vessel stenosis. For TCUS, the brain is imaged using a low-frequency (2-4MHz) US phased-array transducer which is scanning through the temporal bone window of the skull. TCUS generates challenging images with spatially large speckle patterns, low contrast, missing midbrain boundary information as well as a high variety in overall image quality due to varying bone window qualities across different subjects. Nevertheless, TCUS has recently emerged as a promising technique for differential diagnosis and early detection of Parkinson's Disease (PD) [7]. For our registration, we perform two segmentations of the midbrain region in the two image modalities and the registration is performed through registering the segmented region surfaces. Although this approach is not novel in itself [8], we demonstrate that region-based US-MRI registration can be performed using an accurate and robust 3D-TCUS midbrain segmentation method that we proposed previously, despite the difficult nature of 3D-TCUS.

2   Materials and methods

2.1   Data acquisition

The data acquisition for this study was performed in two steps. In the first step, a dataset of transcranial 3D-US (3D-TCUS) on 23 subjects was acquired [9], 11 previously diagnosed PD patients and 11 healthy. Volumes were reconstructed bi-laterally at an isotropic resolution of 0.45mm (Fig. 1, right). The midbrain region was segmented by a blinded expert and a statistical shape model of the midbrain was created for semi-automatic midbrain segmentation, with the aim of computer-aided diagnosis of Parkinson's Disease. The second step was to acquire a 3D US volume of a previously unseen subject, together with an unregistered T1-MRI volume of the same subject, in order to demonstrate the registration feasibility using our US segmentation.

2.2   Registration approach

The registration approach is based on segmentations of the same anatomic region, in both US and MRI modalities. In our case, we use the midbrain, but other regions can be used, if a suitable segmentation method is available in both modalities. Once region surfaces have been obtained using the respective segmentation techniques, a signed-distance-transform (SDT) of the surfaces are calculated in both modalities. The SDT maps of both modalities are then registered using a regular intensity-based rigid registration approach, with sum-of-squared-distances (SSD) as the distance measure (Fig. 1). This approach is similar to chamfer matching, a technique which is reportedly relatively insensitive to noise [10] and is hence able to partly compensate slight inaccuracies of the segmentations.

2.3 Midbrain segmentation in 3D transcranial ultrasound

Recently, we proposed an easy-to-use, robust and accurate semi-automatic method for midbrain segmentation in B-Mode 3D-TCUS [9]. The segmented midbrain region was proposed to serve as a region-of-interest selection (ROI), as mentioned, for a later step of segmenting the substantia nigra (SN) for Parkinson's Disease (PD) diagnosis. The 3D-TCUS segmentation method is based on a statistical shape model (SSM) of the midbrain, which was created using the dataset of 22 subjects. An arbitrary midbrain shape can thus be seen as a linear combination of the average shape S_μ with the M modes of variation S_i. The SSM model is integrated into an explicit Active Surface segmentation framework,

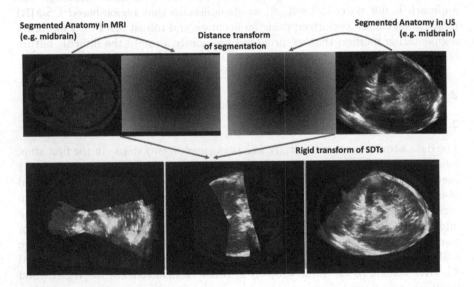

Fig. 1. Illustration of the rigid registration approach for T1-MRI (top left) and 3D-TCUS (top right), using signed distance transforms (SDT) of the segmented surfaces. The bottom row shows an example registration result

in which an active surface energy of the form

$$E(\mathcal{S}) = \int_{int\mathcal{S}} f_i \, dx + \int_{ext\mathcal{S}} f_e \, dx, \quad \mathcal{S}_\alpha = \mathcal{S}_\mu + \sum_{i=1}^{M} \alpha_i \mathcal{S}_i \qquad (1)$$

is iteratively minimized in order to evolve the shape model towards the desired shape configuration. S denotes the segmentation surface, $intS$ and $extS$ denote the interior and exterior region of the surface. As the cost function, we used a localized Chan-Vese mean intensity difference calculation [11], since foreground and background regions of the midbrain cannot be described by global statistics in US images. In order to derive a gradient-descent optimization strategy for iterative shape evolution, the partial derivatives of the shape energy $E(S)$ are calculated with respect to the shape configuration parameters j and a discretized approximation of the iterative energy evolution was derived. In the following formula, N denotes the surface normal and $[.]_k$ denotes the evaluation at vertex k

$$\frac{\partial}{\partial \alpha_j} E(\mathcal{S}_\alpha) = \frac{\partial E}{\partial S} \frac{\partial S}{\partial \alpha_j} = \int_S (f_i - f_e) N \cdot \mathcal{S}_j \, ds \approx \sum_{k=1}^{N} [f_i - f_e]_k \, [N]_k \cdot [\mathcal{S}_j]_k \qquad (2)$$

2.4 Midbrain segmentation in MRI

For the segmentation of the midbrain structure in MRI, we apply the approach of atlas-based segmentation. The principle is to use an atlas that contains a MRI image volume and corresponding labeled anatomical structures. For segmentation, a deformable registration of the atlas to the unknown image, in our case a T1-MRI of the test subject, is performed. Using the calculated deformation maps, the atlas labeling is transformed to the subject's MRI image and a segmentation is obtained. For deformable registration, we use a method based on registration through Markov Random Fields and efficient linear programming (MRFs) [12]. The resulting dense deformation field maps every atlas intensity voxel and hence also voxel-wise labeling information onto the subject's target MRI. As an atlas, we used the freely available SPL brain atlas [13], which is first rigidly registered to the subject's T1-MRI using landmark registration with eight point pairs. After landmark registration is applied as an initialization, the deformable registration is performed. For the deformable registration, Mutual Information (MI) is used as the distance measure.

3 Experiments and results

The proposed US segmentation method was evaluated in [9] and showed a high regional overlap with the manual expert segmentation (median DICE 0.85). The same method was applied for US midbrain segmentation in this work, using the same parameters as in [9]. The MRI atlas-based segmentation was performed using the previously described MRF-based deformable registration method. Both segmentation results were checked qualitatively by an expert and accepted without making any changes. The result for rigid registration of the 3D-TCUS with T1-MRI had to be assessed qualitatively, due to a lack of groundtruth transformation between the two volumes as well as the difficulty to perform a landmark-based registration due to the diffuse nature of 3D-TCUS volumes. Fig. 2 shows that prior to registration, the initialization US volume is clearly mis-aligned to MRI, e.g. at the skull echo boundaries of volumes, which is particularly visible in the axial cut-plane. In the axial slice-view, a slight rotational mis-alignment can be seen. After registration, the translational error is reduced in all three directions, with better correspondence of skull echoes in 3D-TCUS volume with MRI skull boundaries, especially visible in axial, and sagittal view. The caudal part of the hemispheric fissure is well-registered. However, the coronal cut-plane shows that a rotational error along the coronal axis is still present after registration.

4   Discussion and conclusion

From the registration experiment and the qualitative evaluation of the registration performance, it can be seen that a region-based registration is in principle possible, yielding satisfying results, especially in terms of translational accuracy. Using our proposed 3D-TCUS segmentation as well as an atlas-based MRI labeling, we were able to demonstrate a good registration result of both midbrain segmentations, not only in translational accuracy, but also in axial rotation. The coronal rotation inaccuracy stems mainly from the fact that the midbrain structureis too small to give enough geometric support in order to also register structures that are relatively far away, such as the skull boundaries. One way to counteract is to include more structures into the 3D-TCUS segmentation method and to use multiple structures for region-based registration to MRI. Accordingly, we are currently extending the segmentation method to a multi-phase

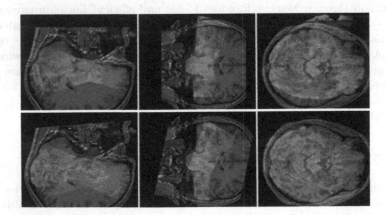

Fig. 2. Results from the region-based registration experiment with initialization (top row) and registration result (bottom row). Ultrasound is overlaid in green

shape model and segmentation framework, both for its diagnostic value as well as to evaluate the increase in registration accuracy. However, in immediate proximity of the midbrain structure, the registration accuracy is already sufficiently high. Given this result, one of our future investigations will be whether it is possible to either initialize a future image-based US-MRI deformable registration method or whether it is even possible to use several segmented structures and their distance transforms directly in order to compute tissue shift, and eventually brain shift, through segmented structures.

References

1. Huang X, Hill NA, Ren J, et al. Dynamic 3D ultrasound and MR image registration of the beating heart. In: Proc MICCAI; 2005. p. 171–8.
2. Winter S, Dekomien C, Hensel K, et al. [Registration of intraoperative 3D ultrasound with preoperative MRI data for computer-assisted orthopaedic surgery]. Z Orthop Unfall. 2007;145:586–90.
3. Blackall JM, Penney GP, King AP, et al. Alignment of sparse freehand 3-D ultrasound with preoperative images of the liver using models of respiratory motion and deformation. IEEE Trans Med Imaging. 2005;24:1405–16.
4. Reinertsen I, Descoteaux M, Siddiqi K, et al. Validation of vessel-based registration for correction of brain shift. Med Image Anal. 2007;11:374–88.
5. Blumenthal T, Hartov A, Lunn K, et al. Quantifying brain shift during neurosurgery using spatially tracked ultrasound. Proc SPIE. 2005;5744:388.
6. Letteboer MM, Willems PW, Viergever MA, et al. Brain shift estimation in image-guided neurosurgery using 3-D ultrasound. IEEE Trans Biomed Eng. 2005;52:268–76.
7. Berg D, Seppi K, Behnke S, et al. Enlarged substantia nigra hyperechogenicity and risk for Parkinson disease: a 37-month 3-center study of 1847 older persons. Arch Neurol. 2011;68:932–7.
8. Feldman M, Tomaszewski J, Davatzikos C. Non-rigid registration between histological and MR images of the prostate: A joint segmentation and registration framework. Proc IEEE CVPR Workshops. 2009;1:125–32.
9. Ahmadi SA, Baust M, Karamalis A, et al. Midbrain segmentation in transcranial 3d ultrasound for parkinson diagnosis. In: Proc MICCAI; 2011. p. 362–9.
10. Borgefors G. Hierarchical chamfer matching: A parametric edge matching algorithm. IEEE Trans Pattern Anal Mach Intell. 1988;10(6):849–65.
11. Lankton S, Tannenbaum A. Localizing region-based active contours. IEEE Trans Image Process. 2008;17(11):2029–39.
12. Glocker B, Komodakis N, Tziritas G, et al. Dense image registration through MRFs and efficient linear programming. Med Image Anal. 2008;12(6):731–41.
13. Talos IF, Wald L, Halle M, et al. Multimodal SPL Brain Atlas Data. http://www.spl.harvard.edu/publications/item/view/1565, last accessed; 2011.

Parallelisierung intensitätsbasierter 2D/3D-Registrierung mit CUDA

Andreas Huppert[1], Thomas Ihme[1], Ivo Wolf[2]

[1]Institut für Robotik, Hochschule Mannheim
[2]Institut für Medizinische Informatik, Hochschule Mannheim
andreas.huppert@gmx.de

Kurzfassung. Die Registrierung von zweidimensionalen, intraoperativen Bilddaten mit präoperativ ermittelten, dreidimensionalen Volumendaten ist eine bekannte Problemstellung mit vielfältigen Anwendungen. Die Anforderung, beispielsweise bei intraoperativer Eingriffsunterstützung möglichst schnell Ergebnisse vorliegen zu haben, legt eine hochparallelisierte Implementierung der dazu nötigen Algorithmen nahe. In diesem Paper wird ein kostengünstiges Verfahren auf Basis von GPGPU-Programmierung mit dem CUDA-Framework beschrieben. Um die Vergleichbarkeit der Umsetzung zu ermöglichen, wird das Registrierungsverfahren unter Verwendung eines Referenzdatensatzes mit bekannten Aufnahmeparametern evaluiert.

1 Einleitung

Grafikkartenprozessoren (Graphic Processing Units, GPUs) übertreffen in ihrer Leistungsfähigkeit klassische Hauptprozessoren potentiell um ein Vielfaches. Voraussetzung ist die effiziente Nutzung der hochparallelen Architektur moderner GPUs. GPGPU-Lösungen (General Purpose Computing on Graphic Processing Units) erleichtern seit einiger Zeit die Implementierung allgemeiner rechen- und datenintensiver Algorithmen. In der medizinischen Bildverarbeitung bietet die Parallelisierung von Bildregistrierungsverfahren mittels solcher GPGPU-Technologien ein hohes Beschleunigungspotential [1].

Unter 2D/3D-Registrierung wird üblicherweise die Registrierung von (intraoperativen) Röntgenaufnahmen, also 2D-Projektionen des Patienten (und nicht etwa allgemeiner 2D-Bilddaten wie z.B. Ultraschallaufnahmen), zu (präoperativen) 3D-Bildvolumina verstanden. Bei der intensitätsbasierten 2D/3D-Registrierung [2] werden aus den 3D-Bilddaten durch Projektion digital rekonstruierte Röntgenaufnahmen (Digitally Reconstructed Radiographs, DRRs) erzeugt und die Projektionsrichtung in einem Optimierungsprozess so angepasst, dass die erzeugten DRRs bestmöglich mit den aufgenommenen Röntgenaufnahmen übereinstimmen. Sowohl die Erzeugung der DRRs als auch der Optimierungsprozess, der in jedem Iterationsschritt die Erzeugung (mindestens) einer DRR erfordert, einschließlich des Bildvergleichs (Metrik) sind rechenintensive Schritte, die eine Parallelisierung nahelegen.

Im Folgenden wird die vollständige Umsetzung eines 2D/3D-Registrierungsverfahrens auf Basis von Röntgenaufnahmen und CT-Volumina erläutert. Von den benötigten Verfahren wurden mit der Generierung der DRRs und der Metrikberechnung nur die rechenintensivsten Teilschritte auf die Grafikkarte ausgelagert und in doppelter Hinsicht parallelisiert: zusätzlich zur Parallelisierung der Berechnung der einzelnen Teilschritte werden mehrere Teilschritte parallel berechnet.

Die Implementierung verwendet das CUDA-Framework von NVIDIA, wodurch spezielle Funktionen, sogenannte Kernels, auf der GPU ausgeführt werden können. Die beschriebene Methodik lässt sich aber in entsprechender Weise auch mit dem herstellerübergreifenden Standard OpenCL umsetzen.

Um die Lösung nicht nur hinsichtlich ihrer Performanz, sondern auch im Hinblick auf ihre Einsatzfähigkeit zu bewerten, wurde sie unter Verwendung einer standardisierten Evaluationsmethode auf einem ebenfalls standardisierten Datensatzes [3] evaluiert, wodurch eine Vergleichbarkeit mit anderen Implementierungen ermöglicht wird.

2 Material und Methoden

Es wird eine Transformation gesucht, für die das Röntgenbild (Abb. 1(a)) und die simulierte Projektion des CT-Volumens (Abb. 1(b)) eine möglichst hohe Übereinstimmung zeigen. Dadurch lässt sich die Position und Orientierung des abgebildeten Körpers zum Zeitpunkt der Röntgenaufnahme im Koordinatensystem des CT-Volumens bestimmen.

Die verwendeten bildgebenden Verfahren basieren auf Röntgenstrahlung, bilden also in erster Linie Knochenstrukturen ab. Daher ist es ausreichend sich auf rigide Transformationen zu beschränken. Nach korrekter Simulation der geometrischen Gegebenheiten und Kalibrierung des Röntgensystems müssen somit

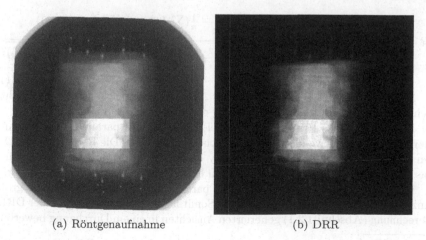

(a) Röntgenaufnahme   (b) DRR

Abb. 1. Zu registrierende Daten mit markierten Regions of Interest (ROI)

noch die sechs Parameterwerte für Rotation und Translation des Körpers im Raum bestimmt werden.

2.1 DRR-Berechnung

Die digitale Rekonstruktion von Röntgenaufnahmen aus dem gegebenen präoperativen CT-Volumen erfolgt mit einem Raycasting-Verfahren. Raycasting-Verfahren sind sehr gut parallelisierbar, weil die Strahlenaussendung für jeden Bildpixel vollkommen unabhängig voneinander geschehen kann. Deswegen existieren für diese Technik des Volume Renderings bereits CUDA-beschleunigte Algorithmen (CUDA-SDK[1], die in erster Linie nur noch auf eine möglichst hohe Ähnlichkeit zu echten Röntgenaufnahmen hin angepasst werden mussten. Das verwendete Verfahren legt das Volumen im Texture Memory der Grafikkarte ab, so dass für das Sampling entlang des Sichtstrahls die nativ auf der Grafikkarte implementierte lineare Interpolation verwendet werden konnte. Die Basisimplementierung, welche eine perspektivisch korrekte DRR-Abbildung erzeugte, wurde in der Folge angepasst, um die gleichzeitige Berechnung mehrerer Ansichten auf das Volumen zu ermöglichen. Der Kernel legt also entsprechend der Menge an bereitgestellten Transformationen eine Anzahl an DRR-Ansichten im Grafikspeicher ab.

2.2 Metrik

Als Ähnlichkeitsmaß für die Übereinstimmung von Röntgenaufnahme (I_R) und DRR-Ansichten (I_DRR) wurde mit der normalisierten Kreuzkorrelation ein intensitätsbasiertes Verfahren gewählt (Gleichung 1). Das Verfahren ist invariant gegenüber globalen Helligkeitsunterschieden und eignet sich daher gut für Bilddaten gleicher Modalität wie im vorliegenden Fall.

$$R = -1 \frac{\sum\limits_{x,y}\left(I_\mathrm{R}(x,y)\cdot I_\mathrm{DRR}(x,y)\right) - \frac{1}{n}\left(\sum\limits_{x,y}I_\mathrm{R}(x,y)\cdot\sum\limits_{x,y}I_\mathrm{DRR}(x,y)\right)}{\sqrt{\sum\limits_{x,y}I_\mathrm{R}(x,y)^2 - \frac{1}{n}(\sum\limits_{x,y}I_\mathrm{R}(x,y))^2}\sqrt{\sum\limits_{x,y}I_\mathrm{DRR}(x,y)^2 - \frac{1}{n}(\sum\limits_{x,y}I_\mathrm{DRR}(x,y))^2}}$$

$$(1)$$

Abhängig von der Bildgröße und der Anzahl zu vergleichenden Bilder, lohnt sich die Parallelisierung der Berechnung der einzelnen Summanden.

Dabei wurde das Prinzip der Parallel Reduction auf parallelisierte Teilsummenbildung [4] angewendet und entsprechend angepasst. Die Reduktion der Daten erfolgt im schnellen Shared Memory der Grafikkarte. Summen, welche nur das Röntgenbild berücksichtigen, werden einmalig auf der CPU vorberechnet.

In unserer Implementierung können parallel die Metrikwerte für eine große Anzahl an Ansichten berechnet werden. Somit lassen sich alle während der DRR-Berechnung (Abschnitt 2.1) generierten Ansichten in einem Durchgang bewerten.

---

[1] http://developer.nvidia.com/cuda-cc-sdk-code-samples#volumeRender

Weil somit die komplette Bildverarbeitung auf der Grafikkarte stattfindet und nach der Initialisierung nur noch Transformations- sowie Metrikdaten übertragen werden müssen, lässt sich der Aufwand für Speichertransfers – ein häufiger Flaschenhals der GPGPU-Programmierung – gering halten.

2.3 Optimierer

Zur Bestimmung der optimalen Transformation kommt ein parallelisiertes Gradientenverfahren zum Einsatz, um (lokale) Optima im sechsdimensionalen Parameterraum zu finden. Die Implementierung orientiert sich an [5]. Es wird in jedem Schritt die aktuelle Ansicht sowie für jeden Parameter jeweils zwei Ansichten mit geringfügig veränderten Werten berechnet. Anschließend wird im Parameterraum ein normierter Schritt in Richtung des steilsten Abstiegs vorgenommen. Kann keine Verbesserung mehr festgestellt werden, arbeitet das Verfahren mit reduzierter Schrittweite weiter. Bei der Evaluierung wurden gute Ergebnisse erzielt, wenn mit Schrittweiten von 1 mm bzw. 1 rad begonnen und diese wiederholt um 1/3 bis zu einem Wert von ca. 0,06 reduziert wurden.

Für jeden Optimierungsschritt ergeben sich durch die Anpassung der Parameter 13 Ansichten, die parallel gerendert und bewertet werden können. Die Anpassung der Parameter anhand der ermittelten Metrikwerte wird aufgrund der geringen Datenkomplexität konventionell auf der CPU durchgeführt.

Wie bei jedem Registrierungsvorgang besteht die Gefahr, dass der Optimierungsvorgang in einem lokalen Optimum endet, das nicht die korrekte Registrierung wiedergibt. Dieser Gefahr kann durch mehrfaches Durchführen der Optimierung mit verschiedenen Startwerten begegnet werden, ein Vorgang, der sich naturgemäß wiederum hervorragend parallelisieren lässt. Die Implementierung bietet daher die Möglichkeit, eine beliebige Anzahl n von Optimierungen mit verschiedenen Startwerten parallel durchzuführen. Die Menge von $n * 13$ Ansichten, die somit gleichzeitig von der GPU verarbeitet werden kann, ist in erster Linie durch den zur Verfügung stehenden Grafikkartenspeicher begrenzt und wird so gewählt, dass die GPU optimal ausgelastet wird.

3 Ergebnisse

Alle Messungen wurden auf einem Rechner mit Intel Core I7 920 CPU (2.66 GHz, 6 GB RAM) durchgeführt. Als CUDA-Device fand eine Geforce GTX 275 mit 896 MB Speicher Verwendung. Zur Evaluierung des Verfahrens wurden die unter [3] beschriebenen Daten (CT-Volumen: 256^3 Voxel, Röntgenbild: 512^2 Pixel, ROI: 147×76 Pixel) eingesetzt, deren korrekte Registrierung sehr genau bekannt ist.

Zur Quantifizierung der durch die Registrierung real auftretenden Abweichungen wurde mit dem mean Target Registration Error (mTRE) ein gängiges Fehlermaß verwendet, das die erwartete mittlere Abweichung in Millimetern in einem definierten Zielgebiet angibt. Durch die Auswertung dieses Wertes zu Beginn und nach Beendigung eines Registrierungslaufs lassen sich Aussagen über

die Qualität des Verfahrens treffen. Für erfolgreiche Registrierungen (definiert
als mTRE < 2 mm) lag der Fehler im Mittel bei 1,14 mm (Abb. 2). Die Capture
Range des Verfahrens lag bei etwa 4-5 mm. Tests ergaben, dass die Metrik ab
einem Wert von ca. -0,994 sehr gut mit dem realen Fehler korreliert. Bei höheren Werten handelt es sich oftmals nur um lokale Optima, was sich in einem
unverhältnismäßig hohem mTRE widerspiegelt.

Der zusätzliche Speedup durch die parallele Berechnung mehrerer Ansichten
des bereits auf der GPU implementierten Renderingverfahrens betrug auf *einer*
GPU den Faktor 1,7. Die Metrikberechnung konnte gegenüber einer zum Vergleich erstellten CPU-seitigen Implementierung um den Faktor 5 beschleunigt
werden (Abb. 3).

Für das gesamte Registrierungsverfahren ergab sich damit eine Halbierung
der Berechnungsdauer, womit die in Abb. 2 beschriebene Registrierung eines
einzelnen maskierten Röntgenbildes ca. 16 Sekunden benötigte.

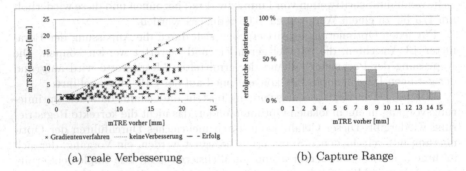

(a) reale Verbesserung   (b) Capture Range

Abb. 2. Ergebnisse des 2D/3D-Registrierungsvorgangs für ein einzelnes Röntgenbild
bei 200 verschiedenen Start-Transformationen. In Diagramm (a) ist die real erreichte
Verbesserung der einzelnen Optimierungen ablesbar. Diagramm (b) zeigt, wie groß der
Anteil erfolgreicher Registrierungen bei zunehmendem Startfehler noch ist

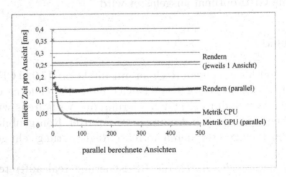

Abb. 3. Beschleunigung durch die parallele Berechnung mehrerer Ansichten auf der
GPU bei angewandter Bildmaske (Auflösung: 147 × 76 Pixel)

4   Diskussion

Es hat sich gezeigt, dass die einzelnen Teilschritte unterschiedliche Anforderungen an die Parallelisierung stellen. Während das Raycasting-Verfahren sehr rechenintensive Threads enthält und die verwendete GPU schon mit wenigen Ansichten auslastet, besteht die Schwierigkeit bei der verwendeten Metrik vor allem darin, eine ausreichend große Menge an Bilddaten bereitzustellen (Abb. 3). Weitere Tests haben ergeben, dass der Speedup der Metrik gegenüber der CPU-Lösung mit steigenden Bildgrößen deutlich zunimmt.

Die Evaluierung ergab, dass die CUDA-beschleunigte Registrierung den verwendeten Datensatz in wenigen Sekunden zuverlässig registrieren kann. Die Qualität der Registrierung liegt in einem Bereich, der üblich für intensitätsbasierte Verfahren mit einer Röntgenaufnahme ist. Trotz des Nachteils, dass aufgrund der Hardware-Architektur mit einfacher Fließkommagenauigkeit gerechnet werden musste, sind die Ergebnisse der vorliegenden Implementierung sogar leicht besser im Vergleich zu den Angaben in [3]. Die Ergebnisse sollten sich durch Verwendung mehrerer Röntgenaufnahmen nochmals deutlich verbessern lassen.

Derzeit wird die Implementierung für Systeme mit mehreren Tesla-Karten erweitert und evaluiert. Der naheliegende Ansatz hierbei ist, die Durchführung der Registrierungen mit verschiedenen Startwerten auf die GPUs zu verteilen. Durch die erhöhte Performance der GPUs bei doppelter Fließkommagenauigkeit ist der Trade-off für eine höhere Genauigkeit der Registrierung hinreichend klein, so dass in Zukunft auch in dieser Hinsicht eine Verbesserung zu erwarten ist.

Literaturverzeichnis

1. Fluck O, Vetter C, Wein W, et al. A survey of medical image registration on graphics hardware. Comput Methods Programs Biomed. 2010; p. online first.
2. Markelj P, Tomaževič D, Likar B, et al. A review of 3D/2D registration methods for image-guided interventions. Med Image Anal. 2010; p. online first.
3. van de Kraats EB, Penney GP, Tomazevic D, et al. Standardized evaluation methodology for 2D-3D registration. IEEE Trans Med Imaging. 2005;24:1177–90.
4. Harris M. Optimizing Parallel Reduction in CUDA. NVIDIA Developer Technology; 2008.
5. Penney GP, Weese J, Little JA, et al. A comparison of similarity measures for use in 2-D-3-D medical image registration. IEEE Trans Med Imaging. 1998;17:586–95.

Ein dämonenartiger Ansatz zur Modellierung tumorinduzierter Gewebedeformation als Prior für die nicht-rigide Bildregistrierung

A. Mang[1], T. A. Schütz[1,3], A. Toma[1,2], S. Becker[1,2], T. M. Buzug[1]

[1]Institut für Medizintechnik, Universität zu Lübeck (UL)
[2]Centre of Excellence for Technology and Engineering in Medicine (TANDEM)
[3]Graduiertenschule für Informatik in Medizin und Lebenswissenschaften, UL
mang@imt.uni-luebeck.de

Kurzfassung. In der vorliegenden Arbeit stellen wir einen Ansatz zur Modellierung tumor-induzierter Gewebedeformation als Prior für Verfahren der nicht-rigiden Bildregistrierung vor. Wir greifen hierfür eine kürzlich vorgeschlagene Strategie, formuliert als ein durch eine weiche Nebenbedingung restringiertes parametrisches Optimierungsproblem, auf und überführen diese in einen dämonenartigen Ansatz. Das vorgestellte Verfahren wird mittels eines variationellen Ansatzes motiviert. Um eine diffeomorphe Abbildung zu gewährleisten wird ein Regridding durchgeführt, sobald die punktweise ausgewertete Funktionaldeterminante der Abbildung unter einen vorgegebenen Schwellwert fällt. Weiter schlagen wir eine auf der Annahme eines diffeomorphen Deformationsmusters basierende Rechenvorschrift zur Erhaltung der Masse der deformierten Zelldichte vor. Die gezeigten numerischen Experimente demonstrieren das Potential des vorgeschlagenen Modells. Der variationelle Formalismus legt nahe, dass sich das Verfahren als generischer Baustein für eine modellbasierte, nicht-rigide Bildregistrierung eignet.

1 Einleitung

Die nicht-rigide Bildregistrierung [1] ist ein etabliertes Werkzeug aus der angewandten Mathematik zur Analyse serieller, multi-modaler und/oder populations-übergreifender Bildgebungsstudien in der Medizin. Im Zentrum der angewandten Forschung steht hierbei eine Extraktion von deskriptiven Bio-Markern, mit dem Ziel vitale Informationen über den Verlauf einer Pathologie zu gewinnen. Ein inhärentes Problem für alle etablierten, intensitätsbasierten Verfahren ist das Vorhandensein von mit dem Verlauf der Pathologie assoziierten Veränderungen in Bild-Morphologie und/oder -Textur. Unter der Annahme, dass sich entsprechende anatomische Strukturen innerhalb der vorliegenden Bilddaten Niveaulinien derselben Topologie (bis auf Messrauschen) abbilden, führt das Vorhandensein von pathologischen Veränderungen neue Isoflächen ein und induziert damit eine Veränderung der Topologie. Entsprechend ist die den intensitätsbasierten Registrieralgorithmen gemeine, fundamentale Forderung der Existenz einer eindeutigen, punktweisen Korrespondenz verletzt: das Templatebild kann nicht mehr als eine durch eine rein räumliche Verrückung verzerrte Repräsentante des Referenzbildes modelliert werden. Eine simple Strategie ist, die von der Pathologie betroffenen Areale auszublenden [2]. Damit ist allerdings die Güte der Registrierung in unmittelbarer Umgebung der Pathologie nicht gesichert. In [3] wurde kürzlich ein eleganter Ansatz zur Bestimmung des durch die Pathologie hervorgerufenen Intensitätsdrifts mittels einer Einbettung der d-dimensionalen Bilddaten in einen $d+1$-dimensionalen Riemannraum vorgeschlagen. Wir verfolgen in der vorliegenden Arbeit eine andere vielversprechende Strategie [4, 5, 6, 7] und schlagen vor, das skizzierte Problem durch eine explizite Modellierung der Pathologie zu umgehen. Das ultimative Ziel ist hierbei, einen generischen Baustein für einen hybriden Ansatz zur modellbasierten Registrierung von Tumorbilddaten zu liefern und *nicht* eine präzise Modellierung patientenindividueller Deformationsmuster. Anwendungsgebiete sind die atlasbasierte Segmentierung und/oder die Generierung von statistischen Pathologieatlanten.

Der wesentliche Beitrag liegt in der Überführung der in [4] vorgeschlagenen Strategie zur Modellierung von tumor-induzierter Gewebedeformation, basierend auf einem parametrischen Optimierungsproblem mit weicher Nebenbedingung, in einen diffeomorphen, dämonenbasierten Ansatz. Damit einhergehend führen wir eine Rechenvorschrift zur Erhaltung der Masse der deformierten Zelldichte ein und erweitern den Ansatz für die Modellierung der raum-zeitlichen Dynamik kanzeröser Zellen durch die Integration unscharfer Gewebekarten.

2 Material und Methoden

2.1 Raumzeitliche Dynamik kanzeröser Zellen

Die Modellierung der raum-zeitlichen Dynamik einer Populationsdichte an kanzerösen Zellen innerhalb des zerebralen Gewebes wird typischerweise über ein Anfangsrandwertproblem (ARWP) erklärt. Die grundlegende und anerkannte Annahme ist hierbei, dass die Ausbreitung der Krebszellen hinreichend gut durch die Prozesse der *Proliferation* und der *Migration* eines Zellverbandes in das umliegende, gesunde Gewebe beschrieben ist. Aus der Lösung des ARWP ergibt sich die gesuchte Populationsdichte $\psi : \Omega_B \times \mathbb{R}_0^+ \to \mathbb{R}_0^+$ mit dem Gebiet $\Omega_B \subset \Omega := (0,1)^d \subset \mathbb{R}^d$, welches das zerebrale Gewebe kennzeichnet. Wir beschränken uns in der vorliegenden Arbeit auf eine isotrope Diffusion mit einer Differenzierung der mittleren Diffusivität zwischen grauer ($\Omega_G \subset \Omega_B$) und weißer ($\Omega_W \subset \Omega_B$) Masse, basierend auf einer unscharfen Gewebekarte mit den Diffusionsraten $\kappa_l > 0$, $l \in \{W, G\}$ [8]. Das Modell der Zellvermehrung ist logistisch, mit der Wachstumsrate $\gamma > 0$ und der oberen Schranke (maximale Zelldichte) $\psi_L > 0$. Eine detaillierte Beschreibung des ARWP ist in [8] zu finden.

2.2 Deformationsmodell

Wir markieren alle Funktionen, die zu einem diskreten Zeitschritt $t^j := jq$, $q = \tau/n$, $j = 1, \ldots, n$ ausgewertet werden, mit einem oberen Index j. Damit ergibt sich die zeitdiskrete Repräsentation $\psi^j(\boldsymbol{x}) := \tilde{\psi}(\boldsymbol{x}, t^j)$, $\psi^j \colon \Omega \to \mathbb{R}_0^+$ der Populationsdichte ψ (Abschnitt 2.1). Der in [4] skizzierte Ansatz zur Bestimmung eines, einer gegebenen Zelldichte ψ^j zugehörigen, Deformationsmusters $\boldsymbol{u}^j \colon \mathbb{R}^d \to \mathbb{R}^d$ kann als Lösung eines inversen Problems interpretiert werden. Gemäß [4] schlagen wir folgendes Modellproblem vor:

Problem 1 *Sei $\psi^j \in L^2(\Omega, \mathbb{R}_0^+)$ zum Zeitpunkt $t^j > 0$, $j \in \mathbb{N}$ gegeben. Finde eine Abbildung $\boldsymbol{u}^j \in L^2(\Omega)^d$, so dass $\mathcal{J} \colon L^2(\Omega)^d \times L^2(\Omega, \mathbb{R}_0^+) \to \mathbb{R}$,*

$$\mathcal{J}[\psi^j, \boldsymbol{u}^j] = \mathcal{S}[\boldsymbol{u}^j] + \alpha \mathcal{D}[\boldsymbol{u}^j, \psi^j] \xrightarrow{\boldsymbol{u}^j} \min \tag{1}$$

mit $\mathcal{S} \colon L^2(\Omega)^d \to \mathbb{R}$, $\mathcal{D} \colon L^2(\Omega)^d \times L^2(\Omega, \mathbb{R}_0^+) \to \mathbb{R}_0^+$ und $\alpha > 0$

Hierbei ist $\mathcal{D}$ ein Datenterm, der die Deformation vorantreibt, und $\mathcal{S}$ eine Regularisierung, die nicht nur sicherstellt, dass Prb. 1 gut gestellt ist, sondern die Lösung $\boldsymbol{u}^j$ darüber hinaus in einem gewissen Sinne glatt ist. Für den Datenterm $\mathcal{D}$ verwenden wir in Anlehnung an [4]

$$\mathcal{D}[\boldsymbol{u}^j, \psi^j] = -\int_\Omega w(\psi^j(\boldsymbol{x}))\, \psi^j(\boldsymbol{u}^j(\boldsymbol{x}))\, \mathrm{d}\boldsymbol{x} \tag{2}$$

Hierbei ist $w(\psi^j(\boldsymbol{x})) := \exp(-p(\psi^j(\boldsymbol{x})/\psi_L)^{-2} - p(2-(\psi^j(\boldsymbol{x})/\psi_L)^2)^{-1})$ [4, 5, 7]. Der Parameter $\psi_L > 0$ entspricht der oberen Schranke aus Abschnitt 2.1. Der Parameter $p > 0$ erlaubt eine lokal-adaptive Steuerung des Deformationsmusters [4, 5, 7]. Entgegen der in [4] vorgeschlagenen Parametrisierung gekoppelt mit einer über einen numerisch delikaten Log-Barrier-Ansatz formulierten Einschränkung des Suchraums, schlagen wir in der vorliegenden Arbeit – der Generalisierung und der Einbettung in einen dämonenbasierten Ansatzes wegen – eine diffusive Regularisierung $\mathcal{S}$ vor. Unter der Annahme $\boldsymbol{u}^j \in C^2(\Omega)^d$ gilt hiermit [9]

$$\mathcal{S}[\boldsymbol{u}^j] = \frac{1}{2} \int_\Omega \sum_{l=1}^d \|\nabla u_l^j(\boldsymbol{x})\|^2\, \mathrm{d}\boldsymbol{x} \tag{3}$$

Mittels Variationsrechnung wird in einem *Optimize-then-Discretize*-Ansatz die Lösung der Optimieraufgabe (1) in die Lösung der Euler-Lagrange-Gleichung

$$\mathcal{A}[\boldsymbol{u}^j](\boldsymbol{x}) = \alpha \boldsymbol{b}^j(\boldsymbol{x}, \psi^j(\boldsymbol{x}), \boldsymbol{u}^j(\boldsymbol{x})) \tag{4}$$

überführt. In (4) repräsentieren $\boldsymbol{b}$ und $\mathcal{A}$ die Gâteaux-Ableitungen des Funktionals $\mathcal{D}$ bzw. $\mathcal{S}$. Für (2) ergibt sich (für ein hinreichend glattes ψ^j) – in Übereinstimmung mit bio-physikalischen Modellieransätzen [6] – der Kraftvektor $\boldsymbol{b}^j(\boldsymbol{x}, \psi^j(\boldsymbol{x}), \boldsymbol{u}^j(\boldsymbol{x})) = -w(\psi^j(\boldsymbol{x})) \nabla(\psi^j(\boldsymbol{u})(\boldsymbol{x}))$ und für (3) der Differentialoperator $\mathcal{A}[\boldsymbol{u}^j](\boldsymbol{x}) = -\Delta \boldsymbol{u}^j(\boldsymbol{x})$. Eine gängige Strategie zur Lösung von (4) ist die Einführung eines artifiziellen Zeitschritts [1, 9]. Wir verfolgen in dieser Arbeit eine andere Stragie: In Anlehnung an einen variationellen Rahmen [1] lässt sich die in [10] vorgestellte Verfahrensweise zur Bestimmung eines Minimierers für ein wie in Prb. 1 geartetes Modellproblem als eine Approximation der stationären Lösung der inhomogenen Diffusionsgleichung

$$\partial_t \boldsymbol{v}^j(\boldsymbol{x}, t) - \Delta \boldsymbol{v}^j(\boldsymbol{x}, t) = \alpha \boldsymbol{b}^j(\boldsymbol{x}, \psi^j(\boldsymbol{x}), \boldsymbol{u}^j(\boldsymbol{x})) \tag{5}$$

mit $v^j(x, 0) = 0$ und $x \in \mathbb{R}^d$, $t > 0$, interpretieren [11]. Dies entspricht der Anwendung einer diffusen Regularisierung auf das Geschwindigkeitsfeld v^j. Der Zusammenhang zwischen v^j und u^j ist durch die substantielle Ableitung $v^j(x, t) = \partial_t u^j(x, t) + (\nabla u^j(x, t))^\mathsf{T} v^j(x, t)$ erklärt. Der Dämonen-Algorithmus nutzt – unter der Annahme $\Omega = \mathbb{R}^d$ – die Tatsache aus, dass die Greensche Funktion $\mathcal{K}(x; \sqrt{2\tau})$ der Diffusionsgleichung einem Gaußkern (parametrisiert über $\tilde{\sigma} = \sqrt{2\tau}$, $\tau > 0$) entspricht und nähert die stationäre Lösung von (5) durch das Alternieren zwischen (i) der Bestimmung eines unrestringierten Updates b^j und (ii) der Annäherung der in (3) gegebenen Regularisierung durch die Faltung (symbolisiert durch *) der aktuellen Iterierten mit der Greenschen Funktion an. Da bei einer Anwendung der Verrückung u^j auf die Zelldichte ψ^j die Erhaltung der Masse nicht gewährleistet ist, führen wir zusätzlich die Rechenvorschrift

$$\psi^j(x) \leftarrow \psi^j(x)/(\det(D\,(x + u^j(x)))) \tag{6}$$

mit der Funktionaldeterminante $\det(D \cdot)$ ein. Die vorgeschlagene Verfahrensweise ist in Alg. 1 zusammengefasst. Entscheidend für die Rechenvorschrift (6) ist, dass die Abbildung $y^j = x + u^j$ regulär, d. h. ein Diffeomorphismus, ist. In Anlehnung an fluidale Ansätze [12] wird ein Regridding durchgeführt sobald eine Singularität im Verrückungsfeld detektiert wird, d.h. die Funktionaldeterminante einen vorgegebenen Schwellwert $\chi > 0$ unterschreitet. Abbruchkriterium ist ein Schwellwert $\varepsilon > 0$ für das Residuum bzw. eine maximale Iterationszahl $n \in \mathbb{N}$.

Algorithmus 1 Modellierung Tumor-induzierter Gewebedeformation.

initialize $v^j(x, 0) = 0$, $t^k = k\tau$, $\hat{u}^j(x, 0) = u^j(x)$, $\hat{\psi}^j(x, 0) = \psi^j(x)$, $k = 0$
while $k \leq n$ & $\|\alpha b^j(x, \hat{\psi}^j(x, t^k), \hat{u}^j(x, t^k)\|_2 > \varepsilon$ **do**
  $v^j(x, t^{k+1}) \leftarrow \mathcal{K}(x; \sqrt{2\tau}) * [v^j(x, t^k) + \alpha b^j(x, \hat{\psi}^j(x, t^k), \hat{u}^j(x, t^k)]$
  $\hat{u}^j(x, t^{k+1}) \leftarrow \hat{u}^j(x, t^k) + \tau[E - \nabla \hat{u}^j(x, t^k)]^\mathsf{T} v^j(x, t^{k+1})$
  if $(\det(D\,(x + \hat{u}^j(x, t^{k+1}))) < \chi)$ **then** regrid
  else
    $\hat{\psi}^j(x, t^{k+1}) \leftarrow \psi^j(x)/(\det(D\,(x + \hat{u}^j(x, t^{k+1}))))$
  endif
  $k \leftarrow k + 1$
end while
$u^j(x) \leftarrow \hat{u}^j(x, t^k)$; $\psi^j(x) \leftarrow \hat{\psi}^j(x, t^k)$

---

3 Ergebnisse

Die Experimente werden in einem zwei-dimensionalen Rahmen vorgestellt, unsere schablonenbasierte C++-Implementierung erlaubt eine d-dimensionale Modellierung. Die Parameter für das Wachstums-Modell (Abschn. 2.1) sind $\psi_L = 1.0$, $\gamma = 0.012/\text{d}$, $\kappa_W = 0.065\,\text{mm}^2/\text{d}$ und $\kappa_G = 0.5\kappa_W$, die für das Deformationsmodell sind $\alpha = 2.0$, $\varepsilon = 10^{-6}$, $\tilde{\sigma} = 1.0$ Pixel und $n = 50$. Abb. 1 zeigt Ergebnisse für die zeitliche Entwicklung des Deformationsmusters (obere Reihe;

$t^j \in \{400, 720, 880\}$ d, $p = 10^{-3}$) und für eine Variation von p (untere Reihe; $t^j = 880$ d). Ein Vergleich zu patientenindividuellen Daten ist in Abb. 2 gegeben.

4 Diskussion

In der vorliegenden Arbeit wurde ein neuartiger Ansatz zur Modellierung tumorinduzierter Gewebedeformation als Prior für die nicht-rigide Registrierung von Bilddaten vorgeschlagen, zwischen denen per Definition kein Diffeomorphismus existiert. Es wurde der in [4] vorgestellte Ansatz, das Deformationsmuster über ein durch eine weiche Nebenbedingungen restringiertes parametrisches Optimierproblem zu bestimmen, aufgegriffen und in eine effiziente, dämonenbasierten Ansätzen entsprechende Strategie überführt. Das vorgeschlagene variationelle Modell stellt im Vergleich zu bio-physikalischen Ansätzen [6, 7] eine effiziente Abkürzung für die modellbasierte Bildregistrierung dar. Da für das vorgestellte Verfahren generell nicht gewährleistet werden kann, dass die berechnete Deformation diffeomorph ist wurde in Anlehnung an fluidale Ansätze [12] ein Regridding Schritt eingeführt, sobald die Funktionaldeterminante einen vorgegebenen

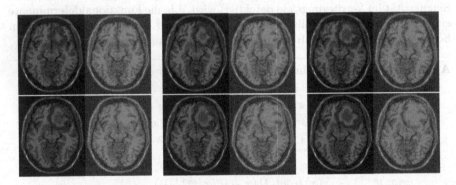

Abb. 1. Illustration der berechneten Gewebedeformation. Obere Reihe: Ergebnisse für die Entwicklung über die Zeit ($t^j \in \{400, 720, 880\}$ d in dieser Reihung). Untere Reihe: Ergebnisse für Parameter $p \in \{10^{-\infty}, 10^{-8}, 10^{-3}\}$ in dieser Reihung

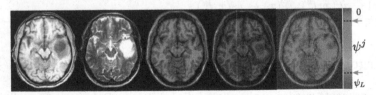

Abb. 2. Vergleich zu patientenindividuellen Daten. Von links nach rechts: T1-gewichteter und T2-gewichteter MR-Datensatz, korrespondierende Schicht des initialen Templatebildes, berechnete Zelldichte und resultierendes Deformationsmuster. Die Farbskala gibt eine Abschätzung der Detektionsschwellwerte in T1- (oranger Pfeil) und T2-gewichteten (grüner Pfeil) Bilddaten

Schwellwert unterschreitet. Eine naheliegende Strategie den Suchraum auf diffeomorphe Abbildungen einzuschränken, die wir aktuell untersuchen, ist anstelle eines Regriddings eine Optimierung auf der Lie-Gruppe der Diffeomorphismen durchzuführen [13]. Weiter wurde im Vergleich zu [4] ein Update zur Erhaltung der Masse eingeführt. Numerische Experimente (Abschnitt 3) demonstrieren das Potential des vorgeschlagenen Modells. Der vorliegende Ansatz liefert im Vergleich zu [4] eine gesteigerte Effizienz, eine Vereinfachung der numerischen Implementierung, eine Verringerung der Modellkomplexität und ermöglicht eine Einbettung in einen aktuellen algorithmischen Rahmen für eine effiziente (diffeomorphe) nicht-rigide Registrierung [10, 11, 13]. Damit ist der Weg für die Etablierung eines hybriden Ansatzes zur simultanen Registrierung und Modellierung, ein Thema dem wir uns aktuell widmen, und damit einhergehend zur Quantifizierung der Güte eines derartig kombinierten Ansatzes, geebnet.

Danksagung. Diese Arbeit wird gefördert durch die Europäische Union und das Land Schleswig-Holstein (AT,SB) [Fördernummer 122-09-024] und die Exzellenzinitiative des Bundes (TAS) [Fördernummer DFG GSC 235/1].

Literaturverzeichnis

1. Modersitzki J. Numerical Methods for Image Registration. Oxf Univ Press; 2004.
2. Henn S, Hömke L, Witsch K. Lesion preserving image registration with application to human brains. Lect Notes Computer Sci. 2004;3175:496–503.
3. Li X, Long X, Wyatt CL. Registration of images with topological change via riemannian embedding. In: IEEE Symp Biomed Imag; 2011. p. 1247–1252.
4. Mang A, Becker S, Toma A, et al. A model of tumour induced brain deformation as bio-physical prior for non-rigid image registration. In: IEEE Symp Biomed Imag; 2011. p. 578–581.
5. Mang A, Becker S, Toma A, et al. Modellierung tumorinduzierter Gewebedeformation als Optimierungsproblem mit weicher Nebenbedingung. Proc BVM. 2011; p. 294–298.
6. Hogea C, Davatzikos C, Biros G. Brain-tumor interaction biophysical models for medical image registration. SIAM J Sci Comput. 2008;30(6):3050–3072.
7. Gooya A, Biros G, Davatzikos C. Deformable registration of glioma images using EM algorithm and diffusion reaction modeling. IEEE Trans Med Imaging. 2011;30(2):375–390.
8. Mang A, Toma A, Schütz TA, et al. Eine effiziente Parallel-Implementierung eines stabilen Euler-Cauchy-Verfahrens für die Modellierung von Tumorwachstum. Proc BVM. 2012.
9. Fischer B, Modersitzki J. Fast diffusion registration. Cont Math. 2002;313:117–129.
10. Thirion JP. Image matching as a diffusion process: an analogy with Maxwell's demons. Med Imag Anal. 1998;2(3):243–260.
11. Cahill ND, Noble JA, Hawkes DJ. A demons algorithm for image registration with locally adaptive regularization. In: Proc MICCAI; 2009. p. 574–581.
12. Christensen GE, Rabbitt RD, Miller MI. Deformable templates using large deformation kinematics. IEEE Trans Image Process. 1996;5(10):1435–1447.
13. Vercauteren T, Pennec X, Perchant A, et al. Diffeomorphic demons: efficient non-parametric image registration. NeuroImage. 2009;45(1):S61–S72.

Image Processing for Detection of Fuzzy Structures in Medical Images

Hartwig Hetzheim[1], Henrik G. Hetzheim[2]

[1]Optische Informationssysteme, DLR Berlin
[2]Medizinische Physik in der Radiologie, DKFZ Heidelberg
hartwig.hetzheim@dlr.de

Abstract. The study of fuzzy structures in medical images is important for operation and radiotherapy planning. To study this, the fuzzy objects will be additionally described by their stochastic properties using the martingale theory in combination with fuzzy measures and fuzzy functions. The detected signal contains implicit stochastic information which is separated to get precise data about the region of interest. The applied methods and algorithms are used for the detection of tumors and nerve branches in MR, CT and PET images.

1 Introduction

In many cases lesions, i.e. tumors and nerve branches have a diffuse structure and the boundaries are fuzzy. To find the required well defined boundary the visual resolution of the gray values is often not sufficient. This is a change of paradigm, we do not only have an interest in the estimation value but also in the stochastic part of the signal. There is much more information in the stochastic part than in the non-stochastic part which can be compared with broadcasting signals, high-frequency signals can carry more information than low-frequency signals. The gray differences between tumors and neighboring normal tissue are very small, the signal is superposed and corrupted by effects of other layers. Because of far-reaching stochastic effects agglomeration is in larger sized tumors more prominent than in smaller ones. The detection procedure begins with the separation of different kinds of stochastic properties and their location. Using the martingale theory [1, 2] the stochastic parts of the signal are separated. Although the image generation is physically different (CT, MRI, PET) the same method can be applied. The model building is demonstrated for CT images. For example a CT image usually contains 14 bit gray levels giving about one million possible combinations between a certain point of the image and its next 8 neighbors. This huge amount of information has to be used to generate, select and combine properties to characterize selected small pieces of tissues like tumors or nerve connections and especially their boundaries. The requirements for our image processing are: knowledge of the model for the generation of the signal creating the image, an adapted mathematics, a relevant approximation and an effective algorithm. For the CT image the detected image signal is a superposition of all acting effects along the way of the X-ray to the detector. In case of MRI the influence of other layers generates disturbances whereas the multiple scattering of the high-energy γ photons induces mainly the blurring in the PET image. The various impacts of the signal components within a tissue layer enables the separation of those signals, which are less influenced from the source to the detector. These can be isolated and utilized to describe the inner regions of the considered tissue. This is possible if the algorithm acts approximately as an inverse function and by applying different algorithm in the correct order. By comparison with results obtained by certified histological treatment the algorithm is adapted and optimized for special cases. If the stochastic properties are detected by iterative methods the interesting boundaries of regions can be determined applying functional dependence. The detected and extracted regions of interest are marked in the image by selected colors.

2 Estimation of stochastic properties

The fundamentals of the estimation include the model building with the generation of the stochastic properties, the mathematical description of the acting effects, the mathematical representation for the generation of stochastic properties, the separation in elementary parts, the methods of their estimation from the given images and a priori knowledge about the disease, histological findings etc.

2.1 Model building

For simplicity the model building is demonstrated here only for CT images with examples given in [3]. The value of a CT pixel is based on the attenuation of the X-rays and by the influence of adjacent points. The influence is a result of the scattering, the diffraction and the refraction of the X-rays in the human tissue. All these effects are combined in non-linear functions, which are investigated for differences in their stochastic structure. As an example the absorption is discussed in more detail. The human body can be divided into different layers. The absorption coefficient in the human body is a parameter representing the influence of incident X-rays with the molecules. This absorption is proportional to the thickness of the layer and depends on the type and the density of the molecules of the layer. Different functions have to be applied, because the molecules and their density are changing within the layer depending on the kind of tissue. The X-rays are described by specific function, which changes after the attenuation in a certain layer. The full vector of properties has to be taken into account to describe the influence of the X-rays from the source to the detector. The model is also applicable for MR or PET images as the relative modification of the signal between the layers is of importance and not the functional calculation depending on the generation of the signal.

2.2   Mathematical description of the effects in the layers

For the contribution of gray values within the tissue layer between the boundaries c and d the Lebesgue integrable function $f(x)$ is given by

$$D\left(c \leqslant x \leqslant d\right) = \int_c^d f\left(x\right) dx \tag{1}$$

After the X-rays penetrate one layer the detected signal can be written as

$$I_1 = \int_0^{x_2} f_1\left(x_1, \eta_1\right) dx_1 \tag{2}$$

where the non-linear function f_1 coupled with the vector η_1, which represents the stochastic properties, acts on the X-ray. The result is going in the next layer, so that the signal going through the following layers is given by the integral

$$I_2 = \int_{x_2}^{x_3} f_2(x_2, \eta_2) dx_2 * I_1 = \int_{x_2}^{x_3} f_2(x_2, \eta_2) dx_2 \int_0^{x_2} f_1(x_1, \eta_1) dx_1 \tag{3}$$

Thereby, we get the signal at the detector after penetrating n layers

$$I_n = \int_{x_{n-1}}^{x_n} f_{n-1}\left(x_{n-1}, \eta_{n-1}\right) dx_{n-1} \cdots \int_{x_2}^{x_3} f_2(x_2, \eta_2) dx_2 \int_0^{x_2} f_1(x_1, \eta_1) dx_1 \tag{4}$$

This describes the intensity obtained at the detector for a selected direction, means for a defined position of the rotating gantry and the patient table. It includes a lot of conditions which are not known a priori. The main problem for solving the equation are the unknown boundaries of the layers, as the measured signal I_n is a superposition of all contributions. More information has to be considered to detect these, such as to find the boundaries of the fuzzy structures of the lesions.

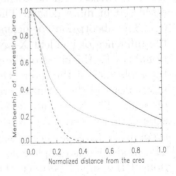

Fig. 1. Plotted are three exemplary functions representing the transition from gray values in a given tissue layer. Those functions satisfy the differential equation of various far-reaching effects as a function of the distance u. Solid is plotted the Erfc function, dotted the function $1 - (1/const) * exp(-const/u)$ and dashed the solution of the Riemann differential equation [4] with the solution $x^{0.5-m} e^{-x} *_1 F_1(0.5 - m - l, -2m+l; x)$. Here $_1F_1$ is the confluent hypergeometric function and m and l are natural numbers

2.3   Methods for isolation of stochastic properties

The martingale theory is a complicated mathematical topic. The fundamental idea is to consider an image as a superposition of lines or stripes along the image. These lines have to be considered in all directions. For all combinations of those lines exist a connection between their gray values. This means that information of a certain point in relation to the neighboring points has to be considered in further pixel points. An extended sampling theorem with the related formulas is given in [5]. For the martingale theory the images are represented by lines in all directions covering the whole space of the image. For each line the ensemble of gray values are decomposed in stochastic parts meaning mathematically to separate the stochastic signal in an unlimited and a limited variation. This decomposition can be done iteratively for various conditions. To understand the martingale, the simplest case can be written as.

$$s(b) = f\left(\langle b\rangle_k - \langle b\rangle_l\right) \tag{5}$$

Here b is a part of the image and $\langle\rangle$ means an averaging like the trivial smoothing operator or a median as the simplest rank filter. More complicated are the non-linear filtering or real rank filters. With this simple form s(b) more complex combinations like

$$s_c = (s(b_1) - s(b_2)) \wedge (s(b_3) - s(b_4)) \tag{6}$$

can be built.

2.4   Generation of new properties by combining properties

The stochastic properties can be represented by fuzzy measures $g(x)$ and fuzzy functions $h(x)$. Both are combined by the fuzzy integral. The formulas are derivative in [6]. The fuzzy measures are coupled by

$$g_\lambda\left(x_i \cup x_j\right) = g_\lambda\left(x_i\right) + g_\lambda\left(x_j\right) + \lambda * g_\lambda\left(x_i\right)g_\lambda\left(x_j\right) \tag{7}$$

where the coupling factor λ is given by $\lambda = (1 + \lambda g(x_1))(1 + \lambda g(x_2)) - 1$ with α being $\{\xi \mid h_\alpha \geqslant \alpha\}$.

The vector components of stochastic properties for each pixel point is a result of the variation of various parameter, like the size of the region of interest, the value of α and other properties determining the value of the fuzzy intergral. The comparison of this vector with the vector obtained for the neighboring pixel point determines a measure for assigning them to a group of similar properties. Sliding this procedure over the whole image generates closed regions with similar properties, see Fig.2 for an example of fuzzy functions.

3   Examples for selection of regions of interest

For PET, MR and CT images the methods above have been applied successfully. In addition the ordering method [3] is included in the following processed figures.

Fig. 2. Example for the calculation of the fuzzy integral $\lambda = (1 + \lambda g(x_1))\,(1 + \lambda g(x_2)) - 1$ where the fuzzy function H_α is given by $\{\xi \mid h_\alpha \geqslant \alpha\}$ and A is a set of variables. The fuzzy function is plotted as a solid line, the cut value α as a dotted line and the fuzzy measure as a dashed line. Moreover, the possibility to generate fuzzy integrals is given by the shaded surface and the fuzzy integral value is plotted as a line. Various fuzzy integrals are written as a vector in order to define a membership value for the selected region

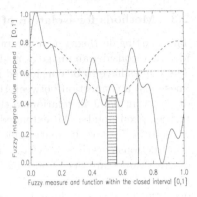

Fig. 3(a) shows an original PET image of a distorted hip. Fig. 3(b) shows a modification of the original image by applying the above described method. Thereby the bladder can be well separated from its surroundings and the bone structure is more pronounced.

A further example of tumor detection in MR images is shown in the following figures. Fig. 4 are 3D representation of a MR image with flat tumor on the ankle given in yellow in Fig. 4(a) and tumors over the whole leg given in magenta in Fig. 4(b). Those tumors were not detected by in a traditional radiological analysis.

4   Discussion of the results

This paper shows that stochastic properties give an essential contribution to detect fuzzy regions in medical images. By means of the martingale theory the stochastic part of the received signal has been separated in its range and

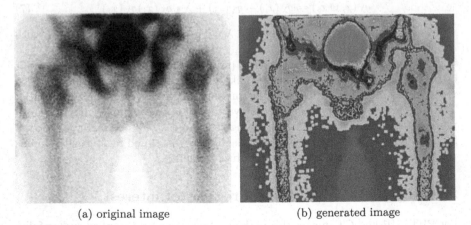

(a) original image   (b) generated image

Fig. 3. Example of a PET image

Fig. 4. 3D representation of MR images for the tumor detection

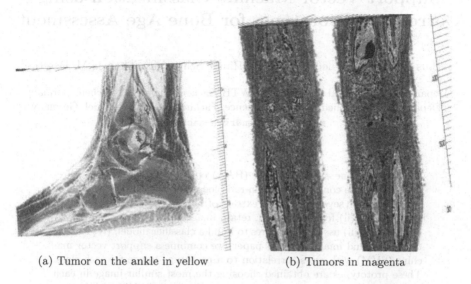

(a) Tumor on the ankle in yellow   (b) Tumors in magenta

influence relative to its neighbors. Furthermore, by using the fuzzy measure and fuzzy integrals for the analysis of medical images, new stochastic properties have been detected and visualized. An adaptive control has been implemented to select the necessary properties within the multiplicity of stochastic properties. In summary, to find applicable stochastic properties in medical images this method can be also applied for CT, PET and MR images, taking into account their different physical processes.

References

1. Wong E. Stochastic processes in information and dynamical systems. McGraw-Hill New York; 1971.
2. Hetzheim H. Interpolation, Filterung und Extrapolation eines Vektor-Markow-Prozesses. Z Elektr Inform Energietechnik. 1976;5:129–40.
3. Hetzheim H, Hetzheim HG. Analysis of stochastic properties in medical images. Proc IIFMBE. 2009; p. 1901–1904.
4. Gradstein IS, Ryschik JM. Table of Integrals, Series, and Products. Physico-matematiczeskoy literatury Moskwa. 1963.
5. Hetzheim H. Interpolative Rekonstruktion von Samplingpunkten und Abschätzung des Fehlers. Z Elektr Inform Energietechnik. 1975;5:48–59.
6. Sugeno M. Theory of fuzzy integrals and its applications. PhD thesis. Japan: Tokyo Institute of Technology; 1974.

Support Vector Machine Classification using Correlation Prototypes for Bone Age Assessment

Markus Harmsen[1], Benedikt Fischer[1], Hauke Schramm[2], Thomas M. Deserno[1]

[1]Department of Medical Informatics, RWTH Aachen University, Aachen, Germany
[2]Department of Applied Computer Science, Fachhochschule Kiel, Kiel, Germany
markus.harmsen@rwth-aachen.de

Abstract. Bone age assessment (BAA) on hand radiographs is a frequent and time consuming task in radiology. Our method for automatic BAA is done in several steps: (i) extract of 14 epiphyseal regions from the radiographs, (ii) for each region, retain image features using the IRMA framework, (iii) use these features to build a classifier model, (iv) classify unknown hand images. In this paper, we combine a support vector machine (SVM) with cross-correlation to a prototype image for each class. These prototypes are obtained choosing the most similar image in each class according to mean cross-correlation. Comparing SVM with k nearest neighbor (kNN) classification, a systematic evaluation is presented using 1,097 images of 30 diagnostic classes. Mean error in age prediction is reduced from 1.0 to 0.9 years for 5-NN and SVM, respectively.

1 Introduction

Bone age assessment (BAA) on hand radiographs is a frequent and time consuming task in diagnostic radiology. In the method developed by Greulich & Pyle [1], the radiologist compares all bones of the hand (Fig. 1) with a standard atlas, whereas according to Tanner & Whitehouse [2], only a certain subset of bones is considered. Different approaches have been developed to automate this

Fig. 1. Epiphysial regions of interest (eROIs) and their corresponding numbers

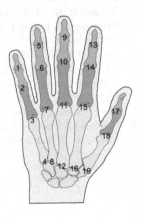

process, including the approach of Fischer et al. [3], in which (i) the epiphyseal/metaphyseal regions (eROIs) are extracted, (ii) using content-based image retrieval (CBIR), similar images to these regions are queried from a database, (iii) classified using the k nearest neighbor (kNN) method and (iv) algebraically combined to propose a bone age.

Although this approach is promising, some weak points have been identified: (i) a fixed amount of k neighbors is used for classification, which – depending on the dataset – may not be optimal; (ii) the classification considers the eROIs to be independent and uses only a (weighted) age average of these regions for age determination; (iii) the gender is disregarded completely, although male and female growth spurts differ significantly; (iv) BAA is performed numerically, based on similar images, and does not use any medical useful classification in respect of growth spurts; and (v) computation is expensive, since the crosscorrelation between all existing reference images is determined.

In the past few years, the support vector machine (SVM) has been introduced into many classification fields and have demonstrated the state of the art performance. For example a combination of SVM with CBIR has been successfully applied to detect malign structures in mammography [4]. Despite of their broad applicability, some essential problems have to be addressed when using SVM. Besides the fundamental choice of attributes, the SVM only classifies binary problems, i.e., a classification into more than two classes is only possible with several SVMs, and the class size has to be chosen carefully.

In this work, our method on automatic CBIR-based BAA is extended by SVM and evaluated critically with respect to the standard kNN classifier.

2 Materials and methods

Our approach is integrated with the image retrieval in medical applications (IRMA) framework (http://irma-project.org), which supports content-based access to large medical image repositories [5]. Global, local, and structural features are supported to describe the image, an eROI, or a constellation of eROIs, respectively [6]. Furthermore, our work is based on Fischer et al. [3].

2.1 ROI extraction

Extracting the eROI has been presented previously [7, 8, 9]. Essentially, a structural prototype is trained where the phalanges and metacarpal bones are represented by nodes, and location, shape as well as texture parameters are modeled with Gaussians. The centers of eROIs are located automatically. Fourteen eROIs are extracted, geometrically oriented into an upright position, and inserted into the IRMA database with reference to the according hand radiography.

2.2 Class prototypes

To address the problem of class size, we have grouped the data related to the growth spurts. According to the ontology defined by Gilsanz & Ratib [10], reference ages can be quantized in steps of 2 m, 4 m, 6 m, and 12 m for the intervals [8 m ... 20 m), [20 m ... 28 m), [2.5 y ... 6 y), and [6 y ... 18 y], respectively, where m and y denotes months and years, respectively. This creates a set of 29 classes with four different ranges. A 30th class for bone ages > 18 years was added. Notice that gender information is so far not used for class building. All eROIs and their according attributes are loaded from the IRMA database and scaled to the range $[-1, +1]$ to avoid attributes in greater numeric ranges dominating those in smaller ranges.

2.3   Feature extraction

The cross-correlation function (CCF) is easy to compute, robust regarding the radiation dose, and has already been used successfully in BAA tasks [3]. The similarity between two eROIs q and p is computed by

$$S_{\text{CCF}}(p,q) = \max_{|m|,|n| \leq d} \left\{ \frac{\sum\limits_{x=1}^{X} \sum\limits_{y=1}^{Y} (p(x-m, y-n) - \overline{p})\,(q(x,y) - \overline{q})}{\sqrt{\left(\sum\limits_{x=1}^{X} \sum\limits_{y=1}^{Y} (p(x-m, y-n) - \overline{p})^2 \right) \left(\sum\limits_{x=1}^{X} \sum\limits_{y=1}^{Y} (q(x,y) - \overline{q})^2 \right)}} \right. \tag{1}$$

where $\overline{p}, \overline{q}$ denote the mean gray values of p, q respectively, and d the warp range for maximum correlation. In our experiments, we set $d = 2$ and use 32×32 pixel scaled version of the eROIS.

For each region R and class C, we select the optimal image I according to mean CCF similarity as our feature prototype

$$F_{R,C} = \max_{I_x \in R, C} \left\{ \frac{1}{n} \cdot \sum_{i=1}^{n} (S_{CCF}(I_x, I_i)) \,|I_i \in R, C, i \neq x \right. \tag{2}$$

We use the IRMA framework to index eROI features extracted from the 30 class prototypes (Fig. 2).

2.4   Creating a classification model

For SVM classification, binary classes are usually presented as two features ranging between zero and one. Hence, the data instance vector used for classification with kNN as well as SVM yields

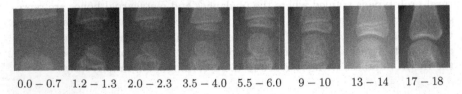

0.0 − 0.7   1.2 − 1.3   2.0 − 2.3   3.5 − 4.0   5.5 − 6.0   9 − 10   13 − 14   17 − 18

Fig. 2. Subset of prototypes for eROI 11 with maximum average similarity in the responding age class clearly indicating the development of epiphyses. The y-translation on age class $5.5 - 6.0$ will be normalized by CCF

$$v_{\text{hand}} = \begin{pmatrix} g_m \\ g_f \\ E_{01} \\ \vdots \\ E_{14} \end{pmatrix}, \quad E_i = \begin{pmatrix} F_{i1} \\ \vdots \\ F_{i30} \end{pmatrix} \tag{3}$$

where g denotes the gender (g_m is 1 if gender is male, 0 otherwise. g_f in analogous), E_i donates the loaded feature vector for the currently referenced hand eROI i with feature parameters F_{i1} till F_{i30} for each class similarity. Notice that all feature parameters F consist of a vector with further numeric values, describing specific image characteristics.

2.5   Age computation

For a hand radiograph with unknown bone age, the eROIs are extracted (cf. Sect. 2.1). For each eROI, the features are extracted (cf. Sect. 2.3), and the data instance vector v_x is built (cf. Sect. 2.4). The SVM and the trained classificatory model is used to classify the new radiograph. For the SVM-based classifier, we used the "one-against-one" approach instead of "one-against-all" due to its good performance and short training time. A comparison of these methods can be found in [11]. The bone age is determined by

$$\text{age} = \frac{1}{2}\Big(\text{upper}\big(\text{class}(v_x)\big) + \text{lower}\big(\text{class}(v_x)\big)\Big) \tag{4}$$

where upper(class(x)) donates the upper age bound of class x and lower(class(x)) the lower age bound of class x analogous.

2.6   Validation experiments

The class prototypes were determined from the 1,097 images of the USC hand atlas. Afterwards, for each hand, the feature vector is generated by measuring the similarity to corresponding region class-prototypes as well as the gender (cf. Sect. 2.4). Now we apply the same feature vectors for kNN and SVM, using k-fold cross-validation for SVM with $k = 5$ and leave-one-out cross-validation for kNN. For SVM, optimal classification parameters will be computed by grid search.

3   Results

In terms of accuracy, the results for kNN range from $12\% - 22\%$ and $13\% - 27\%$. In terms of mean age error they range from $1.38 - 2.65$ years and $1.02 - 2.32$ years for $k = 1$ and $k = 5$, respectively for individual regions. The SVM results in terms of accuracy $21\% - 32\%$ and mean age error $0.99 - 2.34$ years (Tab. 1).

Table 1. Experiment outcome for kNN/SVM and single regions. The second experiment with $k = 5$, as well as SVM, also use the gender. SVM parameters $C = 2048$ and $\gamma = 0.0078125$ have been determined via grid search. Max and min values are bold, some regions have been omitted.

	kNN $k = 1$		kNN $k = 5$		SVM	
Region	Accuracy	Mean error	Accuracy	Mean error	Accuracy	Mean error
1	14.36 %	**2.65**	**13.00 %**	2.32	21.36 %	**2.34**
2	**12.18 %**	2.43	13.55 %	2.00	**20.36 %**	2.32
7	20.09 %	1.63	24.18 %	1.18	31.27 %	1.07
11	**22.00 %**	**1.38**	**27.64 %**	**1.02**	**32.45 %**	**0.99**
15	19.64 %	1.44	25.36 %	1.11	30.09 %	1.11

Table 2. Classification results for multiple regions. A distance of 0 denotes a correct labeled class, whereas a distance of 1 indicates the classifier has labeled a wrong class directly one before or after the actual age class.

Distance	0	1	2	3	4	5	6	7	8	9	10	...	29
kNN hits(%)	26.34	44.76	18.51	6.74	1.82	1.0	0.46	0.27	0.18	0.18	0	...	0
		←— 89.61 —→					←— 10.65 —→						
SVM hits(%)	33.36	38.29	17.59	5.9	1.73	1.82	0.64	0.36	0.18	0.09	0	...	0
		←— 89.24 —→					←— 10.72 —→						

Table 3. Best results from kNN and SVM using different eROIS and parameters. The Clopper-Pearson intervals donate the propotion of labeled hands with an error in the interval $[-2; 2]$ for $\beta = 0.95$.

Classifyer	Accuracy	Mean error	Conf. int.	Used regions	Parameter
kNN	26.34 %	1.00	[0.886; 0.922]	7, 11, 15	$k = 5$
SVM	33.36 %	0.90	[0.903; 0.936]	2, 5, 7, 8, 10, 11, 13	$C = 2048$
					$\gamma = 0.0078125$

The best experimental result for kNN (accuracy 26.27%, mean error 1.00 years) is optained by a subset of 3 regions and $k = 5$. Best results for SVM (accuracy 33.36%, mean error 0.90 years) use a subset of 7 regions (Tab. 3) and therefore outperform kNN as well as the method by Fischer et al., which has a mean error of 0.97 years. Both perform best only on a subset of regions, whereas the SVM can use larger data.

4 Discussion

The overall classification accuracy seems to be low, but most mislabeled classes only have a class distance of 1 or 2 (Tab. 2). Using a larger amount of eROIS for classification, the SVM reaches a mean error of 0.90 years. Therefore SVM outperforms kNN, which has a mean error of 1.00 years (Table 3). The true propotion for our svm conficence intervall is also slighly higher as for the kNN one (Tab. 3, column 4). For this reasons, SVM clearly improves our previous method as it can handle a larger amount of attributes. It's remarkable that our SVM only uses gender and CCF as features and may easily enriched by further features. Computation time for SVM is even lower than for kNN, since the classification model is only build once and then used for all unknown hands. Furthermore using correlation prototypes remarkably improves the performance.

So far, gender is used only as an attribute for classification and not for prototype building, since the classifier should implicit model the fact of different growth spurts for male and female subjects. This should be verified by using the gender to build twice as many prototypes ¬ and therefore increasing the feature space – and repeating the experiments. Another possible improvement might be using prototypes from a standard reference atlas – which is also used in radiology and therefore perfectly match our age classes – instead of computing own prototypes.

References

1. Greulich WW, Pyle SI. Radiographic Atlas of Skeletal Development of Hand Wrist. Stanford CA.: Stanford University Press; 1971.
2. Tanner JM, Healy MJR, Goldstein H, et al. Assessment of Skeletal Maturity and Prediction of Adult Height (TW3) Method. London: WBSaunders; 2001.
3. Fischer B, Welter P, Grouls C, et al. Bone age assessment by content-based image retrieval and case-based reasoning. Proc SPIE. 2011;7963.
4. de Oliveira JEE, Machado A, Chavez G, et al. A. MammoSys: a content-based image retrieval system using breast density patterns. Comput Methods Programs Biomed. 2010;99(3):289–297.
5. Lehmann TM, Gueld MO, Thies C, et al. Content-based image retrieval in medical applications. Methods Inf Med. 2004;43(4):354–61.
6. Deserno TM, Antani S, Long R. Ontology of gaps in content-based image retrieval. J Digit Imaging. 2008;online-first, DOI 10.1007/s10278-007-9092-x.
7. Deserno TM, Beier D, Thies C, et al. Segmentation of medical images combining local, regional, global, and hierarchical distances into a bottom-up region merging scheme. Proc SPIE. 2005;5747(1):546–555.
8. Thies C, Schmidt-Borreda M, Seidl T, et al. A classification framework for content-based extraction of biomedical objects from hierarchically decomposed images. Proc SPIE. 2006;6144:559–568.
9. Fischer B, Sauren M, Gueld MO, et al. Scene analysis with structural prototypes for content-based image retrieval in medicine. Proc SPIE. 2008;6914; online first, DOI 10.1117/12.770541.
10. Gilsanz V, Ratib O. Hand Bone Age: A Digital Atlas of Skeletal Maturity. Berlin: Springer-Verlag; 2005.
11. Hsu CW, Lin CL. A comparison of methods for multi-class support vector machines. IEEE Trans Neural Netw. 2002;13:415–425.

IRMA Code II
A New Concept for Classification of Medical Images

Tim-Christian Piesch[1], Henning Müller[2,3], Christiane K. Kuhl[4],
Thomas M. Deserno[1]

[1]Department of Medical Informatics, RWTH Aachen University
[2]Medical Informatics, Geneva University Hospitals & Univ. of Geneva, Switzerland
[3]Business Information Systems, HES-SO, Switzerland
[4]Department of Diagnostic and Interventional Radiology, University Hospital Aachen
tim.piesch@rwth-aachen.de

Abstract. Content-based image retrieval (CBIR) provides novel options
to access large repositories of medical images. Thus, there are new op-
portunities for storing, querying and reporting especially within the field
of digital radiology. This, however, requires a revisit of nomenclatures
for image classification. The Digital Imaging and Communication in
Medicine (DICOM), for instance, defines only about 20, partly overlapping terms for coding the body region. In 2002, the Image Retrieval in
Medical Applications (IRMA) project has proposed a mono-hierarchic,
multi-axial coding scheme. Although the initial concept of the IRMA
Code was designed for later expansion, the appliance of the terminology
in the practice of scientific projects discovered several weak points. In
this paper, based on a systematic analysis and the comparison with other
relevant medical ontologies such as the Lexicon for Uniform Indexing and
Retrieval of Radiology Information Resources (RadLex), we accordingly
propose axes for medical equipment, findings and body positioning as
well as additional flags for age, body part, ethnicity, gender, image quality and scanned film. The IRMA Code II may be used in the Cross
Language Evaluation Campaign (CLEF) annotation tasks as a database
of classified images to evaluate visual information retrieval systems.

1 Introduction

The Image Retrieval in Medical Applications (IRMA) project aims at providing
a flexible framework for content-based image retrieval (CBIR) applications in
medicine. The IRMA classification scheme is based upon a mono-hierarchic
multi-axial coding system, which includes four axes with three to four positions
(0-9 and a-z). "0" for "unspecified" describes the end of a path of an axis [1].
The four axes contain:

- T (technical) = image modality
- D (directional) = body orientations
- A (anatomical) = body region
- B (biological) = biological system examined.

Table 1. Medical terminologies and their aims [4, 5, 6, 7]. DICOM: Digital Imaging and Communications in Medicine; ICD-10: International Classification of Diseases; MeSH: Medical Subject Headings; RadLex: Lexicon for Uniform Indexing and Retrieval of Radiology Information Ressources; SNOMED CT: Systematized Nomenclature of Medicine Clinical Terms; TNM: Tumor-Nodule-Metastasis Staging; UMLS: Unified Medical Language System

	DICOM	ICD-10	IRMA	MeSH	RadLex	SNOMED	TNM	UMLS
Diagnosis coding		✓				✓		
Literature indexing			✓	✓		✓		✓
Semantic linking			✓	✓		✓		✓
Neoplasia staging							✓	
Radiology reports	✓			✓	✓	✓		
Image classification	✓			✓		✓		
Image retrieval	✓			✓	✓	✓		
Image storage	✓			✓	✓			
CBIR				✓	✓			

The code supports a unique labeling of images and was used in the ImageCLEF annotation tasks, which present a part of the Cross Language Evaluation Campaign (CLEF) [2, 3]. The goal of this project is to provide evaluation of different visual information retrieval systems. However, the appliance of the terminology in the practice of scientific research discovered several weak points:

- pathologies are not enclosed,
- additional parameters such as gender or age are absent,
- missing differentiation between right and left side of the body,
- the defined depth of the hierarchy is not sufficient in parts, e.g. radiographs of single epiphyses of the hand,
- ambiguities due to inconsistencies between is-part-of relations within deeper levels of the hierarchy, for instance the sacrum can be classified as a part of the chord and as well under the term pelvis,
- no coding options for images from the field of genetics and biology (in the course of increasing overlap between bioinformatics and medicine).

In the past years, new ontologies for medical imaging have been developed and substituted existing schemes in research as well as clinical practice (Tab. 1). For instance, the RadLex nomenclature proposed by the Radiological Association of North America (RSNA) provides the radiologist a unified language to organize and retrieve images, imaging reports, and medical records [4]. Furthermore, there are upcoming semantic data platforms such as the LinkedLife Data (http://www.linkedlifedata.com) resource released by the Large Knowledge Collider (LarKC). This is a European project aiming to build a knowledge framework for linking and retrieving large biomedical knowledge databases (currently 26 different ontologies). Taking this into account, the IRMA code is revisited.

2   Material and methods

Designing a new concept for the IRMA code is composed of the following steps:

1. Coding of a provided database of radiological images,
2. Searching images of specific classes determined by the tree structure,
3. Collecting shortcomings within the consisting scheme,
4. Drafting a new basic structure in relation to other medical terminologies,
5. Adjusting the initial version to the new concept, and
6. Evaluating the new version of the IRMA code.

The difficulties, which appeared in the course of manually labeling of new images served to create a defined list of shortcomings.

In order to enhance specific classes of the image database we used the Picture Archiving and Communication System (PACS) database of the Department of Diagnostic and Interventional Radiology of the University Hospital Aachen as well as the medical image search engine called American Roentgen Ray Society (ARRS) GoldMiner® [8].

Based upon experiences gained and shortcomings collected the designing of the new framework includes a revision of the existing main axes. Testing and evaluating the new IRMA classification will be the application within the tasks of the Cross Language Evaluation Campaign (CLEF) and thereby a comparison to former results of this usage [2]. Besides, we plan to implement a mapping between the new IRMA Code and RadLex.

3   Results

The IRMA classification should be unique, clearly arranged and expandable. Especially in regard to the properties uniqueness and expandability it is necessary to modify the basic structure.

3.1   Additional axes

Equipment In image retrieval, the code must reflect the optical appearance of the image. This is majorly determined by artificial objects, such as prostheses, osteosynthetics or electrodes. By means of this axis, images in lower quality and, for instance, an upper ankle joint with plate and screws can be differed from regular images (Fig. 1). Furthermore, one can search the archive for images with special medical implements, for example a tube for respiratory assistance.

Findings So far, pathologies and findings are not modeled within the IRMA code, and the bio-system axis was misused to classify mammograms according to the Breast Imaging Reporting and Data System (BI-RADS) codes. Thus, this axis should be extended by general terms like calcification, necrosis and neoplasias as they can be found in classifications like the Tumor-Node-Metastasis

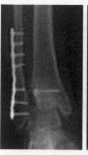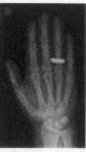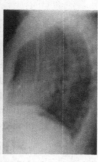

Fig. 1.   Radiographs with equipment and artifacts: (left) Right ankle joint including plate and screws, (middle) Right hand with a ring on the finger, (right) Sagittal view of a chest showing a cardiac pacemaker probe.

(TNM)-classification of Malignant Tumours, which is published by the International Union Against Cancer (UICC). In addition, this axis links the clinical process and thereby confirmed main diagnoses, similar to the International Classification of Diseases (ICD 10) [5]. Particularly with regard to the upcoming projects of computer-aided diagnosis as published by Doi [9] it is necessary to have a particular axis for findings.

Configuration   Similar to artificial objects which are superimposed to the image, patient positioning could impact the entire appearance of the image bitmap. For instance, the fingers of a hand may be closed or spread, and the patient may sit, stand, or lay down. So far, this is partly covered in the direction axis resulting in ambiguous codes.

3.2   Resulting basic structure

The IRMA Code II consists of seven axes each of them with three positions for refinement. For reasons of consistency we adjusted the already existing class titles. In order to illustrate the new coding options there is presented an example of a radiography showing a shoulder after operation with associated codes (Fig. 2). The seven main axes are defined as follows:

- A (anatomy) = body region
- B (bio-system) = general system of the body
- C (configuration) = positioning of the body
- D (direction) = body orientation in the room
- E (equipment) = specific objects and visible equipment (e.g., electrode)
- F (finding) = type of visual observation and/or pathological process
- G (generation) = imaging technique.

3.3   Additional flags

In the previous version of the coding scheme there existed terms (flags) independent of the mono-hierarchic system which gave option to mark images in view of image quality and pathology. In IRMA Code II, pathology is modeled

444   Piesch, Müller, Deserno

as self standing axis. The image quality coding flag remains and was extended by additional options. According to the RadLex terminology modeling "patient identifiers" [4] we integrated flags for age, gender and ethnical group. For instance, coding of age classes – not to be confused with the chronological age, determined by date of birth and date of examination – is important with respect to computer-assisted bone age assessment from plain radiography.

In summary, we suggest the following additional flags, which may be notated in IRMA Code II as an additional axis H of six position:

- Age (0: unspecified; 1: $[0-0.5[$ years, 2: $[0.5-1[$ years, 3: $[1-2[$, etc.);
- Body part (0: unspecified; 1: right; 2: left; 3: both; 4: none);
- Ethnicity (0: unspecified; 1: african-american; 2: asian; 3: caucasian; etc.);
- Gender (0: unspecified; 1: female; 2: male; 3: intersexual);
- Image quality (0: unspecified; 1: poor; 2: acceptable, 3: good, 4: best);
- Scanned film (0: unspecified; 1: true; 2: false).

In IRMA Code I, the "scanned film" feature was set within the axis of imaging technique and complicated it by necessity of a fourth position, which is removed in IRMA Code II unifoming the axis.

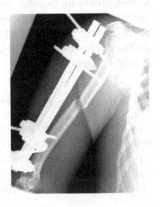

Fig. 2. IRMA II = 463-700-100-120-110-110-111-l13231. The IRMA Code III in form of AAA-BBB-CCC-DDD-EEE-FFF-GGG-HHHHHH is composed of:
A: upper extremity, upper arm, unspecified
B: musculo-sceletal system, unspecified, unspecified
C: elevation, angle < 45-degree, unspecified
D: coronal, anteroposterior, unspecified
E: metal, fixateur externe, unspecified
F: fracture, humerus shaft, unspecified
G: x-ray, plain radiography, overview image
H: Age: l (30-35 years); Body part: right; Ethnicity: Caucasian; Gender: male; Quality: good; Scanned film: true

4   Discussion

As a result of those modifications, IRMA II now has parallels to following axes of RadLex: Examination type, Technique, Exam quality, Image location, Anatomic location and Findings [4]. Concerning the suggested modifications of the basic structure, it has to be figured out to what extend the subclasses can be implemented especially within the axes for (F) findings and (E) equipment. However, the chance of simplifying the axis will also be taken. Fir instance, IRMA Code I definitions for "bregmaticosubmental" or "submentobregmaticofrontal" direction my be replaced by simpler terms. This means that we have to discuss the depth (number of positions) and the hierarchical linking between the subdivisions. Furthermore, mapping the IRMA II classification to other ontologies, for instance RadLex, must be established in order to evaluate and adjust IRMA II to future semantic requirements.

References

1. Lehmann TM, Schubert H, Keysers D, et al. The IRMA code for unique classification of medical images. Procs SPIE. 2003;5033:440–451.
2. Deselaers T, Deserno TM, Müller H. Automatic medical image annotation in ImageCLEF 2007. Overview, results, and discussion. Pattern Recognit Lett. 2008;29(15):1988–95.
3. Deselaers T, Müller H, Clough P, et al. The CLEF 2005 automatic medical image annotation task. Int J Computer Vis. 2007;74(1):51–8.
4. Langlotz CP. RadLex: a new method for indexing online educational materials. RadioGraphics. 2006;26(6):1595–7.
5. Zaiß A, Graubner B, Ingenerf J, et al. Medizinische Dokumentation, Terminologie und Linguistik. In: Lehmann TM, editor. Handbuch der Medizinischen Informatik. 1st ed. Aachen: Hanser; 2002. p. 45–99.
6. Thun S. Medizinische Dokumentation und Kommunikation. In: Johner C, Haas P, editors. Praxishandbuch IT im Gesundheitswesen: Erfolgreich einführen, entwickeln, anwenden und betreiben. 1st ed. München: Hanser; 2009. p. 131–60.
7. Mildenberger P, Eichelberg M, Martin E. Introduction to the DICOM standard. Eur Radiol. 2002 Apr;12(4):920–7.
8. Kahn CE, Jr, Thao C. GoldMiner: a radiology image search engine. Am J Roentgenol. 2007;188(6):1475–8.
9. Doi K. Computer-aided diagnosis in medical imaging: historical review, current status and future potential. Comput Med Imaging Graph. 2007;31(4-5):198–211.

Kategorisierung der Beiträge

Modalität bzw. Datenmaterial
Röntgen, 3, 21, 27, 51, 63, 75, 81, 99, 153, 165, 177, 183, 219, 225, 268, 274, 352, 363, 386, 410, 416, 422, 428, 434
– konventionell, 9, 39, 45, 57, 69, 87, 99, 105, 111, 129, 135, 183, 195, 231, 237, 243, 249, 256, 262, 292, 316, 334, 346, 352, 386, 398, 410
– digital, 183, 207, 298, 386
Endoskopie, 39, 45, 87, 111, 195
Optische Verfahren
– sonstige, 9, 57, 87, 105, 129, 135, 231, 237, 243, 249, 256, 262, 292, 316, 334, 346, 398
Signale (EKG; EEG; etc.), 69
Multimodale Daten, 99, 105, 111, 352, 410
Angiographie, 75, 375, 380
Computertomographie, 15, 33, 45, 141, 147, 171, 183, 189, 201, 207, 268, 280, 286, 304, 310, 328, 340, 352, 375, 392, 404, 416
– hochauflösend, 45, 183, 213, 392, 428
– spiral, 392
Sonographie, 92, 159, 165, 410
– intravaskulär, 21, 165
Kernspintomographie, 27, 63, 75, 81, 153, 177, 219, 225, 268, 274, 363, 410, 422
– funktionell, 225
– hochauflösend, 3, 27, 75, 183, 428
Positron-Emission-Tomographie, 51, 268
– hochauflösend, 428
Single-Photon-Emission-Computertomographie, 352

Dimension der Daten
Signal (1D), 3, 69, 129, 398
Bild (2D), 21, 27, 39, 99, 111, 123, 135, 147, 165, 189, 195, 256, 298, 304, 310, 322, 334, 352, 358, 369, 375, 404, 416, 428, 434
Bildsequenz (2D+t), 3, 33, 39, 45, 57, 87, 105, 123, 129, 135, 159, 165, 207, 231, 237, 243, 249, 292, 316, 375, 380, 386
Volumen (3D), 9, 15, 27, 45, 51, 75, 99, 111, 141, 171, 177, 183, 189, 201, 207, 213, 219, 225, 262, 268, 274, 280, 286, 328, 340, 363, 375, 392, 404, 410, 416, 428

Volumensequenz (3D+t), 63, 81, 92, 105, 117, 141, 153, 183, 363, 422

Pixelwertigkeit
Einkanal, 57, 92, 99, 117, 129, 135, 159, 171, 183, 189, 219, 231, 243, 249, 286, 292, 316, 322, 328, 340, 392, 434
Mehrkanal, 9, 69, 75, 105, 135, 153, 177, 183, 195, 225, 237, 256, 268, 334

Untersuchte Körperregionen
Ganzkörper, 280
Schädel, 15, 27, 63, 81, 123, 153, 159, 171, 177, 189, 225, 268, 363, 380, 410, 422
Wirbelsäule, 274, 286, 310, 328, 416
Extremitäten
– obere, 380, 434
– untere, 75, 298, 352, 380
Thorax, 3, 33, 39, 45, 51, 69, 87, 92, 105, 183, 201, 207, 213, 219, 310, 316, 328, 375, 386
Mamma, 99
Abdomen, 39, 105, 111, 183, 195, 316, 328, 340, 375, 380, 392
Becken, 39

Betrachtetes Organsystem
Systemübergreifend, 57, 69, 123, 171, 310, 340, 392, 410, 440
Immunzelluläres System, 57, 123
Zentrales Nervensystem, 27, 63, 69, 123, 153, 159, 177, 268, 322, 363, 422
Vegetatives Nervensystem, 69
Kardiovaskuläres System, 3, 21, 51, 69, 75, 81, 87, 92, 165, 358, 375, 386
Respiratorisches System, 33, 45, 69, 105, 201, 207, 213, 219, 316, 375
Gastrointestinales System, 195
Muskoloskeletales System, 15, 189, 280, 286, 298

Primärfunktion des Verfahrens
Bilderzeugung und -rekonstruktion, 27, 51, 75, 81, 92, 105, 141, 147, 153, 304, 310, 352, 363, 369, 410, 416

Bildverbesserung und -darstellung, 27, 39, 75, 92, 111, 117, 153, 286, 292, 310, 346, 352, 363, 375, 386, 398, 428

Bildtransport und -speicherung, 440

Merkmalsextraktion und Segmentierung, 3, 9, 15, 21, 27, 33, 57, 69, 75, 87, 92, 105, 159, 177, 183, 189, 195, 201, 213, 219, 225, 231, 237, 243, 256, 262, 268, 274, 280, 286, 322, 328, 369, 375, 410, 428, 434

Objekterkennung und Szenenanalyse, 3, 33, 39, 45, 57, 92, 105, 165, 213, 237, 268, 298, 316, 346, 369, 386, 428

Quantifizierung von Bildinhalten, 9, 45, 57, 81, 87, 92, 135, 165, 171, 231, 243, 363, 369, 380

Multimodale Aufbereitung, 39, 63, 99, 105, 111, 219, 375, 410, 422

Art des Projektes

Grundlagenforschung, 9, 57, 69, 105, 129, 135, 141, 147, 237, 243, 328, 346, 358, 363, 375, 398, 410

Methodenentwicklung, 3, 9, 15, 21, 27, 39, 45, 51, 57, 63, 69, 75, 81, 87, 92, 99, 105, 111, 123, 129, 135, 141, 147, 153, 159, 165, 183, 189, 195, 213, 225, 231, 237, 249, 262, 268, 274, 280, 298, 310, 322, 328, 340, 352, 369, 380, 410, 416, 422, 428

Anwendungsentwicklung, 3, 15, 21, 27, 45, 63, 69, 75, 87, 92, 105, 153, 207, 219, 256, 268, 286, 304, 310, 352, 392, 434

Klinische Diagnostik, 21, 45, 75, 81, 92, 225, 274, 410, 440

Autorenverzeichnis

Aach T, 195, 213, 256, 334
Ahmadi S-A, **410**
Alassi S, **380**

Bammer R, 111
Barendt S, **352**
Barkhausen J, 99
Bartha L, 392
Batra R, 243
Bauer S, **105**, 316
Becker M, 171
Becker S, 63, 123, 422
Behrens A, 195, 256
Bellemann N, 340
Bendl R, 280
Bergmann H, 207
Bernarding J, 27
Berynskyy L, 334
Biesterfeld S, 334
Birkfellner W, 207, 392
Birr S, **404**
Bischof A, 99
Bloch C, 207
Böcking A, 334
Bögel M, **33**
Boelmans K, 225
Boero F, **298**
Boetzel K, 410
Bourier F, 386
Brandt AU, 262
Braumann U-D, 57, 189
Braun J, **1**, 3, 363
Bremser M, **165**
Brost A, 386
Burger M, 51
Buzug TM, 15, 63, 123, 147, 304, 310, 358, 422

Chaisaowong K, 213
Choma MA, 135
Cordes A, **304**
Curio G, **2**

Danishad A, 27
Dekomien C, 159

Demin C, 334
Deniz E, 135
Denter C, 153
Deserno TM, 135, 434, 440
Diessl N, 243
Dolnitzki J-M, **322**
Dukatz T, 274

Eck S, **9**
Egger J, **274**
Ehrhardt J, 99, 201
Eils R, 231, 243
Elgeti T, 3
Erbe M, **358**

Fahrig R, 33
Faltin P, **213**
Fehlner A, **363**
Fetzer A, **183**
Fiehler J, 225
Figl M, 207
Fischer B, 219, 434
Foert E, 75
Forkert ND, **225**
Forman C, 111
Fortmeier D, **117**, 286
Fränzle A, **280**
Franz AM, 340, **392**
Freisleben B, 274
Frericks B, 75
Friedl S, **87**
Friedrich D, **334**
Fritzsche KH, 177
Fuchs S, 340
Furtado H, **207**

Gaa J, **346**
Gasteiger R, 81
Gedat E, **75**
Gendrin C, 207
Georg D, 207
Gergel I, 45, 346
Gigengack F, 51
Glauche I, 57
Godinez WJ, 231

Gogolin S, 243
Gollmer ST, **15**
Graser B, **92**
Greß O, **249**
Groch A, **39**
Gross S, **195**, **256**
Grüttner M, 358
Guerrero D, 398
Gutbell R, **171**

Haase S, 39, **111**, 316
Habes M, **268**
Hamer J, **310**
Handels H, 99, 117, 201, 225, 286
Harder N, **243**
Harmsen M, **434**
Hautmann H, 45
Heimann T, 92, 183
Herdt E, 87
Herpers R, 165
Herzog H, 268
Hetzheim H, **428**
Hetzheim HG, 428
Hien M, 92
Hierl T, 189
Hirsch S, 3, 363
Hofmann HG, 33
Hornegger J, 33, 39, 105, 111, 141, 292, 316, 386
Hummel J, 392
Huppert A, **416**

Ihme T, 416

Jaiswal A, **231**
Janiga G, 81
Jiang X, 51
Jin C, 334
Jonas S, **135**

Kadas EM, **262**
Kadashevich I, 27
Karamalis A, 21
Katouzian A, **21**
Kauczor H-U, 392
Kaufhold F, 262
Kenngott H, 39
Khokha MK, 135
Kilgus T, 39, 111, 340
Kirsch R, 75

Kirschner M, **328**
Klatt D, 3
Klein M, 256
Klein T, 410
Kleine M, **147**
Kluck C, 219
Koch M, 386
Köhler B, **81**
Köhler T, **292**
König R, 243
König S, 87
Köstler H, 380
Kondruweit M, 87
Kops ER, 268
Kowarschik M, 380
Kratz B, 310
Kraus T, 213
Krefting D, 3
Krüger J, **99**
Kuhl CK, 440
Kurths J, 69
Kurzendorfer T, **386**
Kurzidim K, 386
Kuska J-P, 57

Laine A, 21
Lehmann MJ, 231
Levakhina YM, 304
Libuschewski P, **237**
Lipinski H-G, 129, 268, 369
Ludborzs C, 57
Lüttmann SO, 129

Maclaren J, 27
Maier-Hein L, 39, 111, 340, 392, 398
Maier A, 33
Malberg H, 69
Mang A, **63**, **123**, **422**
Mastmeyer A, 117, **286**
Mayer M, 292
Meinzer H-P, 39, 45, 92, 177, 183, 340, 346, 392, 398
Menzel M, 45
Mersmann S, **398**
Meyer B, 75
Michelson G, 292
Mittag U, 165
Modersitzki J, 51, 352
Mönch J, 404
Mohajer M, 75

Morariu CA, 195
Müller H, 440
Müller J, 147, 310
Müller S, 153
Müller-Ott K, 9
Münchau A, 225

Navab N, 21, 45, 410
Neher PF, **177**
Neugebauer M, 81
Nimsky C, 274

Paul F, 262
Pawiro SA, 207
Penzel T, 69
Piesch T-C, **440**
Plate A, 410
Pohl T, 380
Polthier K, 262
Pompe T, 57
Posch S, 249
Preim B, 81, 375, 404

Radeleff BA, 392
Radeleff BR, 340
Rauch H, 92
Régnier-Vigouroux A, 123
Reichl T, **45**
Reicht I, 177
Reisert M, 177
Riedl M, 69
Rippe K, 9
Ritschel K, **159**
Rittweger J, 165
Roeder I, 57
Röttger D, **153**
Rohr K, 9, 231, 243
Rude U, 380
Rühaak J, 219
Ruppertshofen H, 298
Ruthotto L, **51**

Sack I, 1, 3, 363
Sattel TF, 358
Schäfers KP, 51
Scheibe P, 57, **189**
Scherf N, **57**
Schlemmer H-P, 39, 392, 398
Schmidt-Richberg A, **201**, 225
Schnaars A, **375**
Schramm H, 298, 434
Schütz TA, 63, 123, 422
Schulz C, 262

Schulze P, 27
Seitel A, **340**, 392
Servatius M, 340, 392
Sommer CM, 392
Sommerfeld D, 404
Soza G, 375
Speck O, 27, 81
Spoerk J, 207
Stieltjes B, 177
Stock M, 207
Strehlow J, **219**
Strobel N, 386
Stucht D, **27**
Sudyatma N, 369
Swarat D, 129, **369**

Thierbach K, 57
Tietjen C, 375
Timm C, 237
Tischendorf JJ, 195
Toma A, 63, **123**, 422
Tzschätzsch H, **3**

Voigt C, 189

Wagner M, 39
Wagner T, **129**, 369
Wasza J, 105, **316**
Weber C, 207
Weber T, 165
Wegner I, 45, 346
Weichert F, 237
Werner R, 201
Wesarg S, 171, 328
Wessel N, **69**
Westermann F, 243
Weyand M, 87
Wiemann M, 129, 369
Wilms M, 201
Winter S, 159, 322
Wittenberg T, 87
Wörz S, 9
Wolf I, 416
Wolters CH, 51
Wu H, **141**
Wüstling P, 189

Yang S, 27
Yuan L, 334

Zaitsev M, 27
Zhang Y, 334

Stichwortverzeichnis

Ähnlichkeit, 304
Aktive Kontur, 57, 410
Anatomie, 262
Artefakt, 195, 262, 310
Atlas, 63
Auflösung, 27, 111, 189
Augmented Reality, 45, 340, 386
Ausbildung, 404
Automat, 262

B-Spline, 213, 352
Bewegung, 27, 105, 292, 352, 386
Bewegungsanalyse, 3, 87, 105, 243, 316
Bewegungsunterdrückung, 51
Bilddatenbank, 195, 440
Bildfusion, 99, 111, 219
Bildgenerierung, 358
Bildqualität, 27, 292, 304
Bildverbesserung, 237
Bioinformatik, 9, 57, 243
Biomechanik, 105

Clusteranalyse, 21
Computer, 369
Computer Aided Diagnosis (CAD), 21, 99, 153, 195, 225, 274, 334, 410, 428, 440
Computer Assisted Radiology (CAR), 386, 392
Computer Assisted Surgery (CAS), 45, 171, 386, 392
Content Based Image Retrieval (CBIR), 440

Datenbank, 256
Deformierbares Modell, 9, 15, 117, 328, 422
Detektion, 33, 428
Diffusion, 63, 123, 129, 153, 177, 286
Dynamik, 123, 129

Echtzeit, 117, 358
Elastische Registrierung, 105, 213, 219
Erweiterte Realität, 340
Evaluierung, 15, 45, 219, 274, 358, 392

Farbmodell, 195

Filterung, 3, 231, 292
Finite Elemente Modell (FEM), 123
Fourier-Transformation, 75, 87
Frequenzanalyse, 87
Fusion, 39
Fuzzy Logik, 237, 428

Geometrie, 358
Gradient, 165, 322, 358, 416

Haptik, 117, 286
Hardware, 358, 363, 392
Histogramm-Transformation, 310
Hochgeschwindigkeitskamera, 87
Hybrides Modell, 123

Image Retrieval, 434, 440
Interpolation, 183, 310

Kalibrierung, 111, 346, 398
Kantendetektion, 3, 33, 147, 165, 369
Klassifikation
– statistisch, 165, 225, 334, 434
Klinische Evaluierung, 75, 225
Kodierung, 440
Kontur, 165, 274
Koordinatentransformation, 111
Korrespondenzbestimmung, 15, 99, 231, 386
Kreuzmetrik, 416

Landmarke, 219, 274
Lineare Regression, 165
Lokale Adaption, 9
Lokalisation, 9, 15

Matching, 39, 231, 274, 386, 416
Merkmalskarte, 159, 195
Minimalinvasive Chirurgie, 39, 111, 171
Modellierung, 63, 123, 422
Multiskalen, 21, 256
Mutual Information, 304

Navigation, 45, 340, 386, 392
Numerik, 63, 123

Oberfläche, 39, 111, 213, 316
Objekterkennung, 33, 298, 369, 428

Objektverfolgung, 33, 45, 129, 243, 249, 386
Operationsplanung, 171
Optimierung, 183, 237, 352, 422

Partialvolumeneffekt, 3, 189
Perfusion, 159
Picture Archiving and Communication System (PACS), 440
Point-Distribution-Modell, 15, 316, 328
Prädiktion, 249

Quantisierung, 165, 358

Radon-Transformation, 147
Rauschen, 292, 428
Region of Interest (ROI), 3, 9, 15, 33, 165, 213, 274, 316, 416
Registrierung, 45, 51, 57, 105, 165, 207, 225, 292, 410, 416, 422
– elastisch, 105, 213, 219
Regression, 165
Rekonstruktion, 189, 310, 352
– 3D, 39, 75, 189
Rendering, 292

Schwellwertverfahren, 3, 15, 189, 310
Simulation, 123, 171, 304
Sprache, 39

Template Matching, 99, 386
Textur, 105, 428
Therapie, 340
Tissue Engineering, 123
Topologie, 105, 422
Tracking, 45, 57, 105, 231, 243, 249, 346, 392
Transformation
– sonstige, 416
Translation, 358
Tumorstaging, 440

Validierung, 219, 304, 358
Video, 45, 105, 159, 165
Virtuelle Realität, 117
Visualisierung
– 2D, 87, 375
– 2D+t, 87, 316, 375
– 3D, 153, 171
Volume Rendering, 45, 117, 416
Vorverarbeitung, 292

Wavelet-Transformation, 21, 147, 237
World Wide Web (WWW), 404

Zeitreihe, 69, 129, 159, 231, 237, 249
Zellulärer Automat, 123